ADRENAL DISORDERS

CONTEMPORARY ENDOCRINOLOGY

P. Michael Conn, SERIES EDITOR

ADRENAL DISORDERS

Edited by

ANDREW N. MARGIORIS, MD

Department of Clinical Chemistry,
University of Crete School of Medicine,
Heraklion, Crete

and

GEORGE P. CHROUSOS, MD

Pediatric and Reproductive Endocrinology Branch,
National Institute of Child and Human
Development, National Institute of Health,
Bethesda, MD

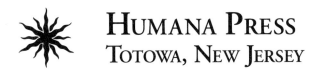

HUMANA PRESS
TOTOWA, NEW JERSEY

© 2001 Humana Press Inc.
999 Riverview Drive, Suite 208
Totowa, New Jersey 07512

For additional copies, pricing for bulk purchases, and/or information about other Humana titles, contact Humana at the above address or at any of the following numbers: Tel: 973-256-1699; Fax: 973-256-8341; E-mail: humana@humanapr.com; Website: http://humanapress.com

Production Editor: Jason S. Runnion
Cover design by Patricia F. Cleary

All articles, comments, opinions, conclusions, or recommendations are those of the author(s), and do not necessarily reflect the views of the publisher.

This publication is printed on acid-free paper. ∞
ANSI Z39.48-1984 (American National Standards Institute)
Permanence of Paper for Printed Library Materials.

Printed in the United States of America.   10 9 8 7 6 5 4 3 2 1

Endocrinology of Aging/edited by Andrew N. Margioris and George P. Chrousos
CIP

PREFACE

Four hundred and fifty years ago, Eustachius described the adrenal glands in his Atlas of Anatomy. Two centuries later, Winslow gave a more complete description, and a hundred years later, only in the middle of last century, the physiological significance of the adrenal glands became apparent, with the description of adrenal insufficiency by Addison and the conclusive experimental evidence produced by Brown-Sequard. Up to the 1930s, the products of the adrenal cortex and their roles were completely unknown. In 1950, the Nobel prize in Medicine or Physiology was awarded to Kendal, Reichstein, and Hench for the isolation, identification, and first therapeutic use of cortisone. It is tempting to compare the pace of data acquisition and concept generation in the adrenal field to that of the technological development of humanity. Indeed, new and exciting concepts in the field of adrenal physiology and pathophysiology have been emerging in an exponential fashion. This tremendous influx of new knowledge is without parallel in the history of adrenal gland studies. Our aim in editing *Adrenal Disorders* was first to select from the existing huge pool of novel information the most relevant to clinical practice and second to incorporate this knowledge into the existing body of clinical knowledge. We have recruited experts who have been active contributors, with the conviction that the best scientist to explain a new concept is frequently the one involved in its generation.

The first part of *Adrenal Disorders* concerns new developments in our understanding of the physiology of the adrenal cortex and medulla. In the first section of this part of the book, we have included chapters on ontogeny, on steroidogenesis, and on the generation of adrenal zonation. The second section deals with the newer concepts regarding the secretion and metabolism of adrenal products. Thus, we have included chapters on the pharmacology and catabolism of glucocorticoids, on the physiologic role of 11β-hydroxysteroid dehydrogenase system, on adrenal androgens, and on StAR protein. Finally, we have included two chapters on the physiology of the adrenal medulla and the significance of the intra-adrenal paracrine/autocrine regulatory networks, composed of locally produced cytokines, neuropeptides, steroids, and catecholamines.

The second part of *Adrenal Disorders* concerns new developments in our understanding of the diseased adrenals. The first section deals with disturbances in the homeostasis of cortisol production. In the first chapter, a concise overview of hyper- and hypocortisolism is given. Two chapters follow that present new data on ACTH resistance and the ectopic ACTH syndromes. The ensuing chapters analyze the different Cushing's and pseudo-Cushing's syndromes and their differential diagnoses, including the combined CRH/dexamethasone test, bilateral simultaneous inferior petrosal sinus sampling, and the desmopressin test. The second section is devoted to new concepts regarding adrenal tumors, including the roles of oncogenes/tumor suppressor genes in adrenocortical tumorigenesis, and novel, albeit yet unsatisfactory therapeutic approaches in adrenal cancer, as well as a chapter on adrenal incidentalomas. The third section includes chapters on hereditary adrenal diseases, including congenital adrenal hyperplasia, micronodular adrenal disease, congenital lipoid adrenal hyperplasia, congenital adrenal hypoplasia, and two chapters with novel, integrated information on the involvement of the adrenals in two systemic conditions, HIV-1 infection, and generalized obesity. The next section deals with mineralocorticoids and the syndromes of mineralocorticoid excess and aldosterone synthase deficiency. *Adrenal Disorders* ends with an extensive chapter describing newer developments in the field of adrenomedullary tumors.

The editors are indebted to the authors for their hard work and willingness to write the chapters of this book. We recognize today's importance of dedicating most of an investigator's effort to the production and publication of primary data, and this doubles our gratefulness. Thanks to the authors, *Adrenal Disorders* is current, which will hopefully make it useful to other adrenal investigators and to colleagues who apply the knowledge presented in their research, teaching, or clinical practice.

Andrew N. Margioris, MD
George P. Chrousos, MD

CONTENTS

CONTRIBUTORS

BRUNO ALLOLIO, MD, *Medizinishe Universitätsklinik Wurzburg, Wurzburg, Germany*

FUTOSHI ARAKANE, MD, PhD, *Department of Obstetrics and Gynecology, Center for Research on Reproduction and Women's Health, University of Pennsylvania Medical Center, Philadelphia, PA*

XAVIER BERTAGNA, MD, *Groupe d'Etude en Physiopathologie Endocrinienne, Institut Cochin de Génétique Moléculaire, Université René Descartes, Paris, France*

PER BJÖRNTORP, MD, PhD, *Department of Heart and Lung Diseases, Sahlgrenska University Hospital, Göteborg, Sweden*

STEFAN R. BORNSTEIN, MD, *Pediatric and Reproductive Endocrinology Branch, National Institute of Child Health & Human Development, NIH, Bethesda, Maryland*

LANE K. CHRISTENSON, PhD, *Department of Obstetrics and Gynecology, Center for Research on Reproduction and Women's Health, University of Pennsylvania Medical Center, Philadelphia, PA*

GEORGE P. CHROUSOS, MD, *Pediatric and Reproductive Endocrinology Branch, National Institute of Child and Human Development, Bethesda, MD*

NADIA DAKINE, MD, *Laboratoire de Neuroendocrinologie, INSERM, Institut Jean Roche, Université de la Méditerranée, Marseille, France*

ERENE DERMITZAKI, MD, *Departments of Clinical Chemistry and Pharmacology, School of Medicine, University of Crete, Heraklion, Greece*

ROBERT G. DLUHY, MD, *Harvard Medical School, Brigham and Women's Hospital, Boston, MA*

DANIEL S. DONOVAN JR., MD, *College of Physicians and Surgeons of Columbia University, New York, NY*

ANTHONY G. DOUFAS, MD, *Endocrine Unit, University of Athens Medical School, Evgenidion Hospital, Athens, Greece*

MONIKA EHRHART-BORNSTEIN, MD, *Department of Internal Medicine III, University of Leipzig, Leipzig, Germany*

GRAEME EISENHOFER, MD, *Clinical Neuroscience Branch, National Institute of Neurological Disorders and Stroke, National Institute of Health, Bethesda, MD*

TED FRIEDMAN, MD, *National Institute of Child Health and Human Development, Bethesda, MD*

RICHARD D. GORDON, MD, PhD, FRACP, *University Department of Medicine, Greenslopes Private Hospital, Brisbane, Australia*

ACHILLE GRAVANIS, MD, *Department of Clinical Chemistry, University of Crete School of Medicine, Heraklion, Crete, Greece*

MICHEL GRINO, MD, PhD, *Laboratoire de Neuroendocrinologie, INSERM, Institut Jean Roche, Université de la Méditerranée, Marseille, France*

W. W. DE HERDER, MD, PhD, *Department of Internal Medicine III, University Hospital Rotterdam, Rotterdam, Netherlands*

DOMINIC HOMAN, MD, *University of Michigan Medical School, Ann Arbor, MI*

CALEB B. KALLEN, MD, *Department of Obstetrics and Gynecology, Center for Research on Reproduction and Women's Health, University of Pennsylvania Medical Center, Philadelphia, PA*

YVES DE KEYZER, MD, *Groupe d'Etudes en Physiopathologie Endocrinienne, Institut Cochin de Génétique Moléculaire, Université René Descartes, Paris, France*

MARIANTHI KIRIAKIDOU, MD, *Department of Obstetrics and Gynecology, Center for Research on Reproduction and Women's Health, University of Pennsylvania Medical Center, Philadelphia, PA*

CHRISTIAN A. KOCH, MD, *Developmental Endocrinology Branch, National Institute of Child and Human Development, Bethesda, MD*

S. W. J. LAMBERTS, MD, PhD, *Department of Internal Medicine III, University Hospital Rotterdam, Rotterdam, The Netherlands*

JACQUES W. M. LENDERS, MD, *Department of Medicine, University Hospital Nijmegen, The Netherlands*

ANDREW N. MARGIORIS, MD, *Department of Clinical Chemistry, University of Crete School of Medicine, Heraklion, Crete, Greece*

GEORGE MASTORAKOS, MD, *Endocrine Unit, University of Athens Medical School, Evgenidion Hospital, Athens, Greece*

WALTER L. MILLER, MD, *Department of Pediatrics, University of California, San Francisco, CA*

MARIA I. NEW, MD, *Division of Pediatric Endocrinology, New York Hospital-Cornell Medical Center, New York, NY*

CHARLES OLIVER, MD, *Laboratoire de Neuroendocrinologie, INSERM, Institut Jean Roche, Université de la Méditerranée, Marseille, France*

KAREL PACACK, MD, *Clinical Neuroscience Branch, National Institute of Neurological Disorders and Stroke, National Institute of Health, Bethesda, MD*

ODILE PAULMYER-LACROIX, MD, *Laboratoire de Neuroendocrinologie, INSERM, Institut Jean Roche, Université de la Méditerranée, Marseille, France*

MICHAEL PETER, MD, *Division of Pediatric Endocrinology, Department of Pediatrics, Christian-Albrechts-University of Kiel, and Sanitas Ostseeklinik Boltenhagen, Germany*

AGNÈS PICON, MD, *Groupe d'Etudes en Physiopathologie Endocrinienne, Institut Cochin de Génétique Moléculaire, Université René Descartes, Paris, France*

STACI E. POLLACK, MD, *Department of Obstetrics and Gynecology, Center for Research on Reproduction and Women's Health, University of Pennsylvania Medical Center, Philadelphia, PA*

MARIE RAFFIN-SANSON, MD, PhD, *Groupe d'Etudes en Physiopathologie Endocrinienne, Institut Cochin de Génétique Moléculaire, Universite Rene Descartes, Paris, France*

MEERA S. RAMAYYA, MBBS, DCH, MS, *Department of Surgery, University of Washington School of Medicine and Children's Hospital and Regional Medical Center, Seattle, WA*

MARTIN REINCKE, MD, *Medical Department, University Hospital of Freiburg, Freiburg, Germany*

ROLAND ROSMOND, MD, PhD, *Department of Heart and Lung Diseases, University of Göteborg, Sahlgrenska University Hospital, Gotëborg, Sweden*

DAVID E. SCHTEINGART, MD, *Internal Medicine, University of Michigan Medical School, Ann Arbor, MI*

JONATHAN SECKL, MD, *Molecular Endocrinology Unit, Molecular Medicine Centre, University of Edinburgh, Western General Hospital, Edinburgh, Scotland, UK*

WOLFGANG G. SIPPEL, MD, *Division of Pediatric Endocrinology, Department of Pediatrics, Universitäts-Kinderklinik, Kiel, Germany*

CONSTANTINE A. STRATAKIS, MD, DMSc, *Developmental Endocrinology Branch, Section on Pediatric Endocrinology, National Institute of Child Health & Human Development, Bethesda, MD*

JEROME F. STRAUSS III, MD, PhD, *Department of Obstetrics and Gynecology, Center for Research on Reproduction and Women's Health, University of Pennsylvania Medical Center, Philadelphia, PA*

TERUO SUGAWARA, MD, *Department of Obstetrics and Gynecology, Center for Research on Reproduction and Women's Health, University of Pennsylvania Medical Center, Philadelphia, PA*

N. THALASSINOS, MD, *Department of Endocrinology, Evangelismos Hospital, Athens, Greece*

S. TSAGARAKIS, MD, PhD, *Department of Endocrinology, Evangelismos Hospital, Athens, Greece*

CONSTANTINE TSIGOS, MD, PhD, *National Institute of Child Health and Human Development, NIH, Bethesda, MD*

MARIA VENIHAKI, MD, *Departments of Clinical Chemistry and Pharmacology, School of Medicine, University of Crete, Heraklion, Greece*

HIDEMICHI WATARI, MD, PhD, *Department of Obstetrics and Gynecology, Center for Research on Reproduction and Women's Health, University of Pennsylvania Medical Center, Philadelphia, PA*

MICHIKO WATARI, MD, *Department of Obstetrics and Gynecology, Center for Research on Reproduction and Women's Health, University of Pennsylvania Medical Center, Philadelphia, PA*

PERRIN C. WHITE, MD, *Division of Pediatric Endocrinology, Department of Pediatrics, University of Texas Southwestern Medical Center, Dallas, TX*

G. W. WOLKERSDÖRFER, MD, *National Institute of Child Health & Human Development, NIH, Bethesda, MD*

I

THE ADRENAL GLAND: *PHYSIOLOGY*

1

Ontogeny of the Hypothalamo-Pituitary-Adrenal Axis

Michel Grino, Nadia Dakine,
Odile Paulmyer-Lacroix, and Charles Oliver

CONTENTS

INTRODUCTION

In adult mammals, glucocorticoids play an important role in maintaining homeostasis under basal conditions and during exposure to stress. In developing rats, during the first 10 d after birth, basal circulating corticosterone levels are reduced and the adrenal response to stress is blunted. These low-circulating glucocorticoid levels are believed to be essential for normal brain and behavioral development. Rats treated with gluco-corticoids during the first week of life have permanently reduced brain weight, neuronal, glial, and myelin alterations, as well as behavioral changes.

In this chapter, we will examine the pre- and postnatal ontogeny of the various components of the hypothalamo-pituitary-adrenal (HPA) axis and discuss the mechanisms involved in their regulation.

REGULATION OF THE HPA AXIS IN FETUSES

Adrenal glands of fetuses synthesize and secrete corticosterone as early as embryonic day 13 (E13) *(1)*. Plasma corticosterone levels rise progressively from E16 to E19, decreasing progressively thereafter. The pattern of plasma ACTH levels parallels that of corticosterone, indicating that the observed adrenal hyperactivity during late gestation is driven by an increased ACTH secretion from the corticotrophs *(2)*. Anterior pituitary proopiomelanocortin (POMC, the precursor of ACTH) mRNA is first detected at E15 *(3)*; it rises steadily between E17 and E21 *(4)*, whereas the pituitary content of ACTH

From: *Contemporary Endocrinology: Adrenal Disorders*
Edited by: A. N. Margioris and G. P. Chrousos © Humana Press, Totowa, NJ

increases between E17 and E19, decreases on E20, before showing a further elevation *(2)*. The transient reduction in pituitary ACTH content may be caused by the high ACTH secretion into the circulation. The activity of anterior pituitary corticotrophs during late gestation is believed to be regulated by both hypothalamic ACTH secretagogues and by glucocorticoids. In vitro, in E15 whole pituitaries explants, CRF stimulates POMC-derived peptide secretion and POMC gene transcription, this effect being inhibited by the synthetic glucocorticoid dexamethasone *(5,6)*. CRF or AVP stimulate ACTH release from superfused pituitary glands collected on E17, E19, and E21 *(7)*. Encephalectomy of fetuses decreases the circulating ACTH and corticosterone levels at term and induces an atrophy of the adrenals *(8)*. In E21 fetuses, CRF and/or AVP injection is followed by an increase in plasma ACTH and corticosterone *(9)*. Using passive immunization techniques, Boudouresque et al. *(2)* have demonstrated that CRF and AVP play a role in the regulation of ACTH and corticosterone production as early as E17. The glucocorticoid regulation of anterior pituitary corticotrophs appears to be functional during late gestation because maternal administration of dexamethasone reduces both plasma ACTH levels and adrenal growth in fetuses *(10)*. Immunoreactive CRF has been localized in the lateral area of the central portion of hypothalamus on E15.5, in the putative paraventricular nucleus (PVN) on E16.5 and in the anterior region of median eminence on E18 *(11,12)*. When measured by radioimmunoassay in hypothalamic extracts, CRF has been shown to increase gradually from E17 to E21 *(13)*. Using *in situ* hybridization, we first detect CRF mRNA on E17 in the putative PVN. From then on, the levels of CRF mRNA increase progressively until E19, then decrease sharply until the day of birth *(4)*. The changing mRNA/peptide ratio observed during late gestation in the rat could be caused either by differences in peptide synthesis, storage, and release, or to developmental changes in the posttranslational processing of CRF precursor to mature peptide. Unfortunately, only few data are available regarding the regulation of CRF mRNA biosynthesis and processing during fetal life. Baram and Schultz *(14)* have reported that pharmacological fetal adrenalectomy, obtained by treating the mother with metyrapone, does not increase CRF mRNA levels in the PVN of E17–18 fetuses. However, Dupouy et al. *(10)* have demonstrated that administration of dexamethasone to the mother, beginning at day 15 of gestation, induces a drastic decrease of hypothalamic CRF content in E21 fetuses. Lesage et al. have recently shown that chronic morphine treatment of pregnant rats, which increases circulating corticosterone, results in a significant decrease of hypothalamic CRF concentration in the newborn, this effect being reversed after maternal adrenalectomy *(15)*. These observations suggest that, during late gestation, glucocorticoids may regulate CRF biosynthesis at a posttranscriptional level. AVP mRNA is detectable in the putative PVN from E18 increasing steadily thereafter, a pattern also observed for immunoreactive AVP *(16,17)*.

The way by which CRF and AVP reach the pituitary is different in fetuses compared to adults. Indeed, the neurovascular link between the median eminence and the pituitary is not fully developed before the end of the second postnatal week *(18)*. Some vascular connections between the median eminence and the anterior pituitary gland have been demonstrated at E12 *(19)* and E18 *(20)*. Nevertheless, there is no clear anatomical proof of neurovascular communication between CRF neurosecretory axons and the primary portal capillary plexus before E18 *(11,12)*. This suggests that, at earlier stages, endogenous CRF may enter the hypophysial portal circulation after intracellular diffusion in hypothalamic tissue. Indeed, Ugrumov et al. *(21)* have shown that neurosecretory axons are present in the external zone of the median eminence of E14 fetuses, although they are not connected with the primary portal capillary plexus prior to the 18th or 20th day of pregnancy.

REGULATION OF THE HPA AXIS DURING THE EARLY POSTNATAL PERIOD

Plasma ACTH and corticosterone are elevated during the day of birth (P0) and decrease sharply at P1. It has been suggested that this increase of glucocorticoids at birth may be necessary for the adaptation to ex-utero life *(22)*. However, plasma ACTH and corticosterone levels are low during the first 10 d of life and increase thereafter to reach adult–like values around P21 *(23)*. The increase in circulating corticosterone that occurs after P10 is clearly related to a suppression of its metabolic clearance rate, primarily because of a decrement in the apparent volume of distribution which, in turn, may result from the concurrent rise in plasma corticosteroid-binding globulin concentrations *(24)*. It has also been suggested that the low levels of corticosterone during the first 10 d of life is also the result of a decreased sensitivity of the adrenal gland to the stimulatory effect of ACTH. Indeed, in young rats, the effect of ACTH injection on corticosterone secretion is much weaker compared to older animals *(25)*. This phenomenon appears to be related to the low-circulating ACTH levels during the same period. Twice-daily injections of a physiological dose of ACTH between P2–P7 increase the adrenal responsiveness to a single-ACTH injection at P8 *(26)*. Similarly, daily injection of a pharmacological dose of ACTH between P5–P7 increased the adrenocortical response to insulin-induced hypoglycemia at P8 *(27)*. In addition to ACTH, other peptides derived from the processing of the POMC molecule may play a role in the activation of the biosynthetic pathway of corticosterone. Indeed, a potentiation of the steroidogenic activity of ACTH by γ_3-MSH has been demonstrated in vivo in adult rats *(28)*, and in vitro in rat *(29)* and human *(30)* perifused adrenal cells. In addition, in the developing rat, pretreatment with Lys-γ_3-MSH potentiates the effect of an acute ACTH injection *(31)*. Several mechanisms may account for the decreased corticosterone biosynthesis in young rats. The density of adrenal-ACTH binding sites parallels the concentration of circulating ACTH, reaching its lowest number 1 wk after birth *(32)*. Similarly, both basal- and ACTH-stimulated adenylate cyclase activity are low in the adrenals of P7 rats, as compared with fetuses or older (P14) animals *(33)*. One contributing cause for this phenomenon may be associated with the low amount of the stored cholesterol in the adrenals. It has been hypothesized that the supply of cholesterol from the cholesterol ester store in the lipid droplets to mitochondria is a rate-limiting factor in the conversion of cholesterol to steroid hormones *(34)*. Enzymes involved in the biosynthesis of corticosterone (the side-chain cholesterol cleaving enzyme (P450scc), the 3β-hydroxysteroid deshydrogenase/isomerase (3β-HSD), the 11β-hydroxylase (P450c11), and P450 21α-hydroxylase (P450c21) show a different pattern of evolution in the adrenal of the developing rat. Although the levels of P450scc and P450c11 are stable, the levels of 3β-HSD and the activity of P450c21 are strongly reduced in the adrenals of 10-d-old rats *(35)*. Interestingly, ACTH increases the availability of cholesterol stores, promotes the inhibition of cholesterol esterification and the activation of P450scc and 3β-HSD, whereas γ_3-MSH activates the neutral cholesterol ester hydrolase *(35–37)*. Taken together, these observations strongly suggest that the immaturity of the adrenal gland of the developing rat is caused by the decreased basal and stimulated enzymatic activity, which, in turn, may result from low-pituitary ACTH synthesis and secretion.

The decreased rate of ACTH synthesis may be caused by immaturity of either the anterior pituitary gland or the hypothalamic factors that control ACTH synthesis and release. The relative proportion of unprocessed POMC, ACTH-related peptides and $_{1–39}$ACTH may be altered in the developing rat. Indeed, the percentage of high molecular-weight ACTH is high during fetal and early postnatal life *(23,38)*. The percentage of corticotroph cells in the anterior pituitary is twice that of the adults at P2 and decreases below adult values between P7–P11. This is followed by a recovery at P15 *(39)*. POMC mRNA levels are low from P1–P5 and increase thereafter *(4)*. The decreased POMC gene transcription observed in the young rat may be consecutive to an increased negative glucocorticoid feedback. Although plasma levels of corticosterone are low, the concentration of circulating corticosteroid binding globulin is also reduced, leading to increased delivery of the hormone to target tissues, especially to corticotrophs where it may contribute to the increased feedback observed *(40)*. Alternatively, the corticotroph cells may be less sensitive to the stimulatory effect of CRF and/or AVP. In vitro, CRF-stimulated ACTH release is comparable between pituitaries obtained from P7 or P14 rats *(41)*. Indeed, CRF stimulates POMC gene transcription to the same extent in P1 as in P10 pituitary explants; pretreatment with dexamethasone blocks the CRF effect *(6)*. Hary et al. *(42)* have shown that AVP stimulates ACTH secretion and potentiates the effect of CRF from superfused pituitaries of P8 animals. In addition, in P8 rats, plasma ACTH levels elevated by insulin-induced hypoglycemia are reduced after passive immunization against AVP *(27)*. Taken together, these observations indicate that the corticotrophs of the developing rat are normally sensitive to the stimulatory effect of CRF and AVP. This suggests that the immaturity of the HPA axis may lie at the hypothalamic or suprahypothalamic level.

Hypothalamic CRF mRNA levels are low between P1–P5 *(4)*. Surprisingly, during the same period, the immunoreactive CRF in the hypothalamus increases steadily *(13,17)*, suggesting that the decreased CRF synthesis is accompanied by a *decreased* rate of CRF secretion. The decreased CRF synthesis and secretion could be consecutive to an *increased glucocorticoid negative feedback,* as was aforementioned. It should be noted, however, that the number of glucocorticoid receptors is low in the brain of the developing rat while the mineralocorticoid receptors are present at much higher concentrations, and thus are able to bind low doses of corticosterone *(43)*. Yi et al. *(44)* have found that chronic local implants of cannulae containing a glucocorticoid antagonist did not increase CRF mRNA concentrations in the PVN during the first postnatal week. We have demonstrated that the postadrenalectomy (ADX) increase in anterior pituitary POMC mRNA is reduced in P7 rats compared to P14 animals. Concomitantly, ADX does not change the expression of the *CRF* gene in the PVN of P7 rats. Chronic CRF treatment of ADX P7 animals is able to normalize the post-ADX increase of POMC mRNA levels *(41)*. In addition, the ADX-induced increase in Fos-like immunoreactivity, a sensitive marker of neuronal activation, is attenuated in the PVN of P11 rats, compared to P3 and P18 animals *(45)*. These observations suggest that the mechanism regulating hypothalamic *CRF* gene expression is not mature enough during the first week of life. This phenomenon may, at least in part, explain the low

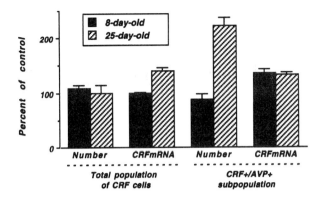

Fig. 1. Summary of the changes in the number of CRF-expressing cells and in the level of CRF mRNA in the total population of CRF-synthesizing cell bodies and in the CRF⁺/AVP⁺ subpopulation in developing rats subjected to insulin-induced hypoglycemia. Values are the mean ± SE ($n = 5$) of data expressing the stress-induced changes as a percentage of control values (control = 100%). * $P<0.05$ vs vehicle-injected rats. (Reproduced from **ref.** *51.*)

response to stress during this period of life. However, we have observed that AVP mRNA levels in PVN reach adult-like values at P3, and that ADX upregulates AVP gene expression in the parvocellular PVN in P7 animals *(16)*. This finding is surprising because it is known that, in the parvocellular PVN of the adult rat, AVP is synthesized in a subpopulation of CRF cell bodies (so-called CRF⁺/AVP⁺) and that exposure to stress induces an increment of *CRF* and *AVP* gene expression and synthesis *(46–49)* increasing the percentage of CRF⁺/AVP⁺ cell bodies *(47,49,50)*. However, we have recently demonstrated that, in P8 rats, insulin-induced hypoglycemia does not stimulate *CRF* gene expression in CRF⁺/AVP⁻ neurons, but induces an increase of CRF mRNA levels in the CRF⁺/AVP⁺ subpopulation (Fig. 1). Concomitantly, the percentage of CRF⁺/AVP⁺ cells is not changed *(51)*. These data suggest that the CRF⁺/AVP⁻ cells do not reach maturity at P8, and, hence, are not able to fully respond to stress.

The factors that regulate CRF and AVP synthesis and secretion are not completely understood. There is evidence that excitatory amino acids *(52)* and central biogenic amines such as catecholamines *(53)* and serotonin *(54)* stimulate CRF and AVP secretion in the adult rat. In P7 rats, administration of N-methyl-D,L-aspartic acid (NMA), quisqualic acid, or kainic acid (KA) induces a rapid and potent stimulation of ACTH secretion. The effect of NMA and KA is blocked following passive immunization against CRF, suggesting that exogenously administered excitatory amino acids act through modulation of hypothalamic CRF secretion *(55)*. The serotoninergic innervation of the hypothalamus, in particular that of PVN, occurs, as early as E19 *(56)*. By comparison, the catecholaminergic innervation of the PVN is not mature until the end of the second week of life. Indeed, phenylethanolamine N-methyltransferase-positive fibers appear on P1 and increase progressively from P1–7. A marked increase occurs from P7–14, at which time an adult-like pattern is established *(57)*. The synthesis or accumulation of catecholamines drops from E20 until P9 and returns to high levels by P21 *(58)*. Nevertheless, data obtained in vivo indicate that catecholamines may participate in the regulation of HPA axis in the developing rat. Indeed, the increase in ACTH secretion during insulin-induced hypoglycemia is significantly reduced after blockade

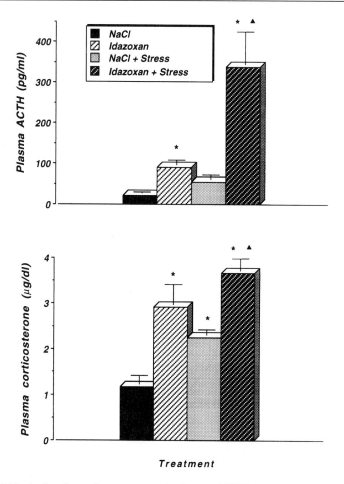

Fig. 2. Effect of blockade of α_2-adrenoceptors on plasma ACTH (upper panel) and corticosterone (lower panel) responses to ether vapors. Rats were injected with 2.5 μg/g idazoxan or vehicle (NaCl) alone. Forty-five min later, they were exposed to ether vapors during 2 min or left undisturbed, and killed 15 min thereafter. One group of rats was injected with vehicle alone, left undisturbed, and killed 60 min later (controls). *, $P<0.05$ vs control; ▲, $P<0.05$ vs idazoxan-injected unstressed rats or NaCl-injected stressed rats. (Reproduced with permission from **ref.** *60*).

of β-adrenoceptors in P8 rats. No additive effect has been detected following pretreatment with an anti-AVP antiserum and the blockade of β-adrenoreceptors, suggesting that the stimulatory effect of catecholamines during insulin-induced hypoglycemia at this age is mediated via a modulation of hypothalamic AVP secretion *(59)*. In addition to β-adrenoreceptors, α_2-adrenoceptors could be involved in regulating the HPA axis during development. We have reported that blockade of α_2-adrenoreceptors induces an increase of both basal and stress-induced ACTH secretion in P8 rats (Fig. 2) *(60)*. Kovacks and Makara *(61)* have suggested that, in the adult rat, in response to activation of α_2-adrenoceptors a corticotropin-release inhibiting substance is released from the PVN. Interestingly, under our experimental conditions, the effect of α_2-adrenoceptors blockade was not modified after passive immunization against CRF or AVP, suggesting that α_2-adrenoceptors blockade induces increased secretion of a corticotropin-releasing factor independent from CRF and AVP or decreased release of a corticotropin-inhibiting factor, both being released from the PVN.

SUMMARY

The HPA axis of the developing rat shows a biphasic pattern of evolution, with an intense activity during the late fetal period and reduced basal- and stress-induced ACTH and corticosterone secretion during the early postnatal period. Several phenomena, such as an immaturity of the adrenal glands, an increased negative glucocorticoid feedback, or an immaturity of the regulation of the hypothalamic ACTH secretagogues could account for the reduced activity of the HPA axis during the immediate postnatal period. The adaptive significance of glucocorticoid hypersecretion during the late fetal period is as yet unexplained. As aforementioned, low-circulating glucocorticoid levels during the first 2 wk of life are believed to be essential for normal brain and behavioral development.

REFERENCES

1. Ross TB. Steroid synthesis in embryonic and fetal rat adrenal tissue. Endocrinology 1967; 81:716–728.
2. Boudouresque F, Guillaume V, Grino M, Strbak V, Chautard T, Conte-Devolx B, Oliver C. Maturation of the pituitary-adrenal function in rat fetuses. Neuroendocrinology 1988; 48:417–422.
3. Hindelang C, Felix JM, Laurent FM, Klein MJ, Stoeckel ME. Ontogenesis of proopiomelanocortin gene expression and regulation in the rat pituitary intermediate lobe. Mol Cell Endocrinol 1990; 70:225–235.
4. Grino M, Young III WS, Burgunder J-M. Ontogeny of expression of the corticotropin-releasing factor gene in the hypothalamic paraventricular nucleus and of the proopiomelanocortin gene in rat pituitary. Endocrinology 1989; 124:60–68.
5. Lugo DI, Pintar JE. Ontogeny of basal and regulated secretion from POMC cells of the developing anterior lobe of the rat pituitary gland. Dev Biol 1996; 173:95–109.
6. Scott RE, Pintar JE. Developmental regulation of proopiomelanocortin gene expression in the fetal and neonatal rat pituitary. Mol Endocrinol 1993; 7:585–596.
7. Dupouy JP, Chatelain A. In vitro effects of corticosterone, synthetic ovine corticotropin-releasing factor and arginine vasopressin on the release of adrenocorticotrophin by fetal rat pituitary glands. J Endocrinol 1984; 101:339–344.
8. Dupouy JP, Chatelain A. La fonction corticotrope dans la période périnatale: ontogénèse et régulation. J Physiol (Paris) 1981; 77:955–968.
9. Deloof S, Montel V, Chatelain A. Effects of rat corticotropin-releasing factor, arginine vasopressin and oxytocin on the secretions of adrenocorticotrophic hormone and corticosterone in the fetal rat in late gestation: in vitro and in vivo studies. Eur J Endocrinol 1994; 130:313–319.
10. Dupouy JP, Chatelain A, Boudouresque F, Conte-Devolx B, Oliver C. Effects of chronic maternal dexamethasone treatment on the hormones of the hypothalamo-pituitary adrenal axis in the rat fetus. Biol Neonate 1987; 52:216–222.
11. Bugnon C, Fellmann D, Gouget A, Cardot J. Ontogeny of the corticoliberin neuroglandular system in rat brain. Nature 1982; 298:159–161.
12. Daikoku S. Immunohistochemical studies of hypophysiotrophic hormone-containing neurons in developing rat hypothalamus. In: Elendorff F, Gluckman PD, Parvisi I, eds. Fetal Neuroendocrinology. Perinatology, New York, 1984, pp. 87–89.
13. Chatelain A, Boudouresque F, Chautard T, Dupouy JP, Oliver C. Corticotrophin-releasing factor immunoreactivity in the hypothalamus of the rat during the perinatal period. J Endocrinol 1988; 119:59–64.
14. Baram TZ, Schultz L. CRH gene expression in the fetal rat is not increased after pharmacological adrenalectomy. Neurosci Lett 1992; 142:215–218.
15. Lesage J, Grino M, Bernet F, Dutriez-Casteloot I, Montel V, Dupouy JP. Consequences of prenatal morphine exposure on the hypothalamo-pituitary-adrenal axis in the newborn rat: effect of maternal adrenalectomy. J Neuroendocrinol 1998; 10:331–342.

16. Grino M, Burgunder J-M. Ontogeny of expression and glucocorticoid regulation of the arginine vasopressin gene in the rat hypothalamic paraventricular nucleus. J Neuroendocrinol 1992; 4:71–77.

17. Rundle SE, Funder JW. Ontogeny of corticotropin-releasing factor and arginine vasopressin in the rat. Neuroendocrinology 1988; 47:374–378.

18. Glydon R St J. The development of the blood supply of the pituitary in the albino rat, with special reference to the portal vessels. J Anat 1957; 91:237–244.

19. Szabo K, Csanyi K. The vascular architecture of the developing pituitary-median eminence complex in the rat. Cell Tiss Res 1982; 224:563–577.

20. Halasz BB, Kasaras B, Lengvari I. Ontogenesis of the neurovascular link between the hypothalamus and the anterior pituitary in the rat. In: Knigge KM, Scott DE, Weindl AD, eds. Brain Endocrine Interaction. Karger, Basel, 1972, pp. 27–34.

21. Ugrumov MV, Ivanova IP, Mitskevich MS, Liposits SZ, Setalo G, Flerko B. Axovascular relationship in developing median eminence of perinatal rats with special reference to luteinizing hormone-releasing hormones projections. Neuroscience 1985; 16:897–906.

22. Nagaya M, Widmaier EP. Twenty-four hour profiles of glucose, corticosterone and adrenocorticotropic hormone during the first postnatal day in rats. Biol Neonate 1993; 64:261–268.

23. Boudouresque F. Thèse, Montpellier (France) 1987.

24. Schroeder RJ, Henning SJ. Roles of plasma clearance and corticosteroid-binding globulin in the developmental increase in circulating corticosterone in infant rats. Endocrinology 1989; 124:2612–2618.

25. Guillet R, Saffran M, Michaelson SM. Pituitary-adrenal responses in neonatal rats. Endocrinology 1980; 106:991–994.

26. Nagaya M, Widmaier EP. ACTH and stress accelerate maturation of adrenocortical function in neonatal rats. Endocr J 1993; 1:247–252.

27. Muret L, Priou A, Oliver C, Grino M. Stimulation of adrenocorticotropin secretion by insulin-induced hypoglycemia in the developing rat involves arginine vasopressin but not corticotropin-releasing factor. Endocrinology 1992; 130:2725–2732.

28. Pedersen RC, Brownie A, Ling N. Proadrenocorticotropin/endorphin derived peptides: coordinate action on adrenal steroidogenesis. Science 1980; 208:1044–1046.

29. Al Dujaili EAS, Hope J, Estivariz FE, Lowry PJ, Edwards CRW. Circulating human pituitary pro-gamma-melanotropin enhances the adrenal response to ACTH. Nature 1981; 291:156–159.

30. Farese RV, Ling NC, Salvi MA, Larson E, Trudeau WL. Comparison of effects of adrenocorticotropin and Lys gamma3-melanocyte stimulating hormone on steroidogenesis, adenosine 3'5' monophosphate production, and phospholipid metabolism in rat adrenal fasciculata reticularis cells in vitro. Endocrinology 1983; 112:129–132.

31. Oliver C, Boudouresque F, Lacroix O, Anglade G, Grino M. Effect of POMC-derived peptides on corticosterone secretion during the stress hyporesponsive period in the rat. Endocr Reg 1994; 28:67–74.

32. Chatelain A, Durand P, Naaman E, Dupouy JP. Ontogeny of ACTH (1–24) receptors in rat adrenal glands during the perinatal period. J Endocrinol 1989; 123:421–428.

33. Chatelain A, Naaman E, Durand P, Lepretre A, Dupouy JP. Development of adenylate cyclase activity in rat adrenal glands during the perinatal period. J Endocrinol 1990; 126:211–216.

34. Boyd GS, Trzeciak WH. Cholesterol metabolism in the adrenal cortex: studies on the mode of action of ACTH. Ann NY Acad Sci 1973; 212:361–377.

35. Nagaya M, Arai M, Widmaier EP. Ontogeny of immunoreactive and bioactive microsomal steroidogenic enzymes during adrenocortical development in rats. Mol Cell Endocrinol 1995; 114:27–34.

36. Pedersen RC, Brownie AC. Gamma$_3$-melanotropin promotes mitochondrial cholesterol accumulation in the rat adrenal cortex. Mol Cell Endocr. 1987; 50:149–156.

37. Mahaffee D, Reitz RC, Ney RL. The mechanism of action of adrenocorticotropic hormone: the role of mitochondrial cholesterol accumulation in the regulation of steroidogenesis. J Biol Chem 1974; 249:227–232.

38. Chatelain A, Dupouy JP. Adrenocorticotrophic hormone in the anterior and neurointermediate lobes of the rat during the perinatal period: polymorphism, biological and immunological activities of ACTH. Biol Neonate 1985; 47:235–248.

39. Childs GV, Ellison DG, Ramaley JA. Storage of anterior lobe adrenocorticotropin in corticotropes and a subpopulation of gonadotropes during the stress-nonresponsive period in the neonatal male rat. Endocrinology 1982; 110:1676–1692.

40. Sakly M, Koch B. Ontogenetical variations of transcortin modulate glucocorticoid receptor function and corticotropic activity in the pituitary gland. Horm Metab Res 1983; 15:92–96.

41. Grino M, Burgunder J-M, Eskay RL, Eiden LE. Onset of glucocorticoid responsiveness of anterior pituitary corticotrophs during development is scheduled by corticotropin-releasing factor. Endocrinology 1989; 24:2686–2692.

42. Hary L, Dupouy JP, Chatelain A. ACTH secretion from isolated hypophysial anterior lobes of male and female newborn rats: effects of corticotrophin-releasing factor, arginine vasopressin and oxytocin alone or in combination. J Endocrinol 1993; 137:123–132.

43. Rosenfeld P, van Eekelen JAM, Levine S, de Kloet ER. Ontogeny of corticosteroid receptors in the brain. Cell Mol Neurobiol 1993; 13:295–318.

44. Yi SJ, Masters JN, Baram TZ. Effects of a specific glucocorticoid receptor antagonist on corticotropin-releasing hormone gene expression in the paraventricular nucleus of the neonatal rat. Dev Brain Res 1993; 73:253–259.

45. Wintrip N, Nance DM, Wilkinson M. Anomalous adrenalectomy-induced Fos-like immunoreactivity in the hypothalamic paraventricular nucleus of stress-hyporesponsive rats. Dev Brain Res 1993; 76:283–287.

46. Lightman SL, Young III WS. Corticotrophin-releasing factor, vasopressin and pro-opiomelanocortin mRNA responses to stress and opiates in the rat. J Physiol (Lond) 1988; 403:511–523.

47. Bartanusz V, Jezova D, Bertini LT, Tilders FJH, Aubry J-M, Kiss JZ. Stress-induced increase in vasopressin and corticotropin-releasing factor expression in hypophysiotrophic paraventricular neurons. Endocrinology 1993; 132:895–902.

48. Priou A, Oliver C, Grino M. In situ hybridization of arginine vasopressin (AVP) heteronuclear ribonucleic acid reveals increased AVP gene transcription in the rat hypothalamic paraventricular nucleus in response to emotional stress. Acta Endocrinol (Copenh) 1993; 128:466–472.

49. Paulmyer-Lacroix O, Anglade G, Grino M. Insulin-induced hypoglycemia increases colocalization of corticotrophin-releasing factor and arginine vasopressin mRNAs in the rat hypothalamic paraventricular nucleus. J Mol Endocrinol 1994; 13:313–320.

50. de Goeij DCE, Jezova D, Tilders FJH. Repeated stress enhances vasopressin synthesis in corticotropin-releasing factor neurons in the paraventricular nucleus. Brain Res 1992; 577:165–168.

51. Paulmyer-Lacroix O, Anglade G, Grino M. Stress regulates differently the arginine vasopressin (AVP)-containing and the AVP-deficient corticotropin-releasing factor-synthesizing cell bodies in the hypothalamic paraventricular nucleus of the developing rat. Endocrine 1994; 2:1037–1043.

52. Joanny P, Steinberg J, Oliver C, Grino M. Glutamate and N-methyl-D-aspartate stimulate rat hypothalamic corticotropin-releasing factor secretion *in vitro*. J Neuroendocrinol 1997; 9:93–97.

53. Grino M, Guillaume V, Conte-Devolx B, Szafarczyk A, Joanny P, Oliver C. Role of central catecholamines in the control of CRF and ACTH secretion. Van Loon GR, Kvetnansky R, Mc Carty R, Axelrod J, eds. Stress: Neurochemical and Humoral Mechanisms. Gordon and Breach, New York, 1989, pp. 355–367.

54. Dinan TG. Serotonin and the regulation of hypothalamic-pituitary-adrenal axis function. Life Sci 1996; 58:1683–1694.

55. Chautard T, Boudouresque F, Guillaume V, Oliver C. Effect of excitatory amino acids on the hypothalamo-pituitary adrenal axis in the rat during the stress-hyporesponsive period. Neuroendocrinology 1993; 57:70–78.

56. Lidov HGW, Molliver ME. An immunohistochemical study of serotonin neuron development in the rat: ascending pathways and terminal fields. Brain Res Bull 1982; 8:389–430.

57. Katchaturian H, Sladeck Jr JR. Simultaneous monoamine histofluorescence and neuropeptide immunocytochemistry. III. Ontogeny of catecholamines varicosities and neurophysin neurons in the rat supraoptic and paraventricular nuclei. Peptides 1980; 1:77–95.

58. Borisova NA, Sapronova AY, Proshlyakova EV, Ugrumov MV. Ontogenesis of the hypothalamic catecholaminergic system in rats: synthesis, uptake and release of catecholamines. Neuroscience 1991; 43:223–229.

59. Grino M, Oliver C. Ontogeny of insulin-induced hypoglycemia stimulation of adrenocorticotropin secretion in the rat: role of catecholamines. Endocrinology 1992; 131:2763–2768.

60. Grino M, Paulmyer-Lacroix O, Faudon M, Renard M, Anglade G. Blockade of α_2 adrenoceptors stimulates basal and stress-induced adrenocorticotropin secretion in the developing rat through a central mechanism independent from corticotropin-releasing factor and arginine vasopressin. Endocrinology 1994; 135:2549–2557.

61. Kovacs KJ, Makara GB. Factors from the paraventricular nucleus mediate inhibitory effect of alpha-2-adrenergic drugs on ACTH secretion. Neuroendocrinology 1993; 57:346–350.

2

Adrenal Organogenesis and Steroidogenesis

Role of Nuclear Receptors Steroidogenic Factor-1, DAX-1, and Estrogen Receptor

Meera S. Ramayya

CONTENTS

INTRODUCTION

Steroid hormone biosynthesis by the fetal adrenal gland is crucial to the integrity and continuation of pregnancy, growth of the fetal and maternal tissues, as well as perinatal homeostatic adaptation for extrauterine survival. The adrenal cortex in the primate undergoes a remarkable morphological and functional remodeling such that the fetal adrenal cortex transforms into an adult adrenal cortex capable of independent glucocorticoid and mineralocorticoid biosynthesis. This architectural and functional transition from a fetal to an adult adrenal cortex ensures self-sufficient existence of the neonate.

The fetal zone of the adrenal cortex, which is unique to the fetal adrenal, atrophies soon after birth *(1–5)*. This predominant zone, which forms 80–90% of the fetal adrenal cortex synthesizes dehydroepiandrosterone sulfate (DHEA-S), the precursor hormone for estrogen biosynthesis by the placenta *(6–9)*. During late gestation, placental estrogen promotes fetal adrenal cortisol biosynthesis, which supports the growth and maturation of various fetal tissues including the lung, thyroid, liver, and the gut *(9,10)*. This placental estrogen is also instrumental in regulating fetal cortisol levels throughout pregnancy. In addition to feto-placental steroidogenesis, estrogen plays a critical role in the maintenance of pregnancy, regulation of maternal cardiovascular system, control of uteroplacental blood flow and neovascularization of the placenta, maintenance of uterine quiescence, and progesterone-mediated immunosuppression to allow implantation of the embryo in the uterus *(9)*.

From: *Contemporary Endocrinology: Adrenal Disorders*
Edited by: A. N. Margioris and G. P. Chrousos © Humana Press, Totowa, NJ

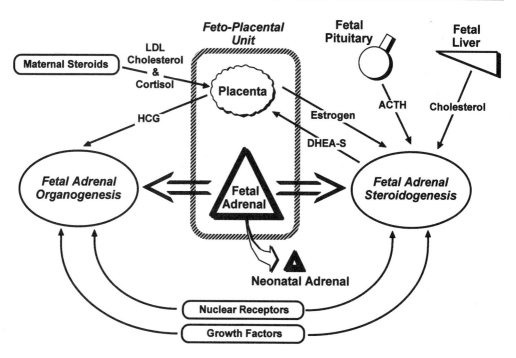

Fig. 1. Fetal adrenal remodeling and steroidogenesis. Fetal adrenal organogenesis and steroidogenesis is governed by factors derived from the mother, the fetus and the fetoplacental unit. These factors include placental chorionic gonadotropin and estrogens, fetal pituitary adrenocorticotropic hormone, and fetal adrenal generated DHEA-S, growth factors, and nuclear receptors. LDL and cholesterol from the mother and the fetal liver provide the substrate for steroid biosynthesis by the fetal adrenal. The placenta developmentally regulates the metabolism of cortisol of maternal origin and in doing so plays an important role in the functional maturation of the fetal adrenal and the HPA axis. (Derived from refs. *7* and *9*).

The steroidogenesis and growth of the fetal adrenal cortex are regulated by endocrine, paracrine and autocrine factors (Fig. 1). These include placental chorionic gonadotropins *(4,5,11–13)* the fetal pituitary adrenocorticotropic hormone (ACTH) *(4,7,13–18)*, the local adrenal cortical growth factors *(19)* such as basic fibroblast growth factor (bFGF) *(20–25)*, epidermal growth factor (EGF) *(26)*, and its homolog—transforming growth factor α (TGFα) *(19)*, insulin-like growth factors 1 and 2 (IGF-1 and IGF-2) *(27–32)*, transforming growth factor β (TGF-β) family of peptides including activin, inhibin, and TGF-β1 *(33–40)*, as well as nuclear receptors—steroidogenic factor 1 (SF-1) *(41–47)*, and *d*osage-sensitive sex reversal-*a*drenal hypoplasia congenita critical region on the *X*-chromosome gene 1 (*DAX-1*) *(48,49)*, and estrogen receptor (ER), which mediates the actions of estrogen *(50,51)*.

Steroidogenic factor 1 (SF-1) is a tissue- and cell-specific orphan nuclear receptor that is pivotal to the transcriptional regulation of several genes encoding steroidogenic enzymes *(52–61)*. Targeted disruption of *SF-1* gene in the mouse has demonstrated that this gene is crucial to adrenal and gonadal development in this species *(41,43,62)*. The newborn mice with the targeted disruption of the *SF-1* gene had adrenal insufficiency secondary to agenesis of the adrenal glands. These newborn mice were rescued following replacement therapy with glucocorticoids and mineralocorticoids. This postnatal picture is similar to the clinical picture of neonates and infants with non-*X*-linked congenital adrenal hypoplasia. Similar to the *SF-1*-gene-disrupted mice, infants with this disorder have aplastic adrenal glands. Recently, a patient was described with a heterozygous mutation located in the "P" box of the DNA-binding domain of the *hSF-1* gene, which resulted in congenital adrenal hypoplasia, adrenal insufficiency, and *XY* sex reversal *(63)*. Thus, similar to its role in the mouse, *SF-1* has a pivotal role in human adrenal and gonadal development.

DAX-1 is also an orphan nuclear receptor, which plays key roles in the development of adrenal gland and the gonads *(48,49,64)*. Studies on patients with *X*-linked adrenal hypoplasia congenita (AHC) with hypogonadotropic hypogonadism (HH) have shown that these patients have mutations and deletions in the *DAX-1* gene *(65–69)*. Targeted disruption of *DAX-1* gene in mice revealed that, similar to the adrenal glands in children with *DAX-1* gene mutations resulting in AHC, the adrenal glands of these mice had persistent fetal adrenal cortical zone. However, unlike the syndrome of *X*-linked AHC in humans, these mice did not require steroid replacement for survival as their adrenal glands had normal zona glomerulosa and fasciculata *(70)*.

SF-1 and *DAX-1* are both expressed in the tissues of hypothalamic-pituitary-adrenal/gonadal axis *(71)*. In addition, recent studies have demonstrated that these two receptors may interact to direct steroidogenesis by regulating the expression of crucial target genes, such as steroidogenic acute regulatory protein (StAR) *(72)*.

Thus, the development of the fetal adrenal gland and its transition into an adult gland capable of supporting independent existence of the organism is a complex process that involves a multitude of factors. In this chapter, in addition to a brief review of the current literature on adrenal organogenesis and steroidogenesis, the roles of nuclear receptors SF-1, DAX-1, and ER in these processes are discussed. For recent excellent reviews on fetal adrenal and placental steroidogenesis, the reader is referred to the papers on these topics by Pepe and Albrecht *(8,9)* and Mesaino and Jaffe *(7)*.

FETAL ADRENAL ORGANOGENESIS AND STEROIDOGENESIS

Fetal adrenal development and steroidogenesis are well-orchestrated and temporally regulated processes. The development of fetal adrenal relies on cellular hyperplasia, hypertrophy, migration, and apoptosis *(7,13,16,38,73–78)*. Steroidogenesis by the fetal adrenal is dependent on maternal factors, the feto-placental unit, and most importantly, on the placental estrogen biosynthesis from precursor fetal DHEA-S *(9,79)*. This placental estrogen sustains and maintains the pregnancy, modulates DHEA-S production by the fetal adrenal, and regulates the function of the fetal hypothalamic-pituitary-adrenal-axis (HPAA). Thus, the fetal adrenal organogenesis and steroidogenesis are closely interlinked and coordinated to ensure the maturation and function of the fetal adrenal cortex.

Fetal and Neonatal Organogenesis

To determine the developmental pattern of the human adrenal gland, Sucheston and Cannon *(80)* studied adrenal glands from 58 autopsy specimens ranging in age from 1 mo to 69 yr. Their study revealed that the adrenal gland in the human is derived from celomic epithelium at 3–4 wk of gestational age. Between 4–10 wk of gestation, these celomic epithelial cells proliferate, migrate, and differentiate into two distinct zones, the inner fetal zone, which forms 80–90% of the cortex and the outer definitive zone, which forms the rest of the fetal adrenal cortex. Most of the fetal adrenal growth and remodeling that starts around the tenth week of intrauterine life and continues until 1 yr of postnatal age. Between 28–30 wk of gestation, the zona glomerulosa, outer zona fasciculata, fetal cortex, and medulla are delineated. Soon after birth, the fetal zone atrophies and disappears by 3 mo of postnatal life. During the second year of life, a poorly organized zona reticularis is discernable and attains its permanent characteristics by 11–12 yr of age. The fetal adrenal does not have an adrenal medulla as a distinct entity. The adrenal medulla appears in the first few postnatal weeks following the involution of the fetal zone. By the fourth week of postnatal life, the chromaffin cells cluster at the center of the gland, and it is not until 12–18 mo of age that the infant has the medulla with the adult-type architecture (81). The adrenal gland attains its adult architecture by 15 yr of age.

Johannisson studied 57 human fetal adrenal cortices at various gestational ages by both light and electron microscopy (73). Adrenal glands from three full-term anencephalics were included in these 57 cases. These studies show that in 1–1.5-cm fetus, corresponding to a gestational age of 5–6 wk, the adrenocortical cells are immature and show poor differentiation of the endoplasmic reticulum, the Golgi apparatus, and the mitochondria. Between 6–7 wk of gestation, these cells form two distinct zones—an outer zone and an inner zone. Although the cells of the outer zone remain immature, those of the inner zone show an increase in the cytoplasmic organelles, which indicates both a functional and structural differentiation and maturation. During the second trimester, a transitional zone located between the outer and inner zone appears, and it consists of two types of "dark" cells with differences in the agranular endoplasmic reticulum. In the second and third trimester of pregnancy, the definitive zone cells show maturation, which correlates with increasing functional activity of this zone. The cells of this transitional zone are capable of synthesizing cortisol and are the precursor cells of the zona fasciculata of the adult adrenal (13).

The cellular processes of, hyperplasia, cell-migration, hypertrophy, and apoptosis govern the growth and remodeling of the human adrenal gland (Fig. 2). By the eighth week of gestation, when the two zones of the fetal adrenal are discernible, cellular mitosis and hyperplasia are limited to the definitive zone (73). This zone is thought to be the germinal/stem-cell compartment, which gives rise to inner cortical zones. Studies by Keene and Hewer, Crowder, and Jirasek show that cells from the definitive zone migrate in a centripetal fashion to invade the outer layers of the fetal zone (1,81,82). However, recent studies by Morley et al. in the mouse embryo using mouse 21-hydroxylase/β-galactosidase transgene experiments show that in this species the centripetal migration of cells in the fetal adrenal is only established in the later stages of embryonic life or early postnatal life (78).

In contrast to the definitive zone, the fetal zone shows mostly hypertrophy and minimal mitosis, forms the bulk of the fetal adrenal gland, and accounts for 80% of its weight. Unlike other species, the fetal adrenal in the humans and other higher primates shows maximal rate of growth during mid- and late gestation. Most of this growth occurs in the inner fetal zone of the adrenal cortex. By 20 wk of gestation, the fetal adrenal weight is similar to that of the fetal kidney. By 30 wk, the gland rapidly enlarges and becomes 10–20 times the size of the adult adrenal gland. Between 30 wk and term, it doubles in size and weighs 3–4 grams at birth (1,82). In addition to cellular

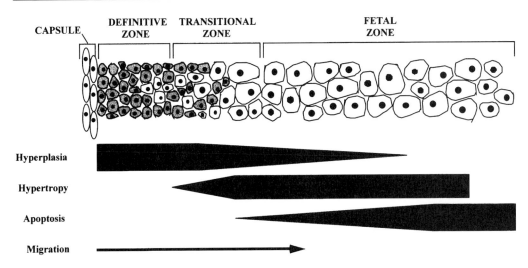

Fig. 2. Schematic representation of the structure and growth of various zones of the primate fetal adrenal cortex at mid-gestation. Hyperplasia occurs mainly in the definitive zone, hypertrophy occurs mainly in the fetal zone, apoptosis occurs mostly in the central region of the fetal zone and cell migration occurs from the periphery to the center of the gland. (Adapted from ref. *27*).

hyperplasia, centripetal migration, and hypertrophy, apoptosis also contributes to the remodeling of fetal adrenal into an adult organ. Both morphologic and DNA-based techniques show that apoptosis, which occurs mainly in the central part of the cortex, is more marked in the fetal zone as compared to the definitive zone *(38,82)*. During the first postnatal week, the fetal zone undergoes rapid involution and disappears by the third month of postnatal life. As the fetal zone involutes by apoptosis, the fetal definitive and transitional zones form the zona glomerulosa and fasciculata, respectively *(13)*. The innermost cells of the transitional zone form the zona reticularis of the adult adrenal cortex. This remodeling continues all through the first year of life.

The growth, development, and function of the fetal adrenal cortex is governed not only by the various cellular processes, aforementioned, but also by the feto-placental steroidogenesis regulated by endocrine factors, a multitude of paracrine growth factors, and autocrine nuclear receptors.

Fetal Adrenal Steroidogenesis

The complex coordination of fetal adrenal, placental, and maternal steroidogenesis is the hallmark of the feto-placental unit. The feto-placental unit ensures the survival and maturation of the fetus. Several studies have shown that baboon and human pregnancy share a great degree of similarity in the structure, function, and steroidogenesis of the feto-placental unit *(8,9,83–86)*. Therefore, studies on regulation of placental and fetal steroidogenesis in primate pregnancy provide an excellent model to understand temporal events related to steroidogenesis of the human feto-placental unit. The discussion that follows is based on in vitro and in vivo studies on primate and human pregnancy.

Morphological features of steroidogenesis in the fetal adrenal cells is first observed at 6–8 wk of gestational age *(7,74)*. The temporal relationship between ambiguous external genital development in female infants with congenital adrenal hyperplasia because of 21-hydroxylase deficiency and the development of the fetal adrenal cortex indicates that the feedback loop of the fetal HPAA is functional prior to the tenth week of gestational life. Between 8–10 wk of gestation, the fetal zone, which forms 80% of the fetal adrenal cortex, synthesizes DHEA-S, the main precursor of estrogen synthesis by the placenta *(79)*. This placental estrogen is crucial to the maintenance of pregnancy, the maturation of the fetal and maternal tissues, and immunosuppression leading to implantation of the placenta and the fetus *(9)*.

Estrogen also plays a very significant role in placental and fetal steroidogenesis through stimulation of placental progesterone production, modulation of DHEA-S production by the fetal adrenal, and regulation of the HPPA, all of which ensure integrity of the pregnancy and neonatal self-sufficiency *(87)*.

In addition to estrogen, fetal steroidogenesis is essential for the maintenance of pregnancy and maturation of fetal organs *(9,10,19)*. In humans as in the other primates, there is substantial transplacental transfer of maternal cortisol to the fetus throughout gestation. The fetal cortisol level is dependent on the fetal cortisol production and metabolic clearance rate, the transplacental transfer of maternal cortisol, as well as the estrogen-mediated conversion of cortisol to cortisone by both the fetus and the placenta. Whereas the fetal zone is the principal site of DHEA-S synthesis, the outer definitive zone of the fetal adrenal mainly produces cortisol *(16,88)*. The fetal cortisol level, which increases with gestational age, plays a significant role in the maturation of the fetal organs *(8)*.

The uptake of maternal low-density lipoproteins by the syncytiotrophoblast provides the substrate necessary for placental steroidogenesis *(89,90)*. The placental synthesis of pregnenalone and progesterone from this maternal cholesterol, is regulated by the estrogen derived from fetal DHEA-S. During early and midgestation, the fetus obtains its cortisol from maternal sources, either through transplacental transfer of maternal cortisol or through the conversion of placental progesterone to cortisol by the fetal adrenal. The fetal zone of the adrenal cortex produces the DHEA-S under the regulation of fetal ACTH *(16,88,91)*. Carr and Simpson *(92)* have demonstrated that in the fetus, the liver produces significant amounts of cholesterol, which is provided as circulating LDL substrate to the adrenal for steroidogenesis. The fetal zone produces DHEA-S from this cholesterol. These investigators have proposed that the positive feedback system that includes the fetal liver, fetal adrenal, and the placenta is responsible for the exponential increase in steroidogenesis by the fetoplacental unit *(90)*. The fetal DHEA-S forms the main substrate for estrogen biosynthesis through placental aromatization of fetal DHEA-S to estrogen *(7,93)*. This fetal DHEA-S-based estrogen production by the placenta is a delicately balanced mechanism. Studies in baboon pregnancy show that estrogen exerts a negative feedback control on the fetal DHEA-S synthesis by suppressing the fetal adrenal responsiveness to ACTH *(83,94,95)*.

Estrogen upregulates both low-density lipoprotein (LDL) receptor and *P450scc* enzyme expression in the placenta, thus increasing placental syncytiotrophoblast LDL uptake and *p450scc* activity *(85,96)*. These estrogen-mediated actions are developmentally regulated in an autocrine and/or paracrine manner in the placenta. Thus, although in early and midgestational periods the fetal adrenal does not significantly contribute to direct cortisol synthesis, it does so indirectly by producing DHEA-S.

In contrast, during late gestation and prior to birth, the fetal adrenal is the major source of cortisol biosynthesis *(88)*. The major substrate for cortisol synthesis by the fetal adrenal is LDLs derived from the fetal liver *(97)*. In addition, placental progesterone also contributes to this cortisol biosynthesis by the fetal adrenal, although in late gestation the conversion of placental progesterone to cortisol is minimal *(98)*. The estrogen-induced regulation of placental and fetal 11β-hydroxysteroid dehydrogenase (11βHSD) increases with advancing age and leads to increased oxidation of cortisol to cortisone, thereby effectively decreasing fetal cortisol levels. This, in turn, regulates the fetal HPAA resulting in an increase in ACTH-stimulated cortisol synthesis by the fetal adrenal. In addition, estrogen through regulation of 11βHSD and cortisol synthesis, plays an important role in the maturation of the hypothalamic-pituitary adrenal axis *(9,99,100)* (Fig. 3).

The differences in steroid biosynthesis by the fetal zone and definitive zone are based on the temporal and spatial expression of branch-point enzymes *P450 17α-hydroxylase/17,20 lyase (P450c17)* and 3β-hydroxysteroid dehydrogenase (3βHSD) *(7,16,101,102)* (Fig. 4a, b). The differential expression of these enzymes in the fetal zone and the definitive zone determines whether the fetal adrenal gland converts pregnenalone to DHEA-S or cortisol. *In situ* hybridization, as well as immunocytohistochemistry studies, show that, all through gestation *P450scc* is expressed in all of the fetal adrenal cortex. Throughout gestation, the fetal zone does not show expression of 3βHSD in vivo, but does show *p450c17* expression. Interestingly, the cells of this zone do show expression of this enzyme when they are exposed to supraphysiological doses of ACTH in vitro. In contrast, the definitive zone cells do not express *p450c17* enzyme, but between 22–24 wk of gestation show 3βHSD expression. By 28 wk, this enzyme is expressed in the entire definitive zone and extends into the transitional zone. Thus, the fetal zone mainly produces DHEA-S and is unable to synthesize cortisol due to a lack or block of 3βHSD. On the other hand, the cortisol synthesis, which mainly occurs during late gestation and near-term, is limited to the definitive zone. Thus, the temporal expression of steroid hydroxylase enzymes in the definitive, transitional, and fetal zones of the adrenal cortex is central to steroidogenesis by these zones *(103,104)*.

MOLECULAR MECHANISMS

The twin processes of adrenal organogenesis and steroidogenesis are both governed by underlying molecular mechanisms that not only regulate the growth and function of the fetal adrenal, but also have a pivitol role in the remodeling of the fetal adrenal into a self-sufficient and life-sustaining adult adrenal cortex. Endocrine, paracrine, and autocrine factors are central to these molecular mechanisms. These factors include human chorionic gonadotropin (HCG) and ACTH, several growth factors including bFGF, EGF, TGF-α, IGF-1 and -2), and members belonging to the TGF-β family of proteins including activin, inhibin, and TGF-β1, and the nuclear receptors *SF-1, DAX-1,* and *ER*.

HCG and ACTH

The growth of the fetal adrenal in the first trimester of pregnancy is regulated by HCG *(4,5)*. Although evidence suggests that the HPAA axis is functional by about the tenth week of intrauterine life, HCG appears to play a significant role in adrenal growth during early gestation. In vitro studies by Seron-Ferre et al. on fetal adrenals between 12–17 wk gestational age show that HCG significantly increased DHEA-S secretion *(11,16)*. Furthermore, studies in anencephalic fetuses have shown that the adrenal gland

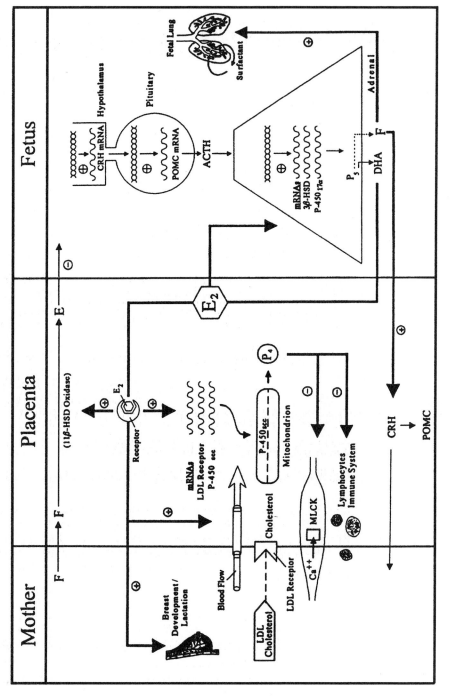

Fig. 3. Schematic representation of the actions of placental and fetal adrenal steroid hormones in primate pregnancy. (Reproduced with permission from ref. 9).

18

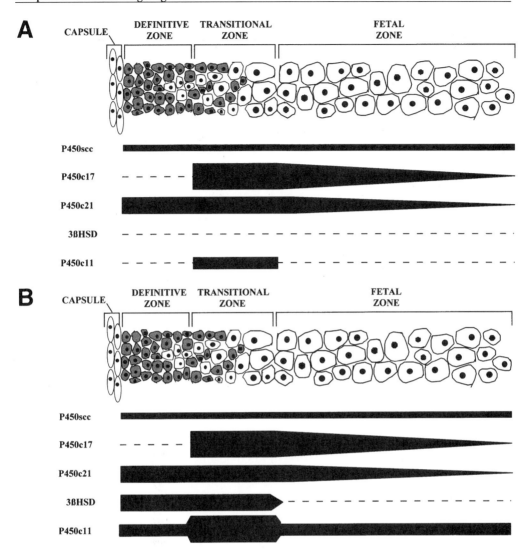

Fig. 4. Schematic representation of localization and relative abundance of expression of p450scc, p450c17, p450c21, 3βHSD and p450c11 in mid- and late gestation primate fetal adrenal cortex. Thickness of line indicates the level of expression of the enzyme. Dashed line indicates lack of expression of the enzyme. P450c17 is not expressed in the definitive zone and 3βHSD is not expressed in the fetal zone. 3βHSD is expressed only in the definitive and transitional zone late in gestation. (Adapted from ref. *7*).

develops normally up to the fifth month of gestation *(105),* thus supporting the role of HCG in early fetal adrenal cortical development.

ACTH plays a pivotal role in the growth, differentiation, and steroidogenesis of the fetal adrenal cells *(11,13,15–18,88,106–111).* After the twentieth week of gestational age, ACTH-mediated effects are of paramount importance in further growth of the fetal adrenal *(88).* Studies of anencephalic fetuses shows that after the first 15 wk of gestation in the absence of ACTH, the fetal zone of the adrenal gland fails to develop, which results in a marked decrease in maternal estrogen levels. The growth of anencephalic fetal adrenals can be partially restored by administration of ACTH to these fetuses *(73)*. In contrast, syndromes of excessive ACTH production such as Cushing's disease caused by ACTH producing tumors of the pituitary and congenital adrenal hyperplasia caused by steroidogenic enzyme deficiencies lead to hyperplastic adrenal glands. Although in vitro studies show that ACTH is not a direct mitogen for adrenocortical cells grown in culture *(110,112)*, it indirectly influences the growth of these cells in vivo *(113–115)*. These indirect effects of ACTH on fetal adrenal glands are governed by growth factors, which, in addition to mediating the effects of ACTH, also act directly on the fetal adrenal to modulate its growth.

Growth Factors

Several growth factors including, bFGF, EGF, IGF 1 and 2, TGF-α, and members belonging to the TGF-β family of proteins including activin, inhibin, and TGF-β1 play a role in steroidogenesis, growth, and development of the adrenal gland *(19)*. These peptide growth factors are produced both by the placenta and the fetus. In conjunction with ACTH, these growth factors play a role in the differential steroid biosynthesis by the two zones of the fetal adrenal.

Basic Fibroblast Growth Factor

bFGF belongs to a family of mitogenic proteins. Cultured fetal adrenal cells from midgestational human fetus showed that bFGF increases the proliferation of both the definitive and fetal zone cells *(21,22)*, as well as adrenal cortex-derived capillary endothelial cells *(23)*. However, its effect on cells of the definitive zone is twice that on the cells of the fetal zone *(21)*. In addition to direct mitogenic effects on fetal adrenal cells, bFGF has indirect mitogenic effects, which are mediated through ACTH *(25)*. ACTH not only increases the expression of bFGF leading to increased cell proliferation, but it also increases angiogenesis and vascularization of the fetal adrenal cortex *(19)*.

EGF, TGF-α, and EGF Receptor

EGF and TGF-α are paracrine intracellular signaling molecules that belong to a larger family of mitogenic proteins *(116–118)*. These two growth factors share sequence homology, activate the EGF receptor, and have similar biological functions.

Studies have shown that EGF is mitogenic to the midgestational cultured fetal adrenal cortical and definitive zone cells *(21,22)*, but not to cultures of adult bovine adrenal cortical cells *(22,119)*. Both EGF and TGF-α and other EGF receptor ligands mediate their actions through the EGF receptor. Whereas, the expression of EGF, TGF-α, and EGF receptor in human fetal adrenals was detected by RT-PCR, immunostaining only showed the expression of TGF-α and EGF receptor. These studies indicate that in the fetal adrenal instead of EGF, TGF-α may be the main peptide growth factor acting through the EGF receptor *(19,120)*. In vivo studies in late gestational-rhesus monkeys show that treatment with EGF significantly increases the weight and width of the definitive zones, as well as the amount of 3βHSD protein in both the definitive and transitional zones of the fetal adrenal *(121)*. However, this increase in weight is caused by cellular hypertrophy and not hyperplasia. Luger et al. examined the effects of EGF on primate HPAA by giving mouse EGF to rhesus monkeys. They determined that mEGF increased the plasma levels of ACTH and cortisol in a dose-dependent manner. However, further studies showed that EGF stimulates hypothalamic CRH release, but does not directly cause pituitary ACTH secretion *(26)*. Thus, in addition to its direct effects on the fetal adrenal cells, EGF may influence the growth and steroidogenic activity of these cells by increasing the 3βHSD protein and regulating the HPAA.

Insulin-Like Growth Factors 1 and 2

The endocrine, paracrine, and autocrine roles of IGF-1 and IGF-2 in proliferation and differentiation of steroidogenic cells is well established *(30,122)*. Growth hormone regulates IGF-1 levels, which mediates many of the somatotropic effects of growth hormone *(123)*. Northern blot and RT-PCR studies show that IGF-1 and 2, their receptors, as well as binding proteins, are all expressed in human fetal adrenals *(27,32)*. However, *in situ* hybridization studies by Mesiano et al. have shown IGF-1 is expressed only in the adrenal capsule, whereas IGF-2 is expressed by all cortical cells *(124)*. Recent studies on adult bovine adrenal cortical cells show that IGF-1 increases the effects of ACTH on these cells *(28)*. Specifically, in the bovine species, IGF-1 enhances adrenal responsiveness to ACTH by increasing the ACTH receptors *(125)*. Human studies have shown that in addition to increasing the adrenal responsiveness to ACTH, IGF-1 also increases the activity of 17α, 21-, and 11β-hydroxylases, thereby enhancing steroidogenic activity of the adrenal *(31)*.

Whereas IGF-1 has important roles in the postnatal steroidogenic tissues, IGF-2 has a central role in the growth and development of the fetal tissues. In most fetal tissues including the fetal adrenals where IGF-2 is detectable, its level of expression is higher than that of IGF-1 *(27,32)*. ACTH and IGF-2 are closely interlinked in the growth and development of the adrenal cortex. *In situ* hybridization studies show that IGF-2 mRNA is highly expressed in the cortical cells. Studies using cultured fetal adrenal cells have shown that these cells retain their ability to express IGF-2 in response to ACTH *(13,126)*. This effect of ACTH on IGF-2 is limited to the fetal cortex and is not seen in early postnatal period. Whereas ACTH increases IGF-2 expression, IGF-2 increases the responsiveness of the adrenal cortical cells to ACTH. Studies also show that in conjunction with estrogen, IGF-2 promotes ACTH-stimulated DHEA-S synthesis. In addition, it also regulates the steroidogenic enzymes *p450scc, p450c17,* and 3βHSD in the fetal adrenal. These key enzymes are central to both cortisol and androgen biosynthesis by the fetal adrenal *(127)*. Thus, IGF-2 is a key growth factor in the fetal adrenal development and steroidogenesis.

Transforming Growth Factor β Family of Growth Factors:
Activin, Inhibin, and TGF β1

Activin and inhibin are glycoproteins that belong to the TGF β family of proteins *(35)*. These proteins form homo- or heterodimers and are composed of α-, βA-, and βB-subunits. The α-subunit, which is a part of the inhibin molecule only, heterodimerizes with βA- and βB-subunits to form inhibin A and B, respectively. Whereas the subunits βA, βB homodimerize to form activin-A (βAβA) and activin-B (βBβB) they heterodimerize to form activin-AB (βAβB). Immunocytohistochemistry and *in situ* hybridization studies show that all the three subunits—α, β and βB, are expressed in the fetal and adult adrenal cortex *(36,37)*. *In situ* hybridization studies on cultured fetal adrenal cortical cells show that ACTH upregulates the expression of the α, and βA subunit-mRNA whereas, the βB unit mRNA expression is not affected. These data suggest that ACTH stimulates the production of inhibin-A, as well as that of activin-A.

In addition to regulating the secretion of FSH by the pituitary, activin also has a paracrine role in the granulosa cells of the ovary and in the fetal adrenal cortical cells, which are both derived from the celomic epithelial cells. Although both of these tissues show expression of activin, the function of activin in the adrenal cortical and ovarian granulosa cells is not the same. Whereas, recombinant human activin-A promotes granulosa cell proliferation, it inhibits fetal zone cell proliferation (36,37). Activin also increases the ACTH-stimulated production of cortisol by the fetal zone cells, however, it has no effect on DHEA-S production by these cells. In contrast, activin had no effect on growth or steroidogenesis in definitive or adult adrenal cortical cells. Interestingly, recombinant human inhibin had no effect on either the growth or function of these cells. A recent study by Spencer et al. also shows that activin promotes apoptosis in the inner-cortical compartment of the adrenal suggesting that it may be responsible for the involution of the fetal adrenal cortex during the postnatal period (38).

The paracrine/autocrine role of TGF-β1 in the adrenal cortex is well-established. TGF-β1 acts by binding to its specific receptor on the fetal adrenal cells and this binding is upregulated by ACTH (40). In the human fetal adrenal, TGF-β1 appears to be a negative regulator of fetal and definitive zone cell proliferation and steroidogenesis (128). Studies in bovine and ovine adrenal cortical cells show that it decreases the expression of p450scc and 17a-hydroxylase expression in both basal, as well as the ACTH-stimulated cells (33,34). Studies by Stankovic et al. show that this peptide factor inhibits basal, as well as ACTH-stimulated steroid biosynthesis by the fetal adrenal cells including DHEA-S and cortisol production in response to foskolin and dibutyryl cAMP (39). In addition, these authors also show that it interferes with the ACTH-stimulated expression of p45017α mRNA in the cells of the fetal zone and the neocortex. Interestingly, whereas TGF-β1 has no effect on ACTH receptor or p450scc expression, it promotes the ACTH-stimulated expression of 3βHSD (129). Thus, both activin and TGF-β1 are negative paracrine regulators of growth and steroidogenesis in the fetal adrenal cortex.

Nuclear Receptors

SF-1, DAX-1, and ER are members of the nuclear hormone receptor superfamily of proteins that have a common modular architecture (130–133). These nuclear receptors have six functional domains. The A/B domain has a transactivation function and is highly variable in both sequence and length. The C domain is highly conserved and it is the DNA-binding domain (DBD), which is characterized by the presence of two zinc-fingers. The highly variable D domain may have nuclear localization signals and/or a transactivation function. The E domain is complex in function. In addition to ligand binding, it also has specific regions for dimerization, nuclear localization, transactivation, intermolecular silencing, and repression. Although the specific function of the F region remains to be established, research has shown that this region is highly variable. The members of this family are transcription factors, which in addition to maintaining biological function, govern the expression of genes that regulate cellular growth, differentiation, and apoptosis.

SF-1 and DAX-1 are crucial to adrenal organogenesis and steroidogenesis. These nuclear receptors are classified as orphan receptors as their ligands are unknown (134). DAX-1 is a unique member of the nuclear receptor family of proteins. Unlike other members of this family, the transactivating A/B domain, the DNA-binding C domain, and the hinge region or the D domain of the DAX-1 protein are replaced by 3.5 tandem repeats of a 65–67 amino acid motif *(135,136)*. Although DAX-1 differs markedly in its N-terminal domain, it is also included in this family of proteins as it has a well-conserved ligand-binding domain, which is similar to that of other members of this superfamily. ER regulates gene transcription by binding to its ligand estrogen *(137,138)*, although recent studies show that ER can also regulate gene transcription in a ligand-independent manner through the transactivating function located in its A/B domain *(139,140)*.

Steroidogenic Factor 1 (SF-1)

Steroidogenic factor 1 (SF-1) is the mouse homolog of *fushi tarazu* factor 1 *(52,141)*, a cell-specific orphan nuclear receptor in the *Drosophila*, proposed to regulate the expression of *fushi tarazu* (*ftz-F1*) homeobox gene *(142,143)*. The gene encoding SF-1 in the mouse was also named *ftz-F1*. *In situ* hybridization studies in the mouse embryos demonstrated that SF-1 was expressed in the gonads, the diencephalon, the urogenital sinus, and the developing adrenal cortex *(54,60,144,145)*. In the adult animal, this gene is expressed in the steroidogenic cells of the adrenal glands and the gonads *(45,146)*, in the gonadotropic cells of the pituitary *(147,148)*, and in the ventromedial nucleus of the hypothalamus (VMH) *(149,150)*. Targeted disruption of the *ftz-F1* gene in mice established its essential role in the organogenesis of these tissues *(41–43,151)*. Thus, these mice had agenesis of their adrenal glands, gonads, and the VMH, resulting in complete congenital adrenal insufficiency and male-to-female sex reversal.

Homologs of *SF-1* gene have been identified in several species *(52,152–154)* including the human *(155,156)*. It is significant to note that all SF-1 cDNAs identified and characterized to date from various species showed a very high degree of sequence conservation in their various functional domains *(155,156)*. In several species, *ftz-F1* genes encode at two or more transcripts *(154,157–159)*. It is noteworthy that in the mouse four distinct alternatively spliced products are derived from the *ftz-F1* gene *(154)*. These four different transcripts, ELPs 1, 2, 3, and SF-1, are generated by alternative use of nested promoters and splice sites. Functional studies of these transcripts, using cotransfection experiments in NIH-3T3 cells, showed that although ELP 1 isoform, which lacks the AF2 domain, repressed the transcription of a reporter construct containing the SF-1/ELP response element, ELP Isoforms 2 and 3 activated transcription of this construct. Also, the ELP3 isoform in this species, which is expressed in the pituitary, is controled by a promoter different than the one that controls the SF-1 isoform, which is expressed in the steroidogenic tissues. In the zebra fish *(159)*, two isoforms of this receptor function differently. The nontruncated form of this receptor (zFF1A) not only stimulates the gonadotropin β-subunit promoter, but also synergizes with ER to further activate this promoter. The C-terminally truncated version (zFF1B), however, does not synergize with ER to regulate the gonadotropin b-subunit promoter, but it does function as repressor. These data suggest that the isoforms have differential species-specific tissue expression, regulation, and function.

To determine the role of SF-1 in humans, we recently isolated and characterized human steroidogenic factor 1 (hSF-1) by heterologous probing of a λgt11 fetal adrenal cDNA library, using a mouse SF-1 cDNA probe that did not include the region coding for the zinc finger domain *(155)*. The human cDNA sequence showed a high degree of homology (>95%) found in both the bovine and murine sequences. The zinc fingers,

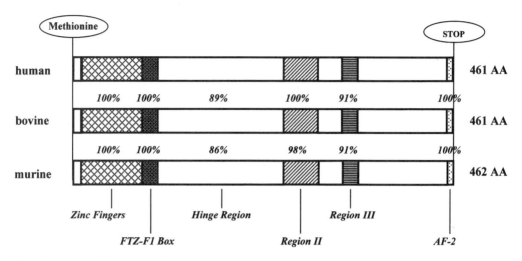

Fig. 5. Functional domains of SF-1 protein and its inter-species homology. The Zinc finger, FTZ-F1 box and AF-2 regions of SF-1 protein show 100% homology between the human, bovine and the murine species. In contrast, the hinge region is only 86% homologous. (Adapted from reference 155).

the FTZ-1 box and the AF2 domains showed 100% conservation of the derived amino acid residues with a lesser degree of homology in the ligand-binding/dimerization domains (Fig. 5).

Following the cloning and sequencing of hSF-1 cDNA, we defined the sites of hSF-1 mRNA expression in human tissues by both Northern blot and *in situ* hybridization analyses *(160)*. These studies revealed high hSF-1 mRNA expression in the adrenal cortex, ovaries, testes, and the spleen. Northern blot analysis of these tissues revealed a main message of 3.5 kb. Interestingly, the spleen showed three additional transcripts of 2.4 kb, 4.4 kb, and 8.0 kb. Specifically, the additional 4.4 kb transcript was also seen in several peripheral tissues, the CNS and several components of the limbic system, as well as the myeloid and lymphoid cancer cell lines. The human gene encoding SF-1 is highly homologous to that of other species, and the pattern of hSF-1 expression in the adrenal glands and gonads is similar to that seen in the mouse and the cow. The expression of SF-1 in the steroidogenic tissues in the human parallels that of the mouse. In the human CNS, unlike in the mouse, the expression of SF-1 mRNA is widespread. This species-specific wide-spread distribution of SF-1 in the human CNS and the strong expression of SF-1 in the reticuloendothelial network of the human spleen suggest that SF-1 may have a more comprehensive role in the human than in other species.

Northern blot analysis of the human placenta did not reveal hSF-1 message after a 16-h exposure, however, a weak signal was noted after 8 wk of exposure. SF-1 message expression in the bovine and human placenta was previously reported, using the highly sensitive RT-PCR technique *(161)*. The apparently low expression of hSF-1 in human placenta suggests that it may not have a major role in placental steroidogenesis. This view is supported by previous studies that demonstrated expression of SF-1 mRNA in BeWo human choriocarcinoma cells only by the highly sensitive RT-PCR technique, nonexpression of the *StAR* gene in the placenta *(162)*, expression of *P450* side-chain-cleavage enzyme in the placenta of SF-1-deficient mice *(43)*, use of SFRE-deficient aromatase promoter 1.1 for placental aromatase gene transcription *(163)*, and regulation of placental *p450scc* gene transcription by a 55-kDa protein that is expressed in the placenta, but not in the adrenal cortex *(164)*. The data from these studies along with our own data suggest that alternative pathways of steroid metabolism or functional homologs of hSF-1 may be operational in human placental steroidogenesis.

In situ hybridization studies of normal architecture adrenal gland showed similar distribution of SF-1 mRNA signal in all the three zones of the adrenal cortex *(160)*. However, within each cortical zone, the signal distribution was heterogeneous. Interestingly, in our *in situ* hybridization studies of a normal nodular variant of the adrenal gland, we detected a very high *SF-1* gene expression in the proliferative nodules. Sasano et al., using immunohistochemistry also demonstrated the heterogeneous distribution of the signal of Ad4BP, the bovine homolog of SF-1, within each of the three cortical zones of normal, neoplastic, and atrophied human adrenal glands *(165)*. These data suggest that, in addition to regulation of steroidogenesis, SF-1 may also have a role in regulating the growth and proliferation of adult adrenal cortical cells.

In situ hybridization studies in the ovary demonstrated that hSF-1 mRNA was abundant in granulosa cells at all stages of follicular development, except for primordial follicles, and was also present in corpora lutea. Both the theca interna and theca externa cells surrounding the graafian follicles also expressed hSF-1 mRNA. hSF-1 mRNA, however, was also seen in atretic follicles, which normally are not steroidogenic. A recent study showed that enhanced SF-1 expression is associated with GC differentiation, and that it inhibits TPA-induced mitosis of these cells *(166)*. Given its role in GC cell differentiation and its increased expression in the adrenal nodules, as seen in our *in situ* hybridization studies, it is conceivable that SF-1 may also govern the fetal adrenal cell proliferation, differentiation, and apoptosis.

In the adult testis, hSF-1 expression was seen in both the interstitial cells and the inner border of the seminiferous tubules, suggesting expression in the steroidogenic Leydig cells and the germinal epithelium. Our results suggest that in the human testis, in addition to steroidogenesis, hSF-1 may also have a role in the function of spermatogenesis.

The data in other species and our human tissue expression studies of this gene suggest that SF-1 isoforms may be present in the human, and it is conceivable that these isoforms have differential tissue expression, function, and regulation. It is therefore also conceivable that mutations, deletions, or rearrangement of the genes encoding hSF-1 or putative hSF-1 isoforms may result in aberrant or truncated proteins with disrupted function leading to defective fetal adrenal organogenesis and steroidogenesis. Ultimately, this could manifest as the clinical syndrome of non-X-linked autosomal recessive congenital adrenal hypoplasia, or dysregulated steroidogenesis. Thus, SF-1 may be pivotal to the organogenesis of the fetal adrenal gland, including its remodeling into a self-sufficient neonatal organ.

Previous studies have revealed that SF-1 plays a pivotal role in the transcriptional regulation of several genes coding for steroidogenic enzymes *(56,61,167–179)*. It is becoming increasingly clear that as a transcription factor SF-1 is crucial to adrenal steroidogenesis at more than one level. In addition to its role as a regulator of steroid hydroxylase enzyme expression, SF-1 also has a role in stimulating the promoter activities of genes encoding the ACTH receptor *(180,181)*, steroidogenic acute regulatory (StAR) protein *(182,183)*, and the scavenger receptor-type class BI (SR-BI)

(184,185). StAR protein is crucial for the translocation of cholesterol from the outer to the inner mitochondrial membrane, which in turn leads to conversion of cholesterol to pregnenolone. The SR-BI/CLA-1 protein binds to high-density lipoproteins (HDL) and mediates the selective transport of lipids from HDL to steroidogenic cells, which provides these cells with the cholesterol for steroidogenesis *(184,187)*. In the human, similar to its expression in the rodents, SR-BI mRNA is highly expressed in the adrenal and the ovary. Interestingly its expression in the fetal adrenal is estimated to be 50 times greater than its expression in the adult adrenal gland. In the fetal adrenal gland, low-density lipoprotein (LDL) rather than HDL is the main source of cholesterol for steroid biosynthesis. Studies have shown that SR-BI also binds to LDL with high affinity (186). In addition to SR-BI receptor, LDL receptor (LDLR) is highly expressed in the fetal adrenal cortex *(184)*. The relative roles of SR-BI and LDLR in providing cholesterol to fetal adrenal cells for steroidogenesis are not known. However, as SR-BI binds to LDL with high affinity, it may also have a significant role in providing LDL to the fetal adrenal for steroidogenesis. Clearly, not only is SF-1 critical for the constitutive activity of the human ACTH receptor-gene promoter, but it also regulates the genes that are important in providing the substrate, cholesterol, for adrenal and gonadal steroid biosynthesis. Furthermore, SF-1 is a global regulator of steroid hydroxy-lase enzymes. Collectively, these studies establish SF-1's role at multiple levels of the HPAA axis and underscore the central role of SF-1 in fetal adrenal steroidogenesis.

SF-1 also plays a critical role in the regulation of genes crucial to development, and maintenance of the reproductive function. SF-1 regulates the genes coding for aromatase *(53,188–192)*, Mullerian inhibiting substance *(193,194)*, oxytocin *(195,196)*, prolactin receptor *(197)*, the α-subunit of the glycoprotein hormones *(198)*, the β-subunit of luteinizing hormone *(199,202)*, gonadotropin-releasing hormone receptor *(203)*. SF-1 may regulate the expression of DAX-1. Recent cotransfection studies in NCI-H295 cells using wild-type and deletional SF-1 mutant expression vectors show that a functional SF-1 response element is present in the DAX-1 promoter, which enhances the activity of this promoter *(204)*. Also, SF-1 and chicken ovalbumin upstream promoter-transcription factor (COUP-TF) modulate the expression of DAX-1 *(205)*. Whereas SF-1 stimulates murine DAX-1 promoter, COUP-TF inhibits its activity.

Recent studies suggest that similar to other members of the nuclear receptor superfam-ily SF-1 also interacts with cofactors such as SRC-1 and CBP/p300 to regulate gene transcription. Most nuclear receptors contain two transactivation domains, called AF1 and AF2 domains, located in the N-terminal and C-terminal regions, respectively *(206)*. Unlike other members of this superfamily, our studies show that in the human, as in other species, SF-1 does not have an AF-1 domain in the N-terminal region *(155)*. However, it has a unique region termed the Ftz-F1 box followed by a proline-rich region located just downstream from the DNA-binding domain. Whereas the Ftz-F1 box facilitates the binding of SF-1 to its response elements in the target DNA *(207)*, the proline-rich region is proposed to contribute to transcriptional activation *(208)*. More recently, Li and colleagues have shown that the Ftz-F1 box together with the proline-rich region termed the FP region, functions in nuclear localization and interaction with basic transcription factor TFIIB and c-*jun* *(209)*. Our studies also show that in the human SF-1, the carboxy-terminal-AF2 domain, which forms an amphipathic α-helix, is conserved. The AF2 region, which is essential for protein–protein interaction between SF-1 and the cofactors *(210, 209, 211)*, is also important in protein kinase-C potentiation of SF-1-regulated reporter gene activity *(212)*. Jacob et al. show that expression of AF2 mutants of SF-1 in the presence of PKA-C drastically inhibited the transcriptional activation of endogenous SF-1 *(212)*. Thus, the AF2 mutant has a dominant negative effect suggesting that the AF2 domain of SF-1 is essential for the activation of SF-1 by cAMP-dependent PKA mediated signaling pathway. Ito et al., using cotransfection experiments in JEG-3 cells, show that although SRC-1 and CBP/p300 act synergistically to potentiate the transcription by SF-1, CBP/p300 in of itself is unable to enhance SF-1 mediated activity of the reporter gene *(213)*. However, Monte et al. show that in NCI-H295 cells the SF-1-mediated activity of *p450scc* gene promoter, which has multiple SF-1 binding sites, is enhanced by CBP/p300. These experiments suggest that SRC-1 is also a cofactor for SF-1 and that the interactions between SF-1 and CBP/p300 are cell and promoter specific *(214)*. The interaction of SF-1 with other proteins, as well as cofactors, may play a significant role in adrenal steroidogenesis. Liu and colleagues have shown that an interaction between SF-1 and Sp1 is necessary for the regulation of the cholesterol side chain cleavage enzyme (*p450scc*) gene expression. This may either be a direct protein–protein interaction between these two transcription factors, or it may be mediated through coactivator CBP/p300 *(215)*. SF-1 and DAX-1 interactions may involve competition for shared coactivator proteins, such as SRC-1 and CBP/p300 *(213,216)*. Thus, the interactions of SF-1 with cofactor proteins expands SF-1's repertoire of strategies for target gene regulation.

DAX-1

Adrenal hypoplasia congenita (AHC) was mapped to *Xp21* by studies in male patients with contiguous gene deletion syndrome *(217–220)*. These patients have complex glycerol kinase deficiency, X-linked AHC, and/or Duchenne muscular dystrophy caused by gene deletions in the *Xp21* locus. Following the isolation of *DAX-1* gene, mutations in this gene were identified in patients with X-linked AHC and hypogonadotropic hypogonadism *(48,221)*. The gene-encoding DAX-1 (*Ahch* gene) consists of two exons separated by an intron. DAX-1 is a unique member of the nuclear receptor family of proteins. Unlike other members of this family it differs markedly in its N-terminal region, which does not have the classical DNA-binding domain. In the DAX-1 protein, the transactivating A/B domain, the DNA-binding C domain and the hinge region or the D domain are replaced by a 3.5 tandem repeats of a 65–67 amino acid motif whereas the ligand-binding domain or the E domain is homologous to the E domain of other family members. Within this E domain are regions II and III that are thought to play important roles in ligand binding, dimerization, and transactivation. These regions are also well-conserved in the DAX-1 protein *(48,135,136,222)*. In addition, similar to other members of this family such as ER, retinoic acid receptor (RAR), retinoic X receptor (RXR), thyroid receptor (TR), and SF-1 *(155,223–226),* the AF2 domain in the carboxy terminal region of DAX-1 is well-conserved *(49)*. Recent studies in patients with X-linked AHC, have revealed truncations or mutations of *DAX-1* gene in this C-terminal region *(216,227,228),* thus establishing its critical role in adrenal organogenesis.

DAX-1 gene expression is tissue specific and this expression is developmentally regulated. It is highly expressed in the fetal and the adult adrenal gland, ovaries, testes, pituitary, and the hypothalamus *(48,49,64,229,230)*. It is significant that SF-1 and DAX-1 show parallel tissue expression, which suggests that these two transcription factors may coregulate adrenal and gonadal organogenesis, as well as steroidogenesis *(71)*.

The mitochondrial StAR protein, which plays a pivotal role in the translocation of cholesterol from the outer to the inner mitochondrial membrane was recently isolated and characterized from LH-induced mouse MA-10 Leydig tumor cells *(231,232)*. In gonadal and adrenal cells, there is a direct correlation between the expression of *StAR* gene and steroidogenic activity *(231)*. Tropic hormones, ACTH and LH, regulate steroid biosynthesis by increasing the translocation of cholesterol from the outer to the inner mitochondrial membrane. Subsequently, the cholesterol side chain cleavage enzyme (*p450scc*), which resides in the inner mitochondrial membrane, catalyses the conversion of cholesterol to pregnenolone. Although the exact mechanism underlying this tropic hormone-stimulated acute steroidogenic response is not clear, recent studies have shown that the tropic hormone-stimulated expression of StAR mRNA and protein was within a time frame concomitant with acute steroid biosynthesis *(231,233)*. Furthermore, recent studies on patients with lipoid congenital adrenal hyperplasia showed that these patients are unable to synthesize adrenal and gonadal steroids due to mutations in the StAR gene, thus confirming the critical role of this gene in steroid biosynthesis *(234,235)*.

Recent studies have shown that DAX-1 blocks steroidogenesis not only by inhibiting the activity of StAR, but also by inhibiting the expression of *p450scc* and 3β-HSD expression *(236)*. Using transient cotransfection experiments, Zazapoulos et al. have recently demonstrated that despite the unique N-terminal region of DAX-1, which does not have any known DNA-binding motif, DAX-1 binds to the StAR promoter to act as a powerful repressor of both basal and cAMP-stimulated activity of the StAR promoter *(72)*. These investigators also show that DAX-1 represses *StAR* gene expression by binding with equal efficiency to both hairpin structures and stems composed of 10–24 nucleotides in the StAR promoter. It is interesting to note that even though the presence of the loop structure in the StAR promoter is crucial to binding of the DAX-1 protein to the promoter, the sequence of the loop itself influences the binding efficiency of DAX-1. Loops rich in thymines or cytosines show increased binding as compared to loops rich in adenines. This study directly links DAX-1 to the StAR protein-mediated regulation of acute steroid biosynthesis in the adrenals and the gonads.

X-linked AHC, is a life-threatening disorder that mostly presents in infancy although it can also present later in childhood. It is characterized by adrenal insufficiency manifesting as glucocorticoid and mineralocorticoid deficiency in males and these infants show a blunted or absent adrenal steroid response to ACTH stimulation. Appropriate replacement therapy with glucocorticoids and mineralocorticoids ensures survival of these children. These children also develop HH at puberty. The permanent zone of the adrenal cortex is absent in AHC, and there is structural disorganization of the adrenal gland. The abnormally large fetal adrenal cells persist resulting in adrenal insufficiency *(48,65,221)*. Studies in families with AHC show that DAX-1 mutations are responsible for both AHC and HH *(66)*. Microdeletions, insertions, point mutations, microduplications, and base substitutions in the *DAX-1* gene resulting in frameshifts and truncated DAX-1 proteins have all been described in patients with isolated AHC and hypogonadotropic hypogonadism. In addition to inherited forms of this disorder, *de novo* mutations of the *DAX-1* gene have also been reported in this disorder *(237)*. Mutations in the *DAX-1* gene have been found both in the unique N-terminal, as well as the C-terminal domains of the DAX-1 protein *(48,49,67,68,238)*. Recent studies have shown that the silencing activity of the DAX-1 protein, which resides in the C-terminal region may be crucial to the pathogenesis of X-linked AHC *(216,228)*. It is significant to note that in patients with AHC all the naturally occurring DAX-1 deletional mutants reported to date show deletions of this silencing domain of the DAX-1 protein. Interestingly, even among patients harboring the same DAX-1 mutation, there is a great degree of variability in expression of adrenal insufficiency including the age of onset and the severity of clinical symptoms. This variability in the clinical expression of the disease could be explained on the basis of the variability of adrenal organogenesis found in patients within the same kindred with the same DAX-1 mutation. Later in life, these children also develop HH. This HH is either caused by a pituitary defect in gonadotropin production or caused by a hypothalamic defect in GnRH production or a combination of the two *(66)*.

Targeted disruption of *DAX-1* gene in the mouse has revealed that the development of the fetal and adrenal cortical zones in the wild-type and the *DAX-1* gene deleted mouse are similar until sexual maturation *(70)*. At puberty in the *DAX-1* gene-deleted adult mouse, the fetal adrenal zone fails to regress. This failure of the fetal zone to regress is similar to the persistence of fetal zone cells in adrenals of patients with DAX-1 mutations. However, unlike these patients, the *DAX-1* gene knockout mice have normal *zona glomerulosa* and *fasciculata* and do not require corticosteroid replacement for survival. Thus, the role of DAX-1 in mice and humans in adrenal organogenesis is not identical.

Estrogen Receptor (ER)

Estrogens have a key role in cell growth, differentiation, and function of diverse tissues, including bone, liver, the cardiovascular system, central nervous system, and the reproductive system. Estrogen actions are mediated through ERs, which are members of the steroid-receptor superfamily *(137,239,240)*. In addition to the previously characterized ER, now called ERα, a homolog of ERα, called ERβ, was recently characterized both in the rat and the human *(241–243)*. These ERs are expressed in a tissue-specific manner. ERα is expressed in the female reproductive system as well as in the placenta *(9)*. In adult humans, ERβ expression was found in the testes, ovary, and pituitary gland *(243–246)*. In the human fetus, semiquantitative RT-PCR revealed that ERβ was highly expressed not only in the ovaries and testes, but also in the spleen and adrenal glands *(247)*. In contrast, the expression of ERα was very low in the fetal spleen and absent in the fetal adrenal. Recent transfection studies show not only that these two subtypes of estrogen receptor signal differently, based on the ligand and the response element, but also that they may have different roles in gene regulation *(248,249)*. These ERs, primarily nuclear proteins, bind to their recognition sites either as homodimers or as ERα and ERβ heterodimers *(137,138,250)*. Studies have shown that ERα can bind to its palindromic DNA recognition sequence both in the presence and in the absence of its ligand, estrogen *(139,251)*. This ligand-independent ERα action is cell- and promoter-specific, and it is attributed to transactivation function 1 (TAF-1), located in the A/B region of the receptor *(139,252–254)*. Transactivation function 2 (TAF-2) of this receptor is located in the carboxy terminal end of the E-domain and is ligand-dependent *(252)*. ER can also modulate its target gene transcription by participating in protein–protein interaction with activator or repressor proteins *(255–258)*.

As discussed earlier in this chapter under the section on steroidogenesis, estrogen is central to fetal steroidogenesis. Through this role, it also regulates fetal adrenal organogenesis and maturation. These actions of estrogen are mediated through its receptor ER isoforms that are expressed both in the placenta and the fetal adrenal.

Steroid Receptor Interactions in the Regulation of Target Genes

Recent studies have demonstrated that the mechanism of steroid-receptor interaction plays a significant role in the regulation of target gene expression. These nuclear hormone receptors use several mechanisms to elicit their actions *(132,259–262)*. They mediate gene transcription by binding to their respective highly conserved and specific enhancer sequences called hormone response elements (HREs), located in the target genes *(130,263)*. Although they primarily recognize specific HREs, these receptors can also bind competitively to other steroid receptor HREs that are similar to their own. Furthermore, they can also bind to overlapping response elements or they can regulate gene transcription through protein–protein interaction with other transcription factors or with a common cofactor *(256,264–267)*. Finally, the generation of protein isoforms, either by alternative splicing of the pre-mRNA or by gene homologs, expands steroid receptors' repertoire of strategies to fine-tune gene expression *(268–270)*.

Oxytocin and c-*fos* gene promoters, which are regulated by a number of steroid receptors, illustrate the mechanism of steroid-receptor interactions in target gene regulation. In rat and human oxytocin genes, a composite hormone response element confers responsiveness to ER, retinoic acid receptor (RAR), thyroid receptor (TR), and orphan nuclear receptors SF-1 and COUP-TF *(196)*. Proto-oncogene c-*fos* functions as a master switch, directs cell proliferation, differentiation, and apoptosis; integrates cytoplasmic signal transduction pathways with gene transcription; and governs signal processing in neuronal cells *(271,272)*. Whereas steroid receptor ER, retinoic acid receptor(s), and vitamin D receptors regulate the c-*fos* gene at a transcriptional level, other steroid receptors, such as the glucocorticoid receptor, interact with the protein products of these proto-oncogenes to regulate gene transcription *(271)*. Similarly, the modulation of murine *DAX-1* gene promoter by SF-1 and COUP-TF is yet another example of coregulation of target genes by nuclear receptors *(205)*. Synergistic interaction between SF-1 and ER in the regulation of the salmon IIβ subunit gene has been recently reported *(199)*. Also, recent studies with SF-1-expressing R2C (Leydig tumor) cells cotransfected with murine StAR promoter luciferase construct, showed increased reporter gene activity with the addition of estradiol *(273)*. These reports point to SF-1 and ER interactions in the regulation of their target genes.

SF-1 and ER Interactions. As aforementioned, star protein regulates the key first step in acute steroidogenic response to tropic hormone stimulation by translocating cholesterol from the outer to the inner mitichondrial membrane. Furthermore, mutations in the *StAR* gene lead to congenital lipoid adrenal hyperplasia. Recent studies on the transcriptional regulation of *StAR* gene have established hSF-1 as a key regulator of basal and cAMP-mediated *StAR* gene expression *(183,274)*. The human StAR promoter has multiple hSF-1 response elements (SFREs), which are essential for cAMP-dependent activation of the *StAR* gene *(161,182,183)*. Mutation of both the proximal and distal sites in the StAR promoter abolishes SF-1-directed StAR activity. In addition, electromobility shift assays reveal that whereas the distal site, which has a SF-1 consensus sequence, binds to SF-1 expressed in COS-1 cells, the mutated distal site does not do so. The proximal site, an ER consensus half-site, also binds to SF-1, but with lesser degree of affinity than the distal site. However, cotransfection studies reveal that the mutated proximal site abolishes SF-1-stimulated StAR promoter activity by 91%, whereas mutated distal site reduced this activity by only 80% *(161)*.

Our transient cotransfection studies done in HeLa cells using the human SF-1 expression vector and human StAR promoter also show that hSF-1 is a regulator of the human StAR promoter through these SFREs. Data from these studies also show that in the absence of either hSF-1 or cAMP, human ERα (hERα) stimulates StAR promoter. These studies suggest that hSF-1 and ER not only independently stimulate the StAR promoter-activity, but also that hSF-1 has a downregulating effect on ER's ability to stimulate StAR promoter activity *(46)*. Thus, hSF-1 and ER may coregulate StAR promoter activity, thereby regulating adrenal steroidogenesis and organogenesis. Furthermore, StAR may not be the only common target gene that hSF-1 and ER coregulate in fetal adrenal steroidogenesis.

Estrogen modulates fetal adrenal steroidogenesis in several ways. Whereas estradiol indirectly increases the fetal adrenal DHEAS production by enhancing the ACTH-stimulated production of this estrogen precursor *(127)*, it directly inhibits the production of DHEAS by downregulating the steroidogenic enzyme *p450c17 (275)*. Interestingly, recent studies have shown that SF-1 is also a transcription factor for the gene encoding this enzyme *(61,173,176,276,277)*. Also, both SF-1 *(41,54)* and ERβ *(247)* are expressed in the fetal adrenal gland. Therefore, SF-1 and ER may potentially coregulate *p450c17* gene expression and modulate DHEA synthesis in the fetal adrenal. In addition, ER also upregulates the expression of *p450scc (278)*, which is also a SF-1 target gene *(167,169,171)*. Therefore, these two receptors may coregulate fetal adrenal steroid biosynthesis at multiple levels.

SF-1 and DAX-1 Interactions. Orphan nuclear receptors SF-1 and DAX-1 are coexpressed in the developing hypothalamus, pituitary, gonads, as well as the adrenal glands *(71)*. *SF-1* and *DAX-1* gene knockout studies in the mouse and mutations of human SF-1 *(63)* and the DAX-1 *(48,221)* genes resulting in the syndrome of non-X-linked and X-linked AHC, respectively, suggest that these two transcription factors are closely connected to the development and function of steroidogenic organs. Recent studies suggest that SF-1 and DAX-1 act in consort to control steroidogenesis by regulating the *StAR* gene promoter *(213)*. Although SF-1 stimulates the StAR promoter activity by binding to the multiple SFREs *(183)*, the DAX-1 protein acts as a repressor of StAR gene activity by binding to hairpin structure and loops in the StAR promoter *(72)*. Furthermore, recent studies using cotransfection experiments and deletion constructs of DAX-1, suggest that DAX-1 inhibits SF-1-mediated transactivation of target genes *(216)*. In addition, these studies also suggest that the carboxy terminal domain of the DAX-1 is responsible for this inhibitory function. These studies also suggest that a protein–protein interaction between SF-1 and DAX-1 or competition for a common coactivator are possible mechanisms responsible for DAX-1 mediated inhibition of SF-1 responsive gene activity.

A large number of the DAX-1 truncated mutants have been identified in patients with X-linked AHC. What is most interesting is that in all these truncated mutants the putative carboxy terminal inhibitory domain is deleted *(216,227)*. Furthermore, two naturally occurring mutations of *DAX-1* gene: one with amino acid substitution (R267P) and the other with single-amino-acid deletion (Δ V269) also showed a reduced DAX-1 inhibitory activity. These patients with DAX-1 mutations resulting in AHC provide compelling evidence that loss of this inhibitory effect of DAX-1 on developmentally regulated target genes may contribute to the pathogenesis of AHC *(228)*. A recent study suggests that DAX-1 recruits N-CoR (nuclear receptor corepressor) to SF-1 *(279)*. Not only do the naturally occurring mutations of *DAX-1* result in the loss of DAX-1-mediated inhibition of SF-1-responsive genes, but these mutations may also lead to markedly diminished recruitment of corepressor(s) to SF-1. Thus, it is conceivable that impaired DAX-1-mediated inhibition of SF-1 responsive genes during development may play a significant role in organogenesis of the adrenal gland and, therefore, the syndrome of AHC.

SUMMARY

The development and remodeling of the fetal adrenal gland and its transition to a self-sufficient adult organ capable of sustaining life is a complex and temporally orchestrated process that is regulated by endocrine, paracrine, and autocrine factors that are derived both from maternal and fetal sources. The twin processes of fetal organogenesis and steroidogenesis are closely intertwined. The key cellular functions of proliferation, differentiation and apoptosis, which govern organogenesis of the fetal adrenal, are all regulated by HCG and ACTH, the growth factors, and the nuclear receptors SF-1, DAX-1, and ER. In addition, the fetoplacental unit, which is pivotal to the fetal adrenal steroidogenesis, is also the source of and at the same time is regulated by these endocrine, paracrine, and autocrine factors. Although the role of HCG and ACTH has been well-known for the past two to three decades, more recent studies have clearly established the seminal role of growth factors and nuclear receptors in both organogenesis and steroidogenesis of the fetal adrenal. Gene knockout studies in mice as well as transient transfection experiments using cell-culture systems have increased and enhanced our understanding of the molecular mechanisms underlying the cellular functions of growth, remodeling as well as steroidogenesis. Furthermore, studies on patients with X-linked AHC, which showed that *DAX-1* gene mutations result in both AHC, as well as hypogonadotropic hypogonadism, and a recent study on a patient with non-X-linked AHC have established the fundamental role of nuclear receptors, DAX-1, and SF-1 in adrenal organogenesis. The increasing body of knowledge about the underlying molecular mechanisms that regulate fundamental cellular functions will enable us in the future to design novel therapies for disorders of the adrenal organogenesis and steroidogenesis.

REFERENCES

1. Keene MFL and Hewer EE. Observations on the development of the human suprarenal gland. J Anat 1927; 61:302–324.
2. Uotila UU. The early embryological development of the fetal and permanent adrenal cortex in man. Anat Res 1940; 76:183–203.
3. Benner MC. Studies on the involution of the fetal cortex of the adrenal glands. Am J Pathol 1940; 16:787–798.
4. Benirschke K. Adrenals in anencephaly and hydrcephaly. Obstet Gynecol 1956; 8:412–425.
5. Lanman JT. The adrenal fetal zone: its occurrence in primates and a possible relationship to chorionic gonadotropin. Endocrinology 1957; 61:684–691.
6. Frandsen VA and Stakemann G. The site of production of oestrogenic hormones in human pregnancy. Hormone excretion in pregnancy with anencephalic fetus. Acta Endocr (Kbh) 1961; 38:383–391.
7. Mesiano S and Jaffe RB. Developmental and functional biology of the primate fetal adrenal cortex. Endocr Rev 1997; 18(3):378–403.

8. Pepe GJ and Albrecht ED. Regulation of the primate fetal adrenal cortex. Endocr Rev 1990; 11(1):151–176.
9. Pepe GJ and Albrecht ED. Actions of placental and fetal adrenal steroid hormones in primate pregnancy. Endocr Rev 1995; 16:608–648.
10. Liggins GC. Adrenocortical-related maturational events in the fetus. Am J Obstet Gynecol 1976; 126(7):931–941.
11. Seron-Ferre M, Lawrence CC, and Jaffe RB. Role of hCG in regulation of the fetal zone of the human fetal adrenal gland. J Clin Endocrinol Metab 1978; 46(5):834–837.
12. Jaffe RB, et al. Regulation of the primate fetal adrenal gland and testis in vitro and in vivo. J Steroid Biochem 1977; 8:479–490.
13. Mesiano S and Jaffe RB. Regulation of growth and the function of the human fetal adrenal. In J.M. Saez, et al., ed. Cellular and Molecular Biology of the Adrenal Cortex, 1992, John Libby and Company: London. p. 235–45.
14. Branchaud CT, et al. Steroidogenic activity of hACTH and related peptides on the human neocortex and fetal adrenal cortex in organ culture. Steroids 1978; 31:557–572.
15. Simonian MH and Gill GN. Regulation of the fetal human adrenal cortex: effects of adrenocorticotropin on growth and function of monolayer cultures of fetal and definitive zone cells. Endocrinology 1981; 108:1769–1779.
16. Jaffe RB, et al. Regulation and function of the primate fetal adrenal gland and gonad. Recent Prog Horm Res 1981; 37:41–103.
17. Di Blasio AM, et al. Maintenance of cell proliferation and steroidogenesis in cultured human fetal adrenal cells chronically exposed to adrenocorticotropic hormone: rationalization of in vitro and in vivo findings. Biol Reprod 1990; 42:683–691.
18. Aberdeen GW, et al. Effect of maternal betamethasone administration at midgestation on baboon fetal adrenal gland development and adrenocorticotropin receptor messenger ribonucleic acid expression. J Clin Endocrinol Metab 1998; 83:976–982.
19. Mesiano S and Jaffe RB. Role of growth factors in the developmental regulation of the human fetal adrenal cortex. Steroids 1997; 62:62–72.
20. Hornsby PJ and Gill GN. Hormonal control of adrenocortical cell proliferation. Desensitization to ACTH and interaction between ACTH and fibroblast growth factor in bovine adrenocortical cell cultures. J Clin Invest 1977; 60:342–352.
21. Crickard K, III CR, and Jaffe RB. Control of proliferation of human fetal adrenal cells in vitro. J Clin Endocrinol Metab 1981; 53:709–796.
22. Hornsby PJ et al. Serum and growth factor requirements for proliferation of human adrenocortical cells in culture: comparison with bovine adrenocortical cells. In Vitro 1983; 19:863–869.
23. Gospodarowicz D, et al. Isolation of fibroblast growth factor from bovine adrenal gland: physiochemical and biological characterization. Endocrinology 1986; 118:82–90.
24. Schweigerer L, et al. Basic fibroblast growth factor: production and growth stimulation in cultured adrenal cortex cells. Endocrinology 1987; 120:796–800.
25. Mesiano S, et al. Basic fibroblast growth factor expression is regulated by corticotropin in the human fetal adrenal: a model for adrenal growth regulation. Proc Natl Acad Sci USA, 1991; 88:5428–5432.
26. Luger A, et al. Interaction of epidermal growth factor with the hypothalamic-pituitary-adrenal axis: potential physiologic relevance. J Clin Endocrinol Metab 1988; 66:334–337.
27. Han VK, et al. Expression of somatomedin/insulin-like growth factor messenger ribonucleic acids in the human fetus: identification, characterization, and tissue distribution. J Clin Endocrinol Metab 1988; 66:422–429.
28. Penhoat A, et al. Characterization of insulin-like growth factor I and insulin receptors on cultured bovine adrenal fasciculata cells. Role of these peptides on adrenal cell function. Endocrinology, 1988; 122:2518–2526.
29. Shigematsu K, et al. Receptor autoradiographic localization of insulin-like growth factor-I (IGF-I) binding sites in human fetal and adult adrenal glands. Life Sci 1989; 45:383–389.
30. D'Ercole AJ. The insulin-like growth factors and fetal growth. In E. Spencer, ed. Modern Concepts of Insulin-Like Growth Factors, 1991, Elsevier: New York, p. 9–23.
31. Pham-Huu-Trung, MT et al. Effects of insulin-like growth factor I (IGF-I) on enzymatic activity in human adrenocortical cells. Interactions with ACTH. J Steroid Biochem Mol Biol 1991; 39:903–909.
32. Ilvesmaki V, Blum WF, and Voutilainen R. Insulin-like growth factor binding proteins in the human adrenal gland. Mol Cell Endocrinol 1993; 97:71–79.

33. Feige JJ, Cochet C, and Chambaz EM. Type beta transforming growth factor is a potent modulator of differentiated adrenocortical cell functions. Biochem Biophys Res Commun 1986; 139:693–700.

34. Rainey WE, Viard I, Mason JI, et al. Effects of transforming growth factor beta on ovine adrenocortical cells. Mol Cell Endocrinol 1988; 60:189–198.

35. Massague J. The transforming growth factor-beta family. Annu Rev Cell Biol 1990; 6:597–641.

36. Spencer SJ, Rabinovici J, and Jaffe RB. Human recombinant activin-A inhibits proliferation of human fetal adrenal cells in vitro. J Clin Endocrinol Metab 1990; 71:1678–1680.

37. Spencer SJ, et al. Activin and inhibin in the human adrenal gland. Regulation and differential effects in fetal and adult cells. J Clin Invest 1992; 90:142–149.

38. Spencer SJ, et al. Proliferation and apoptosis in the human adrenal cortex during the fetal and perinatal periods: implications for growth and remodeling. J Clin Endocrinol Metab 1999; 84:1110–1115.

39. Stankovic AK, Dion LD, and Parker CR Jr. Effects of transforming growth factor-beta on human fetal adrenal steroid production. Mol Cell Endocrinol 1994; 99:145–151.

40. Stankovic AK and Parker CR Jr. Receptor binding of transforming growth factor-beta by human fetal adrenal cells. Mol Cell Endocrinol 1995; 109:159–165.

41. Luo X, Ikeda Y, and Parker KL. A cell-specific nuclear receptor is essential for adrenal and gonadal development and sexual differentiation. Cell 1994; 77:481–490.

42. Luo X, et al. Steroidogenic factor 1 is the essential transcript of the mouse Ftz-F1 gene. Mol Endocrinol 1995; 9:1233–1239.

43. Sadovsky Y, et al. Mice deficient in the orphan receptor steroidogenic factor 1 lack adrenal glands and gonads but express P450 side-chain-cleavage enzyme in the placenta and have normal embryonic serum levels of corticosteroids. Proc Natl Acad Sci USA 1995; 92:10939–10943.

44. Sadovsky Y. Steroidogenic factor-1 (SF-1), a specific transcriptional factor of differentiation and function of steroidogenic cells. Ann Endocrinol (Paris), 1999; 60:247–248.

45. Morohashi K. The ontogenesis of the steroidogenic tissues. Genes Cells 1997; 2:95–106.

46. Ramayya MS, et al. Human steroidogenic factor-1 modulates estrogen receptor-mediated stimulation of StAR promoter activity (abstract) in 5th joint meeting of the European Society for Pediatric Endocrinology and the Lawson Wilkins Pediatric Endocrine Society. 1997. Stockholm, Sweden.

47. Ramayya MS, et al. Human steroidogenic factor-1 and estrogen receptor a co-regulate StAR promoter activity through shared response elements (abstract) in 80th annual meeting of the Endocrine Society. 1998. New Orleans, USA.

48. Zanaria E, et al. An unusual member of the nuclear hormone receptor superfamily responsible for X-linked adrenal hypoplasia congenita. Nature 1994; 372:635–641.

49. Burris TB, Guo W, and McCabe ER. The gene responsible for adrenal hypoplasia congenita, DAX-1, encodes a nuclear hormone receptor that defines a new class within the superfamily. Recent Prog Horm Res 1996; 51:241–259; discussion 259–260.

50. Voutilainen R and Kahri AI. Placental origin of the suppression of 3 beta-hydroxysteroid dehydrogenase in the fetal zone cells of human fetal adrenals. J Steroid Biochem 1980; 13:39–43.

51. Fujieda K, et al. The control of steroidogenesis by human fetal adrenal cells in tissue culture. IV. The effect of exposure to placental steroids. J Clin Endocrinol Metab 1982; 54:89–94.

52. Ikeda Y, et al. Characterization of the mouse FTZ-F1 gene, which encodes a key regulator of steroid hydroxylase gene expression. Mol Endocrinol 1993; 7:852–860.

53. Lynch JP, et al. Steroidogenic factor 1, an orphan nuclear receptor, regulates the expression of the rat aromatase gene in gonadal tissues. Mol Endocrinol 1993; 7:776–786.

54. Ikeda Y, et al. Developmental expression of mouse steroidogenic factor-1, an essential regulator of the steroid hydroxylases. Mol Endocrinol 1994; 8:654–662.

55. Parker KL and Schimmer BP. The role of nuclear receptors in steroid hormone production. Semin Cancer Biol 1994; 5:317–325.

56. Givens CR, et al. Transcriptional regulation of rat cytochrome P450c17 expression in mouse Leydig MA-10 and adrenal Y-1 cells: identification of a single protein that mediates both basal and cAMP-induced activities. DNA Cell Biol 1994; 13:1087–1098.

57. Parker KL and Schimmer BP. Transcriptional regulation of the genes encoding the cytochrome P-450 steroid hydroxylases. Vitam Horm 1995; 51:339–370.

58. Lala DS, et al. A cell-specific nuclear receptor regulates the steroid hydroxylases. Steroids 1995; 60:10–14.

59. Omura T and Morohashi K. Gene regulation of steroidogenesis. J Steroid Biochem Mol Biol 1995; 53:19–25.

60. Morohashi K, et al. Function and distribution of a steroidogenic cell-specific transcription factor, Ad4BP. J Steroid Biochem Mol Biol 1995; 53:81–88.
61. Zhang P and Mellon SH. The orphan nuclear receptor steroidogenic factor-1 regulates the cyclic adenosine 3',5'-monophosphate-mediated transcriptional activation of rat cytochrome P450c17 (17 alpha-hydroxylase/c17-20 lyase). Mol Endocrinol 1996; 10:147–158.
62. Sadovsky Y and Crawford PA. Developmental and physiologic roles of the nuclear receptor steroidogenic factor-1 in the reproductive system. J Soc Gynecol Investig 1998; 5:6–12.
63. Achermann JC, et al. A mutation in the gene encoding steroidogenic factor-1 causes XY sex reversal and adrenal failure in humans [letter]. Nat Genet 1999; 22:125–126.
64. Guo W, Burris TP, and McCabe ER. Expression of DAX-1, the gene responsible for X-linked adrenal hypoplasia congenita and hypogonadotropic hypogonadism, in the hypothalamic-pituitary-adrenal/gonadal axis. Biochem Mol Med 1995; 56:8–13.
65. Muscatelli F, et al. Mutations in the DAX-1 gene give rise to both X-linked adrenal hypoplasia congenita and hypogonadotropic hypogonadism. Nature 1994; 372:672–676.
66. Habiby RL, et al. Adrenal hypoplasia congenita with hypogonadotropic hypogonadism: evidence that DAX-1 mutations lead to combined hypothalmic and pituitary defects in gonadotropin production [see comments]. J Clin Invest 1996; 98:1055–1062.
67. Kinoshita E, et al. DAX-1 gene mutations and deletions in Japanese patients with adrenal hypoplasia congenita and hypogonadotropic hypogonadism. Horm Res 1997; 48:29–34.
68. Nakae J, et al. Three novel mutations and a de novo deletion mutation of the DAX-1 gene in patients with X-linked adrenal hypoplasia congenita. J Clin Endocrinol Metab 1997; 82:3835–3841.
69. Reutens AT, et al. Clinical and functional effects of mutations in the DAX-1 gene in patients with adrenal hypoplasia congenita. J Clin Endocrinol Metab 1999; 84:504–511.
70. Yu RN, et al. Role of Ahch in gonadal development and gametogenesis [see comments]. Nat Genet 1998; 20:353–357.
71. Ikeda Y, et al. Steroidogenic factor 1 and Dax-1 colocalize in multiple cell lineages: potential links in endocrine development. Mol Endocrinol 1996; 10:1261–1272.
72. Zazopoulos E, et al. DNA binding and transcriptional repression by DAX-1 blocks steroidogenesis. Nature 1997; 390:311–315.
73. Johannisson E. The fetal adrenal cortex in the human. Its ultrastructure at different stages of development and in different functional states. Acta Endocrinol Copenh 1968; 58:Suppl 130:7+.
74. McNutt NS and Jones AL. Observations on the ultrastructure of cytodifferentiation in the human fetal adrenal cortex. Lab Invest 1970; 22:513–527.
75. Belloni AS, et al. Cytogenesis in the rat adrenal cortex: evidence for an ACTH-induced centripetal cell migration from the zona glomerulosa. Arch Anat Histol Embryol 1978; 61:195–205.
76. McClellan M and Brenner RM. Development of the fetal adrenals in nonhuman primates: electron microscopy. In MJ Novy and JA Resko, ed., Fetal Endocrinology, 1981, Academic Press, Incorporated: New York, p. 383–403.
77. Hornsby PJ. The regulation of adrenocortical function by control of growth and structure, In D.C. Anderson and J.S.D. Winter, ed., Adrenal Cortex, 1985, Butterworths: London, p. 1–31.
78. Morley SD, et al. Variegated expression of a mouse steroid 21-hydroxylase/beta- galactosidase transgene suggests centripetal migration of adrenocortical cells. Mol Endocrinol 1996; 10:585–598.
79. Siiteri PK and MacDonald PC. The utilization of circulating dehydroisoandrosterone sulfate for estrogen synthesis during human pregnancy. Steroids 1963; 713–730.
80. Sucheston ME and Cannon MS. Development of zonular patterns in the human adrenal gland. J Morphol 1968; 126:477–491.
81. Crowder RE. The development of the adrenal gland in man, with special reference to origin and ultimate location of cell types and evidence in favor of the "cell migration" theory. Contemp Embryol 1957; 251:195–209.
82. Jirasek J. Human Fetal Endocrines. 1981, London: Martinus-Nijhoff, 69–82.
83. Albrecht ED and Pepe GJ. Effect of estrogen on dehydroepiandrosterone formation by baboon fetal adrenal cells in vitro. Am J Obstet Gynecol 1987; 156:1275–1278.
84. Albrecht ED and Pepe GJ. Suppression of maternal adrenal dehydroepiandrosterone and dehydroepiandrosterone sulfate production by estrogen during baboon pregnancy. J Clin Endocrinol Metab 1995; 80:3201–3208.
85. Albrecht ED, Henson MC, and Pepe GJ. Regulation of placental low density lipoprotein uptake in baboons by estrogen. Endocrinology 1991; 128:450–458.

86. Leavitt MG, Albrecht ED, and Pepe GJ. Development of the baboon fetal adrenal gland: regulation of the ontogenesis of the definitive and transitional zones by adrenocorticotropin. J Clin Endocrinol Metab 1999; 84:3831–3835.

87. Pepe GJ and Albrecht ED. Central integrative role of oestrogen in the regulation of placental steroidogenic maturation and the development of the fetal pituitary-adrenocortical axis in the baboon. Hum Reprod Update 1998; 4:406–419.

88. Seron-Ferre M, et al. Steroid production by definitive and fetal zones of the human fetal adrenal gland. J Clin Endocrinol Metab 1978; 47:603–609.

89. Carr BR and Simpson ER. Cholesterol synthesis by human fetal hepatocytes: effect of lipoproteins. Am J Obstet Gynecol 1984; 150 (5 Pt 1): 551–557.

90. Carr BR and Simpson ER. Cholesterol synthesis by human fetal hepatocytes: effects of hormones. J Clin Endocrinol Metab 1984; 58:1111–1116.

91. Voutilainen R and Kahri AI. Functional and ultrastructural changes during ACTH-induced early differentiation of cortical cells of human fetal adrenals in primary cultures. J Ultrastruct Res 1979; 69:98–108.

92. Carr BR and Simpson ER. Lipoprotein utilization and cholesterol synthesis by the human fetal adrenal gland. Endocr Rev 1981; 2:306–326.

93. Bolte E, Wiqvist N, and Diczfalusy E. Metabolism of dehydroepiandrosterone and dehydroepiandrosterone sulphate by the human fetus at midpregnancy. Acta Endocrinol (Copenh), 1996; 52:583–597.

94. Pepe GJ, Waddell BJ, and Albrecht ED. Effect of estrogen on pituitary peptide-induced dehydroepiandrosterone secretion in the baboon fetus at midgestation. Endocrinology 1989; 125:1519–1524.

95. Albrecht ED, et al. Modulation of adrenocorticotropin-stimulated baboon fetal adrenal dehydroepiandrosterone formation in vitro by estrogen at mid- and late gestation. Endocrinology, 1990; 126:3083–3088.

96. Babischkin JS, Pepe GJ, and Albrecht ED. Estrogen regulation of placental P-450 cholesterol side-chain cleavage enzyme messenger ribonucleic acid levels and activity during baboon pregnancy. Endocrinology 1997; 138:452–459.

97. Carr BR, Ohashi M, and Simpson ER. Low-density lipoprotein binding and de novo synthesis of cholesterol in the neocortex and fetal zones of the human fetal adrenal gland. Endocrinology, 1982; 110:1994–1998.

98. Ducsay CA, Stanczyk FZ, and Novy MJ. Maternal and fetal production rates of progesterone in rhesus macaques: placental transfer and conversion to cortisol. Endocrinology 1985; 117:1253–1258.

99. Baggia S, et al. Interconversion of cortisol and cortisone in baboon trophoblast and decidua cells in culture. Endocrinology 1990; 127:1735–1741.

100. Baggia S, Albrecht ED, and Pepe GJ. Regulation of 11 beta-hydroxysteroid dehydrogenase activity in the baboon placenta by estrogen. Endocrinology 1990; 126:2742–2748.

101. Doody KM, et al. 3 beta-hydroxysteroid dehydrogenase/isomerase in the fetal zone and neocortex of the human fetal adrenal gland. Endocrinology 1990; 126:2487–2492.

102. Parker Jr CR, et al. Immunohistochemical evaluation of the cellular localization and ontogeny of 3 beta-hydroxysteroid dehydrogenase/delta 5-4 isomerase in the human fetal adrenal gland. Endocr Res 1995; 21:69–80.

103. Coulter CL, et al. Functional maturation of the primate fetal adrenal in vivo. II. Ontogeny of corticosteroid synthesis is dependent upon specific zonal expression of 3 beta-hydroxysteroid dehydrogenase/isomerase. Endocrinology 1996; 137:4953–4959.

104. Coulter CL and Jaffe RB. Functional maturation of the primate fetal adrenal in vivo: 3. Specific zonal localization and developmental regulation of CYP21A2 (P450c21) and CYP11B1/CYP11B2 (P450c11/aldosterone synthase) lead to integrated concept of zonal and temporal steroid biosynthesis. Endocrinology 1998; 139:5144–5150.

105. Sucheston ME and Cannon MS. Microscopic comparison of the normal and anencephalic human adrenal gland with emphasis on the transient zone. Obstet Gynecol 1970; 35:544–553.

106. Bloch E and Benirschke K. Synthesis in vitro of steroids by human fetal adrenal gland slices. J Biol Chem 1959; 234:1085–1089.

107. Winters AJ, et al. Plasma ACTH levels in the human fetus and neonate as related to age and parturition. J Clin Endocrinol Metab 1974; 39:269–273.

108. Kahri AI. Inhibition of ACTH-induced differentiation of cortical cells and their mitochondria by corticosterone in tissue culture of fetal rat adrenals. Anat Rec 1973; 176:253–271.

109. Kahri AI, Huhtaniemi I, and Salmenpera M. Steroid formation and differentiation of cortical cells

in tissue culture of human fetal adrenals in the presence and absence of ACTH. Endocrinology 1976; 98:33–41.

110. Ramachandran J and Suyama AT. Inhibition of replication of normal adrenocortical cells in culture by adrenocorticotropin. Proc Natl Acad Sci USA 1975; 72:113–117.

111. Fujieda K, et al. The control of steroidogenesis by human fetal adrenal cells in tissue culture. I. Responses to adrenocorticotropin. J Clin Endocrinol Metab 1981; 53:34–38.

112. Masui H and Garren LD. Inhibition of replication in functional mouse adrenal tumor cells by adrenocorticotropic hormone mediated by adenosine 3′:5′-cyclic monophosphate. Proc Natl Acad Sci USA 1971; 68:3206–3210.

113. Farese RV and Reddy WJ. Observations on the interrelations between adrenal protein, Rna and Dna during prolonged Acth administration. Biochim Biophys Acta 1963; 76:145–148.

114. Imrie RC and Hutchison WC. Changes in the activity of rat adrenal ribonuclease and ribonuclease inhibitor after administration of corticotrophin. Biochim Biophys Acta 1965; 108:106–113.

115. Masui H and Garren LD. On the mechanism of action of adrenocorticotropic hormone. Stimulation of deoxyribonucleic acid polymerase and thymidine kinase activities in adrenal glands. J Biol Chem 1970; 245:2627–2632.

116. Carpenter G and Cohen S. Epidermal growth factor. Annu Rev Biochem 1979; 48:193–216.

117. Derynck R. Transforming growth factor alpha. Cell 1988; 54:593–595.

118. Prigent SA and Lemoine NR. The type 1 (EGFR-related) family of growth factor receptors and their ligands. Prog Growth Factor Res 1992; 4:1–24.

119. Gospodarowicz D, et al. Control of bovine adrenal cortical cell proliferation by fibroblast growth factor. Lack of effect of epidermal growth factor. Endocrinology 1977; 100:1080–1089.

120. Smikle CB, et al. Identification of the ligands for the epidermal growth factor receptor in human fetal and adrenal glands. In 10th International Congress of Endocrinology. 1996. San Francisco, USA.

121. Coulter CL, et al. Functional maturation of the primate fetal adrenal in vivo: I. Role of insulin-like growth factors (IGFs), IGF-I receptor, and IGF binding proteins in growth regulation. Endocrinology 1996; 137:4487–4498.

122. Guyda HJ. Concepts of IGF physiology. In E. Spencer, ed. Modern Concepts of Insulin-Like Growth Factors. 1991; Elsevier: New York, p. 99–110.

123. Salmon WD and Daughday WH. A hormonally-controlled serum factor which stimulates $^{35}SO_4$ incorporation by cartilage. J Lab Clin Med 1957; 49:825–836.

124. Mesiano S, Mellon SH, and Jaffe RB. Mitogenic action, regulation, and localization of insulin-like growth factors in the human fetal adrenal gland. J Clin Endocrinol Metab 1993; 76:968–976.

125. Penhoat A, et al. Regulation of adrenal cell-differentiated functions by growth factors. Horm Res 1994; 42:39–43.

126. Voutilainen R and Miller WL. Coordinate tropic hormone regulation of mRNAs for insulin-like growth factor II and the cholesterol side-chain-cleavage enzyme, P450scc [corrected], in human steroidogenic tissues [published erratum appears in Proc Natl Acad Sci USA 1987; Sep; 84(17):6194]. Proc Natl Acad Sci USA, 1987; 84:1590–1594.

127. Mesiano S and Jaffe RB. Interaction of insulin-like growth factor-II and estradiol directs steroidogenesis in the human fetal adrenal toward dehydroepiandrosterone sulfate production. J Clin Endocrinol Metab 1993; 77:754–758.

128. Parker CR Jr, et al. Adrenocorticotropin interferes with transforming growth factor-beta-induced growth inhibition of neocortical cells from the human fetal adrenal gland. J Clin Endocrinol Metab 1992; 75:1519–1521.

129. Lebrethon MC, et al. Regulation of corticotropin and steroidogenic enzyme mRNAs in human fetal adrenal cells by corticotropin, angiotensin-II and transforming growth factor beta 1. Mol Cell Endocrinol 1994; 106:137–143.

130. Beato M. Gene regulation by steroid hormones. Cell 1989; 56:335–344.

131. O'Malley BW and Conneely OM. Orphan receptors: in search of a unifying hypothesis for activation. Mol Endocrinol 1992; 6:1359–1361.

132. Beato M, Herrlich P, and Schutz G. Steroid hormone receptors: many actors in search of a plot. Cell 1995; 83:851–857.

133. Tsai MJ and O'Malley BW. Molecular mechanisms of action of steroid/thyroid receptor superfamily members. Annu Rev Biochem 1994; 63:451–486.

134. Enmark E and Gustafsson JA. Orphan nuclear receptors—the first eight years. Mol Endocrinol 1996; 10:1293–1307.

135. Guo W, et al. Genomic sequence of the DAX1 gene: an orphan nuclear receptor responsible for X-linked adrenal hypoplasia congenita and hypogonadotropic hypogonadism. J Clin Endocrinol Metab 1996; 81:2481–2486.

136. Bae DS, et al. Characterization of the mouse DAX-1 gene reveals evolutionary conservation of a unique amino-terminal motif and widespread expression in mouse tissue. Endocrinology 1996; 137:3921–3927.

137. Kumar V and Chambon P. The estrogen receptor binds tightly to its responsive element as a ligand-induced homodimer. Cell 1988; 55:145–156.

138. Klein H-L, et al. Specific binding of estrogen receptor to the estrogen response element. Mol Cell Biol 1989; 9:43–49.

139. Tzukerman M, et al. The human estrogen receptor has transcriptional activator and repressor functions in the absence of ligand. New Biol 1990; 2:613–620.

140. Reese JC and Katzenellenbogen BS. Examination of the DNA-binding ability of estrogen receptor in whole cells: implications for hormone-independent transactivation and the actions of antiestrogens. Mol Cell Biol 1992; 12:4531–4538.

141. Lala DS, Rice DA, and Parker KL. Steroidogenic factor I, a key regulator of steroidogenic enzyme expression, is the mouse homolog of fushi tarazu-factor I. Mol Endocrinol 1992; 6:1249–1258.

142. Lavorgna G, et al. FTZ-F1, a steroid hormone receptor-like protein implicated in the activation of fushi tarazu. Science 1991; 252:848–851.

143. Ueda H, et al. A sequence-specific DNA-binding protein that activates fushi tarazu segmentation gene expression. Genes Dev 1990; 4:624–635.

144. Ikeda Y, et al. The nuclear receptor steroidogenic factor 1 is essential for the formation of the ventromedial hypothalamic nucleus. Mol Endocrinol 1995; 9:478–486.

145. Ikeda Y. SF-1: a key regulator of development and function in the mammalian reproductive system. Acta Paediatr Jpn 1996; 38:412–419.

146. Morohashi K, et al. Functional difference between Ad4BP and ELP, and their distributions in steroidogenic tissues. Mol Endocrinol 1994; 8:643–653.

147. Ingraham HA, et al. The nuclear receptor steroidogenic factor 1 acts at multiple levels of the reproductive axis. Genes Dev 1994; 8:2302–2312.

148. Asa SL, et al. The transcription activator steroidogenic factor-1 is preferentially expressed in the human pituitary gonadotroph. J Clin Endocrinol Metab 1996; 81:2165–2170.

149. Roselli CE, et al. Expression of the orphan receptor steroidogenic factor-1 mRNA in the rat medial basal hypothalamus. Brain Res Mol Brain Res 1997; 44:66–72.

150. Shinoda K, et al. Developmental defects of the ventromedial hypothalamic nucleus and pituitary gonadotroph in the Ftz-F1 disrupted mice. Dev Dyn 1995; 204:22–29.

151. Luo X, et al. Steroidogenic factor 1 (SF-1) is essential for endocrine development and function. J Steroid Biochem Mol Biol 1999; 69:13–18.

152. Kudo T and Sutou S. Molecular cloning of chicken FTZ-F1-related orphan receptors. Gene, 1997; 197:261–268.

153. Kudo T and Sutou S. Structural characterization of the chicken SF-1/Ad4BP gene. Gene 1999; 231:33–40.

154. Ninomiya Y, et al. Genomic organization and isoforms of the mouse ELP gene. J Biochem (Tokyo) 1995; 118:380–389.

155. Wong M, et al. Cloning and sequence analysis of the human gene encoding steroidogenic factor 1. J Mol Endocrinol 1996; 17:139–147.

156. Oba K, et al. Structural characterization of human Ad4bp (SF-1) gene. Biochem Biophys Res Commun 1996; 226:261–267.

157. Tsukiyama T, et al. Embryonal long terminal repeat-binding protein is a murine homolog of FTZ-F1, a member of the steroid receptor superfamily. Mol Cell Biol 1992; 12:1286–1291.

158. Ziegelbauer-Ellinger H, et al. FTZ-F1-related orphan receptors in Xenopus laevis: transcriptional regulators differentially expressed during early embryogenesis. Mol Cell Biol 1994; 14:2786–2797.

159. Liu D, et al. Teleost FTZ-F1 homolog and its splicing variant determine the expression of the salmon gonadotropin IIbeta subunit gene. Mol Endocrinol 1997; 11:877–890.

160. Ramayya MS, et al. Steroidogenic factor 1 messenger ribonucleic acid expression in steroidogenic and nonsteroidogenic human tissues: Northern blot and in situ hybridization studies. J Clin Endocrinol Metab 1997; 82:1799–1806.

161. Sugawara T, et al. Steroidogenic factor 1-dependent promoter activity of the human steroidogenic acute regulatory protein (StAR) gene. Biochemistry 1996; 35:9052–9059.
162. Sugawara T, et al. Human steroidogenic acute regulatory protein: functional activity in COS-1 cells, tissue-specific expression, and mapping of the structural gene to 8p11.2 and a pseudogene to chromosome 13. Proc Natl Acad Sci USA 1995; 92:4778–4782.
163. Graves KH, et al. Use of transgenic mice to define regions of the human aromatase p450 (p450arom) gene involved in placenta- and gonad-specific expression. In 10th International Congress of Endocrinology (ICE '96). 1996: San Francisco, CA, p. 95.
164. Hum DW, Aza-Blanc P, and Miller WL. Characterization of placental transcriptional activation of the human gene for P450scc. DNA Cell Biol 1995; 14:451–463.
165. Sasano H, et al. Ad4BP in the human adrenal cortex and its disorders. J Clin Endocrinol Metab 1995; 80:2378–2380.
166. Shapiro DB, et al. Steroidogenic factor-1 as a positive regulator of rat granulosa cell differentiation and a negative regulator of mitosis. Endocrinology 1996; 137:1187–1195.
167. Rice DA, et al. A shared promoter element regulates the expression of three steroidogenic enzymes. Mol Endocrinol 1991; 5:1552–1561.
168. Morohashi K, et al. A common transacting factor, Ad4-binding protein, to the promoters of steroidogenic P-450s. J Biol Chem 1992; 267:17,913–17,919.
169. Rice DA, et al. Analysis of the promoter region of the gene encoding mouse cholesterol side-chain cleavage enzyme. J Biol Chem 1990; 265:11,713–11,720.
170. Clemens JW, et al. Steroidogenic factor-1 binding and transcriptional activity of the cholesterol side-chain cleavage promoter in rat granulosa cells. Endocrinology 1994; 134:1499–1508.
171. Chau YM, et al. Role of steroidogenic-factor 1 in basal and 3′,5′-cyclic adenosine monophosphate-mediated regulation of cytochrome P450 side-chain cleavage enzyme in the mouse. Biol Reprod 1997; 57:765–771.
172. Leers S-S, et al. Synergistic activation of the human type II 3beta-hydroxysteroid dehydrogenase/delta5-delta4 isomerase promoter by the transcription factor steroidogenic factor-1/adrenal 4-binding protein and phorbol ester. J Biol Chem 1997; 272:7960–7967.
173. Lund J, et al. Transcriptional regulation of the bovine CYP17 gene by cAMP. Steroids 1997; 62:43–45.
174. White PC and Slutsker L. Haplotype analysis of CYP11B2. Endocr Res 1995; 21:437–442.
175. Clyne CD, et al. Angiotensin II and potassium regulate human CYP11B2 transcription through common cis-elements. Mol Endocrinol 1997; 11:638–649.
176. Bakke M and Lund J. Transcriptional regulation of the bovine CYP17 gene: two nuclear orphan receptors determine activity of cAMP-responsive sequence 2. Endocr Res 1995; 21:509–516.
177. Liu Z and Simpson ER. Steroidogenic factor 1 (SF-1) and SP1 are required for regulation of bovine CYP11A gene expression in bovine luteal cells and adrenal Y1 cells. Mol Endocrinol 1997; 11:127–137.
178. Honda S, Morohashi K, and Omura T. Novel cAMP regulatory elements in the promoter region of bovine P-450(11 beta) gene. J Biochem Tokyo 1990; 108:1042–1049.
179. Crawford PA, et al. Adrenocortical function and regulation of the steroid 21-hydroxylase gene in NGFI-B-deficient mice. Mol Cell Biol 1995; 15:4331–4316.
180. Cammas FM, et al. The mouse adrenocorticotropin receptor gene: cloning and characterization of its promoter and evidence for a role for the orphan nuclear receptor steroidogenic factor 1. Mol Endocrinol 1997; 11:867–876.
181. Marchal R, et al. A steroidogenic factor-1 binding element is essential for basal human ACTH receptor gene transcription. Biochem Biophys Res Commun 1998; 247:28–32.
182. Sugawara T, et al. Regulation of expression of the steroidogenic acute regulatory protein (StAR) gene: a central role for steroidogenic factor 1 [published erratum appears in Steroids 1997 Apr;62(4):395]. Steroids 1997; 62:5–9.
183. Sugawara T, et al. Multiple steroidogenic factor 1 binding elements in the human steroidogenic acute regulatory protein gene 5′-flanking region are required for maximal promoter activity and cyclic AMP responsiveness. Biochemistry. 1997; 36:7249–7255.
184. Cao G, et al. Structure and localization of the human gene encoding SR-BI/CLA-1. Evidence for transcriptional control by steroidogenic factor 1. J Biol Chem 1997; 272:33,068–33,076.
185. Cao G, et al. Developmental and hormonal regulation of murine scavenger receptor, class B, type 1. Mol Endocrinol 1999. 13:1460–1473.

186. Acton SL, et al. Expression cloning of SR-BI, a CD36-related class B scavenger receptor. J Biol Chem 1994; 269:21003–21009.

187. Murao K, et al. Characterization of CLA-1, a human homologue of rodent scavenger receptor BI, as a receptor for high-density lipoprotein and apoptotic thymocytes. J Biol Chem 1997; 272:17,551–17,557.

188. Michael MD, et al. Ad4BP/SF-1 regulates cyclic AMP-induced transcription from the proximal promoter (PII) of the human aromatase P450 (CYP19) gene in the ovary. J Biol Chem 1995; 270:13,561–13,566.

189. Fitzpatrick SL and Richards JS. Identification of a cyclic adenosine 3′,5′-monophosphate-response element in the rat aromatase promoter that is required for transcriptional activation in rat granulosa cells and R2C leydig cells. Mol Endocrinol 1994; 8:1309–1319.

190. Carlone DL and Richards JS. Functional interactions, phosphorylation, and levels of 3′,5′-cyclic adenosine monophosphate-regulatory element binding protein and steroidogenic factor-1 mediate hormone-regulated and constitutive expression of aromatase in gonadal cells. Mol Endocrinol 1997; 11:292–304.

191. Carlone DL and Richards JS. Evidence that functional interactions of CREB and SF-1 mediate hormone regulated expression of the aromatase gene in granulosa cells and constitutive expression in R2C cells. J Steroid Biochem Mol Biol 1997; 61:223–231.

192. Young M and McPhaul MJ. Definition of the elements required for the activity of the rat aromatase promoter in steroidogenic cell lines. J Steroid Biochem Mol Biol 1997; 61:341–348.

193. Shen WH, et al. Nuclear receptor steroidogenic factor 1 regulates the mullerian inhibiting substance gene: a link to the sex determination cascade. Cell 1994; 77:651–661.

194. Giuili G, Shen WH, and Ingraham HA. The nuclear receptor SF-1 mediates sexually dimorphic expression of Mullerian Inhibiting Substance, in vivo. Development 1997; 124:1799–1807.

195. Wehrenberg U, et al. The orphan receptor SF-1 binds to the COUP-like element in the promoter of the actively transcribed oxytocin gene. J Neuroendocrinol 1994; 6:1–4.

196. Wehrenberg U, et al. Two orphan receptors binding to a common site are involved in the regulation of the oxytocin gene in the bovine ovary. Proc Natl Acad Sci USA 1994; 91:1440–1444.

197. Hu Z, et al. Steroidogenic factor-1 is an essential transcriptional activator for gonad-specific expression of promoter I of the rat prolactin receptor gene. J Biol Chem 1997; 272:14,263–14,271.

198. Barnhart KM and Mellon PL. The orphan nuclear receptor, steroidogenic factor-1, regulates the glycoprotein hormone alpha-subunit gene in pituitary gonadotropes. Mol Endocrinol 1994; 8:878–885.

199. Drean YL, et al. Steroidogenic factor 1 and estradiol receptor act in synergism to regulate the expression of the salmon gonadotropin II beta subunit gene. Mol Endocrinol 1996; 10:217–229.

200. Keri RA and Nilson JH. A steroidogenic factor-1 binding site is required for activity of the luteinizing hormone beta subunit promoter in gonadotropes of transgenic mice. J Biol Chem 1996; 271:10,782–10,785.

201. Halvorson LM, Kaiser UB, and Chin WW. The protein kinase C system acts through the early growth response protein 1 to increase LHbeta gene expression in synergy with steroidogenic factor-1. Mol Endocrinol 1999; 13:106–116.

202. Le De-Y, et al. Presence of distinct cis-acting elements on gonadotropin gene promoters in diverse species dictates the selective recruitment of different transcription factors by steroidogenic factor-1. Mol Cell Endocrinol 1997; 135:31–40.

203. Duval DL, Nelson SE, and Clay CM. A binding site for steroidogenic factor-1 is part of a complex enhancer that mediates expression of the murine gonadotropin-releasing hormone receptor gene. Biol Reprod 1997; 56:160–168.

204. Burris TP, et al. Identification of a putative steroidogenic factor-1 response element in the DAX-1 promoter. Biochem Biophys Res Commun 1995; 214:576–581.

205. Yu RN, Ito M, and Jameson JL. The murine Dax-1 promoter is stimulated by SF-1 (steroidogenic factor-1) and inhibited by COUP-TF (chicken ovalbumin upstream promoter-transcription factor) via a composite nuclear receptor-regulatory element. Mol Endocrinol 1998; 12:1010–1022.

206. Evans RM. The steroid and thyroid hormone receptor superfamily. Science 1988; 240:889–895.

207. Ueda H, et al. A novel DNA-binding motif abuts the zinc finger domain of insect nuclear hormone receptor FTZ-F1 and mouse embryonal long terminal repeat-binding protein. Mol Cell Biol 1992; 12:5667–5672.

208. Morohashi K, et al. Activation of CYP11A and CYP11B gene promoters by the steroidogenic cell-specific transcription factor, Ad4BP. Mol Endocrinol 1993; 7:1196–1204.

209. Li LA, et al. Function of steroidogenic factor 1 domains in nuclear localization, transactivation, and interaction with transcription factor TFIIB and c-Jun. Mol Endocrinol 1999; 13:1588–1598.

210. Crawford PA, et al. The activation function-2 hexamer of steroidogenic factor-1 is required, but not sufficient for potentiation by SRC-1. Mol Endocrinol 1997; 11:1626–1635.

211. Hammer GD and Ingraham HA. Steroidogenic factor-1: its role in endocrine organ development and differentiation. Front Neuroendocrinol 1999; 20:199–223.

212. Jacob AL and Lund J. Mutations in the activation function-2 core domain of steroidogenic factor-1 dominantly suppresses PKA-dependent transactivation of the bovine CYP17 gene. J Biol Chem 1998; 273:13,391–13,394.

213. Ito M, Yu RN, and Jameson JL. Steroidogenic factor-1 contains a carboxy-terminal transcriptional activation domain that interacts with steroid receptor coactivator-1. Mol Endocrinol 1998; 12:290–301.

214. Mont'e D, DeWitte F, and Hum DW. Regulation of the human P450scc gene by steroidogenic factor 1 is mediated by CBP/p300. J Biol Chem 1998; 273:4585–4591.

215. Liu Z and Simpson ER. Molecular mechanism for cooperation between Sp1 and steroidogenic factor-1 (SF-1) to regulate bovine CYP11A gene expression. Mol Cell Endocrinol 1999; 153:183–196.

216. Ito M, Yu R, and Jameson JL. DAX-1 inhibits SF-1-mediated transactivation via a carboxy-terminal domain that is deleted in adrenal hypoplasia congenita. Mol Cell Biol 1997; 17:1476–1483.

217. Francke U, et al. Congenital adrenal hypoplasia, myopathy, and glycerol kinase deficiency: molecular genetic evidence for deletions. Am J Hum Genet 1987; 40:212–227.

218. Goonewardena P, et al. Molecular Xp deletion in a male: suggestion of a locus for hypogonadotropic hypogonadism distal to the glycerol kinase and adrenal hypoplasia loci. Clin Genet 1989; 35:5–12.

219. Worley KC, et al. Identification of new markers in Xp21 between DXS28 (C7) and DMD. Genomics 1992; 13:957–961.

220. Worley KC, et al. Yeast artificial chromosome cloning in the glycerol kinase and adrenal hypoplasia congenita region of Xp21. Genomics 1993; 16:407–416.

221. Guo W, et al. Diagnosis of X-linked adrenal hypoplasia congenita by mutation analysis of the DAX1 gene. Jama 1995; 274:324–330.

222. Guo W, et al. Ahch, the mouse homologue of DAX1: cloning, characterization and synteny with GyK, the glycerol kinase locus. Gene 1996; 178:31–34.

223. Danielian PS, et al. Identification of a conserved region required for hormone dependent transcriptional activation by steroid hormone receptors [published erratum appears in EMBO J 1992; Jun;11(6):2366]. Embo J 1992; 11:1025–1033.

224. Tate BF, et al. Distinct binding determinants for 9-cis retinoic acid are located within AF-2 of retinoic acid receptor alpha. Mol Cell Biol 1994; 14:2323–2330.

225. Durand B, et al. Activation function 2 (AF-2) of retinoic acid receptor and 9-cis retinoic acid receptor: presence of a conserved autonomous constitutive activating domain and influence of the nature of the response element on AF-2 activity. Embo J 1994; 13:5370–5382.

226. Leng X, et al. Mouse retinoid X receptor contains a separable ligand-binding and transactivation domain in its E region. Mol Cell Biol 1995; 15:255–263.

227. Nakae J, et al. Truncation at the C-terminus of the DAX-1 protein impairs its biological actions in patients with X-linked adrenal hypoplasia congenita. J Clin Endocrinol Metab 1996; 81:3680–3685.

228. Lalli E, et al. A transcriptional silencing domain in DAX-1 whose mutation causes adrenal hypoplasia congenita. Mol Endocrinol 1997; 11:1950–1960.

229. Tamai KT, et al. Hormonal and developmental regulation of DAX-1 expression in Sertoli cells. Mol Endocrinol 1996; 10:1561–1569.

230. Ikuyama S, et al. Expression of an orphan nuclear receptor DAX-1 in human pituitary adenomas. Clin Endocrinol Oxf 1998; 48:647–654.

231. Clark BJ, et al. Hormonal and developmental regulation of the steroidogenic acute regulatory protein. Mol Endocrinol 1995; 9:1346–1355.

232. Stocco DM and Clark BJ. Regulation of the acute production of steroids in steroidogenic cells. Endocr Rev 1996; 17:221–244.

233. Clark BJ, et al. Inhibition of transcription affects synthesis of steroidogenic acute regulatory protein and steroidogenesis in MA-10 mouse Leydig tumor cells. Endocrinology 1997; 138:4893–4901.

234. Lin D, et al. Role of steroidogenic acute regulatory protein in adrenal and gonadal steroidogenesis. Science 1995; 267:1828–1831.

235. Okuyama E, et al. A novel splicing junction mutation in the gene for the steroidogenic acute regulatory protein causes congenital lipoid adrenal hyperplasia. J Clin Endocrinol Metab 1997; 82:2337–2342.

236. Lalli E, et al. DAX-1 blocks steroid production at multiple levels. Endocrinology 1998; 139:4237–4243.

237. Yanase T, et al. New mutations of DAX-1 genes in two Japanese patients with X-linked congenital adrenal hypoplasia and hypogonadotropic hypogonadism. J Clin Endocrinol Metab 1996; 81:530–535.

238. Meloni A, et al. New frameshift mutation in the DAX-1 gene in a patient with X-linked adrenal hypoplasia and hypogonadotropic hypogonadism. Hum Mutat 1996; 8:183–184.

239. Kumar V, et al. Localization of the oestradiol-binding and putative DNA-binding domains of the human oestrogen receptor. Embo J 1986; 5:2231–2236.

240. Kumar V, et al. Functional domains of the human estrogen receptor. Cell 1987; 51:941–951.

241. Kuiper GG, et al. Cloning of a novel receptor expressed in rat prostate and ovary. Proc Natl Acad Sci USA 1996; 93:5925–5930.

242. Kuiper GG and Gustafsson JA. The novel estrogen receptor-beta subtype: potential role in the cell- and promoter-specific actions of estrogens and anti-estrogens. FEBS Lett, 1997; 410:87–90.

243. Mosselman S, Polman J, and Dijkema R. ER beta: identification and characterization of a novel human estrogen receptor. FEBS Lett 1996; 392:49–53.

244. Wilson ME, Price RH Jr, and Handa RJ. Estrogen receptor-beta messenger ribonucleic acid expression in the pituitary gland. Endocrinology 1998; 139:5151–5156.

245. Shupnik MA, et al. Selective expression of estrogen receptor alpha and beta isoforms in human pituitary tumors. J Clin Endocrinol Metab 1998; 83:3965–3972.

246. Pennie WD, Aldridge TC, and Brooks AN. Differential activation by xenoestrogens of ER alpha and ER beta when linked to different response elements. J Endocrinol 1998; 158:R11–R14.

247. Brandenberger AW, et al. Tissue distribution of estrogen receptors alpha (ER-alpha) and beta (ER-beta) mRNA in the midgestational human fetus. J Clin Endocrinol Metab 1997; 82:3509–3512.

248. Paech K, et al. Differential ligand activation of estrogen receptors ERalpha and ERbeta at AP1 sites [see comments]. Science 1997; 277:1508–1510.

249. Pennisi E. Differing roles found for estrogen's two receptors [news; comment]. Science 1997; 277:1439.

250. Pettersson K, et al. Mouse estrogen receptor beta forms estrogen response element-binding heterodimers with estrogen receptor alpha. Mol Endocrinol 1997; 11:1486–1496.

251. El-Tanani MK and Green CD. Two separate mechanisms for ligand-independent activation of the estrogen receptor. Mol Endocrinol 1997; 11:928–937.

252. Tora L, et al. The human estrogen receptor has two independent nonacidic transcriptional activation functions. Cell 1989; 59:477–487.

253. Berry M, Metzger D, and Chambon P. Role of the two activating domains of the oestrogen receptor in the cell-type and promoter-context dependent agonistic activity of the anti-oestrogen 4-hydroxyta-moxifen. Embo J 1990 9:2811–2818.

254. Tzukerman MT, et al. Human estrogen receptor transactivational capacity is determined by both cellular and promoter context and mediated by two functionally distinct intramolecular regions. Mol Endocrinol 1994; 8:21–30.

255. Halachmi S, et al. Estrogen receptor-associated proteins: possible mediators of hormone-induced transcription. Science 1994; 264:1455–1458.

256. Landel CC, Kushner PJ, and Greene GL. The interaction of human estrogen receptor with DNA is modulated by receptor-associated proteins. Mol Endocrinol 1994; 8:1407–1419.

257. Baniahmad C, et al. Enhancement of human estrogen receptor activity by SPT6: a potential coactivator. Mol Endocrinol 1995; 9:34–43.

258. Hong H, et al. GRIP1, a novel mouse protein that serves as a transcriptional coactivator in yeast for the hormone-binding domains of steroid receptors. Proc Natl Acad Sci USA 1996; 93:4948–4952.

259. Mader S, et al. Multiple parameters control the selectivity of nuclear receptors for their response elements. Selectivity and promiscuity in response element recognition by retinoic acid receptors and retinoid X receptors. J Biol Chem 1993; 268:591–600.

260. Meyer ME, et al. Steroid hormone receptors compete for factors that mediate their enhancer function. Cell 1989; 57:433–442.

261. Meyer ME, et al. A limiting factor mediates the differential activation of promoters by the human progesterone receptor isoforms. J Biol Chem 1992; 267:10,882–10,887.

262. Wahli W and Martinez E. Superfamily of steroid nuclear receptors: positive and negative regulators of gene expression. Faseb J 1991; 5:2243–2249.

263. Glass CK. Differential recognition of target genes by nuclear receptor monomers, dimers, and heterodimers. Endocr Rev 1994; 15:391–407.

264. Berrodin TJ, et al. Heterodimerization among thyroid hormone receptor, retinoic acid receptor, retinoid X receptor, chicken ovalbumin upstream promoter transcription factor, and an endogenous liver protein. Mol Endocrinol 1992; 6:1468–1478.

265. Horwitz KB, et al. Nuclear receptor coactivators and corepressors. Mol Endocrinol 1996; 10:1167–1177.

266. Miner JN and Yamamoto KR. Regulatory crosstalk at composite response elements. Trends Biochem Sci 1991; 16:423–426.

267. Onate SA, et al. Sequence and characterization of a coactivator for the steroid hormone receptor superfamily. Science 1995; 270:1354–1357.

268. Breitbart RE, Andreadis A, and Nadal G-B. Alternative splicing: a ubiquitous mechanism for the generation of multiple protein isoforms from single genes. Annu Rev Biochem 1987; 56:467–495.

269. L'Opez AJ. Developmental role of transcription factor isoforms generated by alternative splicing. Dev Biol 1995; 172:396–411.

270. MacDougall C, Harbison D, and Bownes M. The developmental consequences of alternate splicing in sex determination and differentiation in Drosophila. Dev Biol 1995; 172:353–376.

271. Angel P and Karin M. The role of Jun, Fos and the AP-1 complex in cell-proliferation and transformation. Biochim Biophys Acta 1991; 1072:129–157.

272. Preston GA, et al. Induction of apoptosis by c-Fos protein. Mol Cell Biol 1996; 16:211–218.

273. Sandhoff TW and McLean MP. Identification and functional characterization of multiple steroidogenic factor 1 elements in the rat steroidigenic acute regulatory (StAR) protein gene promoter (Abstract). J Soe Gynecol Invest 1997; 4.

274. Caron P, et al. Combined hypothalamic-pituitary-gonadal defect in a hypogonadic man with a novel mutation in the DAX-1 gene. J Clin Endocrinol Metab 1999; 84:3563–3569.

275. Couch RM, Muller J, and Winter JS. Regulation of the activities of 17-hydroxylase and 17,20-desmolase in the human adrenal cortex: kinetic analysis and inhibition by endogenous steroids. J Clin Endocrinol Metab 1986; 63:613–618.

276. Bakke M and Lund J. Mutually exclusive interactions of two nuclear orphan receptors determine activity of a cyclic adenosine 3',5'-monophosphate-responsive sequence in the bovine CYP17 gene. Mol Endocrinol 1995 9:327–339.

277. Zhang P and Mellon SH. Multiple orphan nuclear receptors converge to regulate rat P450c17 gene transcription: novel mechanisms for orphan nuclear receptor action. Mol Endocrinol 1997;11:891–904.

278. Pepe GJ and Albrecht ED. Activation of the baboon fetal pituitary-adrenocortical axis at midgestation by estrogen: adrenal delta 5-3 beta-hydroxysteroid dehydrogenase and 17 alpha-hydroxylase-17,20-lyase activity. Endocrinology 1991; 128:2395–2401.

279. Crawford PA, et al. Nuclear receptor DAX-1 recruits nuclear receptor corepressor N-CoR to steroidogenic factor 1. Mol Cell Biol 1998; 18:2949–2956.

3

Reappraisal of Adrenal Zonation Theories Based on the Differential Regulation of Apoptosis

G. W. Wolkersdörfer and S. R. Bornstein

CONTENTS

INTRODUCTION

The histological subdivision of the adrenal cortex in three distinctive zones, *zona glomerulosa, zona fasciculata*, and *zona reticularis*, reflects functional and developmental features of the gland. Cell proliferation and death and hereby their stimuli cover this morphologic peculiarity under physiological and pathophysiological conditions, and the balance of both, cell proliferation and death, is a precondition for the organ's integrity and appropriate functioning. Three main theories provide inroads into the exact mechanisms involved in the zonation of the adrenal cortex *(1)*. In light of these theories, it is possible to develop the connection between cell proliferation, functional differentiation, and cell death in the adrenal cortex.

APOPTOSIS

The morphological definition of programmed cell death known as apoptosis refers to a particular biochemical and morphological pattern of the physiological cell death,

From: *Contemporary Endocrinology: Adrenal Disorders*
Edited by: A. N. Margioris and G. P. Chrousos © Humana Press, Totowa, NJ

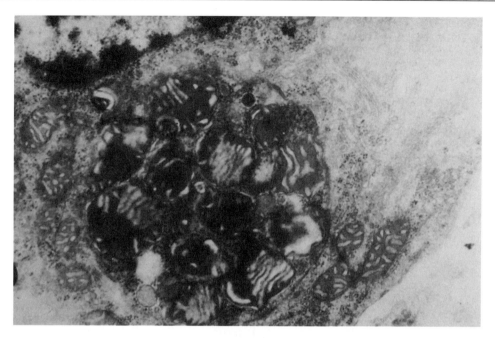

Fig. 1. Apoptosis in the adrenal cortex. The electron micrograph depicts an apoptotic body containing preserved tubulo-vesicular mitochondria, originating from epithelial cells of the cortex. The apoptotic body is membrane engulfed and was phagocytosed by an adrenocortical cell with the characteristic elongated mitochondria containing sickle-forming internal tubuli as defined for the *zona glomerulosa*. Figures 1 and 3 reprinted with permission.

the programmed cell death type I, according to a system introduced in 1973 by Schweichel and Merker *(8)*, and extended by Clarke in 1990 *(9)*. The characteristic morphological features found in apoptotic cells are a condensation of cytoplasm and chromatin, shrinkage of nucleus, and protrusion of plasma and nuclear membranes; a process which finally creates apoptotic bodies, i.e. membrane engulfed cell remnants containing clearly identifiable cyto-organelles *(2)*, Fig. 1. Contrary, necrotic cells show membrane disintegration and irregular chromatin aggregation, lysosomal leakage and diffusion, cell-swelling and lysis, accompanied, and followed by an inflammatory response *(3)*. Investigations in the structure of the adrenal gland profoundly contributed to the understanding of the programmed cell death and its morphologic features in the early 70th *(2, 4–7)*. Therein, clearly distinguishable form injured necrotic cells—single-dying cells exhibiting morphological signs, later referred to as being "apoptosis," were found frequently in inner cortical zones and the *zona reticularis*.

ZONE FORMATION IN THE ADRENAL

Transformation Field Theory

This theory was based on the assumption of two dynamic fields of cell replacement, proliferation and growth *(10–12)*. According to this theory, one field was located at

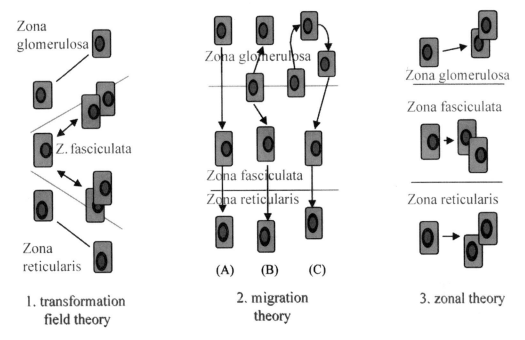

Fig. 2. Three theories of adrenal cortex zonation. Arrows indicate the direction of cell growth and proliferation. **1.** Transformation field theory. Two transformational fields, one between *zona glomerulosa* and *zona fasciculata*, and one between *zona fasciculata* and *zona reticularis*. *Progressive* transformation causes a proliferative increase of the fasciculata zone, *regressive* transformation leads to cell-reduction. **2.** Migration theory. Mitoses and signs of proliferation were mainly found in the *zona glomerulosa* and the outermost *zona fasciculata*. **(A)** Cords running straight from the *zona glomerulosa* toward the medulla. **(B)** Bidirectional migration originating from the *zona intermedia*. **(C)** Cell cords form loops from the outer *zona fasciculata* and the *zona glomerulosa* finally migrating toward the medulla. **3.** Zonal theory. Independent proliferation of all three zones evidenced by a low number of mitoses in all adrenocortical zones.

the transition area between *zona glomerulosa* and *zona fasciculata*, and the other between *zona fasciculata* and *reticularis*. The zonation process took place within these transformation fields, possibly including the entire *zona fasciculata*. Thus, the zonation process might be governed by the *zona fasciculata* and its regulatory mechanisms. Two transformational processes are postulated to be involved, a progressive and a regressive transformation. Progressive transformation described physiologically activated cell replication and proliferation of *fasciculata* cells, and regressive transformation was the counterbalancing decrease in cell numbers by cell death in these fields, leaving *glomerulosa* and *reticularis* cells remaining on its extreme (*see* Fig. 2).

Migration Theory

The migration theory suggests a process where cortex cells proliferate at the outer layers of the adrenal, with the cells growing toward the medulla *(17–19)*. Indeed, S-phase cells had been autoradiographically identified in the *zona glomerulosa* and outermost *zona fasciculata*. A further zone of cell proliferation with high mitotic activity was introduced in rodents *(20–22)*. It is situated between *zona glomerulosa* and *zona fasciculata* and was therefore named *zona intermedia*. Based on the location of the regions with highest mitotic activity, three varying patterns of migration have been suggested. Those patterns are the unidirectional way of cell-migration from *glomerulosa* to *reticularis* [Fig. 2(A)], the bi-directional way starting in the *zona intermedia* towards glomerulosa and reticularis [Fig. 2(B)] and the possibility of loop-forming cell cords originating in the *zona intermedia* and passing through the *zona glomerulosa* toward the medulla [*23, see* Fig. 2(C)]. All of them leave the *zona reticularis* as the main site of cell death *(5,6,24)*. Consistently, varying cell death initiating factors in rats and adrenocorticotropic hormone (ACTH) deprivation *(6,7)* or toxic and hypoxic stress in guinea pigs *(24)* suggested an inducability and regulation of cell death in inner cortical zones.

Zonal Theory

The findings on autoradiographic-labeled mitotic cells in specific regions of cell proliferation are by far not unequivocal. Based on the observation of H^3-thymidine labeled S-phase cells in the rat, mitoses are not only to be found in the outer cortex, but occur all over the cortical layers *(13–16)*. Therefore, it was implicated that the three cortical zones develop independently of each other, using their own regulatory mechanisms. Hence, the development of one zone did not affect the actions of another, and there was no set direction in the pattern of cell proliferation and migration between the zones; thus proliferation, differentiation and functional regulation were thought to be "zonally" (*see* Fig. 2).

APPLYING CELL PROLIFERATION AND APOPTOSIS TO ADRENAL INTEGRITY

The complex process of cell renewal and death is regulated by endocrine, autocrine, and paracrine mechanisms. These, in turn, regulate cell-cycle mediators and transcription factors, which contribute to cell cycle and apoptosis regulation directly *(37,38)*. ACTH affects differentiation and integration of the adrenal tissue. In rats and humans, ACTH was shown to increase the levels of proto-oncogenes, c-*jun*, *jun*-B, c-*fos* and *fos*-B *(39)*, and c-*myc (40)*. Furthermore, an increased cell proliferation in the *zona glomerulosa* was suggested because of elevated fetal growth factor (bFGF) and insulin growth factor (IGF-I) mRNA levels because of ACTH stimulation *(42)*. Similarly, angiotensin II (Ang II) stimulates c-*jun*, c-*fos*, and *jun*-B in bovine and ovine *zona fasciculata* cells *(41)*.

The cell proliferation associated antigen Ki-67 is expressed in the outer *zona fasciculata*, but also in the *zona glomerulosa* and *zona reticularis* of human adrenal glands *(26)*. However, proliferating cell nuclear antigen (PCNA), a polypeptide expressed at peak synthesis during the S-phase of the cell cycle and identified as polymerase delta subunit *(34,35)*, is mainly detectable in the *zona reticularis*. Interestingly, PCNA is also expressed in cells with activated DNA repair mechanisms *(36)*.

Cell-cycle arrest or, if the arrest is not sufficient for DNA repair, apoptosis are regulated through *p53*-tumor-suppressor gene. Inner cortical layers express *p53* in correlation with its downstream effector *p21* after ischemic injury *(31)*. Therefore, it is understandable, that mutations of the *p53*-gene can induce and are associated with neoplastic degeneration in many tumors and in the adrenal gland as well *(32,33)*. Similarly, *p21* blocks cell development in the S-phase and promotes G_1-phase arrest, giving time to repair damaged DNA or to induce apoptosis. In this context and in view of markers associated with proliferation, the expression of *p53* and *p21* suggests a balance between apoptosis, DNA repair, and possibly proliferation in inner cortical zones.

Activated DNA repair mechanisms might be concluded because of very low percentage of nuclei with fragmented DNA in inner zones *(25)*. Internucleosomal fragmentation of DNA is a characteristic of apoptosis, and nuclei with such fragmented DNA occur throughout the whole organ. Although data are different in the absolute numbers of nuclei with labeled fragmented DNA among different research groups, they are consistent at least for the inner cortical zones; and a decrease in percentage of nuclei with fragmented DNA toward the inner zones has been suggested *(26,27)*. Clearly, earlier stages of apoptosis are detectable in all cortical zones through *in situ* end-labeling of fragmented DNA as compared to ultrastructural detection. The differences between zones in the abundance of apoptotic nuclei can suggest distinctive regulatory mechanisms in connection with zonal different expression of cell cycle or proliferation related markers.

Specific cell-cycle markers or proliferation related molecules describe functional moments of a cell's life, which can be completed by analyses of cell and tissue structure. The mitochondria, lysosomes, and Golgi apparatus can be visualized by ultrastructural analysis, which therefore became the standard method in examining the morphological aspects of apoptosis *(43)*. Early works established apoptosis as a physiologic process, but focus on investigation of the innermost cortical zones. Later, apoptosis was confirmed in all zones of the adrenal cortex *(31)* because of condensation of chromatin and cytoplasma, membrane blebbing, and formation of apoptotic remnants. The remnants of apoptosis will be removed through macrophages passing through or residing in the adrenal gland. However, macrophages occur mainly in inner cortical zones. Other mechanisms, therefore, must serve to eliminate apoptotic bodies in outer cortical zones. Indeed, epithelial cells have been discovered to be able to phagocytose apoptotic bodies by themselves in outer cortical zones as the *zona glomerulosa* *(27,* Fig. 1).

AUTOCRINE AND PARACRINE FACTORS IN APOPTOSIS REGULATION AND IMMUNITY

A local renin–angiotensin system in the *zona glomerulosa* *(44–47)* may serve to find balance actions through angiotensin II receptors (AT_2) expressed in the adrenal gland *(49)*. All biologic actions of this system are believed to be mediated via AT_2-type 1 receptors, but also the antiproliferative and apoptosis associated AT_2-type 2 receptor has been found with restriction to the outer cortical zones *(50)*. Conditions with elevation of AT_2 levels therefore might well induce apoptosis within the *zonae glomerulosa et fasciculata*, although there are no experimental data available to date.

In addition to feedback mechanisms within regulatory axis of hormonal systems, the immune system is known to interact with the hypothalamus-pituitary-adrenal (HPA) axis on several levels *(57–60)*. This interaction involves activation of the HPA axis by cytokines and on the other hand, blunting of immunologic activity by glucocorticoids. In addition, immunoadrenal interaction could induce receptor-related apoptosis because of CD 95 (Fas) expression throughout the entire adrenal cortex, a higher expression has been noted at the cortico-medullary transition zone *(27–30)*.

The CD 95 (Fas) ligand is expressed in T cells. In fact, T cells of different subpopulations have been found preferentially in inner cortical zones *(61)*. Moreover, inner

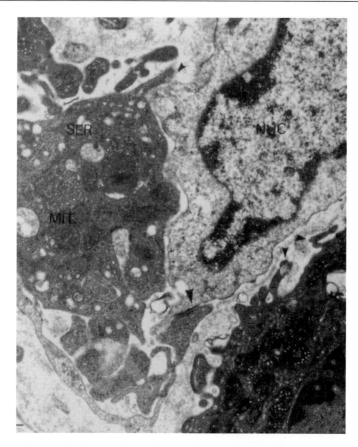

Fig. 3. Electron micrograph demonstrating direct cellular contact between adrenocortical cells and lymphocytes. The adrenocortical cells are characterized by their typical tubulovesicular mitochondria and ample smooth endoplasmic reticulum. The lymphocyte shows a characteristic large nucleus and sparse undifferentiated cytoplasm with few cytoorganelles. The adrenocortical cells show signs of stimulation with large vesicular mitochondria and dilated SER.

adrenocortical cells as of the *zona reticularis* are the only adrenocortical cells that constitutively express major histocompatibility complex (MHC) class II molecules *(71–73)*. MHC class II molecules are activation markers of antigen-presenting cells that interact with T-cell receptor bearing cells *(68)*. Interestingly, the expression of MHC class II molecules is related to the maturation of the adrenal gland during adrenarche and correlates with the gain of full androgen secretory capacity *(62,63)*. The peak activity is achieved in the third decade of life. Because the secretory function and the size of the androgen-producing *zona reticularis* declines in parallel with decreasing adrenal androgen levels after the third decade of life *(64,65)*, the number of resident T lymphocytes within it increase, although in an infiltration-like manner *(66)*. Recent data suggested, that direct cellular contact between adrenocortical cells and T cells mediates an increase in adrenal androgen release *(61,* Fig. 3). Although, MHC class II molecules are less or not expressed in malignant adrenocortical carcinomas *(69,70)*, a direct involvement of MHC class II molecules in the induction of apoptosis via the CD95 (Fas)/CD95 (Fas)-L system could not be proven so far, and the immuno–adrenal interaction via MHC class II molecules remains yet to be fully understood.

Resident monocytes/ macrophages are present within the *zona reticularis* at all stages of life *(56)*. KiM8 expression and the adhesion molecule CD 11 and CD 68 are characteristic for the phagocytic subset of macrophages of the inner adrenalocortical zones. Besides, macrophages and monocytes are established secretory cells of the immune system *(67)* and might, together with lymphocytes, serve to producing and/ or effecting cytokines and their actions. Interleukin 1 (IL-1) and the mitogenic factor interleukin 6 (IL-6) are expressed in abundance in the inner zones of the adrenal cortex *(74,75)*. IL-1 is seen as an apoptosis inhibitor *(76)*. Apoptosis-stimulating cytokines such as TNF-α have also been found in the inner zones of the adrenal cortex. *In situ* hybridization and double immunostaining revealed expression of both TNF-α mRNA and MHC class II by 17α-hydroxylase cytochrome P450 positive cells *(77)*. TNF-α is known as a major mediator of MHC class II expression *(78,79)*.

Late research has established the presence of chromaffin cells in the cortex and cortical cells in the medulla. Ultrastructural analyses have revealed a close relationship between both cell types *(51)*. Thus, catecholamines and neuropeptides produced by chromaffin cells could exert a direct regulatory effect on steroid production in all three zones of the cortex *(52,53)*, possibly facilitated by gap junctions between chromaffin cells and cortical cells *(54)*. The highest density of gap junctions between cortical cells was found in the *zona fasciculata* and *zona reticularis (55)*. Apoptosis, however, would generate single isolated cells with lacking metabolic coupling in these zones.

INTEGRATING THE ZONATION THEORIES WITH APOPTOSIS AND CELL PROLIFERATION

In mice, recent research with the mouse steroid 21-hydroxylase/β-galactosidase transgene showed clonal expansion and migration of cells into a fascicle-like formation towards the medulla *(81)*, corresponding to the migration theory. Cortex stimulation through ACTH causes *zona fasciculata* cell activation and needs controlling mechanisms against neoplastic degeneration or cell hyperproliferation after overactivation. In line with the hypothesis that even functional stages could be balanced by apoptosis are experiments with ACTH deprivation, which demonstrate apoptosis in cells positive for 17α-hydroxylase immunostaining *(82)*. The surviving cells expressed PCNA, but not 17α-hydroxylase, indicating the remaining cells are not specialized in the production of steroid hormones. Although these findings provide some insight, at least in ACTH-dependent layers, proliferation and its markers are, in general, difficult to be connected to any particular zone; and recent research showed DNA synthesis independently in each of the three zones *(84)*.

A low salt diet coupled with the administration of Ang II showed an increase of the *zona glomerulosa* with a diminishing *zona intermedia* in rats *(83)*. This supports the theory of transformation towards the *zona glomerulosa* and the *zona fasciculata* or bi-directional migration in rodents *(84,85)*. Corticotropin releasing hormone (CRH), or the effects of CRH production in the adrenal medulla *(86)*, could stimulate basal proliferation levels in the cortex similar to the morphological appearance of the adrenal cortex in Addison's disease or due to long-term glucocorticoid treatment. Contrary to autoimmune disease or hormonal suppression and hereby zone-related cell loss, cell injury leading to DNA damage, and cell death is not linked to any specific zone *(31)*.

Mechanisms of inducing cell death in the adrenal gland are present, they serve to control cell proliferation and perhaps functional cell hyperactivity, DNA and cell damage, proliferation and homeostasis through trophic hormones, the overall control of the cell cycle, and telomerase-inactivity dependent cell death *(80)*. The occurrence of apoptosis in each zone could suggest a contribution to the regulation of all these processes. Thus, apoptosis serves as a control mechanism in the structural development of the organ, i.e., the zonation process, within the zones or at their periphery. Apoptosis in all zones was demonstrated by the CD 95 (Fas) distribution *(27,30)*, the presence of fragmented nucleolar DNA *(26,27)* and ultrastructural analysis *(27,31)*. In the cortex periphery, very few macrophages were found. Ultrastructural analysis prove that the epithelium is able to remove apoptotic waste. The type 2 AT_2 receptor has been found in the adrenal cortex and is known to affect differentiation and programmed cell death *(87,88)*. Whether type 2 AT_2 receptor affects apoptosis in the adrenal has yet to be proven. There are signs of apoptosis in the inner layers of the adrenal cortex, such as cell shrinkage and the presence of apoptotic remnants. A system consisting of MHC class II expressing adrenocortical cells and corresponding T lymphocytes has been proven to interact directly via cellular contact mechanisms and was shown to induce hormone release *(61)*. The resulting high DHEA concentration would cause a T-lymphocyte subtype shift towards the Th1 function, while glucocorticoids might cause a shift towards Th2 *(89,90)*. CD 95 (Fas) ligand expression in T cells initiated by the interaction with MHC would then trigger the apoptosis process in both the cortical cells and the T lymphocytes, known as activation-induced apoptosis (A1A) *(91,92)*. MHC class II-dependent interaction mediates lymphocyte apoptosis *(93)* and enhances sensitivity to apoptosis mediated by CD 95 (Fas) *(94–96)*. A pool of cytokines could fine-tune the entire system as summarized in Fig. 4.

CONCLUSION AND PERSPECTIVE

The apoptotic markers suggest a new way of analyzing the gland under stress and adverse pathophysiological conditions. Furthermore, new insights may allow integration of old zonation theories with apoptosis and cell proliferation. Apoptosis is a key element in forming the structure of the adrenal and in protecting from neoplastic transformation. Analysis of protein and receptor expression coupled with the presence of MHC class II could prove to be a vital tool in identifying malignant adrenal neoplasms or for screening of incidentaloma *(70,71)* when other forms of histological examination do not give a clear result *(97–99)*.

The new aspects of adrenal physiology provide further concepts in our understanding of adrenal diseases. MHC class II molecules provide a link between the HPA axis and the immune system. As MHC class II and DHEA production decline in parallel in the course of life, there may be effects on the aging process as well *(100,101)*. The immuno–adrenal interaction may give explanations for disorders of the immune system and their specific endocrine features or some conditions in elders.

ACKNOWLEDGMENTS

This work was supported by a grant from Studienstiftung des Deutschen Volkes and BASF Aktiengesellschaft to G. W. Wolkersdörfer.

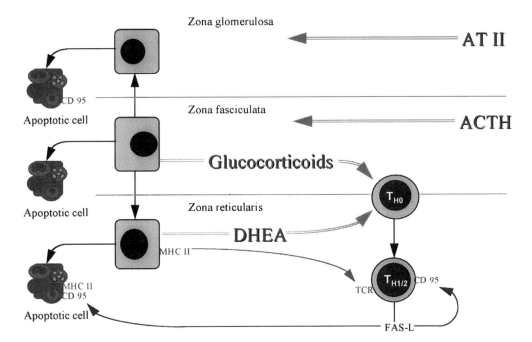

Fig. 4. Differential regulation of apoptosis may be a key factor in adrenal gland zonation. Apoptosis is one mechanism assuring a zone-related regulation of proliferation, growth, migration, and differentiation depending on requirements for zone-specific products. Apoptosis was found in all cortical layers. Receptors such as CD 95 and AT_1-type 2 receptors were found in the adrenal cortex and could trigger apoptosis. Zone-specific products such as glucocorticoids and DHEA support T-cell shift toward Th1 or Th2 function. High-cortical-cell differentiation and the cytokine pool promote MHC class II (MHC II) expression. MHC class II interacts with the T-cell receptor (TCR) perhaps stimulating CD95 (Fas)-Ligand (FAS-L) expression. FAS-L promotes apoptosis in both adrenocortical cells and in T cells. Direct cellular contact provokes adrogen secretion.

REFERENCES

1. Nussdorfer GG. Cytophysiology of the adrenal cortex. Int Rev Cytol 1986; 98.
2. Kerr JFR, Wyllie AH, Macaskill IAM, Currie AR. Apoptosis: a basic biological phenomenon with wide-ranging implications in tissue kinetics. Br J Cancer 1972; 26:239–257.
3. Thompson HJ, Strange R, Schedin PJ. Apoptosis in the genesis and prevention of cancer. Cancer Epidemiol Biomarkers Prev 1992; 1:597–602.
4. Idelman S. Ultrastructure of the mammalian adrenal cortex. Int Rev Cytol 1970; 27:181–281.
5. Kerr JFR. Shrinkage necrosis of adrenal cortical cells. J Pathol 1972; 107:217–219.
6. Wyllie AH, Kerr JFR, Currie AR. Cell death in the normal neonatal rat adrenal cortex. J Pathol 1973; 111:255–261.
7. Wyllie AH, Kerr JFR, Macaskill IAM, Currie AR. Adrenocortical cell deletion: the role of ACTH. J Pathol 1973; 111:85–94.
8. Schweichel JU, Merker HJ. The morphology of various types of cell death in prenatal tissues. Teratology 1973; 7:253–266.
9. Clarke GH. Developmental cell death: morphological diversity and multiple mechanisms: Anat Embryol 1990; 181:195–213.
10. Yoffey JM. Yoffey JM, ed. The Suprarenal Gland 1953; pp. 31–38.
11. Tonutti E. Über die strukturelle Funktionsanpassung der Nebennierenrinde, Endokrinologie 1951; 28:1–15.
12. Chester-Jones I. The Adrenal Cortex. Cambridge Univ Press London and New York. 1957.

13. Swann HG. The pituitary-adrenocortical relationship. Physiol Rev 1940; 20:493–521.

14. Sarason EL. Morphological changes in the rat's adrenal cortex under various experimental conditions. Arch Pathol 1943; 35:373–390.

15. Malendowicz LK, Jachimowicz B. Sex differences in adrenocortical structure and function. Cell Tissue Res 1982; 227:651–659.

16. Carr IA. The human adrenal cortex at the time of death. J Pathol Bacteriol 1959; 78:533–541.

17. Gottschau M. Structur und embryonale Entwicklung der Nebenniere bei Säugetieren. Arch Anat Physiol (Leipzig) 1883; 412–457.

18. Celestino da Costa. Histophysiologie du cortex surrenal. Ann Endocrinol 1951; 12:361–403.

19. Idelman S. General comparative and clinical endocrinology of adrenal cortex. In: Jones IC, ed. Adrenal Cortex 2. Academic London. 1978, pp. 1–199.

20. Sugihara H, Kawai K, Tsuchiyama H. Effects of exogenous ACTH on the rat fetal adrenal cortex: a histochemical and electron-microscopical observation. Acta Pathol Jpn 1977; 27:477–484.

21. Orenberg EK, Glick D. Quantitative histologic distribution of adenosine-3',5-monophosphate in the rat adrenal and effect of adrenocorticotropin. J Histochem Cytochem 1972; 20:923–928.

22. Golder MP, Boyns AR. Distribution of adrenocorticotrophic hormone-stimulated adenylate cyclase in the adrenal cortex. J Endocrinol 1973; 56:471–481.

23. Belloni AS, Mazzocchi G, Meneghelli V, Nussdorfer GG. Cytogenesis in the rat adrenal cortex: evidence for an ACTH-induced centripetal cell migration from the zona glomerulosa. Arch Anat Histol Embryol Norm Exp 1978; 61:195–201.

24. Hoerr NL. The cells of the suprarenal cortex in the guinea-pig. Am J Anat 1931; 48:139–197.

25. Compton MM. A biochemical hallmark of apoptosis: Internucleosomal degradation of the genome. Cancer and Metastasis Reviews 1992; 11:105–119.

26. Sasano H, Imatani A, Shizawa S, Suzuki T, Nagura H. Cell proliferation and apoptosis in normal and pathologic human adrenal. Mod Pathol 1995; 8:11–17.

27. Wolkersdörfer GW, Ehrhart-Bornstein M, Brauer S, Marx C, Scherbaum WA, Bornstein SR. Differential regulation of apoptosis in the normal human adrenal gland. J Clin Endocrinol Metab 1996; 81:4129–4136.

28. Itho N, Yonehera S, Ishii A, et al. The polypeptide encoded by the cDNA for human cell surface antigen Fas can mediate apoptosis. Cell 1991; 66:233–243.

29. Trauth BC, Klas C, Peters AMJ, et al. Monoclonal antibody-mediated tumor regression by induction of apoptosis. Science 1989; 245:301–305.

30. Leithäuser F, Dhein J, Mechtersheimer G, et al. Constitutive and induced expression of APO-1, a new member of the nerve growth factor/tumor necrosis factor receptor superfamily, in normal and neoplastic cells. Lab Invest 1993; 69:415–429.

31. Didenko VV, Wang X, Yang L, Hornsby PJ. Expression of p21 WAF1/CIP1/SDI1 and p53 in apoptotic cells in the adrenal cortex and induction by ischemia/reperfusion injury. J Clin Invest 1996; 97:1723–1731.

32. Reincke M, Karl M, Travis WH, et al. p53 mutations in human adrenocortical neoplasms: immunohistochemical and molecular studies. J Clin Endocrinol Metab 1994; 78:790–794.

33. Lin SR, Lee JY, Tsai HJ. Mutations of the gene in human functional adrenal neoplasms. J Clin Endocrinol Metab 1994; 78:483–491.

34. Mathews MB, Bernstein RM, Franza BR, Jr, Garrels JI. Identity of the proliferating cell nuclear antigen and cyclin. Nature 1984; 309:374–376.

35. Waseem NH, Lane DP. Monoclonal antibody analysis of the proliferating cell nuclear antigen (PCNA). Structural conservation and the detection of a nucleolar form. J Cell Sci 1990; 96:121–129.

36. Shivji KK, Kenny MK, Wood RD. Proliferating cell nuclear antigen is required for DNA excision repair. Cell 1992; 69:367–374.

37. King KL, Cidlowski JA. Cell cycle and apoptosis: common pathways to life and death. J Cell Biochem 1995; 58:175–180.

38. Buttyan R, Zakeri Z, Lockshin R, Wolgemuth D. Cascade induction of c-fos, c-myc and heat shock 70k transcripts during repression of the rat ventral prostate gland. Mol Endocrinol 1988; 2:650–657.

39. Le Houx JG, Ducharme L. In vivo effects of adrenocorticotropin on c-jun, jun-B, c-fos and fos-B in rat adrenal. Endocr Res 1995; 21:267–274.

40. Liu J, Voutilainen R, Kahri AI, Heikkilä P. Expression of the c-myc gene in human adrenals: regulation by adrenocorticotropin in primary cultures. J Endocrinol 1996; 148:523–529.

41. Viard I, Hall SH, Jaillard C, Berthelon MC, Saez JM. Regulation of c-fos, c-jun and jun-B messenger

ribonucleic acids by angiotensin-II and corticotropin in ovine and bovine adrenocortical cells. Endocrinology 1992; 130:1193–1200.

42. Ho MM, Vinson GP. Endocrine control of the distribution of basic fibroblast growth factor, insulinlike growth factor-I and transforming growth factor-beta 1 mRNAs in adult rat adrenals using non-radioactive in situ hybridization. J Endocrinol 1995; 144:379–387.

43. Schwartzman RA, Cidlowski JA. Apoptosis: the biochemistry and molecular biology of programmed cell death. Endo Rev 1993; 14:133–151.

44. Gupta P, Franco-Saenz R, Mulrow PJ. Locally generated angiotensin II in the adrenal gland regulates basal, corticotropin-, and potassium-stimulated aldosterone secretion. Hypertension 1995; 25:443–448.

45. Bahr V, Sander-Bahr C, Hensen J, Oelkers W. Influence of sodium and potassium diets on adrenal vasopressin content and direct effect of vasopressin on aldosterone synthesis in adrenocortical cells. Horm Metab Res 1993; 25:411–416.

46. Mazzochi G, Malendowicz LK, Meneghilli V, Gottardo G, Nussdorfer GG. In-vitro and in-vivo studies of the effects of arginine-vasopressin on the secretion and growth of rat adrenal cortex. Histol Histopathol 1995; 10:359–370.

47. Redmann A, Mobius K, Hiller HH, Oelkers W, Bahr V. Ascorbate depletion prevents aldosterone stimulation by sodium deficiency in guinea pig. Eur J Endocrinol 1995; 133:499–506.

48. Oelkers W, Kohler A, Belkien L, et al. ACTH stimulates plasma renin and angiotensin in man. Clin Sci 61 Suppl 1981; 7:273–275.

49. Murray SA, Oyoyo UA, Pharrams SY, Kumar NM, Gilula NB. Characterization of gap junction expression in the adrenal gland. Endocr Res 1995; 21:221–229.

49. Clauser E, Curnow KM, Davies E, et al. Angiotensin II receptors: protein and gene structures, expression and potential pathological involvements. Eur J Endocrinol 1996; 134:403–411.

50. Shanmugam S, Llorens-Cortes C, Clauser E, Corvoll P, Gasc JM. Expression of angiotensin II AT2 receptor mRNA during development of rat kidney and adrenal gland. Am J Physiol 1995; 258:F922–F930.

51. Bornstein SR, Ehrhart-Bornstein M. Ultrastructural evidence for a paracrine regulation of the rat adrenal cortex mediated by the local release of catecholamines from chromaffin cells. Endocrinology 1992; 131:3126–3128.

52. Ehrhart-Bornstein M, Bornstein SR, Trzeciak WH, et al. Adrenaline stimulates cholesterol side-chain cleavage cytochrome P450 mRNA accumulation in bovine adrenocortical cells. J Endocrinol 1991; 131:R6–8.

53. Bornstein SR, Ehrhart-Bornstein M, Scherbaum WA. Morphological studies of the paracrine interaction between cortex and medulla in the adrenal gland. Micr Res Tech 1997; 36:520–533.

54. Bornstein SR, González-Hernández JA, Ehrhart-Bornstein M, Adler G, Scherbaum WA. Intimate contact of chromaffin and cortical cells within the human adrenal gland forms the cellular basis for important intraadrenal interactions. J Clin Endocrinol Metab 1994; 78:225–232.

55. Munari-Silem Y, Lebrethon MC, Morand I, Rousset B, Saez JM. Gap-junction mediated cell-to-cell communication in bovine and human adrenal cells. A process whereby cells increase their responsiveness to physiological corticotropin concentrations. J Clin Invest 1995; 95:1429–1439.

56. González-Hernández JA, Bornstein SR, Ehrhart-Bornstein M, Gschwend JE, Gwosdow A, Alder G, et al. Macrophages within the human adrenal gland. Cell Tissue Res 1994; 278:201–205.

57. Axelrod J, Reisine TD. Stress hormones: their interaction and regulation. Science 1984; 224:452–459.

58. Chrousos GP. The hypothalamic-pituitary-adrenal axis and immune-mediated inflammation. N Engl J Med 1995; 332:1351–1362.

59. Besedovsky HO, DelRey A. Immune-neuro-endocrine interactions: Facts and hypothesis. Endo Rev 1996; 17:64–102.

60. Ehrhart-Bornstein M, Bornstein SR, Scherbaum WA. Sympathoadrenal system and immune system in the regulation of adrenocortical function. Eur J Neuroendocrinol 1996; 135:19–26.

61. Wolkersdorfer GW, Lohmann T, Marx C, Schroder S, Pfeiffer R, Stahl HD, et al. Lymphocytes stimulate dehydroepiandrosterone production through direct cellular contact with adrenal zona reticularis cells: a novel mechanism of immune-endocrine interaction. J Clin Endocrinol Metab 1999; 84:4220–4227.

62. Marx C, Bornstein SR, Wolkersdorfer GW, Peter M, Sippell WG, Scherbaum WA. Relevance of major histocompatibility complex class II expression as a hallmark for the cellular differentiation in the human adrenal cortex. J Clin Endocrinol Metab 1997; 82:3136–3140.

63. Orentreich N, Brind JL, Rizer RL, Vogelman JH. Age changes and sex differences in serum dehydro-epiandrosterone sulfate concentrations throughout adulthood. J Clin Endocrinol Metab 1984; 59:551–555.

64. Labrie F, Belanger A, Cusan L, Gomez JL, Candas B. Marked decline in serum concentrations of adrenal C19 sex steroid precursors and conjugated androgen metabolites during aging. J Clin Endocrinol Metab 1997; 82:2396–2402.

65. Parker CR Jr, Mixon RL, Brissie RM, Grizzle WE. Aging alters zonation in the adrenal cortex of men. J Clin Endocrinol Metab 1997; 82:3898–3901.

66. Hayashi Y, Hiyoshi T, Takemura T, Kurashima C, Hirokawa K. Focal lymphocytic infiltration in the adrenal cortex of the elderly: immunohistological analysis of infiltrating lymphocytes. Clin Exp Immunol 1989; 77:101–105.

67. Nathan CF. Secretory products of macrophages. J Clin Invest 1987; 79:319–326.

68. Germain RN. MHC-dependent antigen processing and peptide presentation: Providing ligands for T lymphocyte activation. Cell 1994; 76:287–299.

69. Marx C, Wolkersdörfer GW, Brown J, Scherbaum WA, Bornstein SR. MHC class II expression- a new tool to assess dignity in adrenocortical tumours. J Clin Endocrinol Metab 1996; 81:4488–4491.

70. Wolkersdörfer GW, Marx C, Brown JW, Scherbaum WA, Bornstein SR. Evaluation of apoptotic parameters in normal and malignant human adrenal. Endocr Res 1996; 22:411–419.

71. Khoury EL, Greenspan JS, Greenspan FS. Adrenocortical cells of the zona reticularis normally express HLA-DR antigenic determinants. Am J Pathol 1987; 127:580–591.

72. McNicol AM. Class II MHC antigen expression in the adrenal cortex. Letter, Lancet 1986; II:1282.

73. Jackson R, McNicol AM, Farquharson M, Foulis AK. Class II MHC expression in normal adrenal cortex and cortical cells in autoimmune addison's disease. J Pathol 1988; 155:113–120.

74. González-Hernández JA, Bornstein SR, Ehrhart-Bornstein M, et al. IL-1 is expressed in human adrenal gland in vivo. Possible role in a local immune-adrenal axis. Clin Exp Immunol 1993; 99:137–141.

75. González-Hernández JA, Bornstein SR, Ehrhart-Bornstein M, Gschwend JE, Gwosdow A, Späth-Schwalbe E, et al. Interleukin-6 messenger ribonucleic acid expression in human adrenal gland in vivo: new clue to a paracrine or autocrine regulation of adrenal function. J Clin Endocrinol Metab 1994; 79:1492–1497.

76. McConkey DJ, Hartzell P, Show SC, Orrenius S, Jondal M. Interleukin 1 inhibits T cell receptor-mediated apoptosis in immature thymocytes. J Immunol 1990; 145:1227–1230.

77. González-Hernández JA, Ehrhart-Bornstein M, Scherbaum WA, Bornstein SR. Human adrenal cells express TNFα-mRNA: Evidence for a paracrine control of adrenal function. J Clin Endocrinol Metab 1996; 81:1–7.

78. Pfitzenmaier K, Scheurich P, Schlüter C, Krönke, M. TNFα enhances HLA-A,B,C and HLA-DR expression in human tumor cells. J Immunol 1987; 138:975–980.

79. Watanabe Y, Jacob CO. Regulation of MHC class II expression. Opposing effects of TNFα on INFγ induced HLA-DR and Ia expression depend on the maturation and differentiation stage of the cell. J Immunol 1991; 146:899–905.

80. Harley CB, Futcher AB, Greider CW. Telomeres shorten during ageing of human fibroblasts. Nature 1990; 345:375–382.

81. Morley SD, Viard I, Chung BC, Ikeda J, Parker KL, Mullins JJ. Variegated expression of a mouse steroid 21-hydroxylase/ β-galactosidase transgene suggests centripetal migration of adrenocortical cells. Mol Endocrinol 1996; 10:585–598.

82. Negoescu A, Labat-Moleur F, Defaye G, Mezin P, Drouet C, Brambilla C, et al. Contribution of apoptosis to the phenotypic changes of adrenocortical cells in primary culture. Mol Cel Endocrinol 1995; 110:175–184.

83. Tian Y, Balla T, Baukal AJ, Catt KJ. Growth responses to angiotensin II in bovine adrenal glomerulosa cells. Am J Physiol 1995; 268:E135–E144.

84. McEwan PE, Lindop GB, Kenyon CJ. In vivo studies of the control of DNA synthesis in the rat adrenal cortex and medulla. Endocrine Res 1995; 21:91–102.

85. Mitani F, Ogishima T, Miyamoto H, Ishimura Y. Localization of P450aldo and P45011 beta in normal and regenerating rat adrenal cortex. Endocrine Res 1995; 21:413–423.

86. Bornstein SR, Ehrhart M, Scherbaum WA, Pfeiffer EF. Adrenocortical atrophy of hypophysectomized rats can be reduced by corticotropin-releasing hormone (CRH). Cell Tissue Res 1990; 260:161–166.

87. Nakajima M, Hutchinson HG, Fujinaga M, Hayashida W, Morishita R, Zhang L, et al. The angiotensin

II type 2 (AT2) receptor antagonizes the growth effects of the AT1 receptor: gain-of-function study using gene transfer. Proc Natl Sci USA 1995; 92:10,663–10,667.

88. Yamada T, Horiuchi M, Dzau VJ. Angiotensin II type 2 receptor mediates programmed cell death. Proc Natl Acad Sci USA 1996; 93:156–160.

89. Blauer KL, Poth M, Rogers WM, Bernton EW. Dehydroepiandrosterone antagonizes the suppressive effects of dexamethasome on lymphocyte proliferation. Endocrinology 1991; 129:3174–3179.

90. Rook GAW, Hernandez-Pando R, Lightman SL. Hormones, peripherally activated prohormones and regulation of the Th1/Th2 balance. Immunol today 1994; 15:301–303.

91. Dhein J, Walczak H, Bäumler C, Debatin K-L, Krammer PH. Autocrine T-cell suicide mediated by APO-1/(FAS/CD95). Nature 1995; 373:438–441.

92. Brunner T, Mogil RJ, LaFace D, Yoo SJ, Mahboubi A, Echeverri F, et al. Cell-autonomous FAS(CD95)/FAS-ligand interaction mediates activation induced apoptosis in T-cell hybridomas. Nature 1995; 373:441–444.

93. Truman JP, Ericson ML, Choqueux-Séébold CJ, Sharron DJ, Mooney NA. Lymphocyte programmed cell death is mediated via HLA class II DR. Int Immunol (England) 1994; 6:887–896.

94. Yoshino T, Cao L, Nishiuchi R, Matsuo Y, Yamadori I, Kondo E, et al. Ligation of HLA class II molecules promotes sensitivity to CD95 (Fas antigen, APO-1)- mediated apoptosis. Eur J Immunol 1995; 25:2190–2195.

95. Newell MK, Vander Wall J, Beard KS, Freed JH. Ligation of major histocompatibility complex class II molecules mediates apoptotic cell death in resting B lymphocytes. Proc Natl Acad Sci 1993; 90:10,459–10,463.

96. Arimilli S, Mumm JB, Nag B. Antigen-specific apoptosis in immortalized T cells by soluble MHC class II-peptide complexes. Immunol Cell Biol 1996; 74:96–104.

97. Weiss ML, Medeiros LJ, Vickery AL. Pathologic features of prognostic significance in adrenocortical carcinoma. Am J Surg Pathol 1989; 13:202–206.

98. Tartour E, Caillou B, Tenenbaum F, Schröder S, Luciani S, Talbot M, et al. Immunohistochemical study of adrenocortical carcinoma. Cancer 1993; 72:3296–303.

99. Oelkers W. Diagnostic puzzle of adrenal "incidentaloma." Eur J Endocrinol 1995; 132:422–428.

100. Hirokawa K, Utsuyama M, Kurashima C. Ageing and immunity. Acta Pathol Jpn 1992; 42:537–548.

101. Kurashima C, Utsuyama M, Kasai M, Hirokawa K. Senescence of immune function in animal models. Biomed Gerontol 1992; 16:160–170.

4 Pharmacology of Glucocorticoids: An Overview

Achille Gravanis and Andrew N. Margioris

Contents

BIOSYNTHESIS

The adult human adrenal is composed of two parts: the cortex, which is the outer part, representing 90% of its weight, and the medulla, or inner part of the gland. The adrenal cortex is made up of three zones: the *zona glomerulosa* (outermost), the *zona fasciculata* (middle), and the *zona reticularis* (innermost, next to the medulla). Glucocorticoids are synthesized mainly in the *zona fasciculata,* which constitutes 75% of the weight of the adrenal gland (Fig. 1).

Cholesterol is the precursor molecule of cortisol synthesis *(1).* Although the cortex is capable for *de novo* cholesterol biosynthesis, most of the cholesterol used for glucocorticoids is taken up from the circulation. However, in the adrenals, uptake of circulating cholesterol or its synthesis *de novo* are interchangeable functions so that blockade of former or the latter does not cause any significant decrease in cortisol or aldosterone production. It should be noted that the circulating cholesterol is carried by low- and high-density lipoproteins for both of which the adrenal cortex has receptors. In humans, low-density lipoproteins are the major source of adrenal cholesterol. In the adrenal cortex, cholesterol is esterified and stored inside cytoplasmic lipid droplets. For glucocorticoid synthesis, the esterified cholesterol is first hydrolyzed by cytoplasmic cholesterol ester hydrolasc and, subsequently, it is transported into the mitochondria by a sterol carrier protein where it is converted to pregnenolone (Fig. 1). This conversion requires NADPH and oxygen and involves: (1) removal of a portion of the side chain of cholesterol (which is attached to its 17th carbon), and (2) addition of a double-bonded oxygen at position 20. Pregnenolone is transferred from the mitochondria to the smooth endoplasmic reticulum where most of it is hydroxylated by the 17α-hydroxylase enzyme into 17α-hydroxypregnenolone, which in turn, is converted to

From: *Contemporary Endocrinology: Adrenal Disorders*
Edited by: A. N. Margioris and G. P. Chrousos © Humana Press, Totowa, NJ

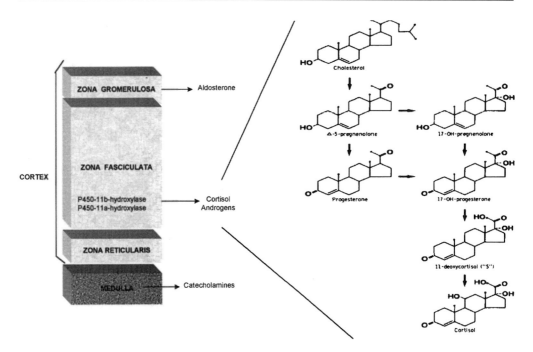

Fig. 1. Biosynthesis of glucocorticoids. Glucocorticoids are synthesized mainly in the *zona fasciculata* of the adrenal gland. The adult human adrenal is composed of two parts: the cortex which is the outer part, representing 90% of its weight, and the medulla, or inner part of the gland. The adrenal cortex is made up of three zones: the *zona glomerulosa* (outermost), the *zona fasciculata* (middle), and the *zona reticularis* (innermost, next to the medulla).

Cholesterol is the precursor molecule of glucocorticoid biosynthesis. Adrenal cortical cholesterol is esterified and converted to pregnenolone. Pregnenolone is hydroxylated by the 17α-hydroxylase enzyme into 17α-hydroxypregnenolone, which in turn, is converted to 17α-hydroxyprogesterone through replacement of a 5,6 double bond by a 4,5 double bond. The latter reaction is catalysed by the 3β-hydroxysteroid dehydrogenase/Δ5-isomerase enzyme complex. A small percentage of pregnenolone is first converted by this enzyme complex to progesterone and then hydroxylated at the 17 position to 17α-hydroxyprogesterone. 17α-hydroxyprogesterone is a strategically located steroid. In the *zona fasciculata,* this compound undergoes two successive hydroxylations: at position 21 by the 21-hydroxylase enzyme resulting in 11-deoxycortisol, then at position 11 by the 11β-hydroxylase enzyme to cortisol.

17α-hydroxyprogesterone through replacement of a 5,6 double bond by a 4,5 double bond. The latter reaction is catalyzed by the 3β-hydroxysteroid dehydrogenase/Δ5-isomerase enzyme complex. For any corticoid to be biologically active, it has to pass this crucial step. A small percentage of pregnenolone is first converted by this enzyme complex to progesterone and then hydroxylated at the 17 position to 17α-hydroxy-progesterone. 17α-hydroxyprogesterone is a strategically located steroid. In the *zona fasciculata,* this compound undergoes two successive hydroxylations. First, it is hydroxylated at position 21 by the 21-hydroxylase enzyme (located in the endoplasmic reticulum) resulting in 11-deoxycortisol (also called compound S). Compound S is then hydroxylated at position 11 by the 11β-hydroxylase enzyme (located inside the mitochondria) to cortisol (also called compound F). In the *zona glomerulosa,* there is no 17α-hydroxylase enzyme present and thus, all available pregnenolone is transformed to progesterone, which in turn, follows the pathway for the synthesis of the mineralocorticoid aldosterone.

Cortisol synthesis and secretion is regulated by the pituitary hormone corticotropin (ACTH), which is secreted into the systemic circulation. ACTH reaches the ACTH receptors located on the surface of adrenocortical cells. The activated receptors initiate a cAMP-dependent increase of transcription of almost all enzymes involved in cortisol biosynthesis, resulting in an increase of cortisol production and secretion. ACTH also exerts a growth-promoting effect on the adrenal cortex. Indeed, constant low levels of ACTH result not only in a decrease of cortisol synthesis and secretion, but also in a gradual atrophy of the adrenal cortex. The production of ACTH by the pituitary corticotrophs is very sensitive to suppression by exogenous glucocorticoids. It should be stressed that manipulation of this system, for therapeutic purposes, should be approached with extreme care because chronic exposure of the pituitary corticotrophs to pharmacological concentrations of glucocorticoids results in pituitary changes and adrenal cortical atrophy and severe impairment of endogenous glucocorticoid production.

PHARMACODYNAMICS

Glucocorticoids exert their effects by binding to a specific glucocorticoid receptor (GR). GR belongs to the superfamily of nuclear steroid receptors *(2)*. This protein of 800 amino acids resides mainly in cytoplasm in an inactive form. The GR protein can be divided into three domains: (a) the glucocorticoid-binding domain located at the carboxy-terminal of the molecule; as its name implies, it is the area where ligands, i.e., glucocorticoids, bind. Deletion of this domain may result in constitutive activation of the receptor in the absence of ligands and (b) the DNA-binding domain is located in the middle part of the protein and contains nine cysteine residues that form a "two-finger" structure stabilized by zinc ions taking the shape of two tetrahedrons; this structure binds to specific sites on the DNA the so-called glucocorticoid-responsive elements (GREs), which mediate the effect of glucocorticoids on the glucocorticoid-responsive genes. Finally, (c) the amino-terminus domain of the receptor is located at the amino-terminal of the molecule in a highly antigenic area; its exact function has not been defined, although there is much evidence suggesting that it is involved in the translocation of the receptor into the nucleus and its subsequent interaction with chromatin.

The inactive form of the glucocorticoid receptor located in the cytoplasm is in the form of a heteromer associated with a number of "chaperon" proteins (Fig. 2), the most important are: (a) heat-shock protein 90 (HSP90); (b) heat-shock protein 70 (HSP70); and (c) the 56-kDa immunophilin, a binding protein of the immunosuppressants cyclosporine and tacrolimus (Fig. 2). The glucocorticoid receptor heteromer is unable to exert any effect by itself. Binding of glucocorticoid hormones to the heteromeric receptor results in dissociation of the chaperon proteins (receptor "activation"), and liberation of its DNA-binding domain that is now available for interaction with the DNA. The activated glucocorticoid-receptor complex then enters the nucleus ("translocation") where two molecules of the activated receptor associate (through two leucine zippers) to form a homodimer that binds to specific glucocorticoid response elements (GRE), i.e., DNA sequences located within the promoter region of the glucocorticoid-

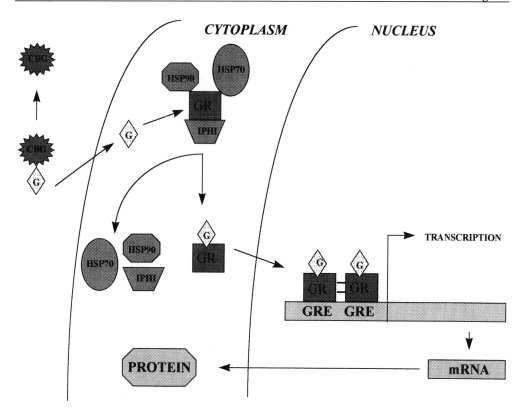

Fig. 2. Mechanism of glucocorticoids action. The inactive form of the glucocorticoid receptor is located in the cytoplasm as an heteromer associated with the heat-shock protein 90 (HSP90), the heat-shock protein 70 (HSP70), and the 56-kDa immunophilin, a binding protein of the immunosupressants cyclosporine and tacrolimus. Binding of a glucocorticoid to its receptor results in the dissociation of the chaperon proteins (receptor activation), and the exposure of its DNA-binding domain, which now is available for interaction with specific areas of DNA. The activated glucocorticoid-receptor complex then enters the nucleus (translocation). Within the nucleus, two molecules of the activated receptor are associated (through two leucine zippers) to form an homodimer, which binds to specific glucocorticoid response elements (GRE), DNA sequences located within the promoter region of GR genes, resulting in altered transcription rates. GREs contain mainly the following nucleotide consensus sequence: GGTACAnnnTGTTCT.

responsive genes, resulting in altered transcription rates. It should be noted that the GREs contain the nucleotide consensus sequence "GGTACAnnnTGTTCT."

Posttranslational splicing of the glucocorticoid receptor genes is very important physiologically. Indeed, alternative splicing of the human glucocorticoid receptor pre-mRNA generates two highly homologous isoforms, termed hGR-α and hGR-β. hGR-α is our ligand-activated transcription factor which, in the hormone-bound state, modulates the expression of the glucocorticoid-responsive genes by binding the GREs. In contrast, hGR-β does not bind glucocorticoids and it is, thus, transcriptionally inactive. However, hGR-β is able to inhibit the effects of hormone-activated hGR-α on the glucocorticoid-responsive genes playing the role of an endogenous inhibitor of glucocorticoid action *(3)*.

Some of the bio-effects of cortisol are attributable to its binding to the receptors of aldosterone (AR). Indeed, AR binds both aldosterone and cortisol with similar affinities.

To avoid any mineralocorticoid effect of cortisol, some tissues produce the enzyme 11β-hydroxysteroid dehydrogenase that can transform cortisol to its 11-keto derivative cortisone that has minimal affinity toward the aldosterone receptor.

In addition to their genomic effects, glucocorticoids also exert several nongenomic effects. The common characteristic of these effects is their extremely rapid onset. It now appears that these glucocorticoid effects are mediated by membrane-bound receptors; the exact mechanism of which is not yet clear. Recent findings suggest the acute effect of glucocorticoids is mediated by cAMP and the subsequent alteration of the actin-based cytoskeleton *(4)*.

PHARMACOKINETICS

Most glucocorticoids are rapidly and readily absorbed from the gastrointestinal tract, as a result of their lipophilic character. Glucocorticoids are also absorbed from synovial and conjunctival tissues *(5)*. It should be noted here that absorption of glucocorticoids through the skin is very inefficient and slow. Consequently, dia-dermal administration of glucocorticoids is not recommended. Indeed, skin application of glucocorticoids should be intended only for local effects. However, excessive and prolonged local application of glucocorticoids may result in enough absorption to cause some systemic effects.

Cortisol and prednisolone possess a hydroxyl group at carbon 11 the presence of which confers glucocorticoid activity to the molecules. Cortisone and prednisone have a keto group at carbon 11 and, thus, they must be hydroxylized first in order to become bioactive. This hydroxylation takes place mainly in the liver. Consequently, the administration of 11-keto corticoids to patients with abnormal liver function should be avoided. For the same reason, topical application of 11-keto corticoids on the skin for local action is ineffective.

Almost 90% of the circulating cortisol is bound to plasma proteins, i.e., to cortisol-binding globulin, an α2-globulin produced by the liver, also called CBG or transcortin and to albumin. CBG binds cortisol with high affinity, but low capacity while albumin binds them with low affinity—but with high capacity because of its high concentration. Under normal conditions, the free (bioactive) fraction is approx 3 to 10% of the circulating cortisol. CBG also binds synthetic glucocorticoids, such as prednisone and prednisolone. However, the potent glucocorticoid compound, dexamethasone, does not bind to CBG and consequently almost 100% of its plasma concentration is in its free form, thus representing one of the most bioactive glucocorticoid agonists. Estrogens may induce the biosynthesis of hormone-binding globulins from the liver, while androgens suppress them. Thus, during estrogen therapy (contraception, hormone replacement therapy, and so on) or pregnancy, the CBG is elevated, resulting in increased levels of total plasma cortisol and normal free hormone. The physiological significance of this elevation is not clear.

The liver and kidneys are major organs where glucocorticoid biotransformation takes place leading to their inactivation by conferring them water-soluble qualities. The biotransformation of glucocorticoids is composed of several steps including reduction of the double bond of position C4–5, reduction of the keto group of the C3, and hydroxylation at the C6 position. About 30% of the inactivated cortisol is metabolized to tetrahydrocortisol and tetrahydrodeoxycortisol, which are then conjugated in the liver through their 3-hydroxyl group with glucuronide or sulfate and excreted in the urine. In humans, biliary and fecal excretion of glucocorticoid metabolites is minimal. Another important cortisol inactivation pathway takes place in the kidneys and results in its conversion to cortisone by the 11-ketosteroid reductase/11β-dehydroxysteroid dehydrogenase enzyme complex. As aforementioned, cortisone in contrast to cortisol does not bind to kidney mineralocorticoid receptor and thus does not exert significant salt-retaining effects.

Inducers or inhibitors of hepatic drug metabolism, such as rifampicin, phenobarbital, and phenytoin may interfere with liver biotransformation of glucocorticoids. Thus, the coadministration of this type of medication may necessitate alteration of the required dose of glucocorticoids.

GLUCOCORTICOID ANTAGONISTS

The prolonged search for a glucocorticoid antagonist finally succeeded with the development of the 11β-aminophenyl-substituted 19-norsteroid RU486, later named mifepristone. This compound has strong antiprogestin activity and initially was proposed as a contraceptive/contragestive agent *(6)*. High doses of mifepristone exert antigluco-corticoid activity by blocking glucocorticoid receptors because mifepristone binds with high affinity to them causing an alteration of its conformation different than that induced by the glucocorticoid agonists. This effect of mifepristone results in stabilization of the hsp/GR complex and, thus, inhibition of the dissociation of hsp chaperon proteins from the GR molecule. There is also some evidence suggesting that binding of the mifepristone to GR results in a reduced DNA binding affinity of the GR/antagonist complex, as well as a reduced transcription of glucocorticoid-responsive genes.

The mean half-life of mifepristone is about 20 h *(7)*. Thus, the apparent half-life of mifepristone is prolonged compared to that of the glucocorticoid agonists as, for instance, that of dexamethasone which has a half-life of only 5 h. Less than 1% of mifepristone is excreted through the urine indicating that the kidneys play a minor role in the clearance of this compound. The long plasma half-life of mifepristone most probably results from an extensive and strong binding to plasma proteins. Indeed, less than 5% of the compound is found in free form when plasma is analyzed by equilibrium dialysis. Mifepristone can bind to albumin and to an a1-acid glycoprotein but has no affinity toward the CBG.

In humans, mifepristone causes generalized glucocorticoid resistance. Mifepristone given orally to several patients with Cushing's syndrome, caused by ectopic ACTH production or adrenal carcinoma, was able to reverse the Cushingoid phenotype, to eliminate carbohydrate intolerance, decrease hypertension, correct thyroid and gonadal hormone suppression, and ameliorate the psychological sequels *(8)*. It should be noted, however, that prolonged exposure to this compound may result in a "paradoxical stimulation" of the hypothalamus-pituitary-adrenal axis (HPAA). To date, the application of mifepristone can only be recommended for inoperable patients with ectopic ACTH secretion or adrenal carcinoma who have failed to respond to other therapeutic manipulations.

Recent experimental studies have elucidated the molecular mechanism by which glucocorticoids regulate gene transcription. Two important functions of glucocorticoids, namely, suppression of the immune system and feedback suppression of the HPAA are mediated through repression of gene transcription. The repression is exerted in part through antagonism between the GR and various transcription factors at the level of response elements in the promoter region of glucocorticoid-sensitive genes. These transcription factors represent potential targets for the development of a new generation of glucocorticoid antagonists. These compounds will antagonize glucocorticoids not at the level of the receptor binding sites, but at the promoter region of the GR genes. Typical candidates are the *Nur77* and NK kappaB transcription factors. Indeed, the recent identification of the orphan nuclear receptor *Nur77* as a mediator of CRH-induced POMC transcription has shown that glucocorticoids may antagonize this positive signal through their binding to GR and prevent the effect of *Nur77,* its specific *Nur*-responsive element on the promoter of the POMC gene *(9)*. The convergence of positive signals mediated by *Nur77* and negative signals exerted by GR offers a novel level of glucocorticoid antagonism. On the other hand, nuclear factor kappa B (NF-kappa B) is an inducible transcription factor that positively regulates the expression of proimmune and proinflammatory genes, whereas glucocorticoids are extremely potent suppressors of immune and inflammatory responses. It is now known that NF-kappa B and the GR interact resulting in a mutual antagonism *(10,11)*. Indeed, functional dissection of the NF-kappa B *p50* and *p65* subunits and deletion mutants of GR indicate that the GR antagonism is specific to the *p65* subunit of NF-kappa B heterodimer, whereas multiple domains of GR are essential to repress *p65*-mediated transactivation.

An alternative mechanism by which to antagonize glucocorticoids is through inhibition of the activation of glucocorticoid receptors. As aforementioned, the GR is a ligand-regulated transcription factor whose ability to bind the hormone depends on its disassociation from the 90-kDa heat-shock protein (hsp90). It is feasible that a form of the glucocorticoid receptor can be generated in which the receptor remains firmly complexed to the hsp90 chaperon protein and, thus, unable to bind the hormone ligand. Indeed, treatment of intact cells with the calmodulin (CaM) antagonist phenoxybenzamine (POBA) results in inhibition of hormone-induced transformation of the GR and blockade of its subsequent nuclear translocation *(12)*. These results point to the potential use of POBA, and possibly other CaM inhibitors, as antagonists of glucocorticoid receptors.

JNK, a c-Jun N-terminal kinase, phosphorylates GR in vitro primarily in Ser-246. Selective activation of JNK in vivo inhibits GR-mediated transcriptional activation, which depends on receptor phosphorylation at Ser-246 *(13,14)*. Thus, JNK inhibits GR transcriptional activation by direct receptor phosphorylation. Phosphorylation of GR by JNK provides mechanisms to ensure the rapid inhibition of GR-dependent gene expression when it conflicts with mitogenic or proinflammatory signals.

Table 1
Mean Pharmacokinetic Values for Oral Administration of Major Glucocorticoids

Compound	Biological Half-Life	Volume of Distribution (lt/kg)	Bound in Plasma (%)	Clearance (ml/min/kg)	Bio-availability (%)	Potency Rel. to Cortisol (%)
Prednisone	12–36	1.0	75	3.6	80	400
Prednisolone	12–36	1.5	95	8.7	82	400
Methylprednisonone	12–36	1.2	78	6.2	82	500
Dexamethasone	36–72	0.8	68	4.0	78	25000
Betamethasone	36–72	1.4	64	2.9	72	25000

Table 2
Systemic Effects of Glucocorticoids

System	Effect	Mechanism(s) of Action
Carbohydrate and protein metabolism	—Increase blood glucose levels.	—Activate liver glucose biosynthesis from aminoacids and glycerol (induce the expression of phosphoenolpyruvate carboxylase, glucose-6-phosphatase) —Protein catabolism to supply aminoacids —Activate lipolysis to supply glycerol —Deposition of glucose to liver glycogen —Decrease peripheral glucose utilization (inhibit glucose transporters)
Lipid metabolism	—Redistribution of body fat (neck, face, supraclavicular)	
	—Lipolysis	—Facilitate the lipolytic effect of β-adrenergic agonists and growth hormone
Electrolyte and water balance	—Decrease total body Ca^{2+} levels	—Decrease Ca^{2+} uptake in the gut and increase Ca^{2+} excretion in the kidney
	—Reabsorption of Na^+, water retention	—Through binding to aldosterone receptors
Cardiovascular	—Hypertension	—Not clear, maybe by increasing the sensitivity of vascular wall to vasoactive agents through stimulation of adrenergic receptor gene expression
Skeletal muscle	—Proximal muscle wasting (steroid myopathy)	—Mostly unknown, maybe through excessive protein catabolism to supply aminoacids for neoglucogenesis
Blood cells	—Decrease number of lymphocytes, monocytes, eosinophils, basophils	—Induce cell apoptosis
	—Increase number of polymorphonuclear lymphocytes	—Stimulate the release from the bone marrow
Immune/ inflammatory response	—Decrease inflammatory response	—Inhibit the production of vasoactive and chemoattractive agents (prostaglandins, histamine, leukotrienes) —Decrease the secretion of lipolytic and proteolytic enzymes —Decrease lymphocyte extravasation and tissue fibrosis (inhibit endothelial leukocyte adhesion molecule-1 ECAM-1 and intracellular adhesion molecule-1 (CAM-1).
	—Decrease immune response	—Inhibit the production and release of cytokines (IL-1, IL-2, IL-3, IL-6; TNF-α, GM-CSF, IFN-γ)

Table 3
Side Effects and Toxicity of Long-Term Administration of
Pharmacological Doses of Glucocorticoids

Toxic Effect	Mechanism(s)
—Increase susceptibility to infection	—Decrease immune response
—Growth retardation in children	—Inhibit the production of GH and somatomedin C
	—Decrease the sensitivity of target cells to GH and somatomedin C
—Osteoporosis and vertebral compression fractures (increase bone resorption)	—Inhibit the activity of osteoblasts
—Osteonecrosis (bone aseptic necrosis)	—Decrease Ca^{2+} uptake in the gut and increase Ca^{2+} excretion in the kidney
	—Decrease osteocalcin and increase PTH
	—Block the bone-sparing effect of calcitonin
—Hypertension	—Reabsorption of Na^+ and water retention in the kidney
	—Increase sensitivity of vascular wall to vasoactive agents
—Hyperglycemia and development of Diabetes Mellitus in susceptible individuals	—Activate liver glucose biosynthesis
	—Decrease peripheral glucose utilization
—Increase incidence of peptic ulcers	—Increase gastric acid output
	—Inhibit the synthesis of mucopolysaccharides that protect gastric mucosa from acid.
—Male: hypogonadism and decreased plasma testosterone	—Suppress the synthesis and secretion of gonadotropins
—Female: anovulation, oligomenorrhea or dysfunctional uterine	
—Steroid myopathy, muscle wasting (more vulnerable patients with asthma or chronic obstructive pulmonary disease)	—Induce excessive protein catabolism
—Posterior subcapsular cataracts	—Covalently bind to lens proteins resulting in destabilization of the protein structure and their oxidation
—Anxiety, depression, psychosis	—Not known, maybe through regulation of brain CRH or neurosteroids synthesis

Suppression of the HPAA is the most common side effect of chronic glucocorticoid therapy. The suppressive effect of glucocorticoids on the HPAA appears within days following the start of glucocorticoid treatment. It has been calculated that any patient who receives glucocorticoids in doses equivalent to 5 mg or more of prednisone daily for more than 2 wk should be considered to have a suppressed HPAA. The time needed for the axis to recover depends on the type of glucocorticoid given, the dose and frequency of administration (i.e., daily vs alternate days), and the length of treatment. In cases of prolonged glucocorticoid administration, the recovery of the HPAA may take up to 1 yr or longer.

Table 4
Glucocorticoid Replacement Therapy in Adrenal Insufficiency

Type of Adrenal Insufficiency	Typical Regimen
—Acute adrenal insufficiency	Hydrocortisone: 100 mg iv, then infusion 100 mg every 8 h, finally 25 mg every 8 h
—Chronic primary adrenal insufficiency	Hydrocortisone: 20 mg po a.m. and 10 mg p.m.
—Secondary adrenal insufficiency	Hydrocortisone: 20 mg po a.m. and 10 mg p.m.
—Congenital adrenal hyperplasia	Hydrocortisone: 0.3 mg/kg po twice daily

Cortisol (hydrocortisone) and cortisone are used only for replacement in patients with adrenal insufficiency. They are not recommended as antiinflammatory agents because of their high-mineralocorticoid activity compared to their relatively low-antiinflammatory activity.

Table 5
Major Indications of Glucocorticoid Therapy

Disease	Typical Regimen
Rheumatic diseases systemic lupus erythimatosus polyarteritis nodosa giant cell arteritis Wegener's granulomatosis	Prednisone: 1 mg/kg/day po in divided doses
—**Nephrotic syndrome**	Prednisone: 1–2 mg/kg/day po for 6 wk
—**Allergic disease** hay fever urticaria serum and drug reactions bee stings contact dermatitis angioneurotic adema	Variable
—**Broncial asthma**	Methylprednisolone: 60–120 mg iv every 6 h, then Prednisone: 40–60 mg/day po
—**Ocular inflammation**	Dexamethasone: 2 drops every 4 h from 0.1% solution
—**Skin eczemas**	Hydrocortisone: 1% ointment locally twice daily
—**Chronic ulcerative colitis, Crohn's disease**	Prednisone: 10–30 mg/day po
—**Sarcoidosis**	Prednisone: 1 mg/kg/day po
—**Thrombocytopenia**	Prednisone: 0.5 mg/kg/day po
—**Stroke and spinal cord injury**	Methylprednisolone: 30 mg/kg iv then infusion for 24 h 5mg/kg
—**Malignancies** Acute lymphocytic leukemia Lymphomas Combination chemotherapy of varioustumors	Variable

Prednisone, prednisolone, and methylprednisolone possess strong antiinflammatory activity, intermediate plasma half-lives, and relatively low-mineralocorticoid activity. They represent the first choice of drugs for chronic antiinflammatory/immunosuppressant therapeutic regimens.

Dexamethasone and betamethasone exhibit maximal antiinflammatory activity, prolonged plasma half-lives, and marked growth-suppressing properties. They represent the best choice in cases where a maximum antiinflammatory therapy is needed acutely.

REFERENCES

1. Margioris A, Gravanis A, Chrousos G. Glucocorticoids and mineralocorticoids. In: Brondy G, Larner J, Minneman K, Neu H, eds. Human Pharmacology: molecular to clinical 2th ed., Mosby, New York, 1994, pp. 473–481.
2. Bamberger CM, Schulte HM, Chrousos GP. Molecular determinants of glucocorticoid receptor function and tissue sensitivity to glucocorticoids. Endocr Rev 1996; 17:245–261.
3. Bamberger CM, Bamberger AM, de Castro M, Chrousos GP. Glucocorticoid receptor beta, a potential endogenous inhibitor of glucocorticoid action in humans. J Clin Invest 1995; 95:2435–2441.
4. Koukouritaki E, Theodoropoulos P, Margioris A, Gravanis A, Stournaras C. Dexamethasone alters rapidly actin polymerization dynamics in human endometrial cells: evidence for non-genomic actions involving cAMP turnover. J Cell Biochem 1996; 64:251–261.
5. Schimmer B, Parker K. Adrenocorticotropic hormone: adrenocortical steroids and their synthetic analogs: inhibitors of the synthesis and actions of adrenocortical hormones. In: Hardman J, Limbird L, eds. The pharmacological basis of therapeutics 9th ed. McGraw-Hill, New York, 1996, pp. 1459–1485.
6. Gravanis A, Schaison G, George M, Satyaswaroop P, Baulieu EE, Robel P. Endometrial and pituitary responses to the steroidal antiprogestin RU486 in post-menopausal women. J Clin Endocrinol Metab 1985; 60:156–163.
7. Kawal SL, Nieman L, Brandon D, Udelsman R, Loriaux DL, Chrousos GP. Pharmacokinetic properties of the antiglucocorticoid and antiprogestin steroid RU 486 in man. J Pharmacol Exp Ther 1987; 241:401–406.
8. Nieman L, Chrousos GP, Kellner C, Spitz IM, Nisula B, Cutler G, et al. Successful treatment of Cushing's syndrome with the glucocorticoid antagonist RU 486. J Clin Endocrinol Metab 1985; 61:536–540.
9. Philips A, Maira M, Mullick A, Chamberland M, Lesage S, Hugo P, Drouin J. Antagonism between Nur77 and glucocorticoid receptor for control of transcription. Mol Cell Biol 1997; 17:5952–5959.
10. Ray A, Prefontaine KE. Physical association and functional antagonism between the p65 subunit of transcription factor NF-kappa B and the glucocorticoid receptor. Proc Natl Acad Sci USA 1994; 91:752–756.
11. McKay LI, Cidlowski JA. Cross-talk between nuclear factor-kappa B and the steroid hormone receptors: mechanisms of mutual antagonism. Mol Endocrinol 1998; 12:45–56.
12. Ning YM, Sanchez ER. In vivo evidence for the generation of a glucocorticoid receptor-heat shock protein-90 complex incapable of binding hormone by the calmodulin antagonist phenoxybenzamine. Mol Endocrinol 1996; 10:14–23.
13. Rogatsky I, Logan SK, Garabedian MJ. Antagonism of glucocorticoid receptor transcriptional activation by the c-Jun N-terminal kinase. Proc Natl Acad Sci USA 1998; 95:2050–2055.
14. Caelles C, Gonzalez-Sancho JM, Munoz A. Nuclear hormone receptor antagonism with AP-1 by inhibition of the JNK pathway. Genes Dev Dec 1997; 11:3351–3364.

5 Glucocorticoid Catabolism and the 11β-Hydroxysteroid Dehydrogenase System

Jonathan R. Seckl

CONTENTS

INTRODUCTION

The adrenal cortex synthesizes and secretes steroid hormones including glucocorticoids (cortisol, corticosterone) and mineralocorticoids (aldosterone). These adrenocorticosteroids perform a broad range of metabolic and other functions underpinning many aspects of homeostasis and the response to stress *(1)*. Receptors for steroids are intracellular, located in the nucleus or cytoplasm, and are members of the nuclear hormone receptor superfamily of ligand-activated transcription factors. Corticosteroids are highly lipophilic compounds and thus readily enter cells to access their receptors that are of two types, mineralocorticoid receptors (MRs or type I receptors), and glucocorticoid receptors (GRs or type II receptors). GRs are expressed in most cells, whereas MRs show a distribution limited to aldosterone target tissues (distal nephron, colon, salivary gland) and a few nonaldosterone target sites, notably the heart and hippocampus *(2)*. However, in vivo, more functional receptor types can be distinguished than are accounted for by the products of the two known receptor genes. In particular, whereas MRs in the kidney selectively bind aldosterone, structurally identical MR in the hippocampus and heart are preferentially occupied by glucocorticoids in vivo. It was the investigation

From: *Contemporary Endocrinology: Adrenal Disorders*
Edited by: A. N. Margioris and G. P. Chrousos © Humana Press, Totowa, NJ

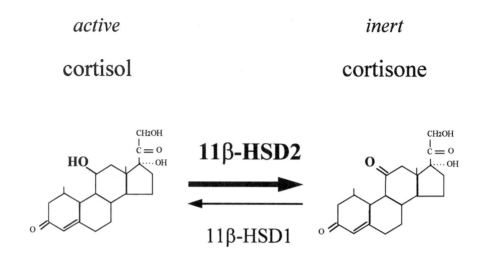

active   *inert*

cortisol   cortisone

Fig. 1. 3 line caption to come.

of this so-called "MR paradox" that first illuminated the role of 11β-hydroxysteroid dehydrogenase (11β-HSD) as a crucial determinant of glucocorticoid regulation at the cellular level.

THE MR PARADOX

In normal subjects the circulating levels of cortisol are 100- to 1000-fold higher than those of aldosterone, on a molar basis. Even allowing for the sequestration of up to 95% of cortisol by plasma proteins, notably corticosterone-binding globulin (CBG), "free" cortisol levels are at least 10-fold higher than those of aldosterone. Because purified or recombinant MRs bind cortisol, corticosterone, and aldosterone with similar high-affinity in vitro, it is not surprising that MRs in the hippocampus and heart are largely occupied by glucocorticoids in vivo. However, MRs in the distal nephron of the kidney and other aldosterone target tissues (salivary gland, sweat gland, colon) selectively bind aldosterone in vivo in spite of the high concentrations of cortisol. The solution to this apparent paradox was uncovered in 1988 by two separate groups in Edinburgh and in Melbourne and lies in the action of 11β-HSD type 2 *(3,4)*. This enzyme rapidly inactivates cortisol and corticosterone to their inert 11-keto derivatives, cortisone and 11-dehydrocorticosterone, which cannot bind MR (Fig. 1). Thus, only aldosterone, which is protected from 11β-HSD-2 by its *(11–18)* hemi-acetal bridge structure, is able to gain access to MR in cells coexpressing 11β-HSD-2. In patients with the rare syndrome of AME, 11β-HSD-2 activity is markedly reduced and cortisol is able illicitly to occupy and activate renal MR causing sodium retention, hypokalemia, and hypertension, a situation dubbed "Cushing's disease of the kidney" *(5)*. Similarly, when 11β-HSD inhibitors, such as licorice and its derivatives (glycyrrhetinic acid, glycyrrhizic acid, and carbenoxolone), are administered, they cause "apparent mineralo-corticoid excess," because of endogenous glucocorticoids occupying renal MR *(6)*. Definitive proof of this mechanism came with the recent identification of loss of function mutations in the 11β-*HSD-2* gene in patients with AME *(7)*. Thus, the exquisitely high affinity and exclusive 11β-dehydrogenase action of 11β-HSD-2 makes this enzyme uniquely suited to exclude cortisol from colocalized receptors. Subtle variations in AME phenotypes have been identified *(8)*, based largely upon the downstream patterns of metabolism of cortisol and cortisone, but mutations in the 11β-*HSD-2* gene may underlie both types of the syndrome.

11β-HSD-2 deficiency is also an obvious candidate mechanism for more common forms of hypertension than AME. In patients with essential hypertension, some data suggest increased urinary cortisol to cortisone metabolites *(9)* and prolongation of the half-life of 11[^{3}H]cortisol occurs in a subgroup *(10)*, but others have not replicated these results *(11)*. Linkage to the 11β-HSD-2 locus on 16q22.1 has been reported in one population with hypertensive renal disease *(12)*, but confirmation in other hypertensive populations has yet to be documented. Thus, the role, if any, of 11β-HSDs, in essential hypertension remains unresolved.

11β-HSD-2 IN THE FETUS AND PLACENTA

It should be noted, however, that some clinical features of patients with AME are not fully explained only by the loss of 11β-HSD-2 activity in aldosterone target tissues. These include apparent deficiency of 5β-reductase, bone abnormalities, and low birth-weight. The first may correlate with the documented defects in 11β-HSD-2 in aldosterone target organs such as kidney *(11)*, and the bony effects may reflect chronic hypokalemia. However, birth weight reductions occurs before renal function takes precedence over placental excretion.

11β-HSD-2 is also highly expressed in the placenta *(13)*, as well as in many fetal tissues until midgestation *(14,15)*. Whereas the function of the enzyme in these sites is less clear (MRs are hardly expressed until very late in gestation in the fetus and barely, if at all, in placenta), it has been hypothesized that 11β-HSD-2 protects fetal GR-bearing cells from potential deleterious effects of the high levels of glucocorticoids (of maternal or fetal origin) *(13)*. The placenta has been suggested to act as a "barrier" to maternal glucocorticoids in many mammalian species, producing a low glucocorticoid environment for the fetus, with the majority of fetal glucocorticoids emanating from its own adrenal glands until term *(16)*. Direct evidence for such a placental "barrier" role for 11β-HSD-2 has recently been presented in humans *(17)*. However, the biological importance of this phenomenon has not been fully elucidated. One intriguing notion is that the feto-placental barrier to glucocorticoids may attenuate glucocorticoid access to placental and, indeed, fetal GR. Excessive exposure of the fetus to glucocorticoids is known to reduce birthweight and alter the maturation rates of a variety of organs *(18)*. This is, of course, exploited therapeutically to accelerate the maturation of the lung and gastrointestinal system when premature delivery is threatened, but other organs (brain, kidney) may not be so beneficially affected by glucocorticoids. In rats, placental 11β-HSD activity correlates with late gestation fetal weight *(19)*. Recent studies suggest that if pregnant rats are given dexamethasone, a synthetic glucocorticoid that is a poor substrate for 11β-HSD-2, or the enzyme inhibitor, carbenoxolone, the offspring show reduced birthweight and exhibit permanent elevations of blood pressure, blood glucose, and plasma glucocorticoid levels throughout the life-span. These results suggest that feto-placental 11β-HSD-2 may modulate glucocorticoid-mediated fetal "programming"

(20,21), most notably in the last trimester of pregnancy *(22).* Key target mechanisms of prenatal programming of adult hyperglycemia, including the role of induction of phosphoenolpyruvate carboxykinase in the liver, the rate-limiting enzyme in hepatic gluconeogenesis, have been advocated by studies in rodents *(22,23)* and would accord with observations of increased fasting gluconeogenesis in humans with noninsulin-dependent diabetes mellitus. Interest in such programming phenomena has recently been stimulated by human epidemiological studies associating lower, but still normal birthweights with a substantially increased risk of cardiovascular and metabolic disorders, including hypertension and noninsulin-dependent diabetes mellitus, in subsequent adult life *(24,25).* Indeed, some evidence suggest that placental 11β-HSD-2 activity correlates with birthweight in humans *(26),* although other studies have not supported this notion *(11).* The source of the glucocorticoid excess (fetal or maternal) and the location and degree of 11β-HSD-2 inhibition required for these effects have yet to be established.

11β-HSD-1

Whereas the biological functions of 11β-HSD-2 are increasingly well recognized, at least in aldosterone target tissues, the role of the more widely expressed 11β-HSD-1 isozyme is less understood. This not only reflects the potential for metabolism of substrates other than corticosteroids, because the enzyme also functions as a carbonyl reductase of xenobiotics, including important carcinogens *(27,28),* but also the uncertainty over the predominant reaction direction of this isozyme. However, recent studies in *intact* cells and whole organs, suggest the enzyme is a predominant 11β-reductase *(29–31).* Crucially, mice bearing targeted disruption of the 11β-*HSD-1* gene are unable to regenerate corticosterone from inert 11-dehydrocorticosterone *(32),* suggesting this isozyme is the sole enzyme responsible for the regeneration of cortisol from inert cortisone.

So what might be the function of 11β-HSD reductase? Recently, it has been hypothesized that this might amplify glucocorticoid action within particular target cells to maintain basal metabolic function in the face of the diurnal nadir of glucocorticoid secretion and to potentiate adaptive responses to stress *(33,34).* Certainly, plentiful 11-keto substrates circulate in humans and rodents, with levels of cortisone (11-dehydrocorticosterone) of around 50–100 n*M,* most of which is available for conversion by 11β-HSD-1 into active forms as 11-keto steroids are poorly bound by CBG. Recently, a series of studies have suggested that such glucocorticoid amplification might be of physiological importance. 11β-HSD inhibitors attenuate glucocorticoid actions such as antagonism of insulin sensitivity and promotion of gluconeogenesis, both in experimental animals and humans *(34).* Indeed, the 11β-HSD-1 null mouse appears to be deficient in hepatic gluconeogenic responses and, presumably in consequence, resists hyperglycemia on stress and with obesity *(32).* Similarly, the enzyme has been proposed to amplify glucocorticoid action in fat *(35)* and may potentiate neurotoxicity in the brain *(33).* The details of these processes need to be defined further, not only in animal models, but also at the crucial level of human biology and disease, including patients with noninsulin-dependent diabetes mellitus, centripetal obesity, and neurodegenerative disorders.

Occasional clinical cases of possible 11β-HSD-1 reductase deficiency have been reported *(36)*. Although these individuals manifest appropriate clinical signs and bio-chemistry for hepatic 11β-reductase deficiency (ACTH-stimulated hypercortisolism—presumed to compensate for lack of hepatic regeneration of cortisone to cortisol—without features of Cushing's syndrome, hirsutism, and acne owing to concomitant ACTH driven excess of adrenal androgen secretion, reduced urinary cortisol to cortisone metabolites), final proof of the phenotype and documentation of mutations in the 11β-*HSD-1* gene have yet to be presented. Whether this reflects the difficulties of defining the precise biochemical phenotype or the presence of an alternative 11β-reductase gene in humans, but not mice, remains unresolved. There is clearly a requirement for the development of selective 11β-HSD-1 reductase inhibitors. These will allow determina-tion of 11β-HSD-1 in glucocorticoid and xenobiotic physiology in humans. Moreover, such agents may be efficacious in patients with noninsulin-dependent diabetes mellitus, obesity, and neurodegenerative disorders associated with hypercortisolism, presenting an exciting area for future study.

REGULATION OF 11β-HSDs

Considerable data address the control of 11β-HSDs *(11,37)*. The 11β-*HSD-1* gene promoter has been isolated *(38)*. Several tissue-specific transcriptional start sites have been described, although only the major (liver) promoter can encode clearly active translated products. A promoter in intron 1 is used in kidney and encodes a truncated and apparently inactive form (11β-HSD-1B) *(39)*. The 11β-*HSD-1* gene shows tissue-specific regulation by glucocorticoids, sex steroids, insulin, and many other endocrine factors. The effects of sex steroids are, in part, mediated by actions upon the sex-specific patterns of growth-hormone secretion. Both glucocorticoids and insulin appear directly to influence 11β-*HSD-1* gene transcription *(40)*, effects that are, in part, mediated via the C/EBP family of transcription factors *(41)*. 11β-*HSD-2* gene expression is also regulated. During midgestational development, there is widespread loss of 11β-HSD-2 mRNA expression and activity in many fetal tissues, whereas dramatic upregulation occurs in the rodent corpus luteum and to a lesser degree in the primate placenta near term *(42,43)*. Initial study of the 11β-HSD-2 promoter has been reported *(44)*, but detailed analysis of the molecular mechanisms involved remains to be undertaken.

TISSUE FUNCTIONS

Comprehensive analysis of the tissue-specific functions of the 11β-HSD system has been addressed above (11β-HSD-1 in liver and fat; 11β-HSD-2 in kidney and placenta) and elsewhere *(11,37,45)*. Selected additional putative actions are outlined below to illustrate the broad applications of the enzyme system to physiology and disease and to underline some lacunae in our current knowledge and understanding.

Brain

Glucocorticoids have myriad actions in the central nervous system (CNS), including effects upon neurotransmission, behavior, and neuronal birth and survival. 11β-HSD-1 is widely expressed in neurons and appears to function in the 11β-reductase direction *(33)*. This amplifies glucocorticoid action and promotes the neurotoxicity of glucocorticoid excess, at least in vitro. Whether such activity contributes to neuropathologies associated with hypercortisolemia (e.g., depression, Alzheimer's disease, and other age-related cognitive dysfunction) remains an intriguing, but unexplored point. Aldosterone also exerts selective central effects (not mimicked by glucocorticoids) upon blood pressure and salt appetite. Intriguingly, central administration of 11β-HSD inhibitors, using doses that are ineffective when given peripherally, also produces hypertension *(46)*, suggesting an aldosterone-selective MR system exists in the brain. 11β-HSD-2 mRNA expression has been localized in a few specific regions of the rat CNS *(47)*, notably around the cerebral ventricles in areas putatively associated with the control of sodium homeostasis (subcommissural organ) and cardiovascular regulation (nucleus tractus solitarius). Although colocalization with MR has not been reported, these loci are reasonable candidates to mediate the selective central actions of aldosterone.

Immune Systems

Lymphocytes express 11β-HSD that appears to be a dehydrogenase *(48)*. Inhibition of enzyme activity reduces type 1 and increases type 2 cytokine production by activated T cells. Perhaps, in consequence, 11β-HSD inhibitors attenuate rodent contact hypersensitivity responses and increase host susceptibility to pathogens, such as Listeria monocytogenes in vivo *(48,49)*. Patients with active tuberculosis, but not those with treated TB or other respiratory disorders, show an increased ratio of urinary cortisol metabolites, suggesting either loss of 11β-HSD-2 or gain of 11β-HSD-1 activity *(50)*. The former seems more likely and may fit with local glucocorticoid excess mediated attenuation of host responses, with potential advantages for pathogen survival. However, the 11β-HSD isozyme(s) and the reaction direction(s) involved in each specific cell type in the relevant lymphoid and other target organs, have yet to be defined. Such data are crucial for any sensible interpretation of these intriguing findings.

Gonads

11β-HSD activity has been localized to ovary and testis. In humans, 11β-dehydrogenase has been reported to predominate in granulosa cells in culture and associates (negatively) with success in in vitro fertilization *(51)*. More recent data, however, suggest complex tissue and time-specific changes in both isozymes in granulosa cells, with nonluteinized granulosa cells expressing high levels of 11β-HSD-2 mRNA, but not 11β-HSD-1. Conversely, luteinizing granulosa cells abundantly express 11β-HSD-1, but not 11β-HSD-2 *(52)*. Neither isozyme is detectable in the ovarian stroma. The implications are for a low glucocorticoid environment prior to ovulation, but high glucocorticoid levels after follicular rupture. The role of such elevated local glucocorticoid levels in attenuating inflammatory responses to the tissue breakdown at ovulation has been advocated. In the testis, matters are less clear-cut. Rat and human Leydig cells highly express 11β-HSD-1 (but not 11β-HSD-2), which correlates directly with reproductive competence in rats. It has been proposed that such 11β-HSD actively prevents glucocorticoid inhibition of testosterone production, by catalyzing effective dehydrogenation, analogous to the actions of 11β-HSD-2 in the distal nephron *(53)*. However, this notion does not conform with the low affinity of 11β-HSD-1 for glucocorticoids, nor with the predominant reductive direction of 11β-HSD-1 in most intact cells and organs, nor with the apparently normal fertility of 11β-HSD-1 null mice, though even wild-type mice lack 11β-HSD-1 expression in the testis.

OTHER TISSUES

Roles for 11β-HSD-1 have been proposed in modulating glucocorticoid effects upon lung maturation and inflammation *(30,54)*, in hypothalamic-pituitary function *(33)*, in vascular tone *(55)*, and in adipose cell biology *(35)*. Many are, as yet, ill-defined, and are the subject of intense research and interest. The notion that intracellular glucocorticoid concentrations are determined more by "intracrine" regeneration of glucocorticoids from inert circulating 11-keto forms than by active cortisol in the circulation is intriguing. This idea has been lent substantial support by the phenotype of the 11β-HSD-1 knockout mouse *(32)*, which exhibits apparently deficient glucocorticoid-associated metabolic processes in its liver in the face of mildly elevated plasma levels of active glucocorticoids, themselves presumably a result of deficient 11β-reductase amplification of the negative feedback signal in the pituitary, hypothalamus, and hippocampus.

CLINICAL INVESTIGATION

Study of patients suspected to have disorders of cortisol metabolism has advanced with the development of gas chromatography with mass spectrometry methodologies in recent years, permitting precise detailing of the urinary concentrations of all the major metabolites of cortisol *(56)* with 11β-HSD deficiencies defined by altered ratios of cortisol to cortisone metabolites in the urine. Conventional assessment has examined the ratios of conjugated cortisol and cortisone metabolites. However, these do not permit distinction between the tissue-specific activities of the enzymes and do not reflect all forms of 11β-HSD deficiency, such as abnormalities of 11β-HSD activity in the liver *(57)*. Other tests include measurements of the ratio of cortisol to cortisone in blood, which is rather imprecise, determination of the metabolism of cortisol labeled at the 11-position with tritium in vivo, which examines 11β-HSD-2 dehydrogenation, but not reduction and involves infusion of radioactive tracers, and by the oral administration of cortisone with measurement of the consequent rise in plasma cortisol, which tests 11β-reductase albeit at "first-pass" not steady state. Recent advances include the recognition that urinary "free" or unconjugated cortisol to cortisone ratios are a good measure of renal 11β-HSD-2 activity *(57)*, whereas urinary tetrahydrocortisol, allo-tetrahydrocortisol, and tetrahydrocortisone derivatives may be more a reflection of liver metabolism by 5a- and 5β-reductases and 11β-HSD-1. Complications of analyses, such as sex differences in such indices and even seasonal variation suggesting increased cortisol metabolism by 11β-HSD-1 in the liver in winter *(58)*, are becoming recognized, and clearly the interpretation of urinary steroid tests should be undertaken with some care.

THE BROADER PERSPECTIVE

The roles of the 11β-HSDs to modulate glucocorticoid access to intracellular receptors at a cell-specific level is not exceptional, but appears to be more the rule for the steroid-thyroid hormone nuclear hormone receptor superfamily. For example, monodeiodinase isozymes "upstream" of thyroid hormone receptors may either activate or terminally inactivate the "prohormone" thyroxine to T3 or reverse T3, respectively, thus determining receptor activation. Similarly, aromatase and 5-alpha-reductase provide site-specific activation of sex steroids for estrogen and androgen receptors in a variety of tissues.

Thus the 11β-HSDs (type 1 amplifying glucocorticoid action, type 2 inactivating gluco-corticoids in aldosterone-specific tissues) illustrate a broader biological principle of prereceptor metabolism, which increases the complexity of tissue-specific control of steroid action in complex organisms. Key future directions must include the understanding of the role of 11β-HSD-2 in fetus and placenta and the biological importance of 11β-HSD-1 in corticosteroid and xenobiotic metabolism. This evolving area of endeavour clearly shows considerable promise for understanding of pathogenesis and the development of novel therapies.

ACKNOWLEDGEMENTS

Work in the author's laboratory is generously funded by a Wellcome Trust Programme grant, a Wellcome Trust Senior Research Fellowship (JRS), and grants from the Wellcome Trust, Medical Research Council, and the Scottish Hospital Endowments Research Trust.

REFERENCES

1. Miller WL, Tyrrell JB. The adrenal cortex. In: Endocrinology and Metabolism, 3rd ed., 1995, pp. 555–711.
2. Evans RM. The steroid and thyroid hormone receptor superfamily. Science 1988; 240:889–895.
3. Edwards CRW, Stewart PM, Burt D, Brett L, McIntyre MA, Sutanto WS, et al. Localization of 11β-hydroxysteroid dehydrogenase-tissue specific protector of the mineralocorticoid receptor. Lancet 1988; ii:986–989.
4. Funder JW, Pearce PT, Smith R, Smith AI. Mineralocorticoid action: target tissue specificity is enzyme, not receptor, mediated. Science 1988; 242:583–585.
5. Stewart PM, Corrie JET, Shackleton CHL, Edwards CW. Syndrome of apparent mineralocorticoid excess: a defect in the cortisol-cortisone shuttle. J Clin Invest 1988; 82:340–349.
6. Stewart PM, Valentino R, Wallace AM, Burt D, Shackleton CHL, Edwards CRW. Mineralocorticoid activity of liquorice: 11β-hydroxysteroid dehydrogenase deficiency comes of age. Lancet ii:821–824.
7. Mune T, Rogerson FM, Nikkilä H, Agarwal AK, White PC. Human hypertension caused by mutations in the kidney isozyme of 11β-hydroxysteroid dehydrogenase. Nature Genet 1995; 10:394–399.
8. Mantero F, Tedde R, Opocher G, Fulgheri PD, Arnaldi G, Ulick S. Apparent mineralocorticoid excess type-Ii. Steroids 1994; 59:80–83.
9. Soro A, Ingram MC, Tonolo G, Glorioso N, Fraser R. Evidence of coexisting changes in 11beta-hydroxysteroid dehydrogenase and 5beta-reductase activity in subjects with untreated essential hypertension. Hypertension 1995; 25:67–70.
10. Walker BR, Stewart PM, Shackleton CHL, Padfield PL, Edwards CRW. Deficient inactivation of cortisol by 11β-hydroxysteroid dehydrogenase in essential hypertension. Clin Endocrinol 1993; 38:221–227.
11. White PC, Mune T, Agarwal AK. 11beta-Hydroxysteroid dehydrogenase and the syndrome of apparent mineralocorticoid excess. Endocrine Rev 1997; 18:135–156.
12. Watson B, Jr., Bergman SM, Myracle A, Callen DF, Acton RT, Warnock DG. Genetic association of 11beta-hydroxysteroid dehydrogenase type 2 (HSD11B2) flanking microsatellites with essential hypertension in blacks. Hypertension 1996; 28:478–482.
13. Murphy BEP, Clark SJ, Donald IR, Pinsky M, Vedady DL. Conversion of maternal cortisol to cortisone during placental transfer to the human fetus. Am J Obstet Gynecol 1974; 118:538–541.
14. Stewart PM, Murry BA, Mason JI. Type 2 11β-hydroxysteroid dehydrogenase in human fetal tissues. J Clin Endocrinol Metab 1994; 78:1529–1532.
15. Brown RW, Diaz R, Robson AC, Kotelevtsev Y, Mullins JJ, Kaufman MH, et al. The ontogeny of 11β-hydroxysteroid dehydrogenase type 2 and mineralocorticoid receptor gene expression reveal intricate control of glucocorticoid action in development. Endocrinology 1996; 137:794–797.
16. Beitens IZ, Bayard F, Ances IG, Kowarski A, Migeon CJ. The metabolic clearance rate, blood

production, interconversion and transplacental passage of cortisol and cortisone in pregnancy near term. Pediatr Rers 1973; 7:509–519.

17. Benediktsson R, Calder AA, Edwards CRW, Seckl JR. Placental 11β-hydroxysteroid dehydrogenase type 2 is the placental barrier to maternal glucocorticoids: ex vivo studies. Clin Endocrinol 1997; 46:161–166.

18. Seckl JR. Glucocorticoids, feto-placental 11beta-hydroxysteroid dehydrogenase type 2 and the early life origins of adult disease. Steroids 1997; 62:89–94.

19. Benediktsson R, Lindsay R, Noble J, Seckl JR, Edwards CRW. Glucocorticoid exposure in utero: a new model for adult hypertension. Lancet 1993; 341:339–341.

20. Lindsay RS, Lindsay RM, Edwards CRW, Seckl JR. Inhibition of 11β-hydroxysteroid dehydrogenase in pregnant rats and the programming of blood pressure in the offspring. Hypertension 1996; 27:1200–1204.

21. Lindsay RS, Lindsay RM, Waddell B, Seckl JR. Programming of glucose tolerance in the rat: role of placental 11β-hydroxysteroid dehydrogenase. Diabetologia 1996; 39:1299–1305.

22. Nyirenda MJ, Lindsay RS, Kenyon CJ, Burchell A, Seckl JR. Glucocorticoid exposure in late gestation permanently programs rat hepatic phosphoenolpyruvate carboxykinase and glucocorticoid receptor expression and causes glucose intolerance in adult offspring. J Clin Invest 1998; 101:2174–2181.

23. Desai M, Byrne CD, Zhang JL, Petry CJ, Lucas A, Hales CN. Programming of hepatic insulin-sensitive enzymes in offspring of rat dams fed a protein-restricted diet. Am Physiol Gastrointest Liver Physiol 1997; 35:G1083–G1090.

24. Barker DJP. Mothers, babies and disease in later life. 1994; 180.

25. Curhan GC, Chertow GM, Willett WC, Spiegelman D, Colditz GA, Manson JE, et al. Birth weight and adult hypertension and obesity in women. Circulation 1996; 94:1310–1315.

26. Stewart PM, Rogerson FM, Mason JI. Type 2 11β-hydroxysteroid dehydrogenase messenger RNA and activity in human placenta and fetal membranes: its relationship to birth weight and putative role in fetal steroidogenesis. J Clin Endocrinol Metab 1995; 80:885–890.

27. Maser E, Richter E, Friebertshauser J. The identification of 11-beta-hydroxysteroid dehydrogenase as carbonyl reductase of the tobacco-specific nitrosamine 4-(Methylnitrosamino)-1-(3-Pyridyl)-1-buta-none. Europ J Biochem 1996; 238:484–489.

28. Maser E. Stress, hormonal changes, alcohol, food constituents and drugs: Factors that advance the incidence of tobacco smoke-related cancer? Trends in Pharmacolog Sci 1997; 18:270–275.

29. Jamieson PM, Chapman KE, Edwards CRW, Seckl JR. 11β-hydroxysteroid dehydrogenase is an exclusive 11β-reductase in primary cultured rat hepatocytes: effect of physicochemical and hormonal manipulations. Endocrinology 1995; 136:4754–4761.

30. Hundertmark S, Buhler H, Ragosch V, Dinkelborg L, Arabin B, Weitzel HK. Correlation of surfactant phosphatidylcholine synthesis and 11beta-hydroxysteroid dehydrogenase in the fetal lung. Endocrinology 1995; 136:2573–2578.

31. Jamieson PM, Walker BR, Chapman KE, Seckl JR. 11β-hydroxysteroid dehydrogenase type 1 is a predominant reductase in the intact perfused rat liver. J Endocrinol 2000; 165:685–692.

32. Kotelevtsev Y, Holmes MC, Burchell A, Houston PM, Schmoll D, Jamieson PM, et al. 11β-hydroxysteroid dehydrogenase type 1 knockout mice show attenuated glucocorticoid inducible responses and resist hyperglycaemia on obesity or stress. Proc Natl Acad Sci USA 1997; 94:14,924–24,929.

33. Seckl JR. 11β-hydroxysteroid dehydrogenase in the brain: a novel regulator of glucocorticoid action? Front Neuroendocrinol 1997; 18:49–99.

34. Walker BR, Connacher AA, Lindsay RM, Webb DJ, Edwards CRW. Carbenoxolone increases hepatic insulin sensitivity in man: a novel role for 11-oxosteroid reductase in enhancing glucocorticoid receptor activation. J Clin Endocrinol Metab 1995; 80:3155–3159.

35. Bujalska I, Kumar S, Stewart PM. Central obesity: "Cushing's disease of the omentum." Lancet 1997; 349:1210–1213.

36. Phillipov G, Palermo M, Shackleton CHL. Apparent cortisone reductase deficiency: a unique form of hypercortisolism. J Clin Endocrinol Metab 1996; 81:3855–3860.

37. Seckl JR. 11β-hydroxysteroid dehydrogenase isoforms and their implications for blood pressure regulation. Europ J Clin Invest 1993; 23:589–601.

38. Moisan M-P, Edwards CRW, Seckl JR. Differential promoter usage by the rat 11β-hydroxysteroid dehydrogenase gene. Molec Endocrinol 1992; 1082–1087.

39. Obeid J, Curnow KM, Aisenberg J, White PC. Transcripts originating in intron 1 of the HSD11 (11β-

hydroxysteroid dehydrogenase) gene encode a truncated polypeptide that is enzymatically inactive. Molec Endocrinol 1993; 7:154–160.

40. Voice M, Seckl JR, Edwards CRW, Chapman KE. 11β-hydroxysteroid dehydrogenase type 1 expression in 2S-FAZA hepatoma cells is hormonally-regulated: a model for the study of hepatic corticosteroid metabolism. Biochem J 1996; 317:621–625.

41. Chapman KE, Kotelevstev YV, Jamieson PM, Williams LJS, Mullins JJ, Seckl JR. Tissue-specific modulation of glucocorticoid action by the 11β-hydroxysteroid dehydrogenases. Biochem Soc Trans, 1997; 25:583–587.

42. Waddell B, Benediktsson R, Seckl JR. 11β-hydroxysteroid dehydrogenase type 2 in the rat corpus luteum: induction of mRNA expression and bioactivity coincident with luteal regression. Endocrinology 1996; 137:5386–5391.

43. Pepe GJ, Babischkin JS, Burch MG, Leavitt MG, Albrecht ED. Developmental increase in expression of the messenger ribonucleic acid and protein levels of 11beta-hydroxysteroid dehydrogenase types 1 and 2 in the baboon placenta. Endocrinology 1996; 137:5678–5684.

44. Agarwal AK, White PC. Analysis of the promoter of the NAD + dependent 11beta-hydroxysteroid dehydrogenase (HSD11K) gene in JEG-3 human choriocarcinoma cells. Mol Cell Endocrinol 1996; 121:93–99.

45. Monder C, White PC. 11β-hydroxysteroid dehydrogenase. Vitam Horm 1993; 47:187–271.

46. Gomez-Sanchez EP, Gomez-Sanchez CE. Central hypertensinogenic effects of glycyrrhizic acid and carbenoxolone. Am J Physiol 1992; 263:E1125–E1130.

47. Roland BL, Li KXZ, Funder JW. Hybridization histochemical localization of 11β-hydroxysteroid dehydrogenase type 2 in rat brain. Endocrinol 1995; 136:4697–4700.

48. Hennebold JD, Ryu SY, Mu HH, Galbraith A, Daynes RA. 11β-Hydroxysteroid dehydrogenase modulation of glucocorticoid activities in lymphoid organs. Am J Physiol—Regul Integrat Compar Physiol 1996; 270:R1296–R1306.

49. Hennebold JD, Mu HH, Poynter ME, Chen XP, Daynes RA. Active catabolism of glucocorticoids by 11beta-hydroxysteroid dehydrogenase in vivo is a necessary requirement for natural resistance to infection with Listeria monocytogenes. Int Immunol 1997; 9:105–115.

50. Baker RW, Zumla A, Rook GAW. Tuberculosis, steroid metabolism and immunity. QJM—Month Assoc Phys 1996; 89:387–394.

51. Michael AE, Gregory L, Walker SM, Antoniw JW, Shaw RW, Edwards CRW, et al. Ovarian 11β-hydroxysteroid dehydrogenase: potential predictor of conception by in vitro fertilization and embryo transfer. Lancet 1993; 342:711–712.

52. Tetsuka M, Thomas FJ, Thomas MJ, Anderson RA, Mason JI, Hillier SG. Differential expression of messenger ribonucleic acids encoding 11 beta-hydroxysteroid dehydrogenase types 1 and 2 in human granulosa cells. J Clin Endocrinol Metab 1997; 82:2006–2009.

53. Monder C, Miroff Y, Marandici A, Hardy MP. 11β-hydroxysteroid dehydrogenase alleviates glucocorticoid-mediated inhibition of steroidogenesis in rat Leydig cells. Endocrinol 1994; 134:1199–1204.

54. Rook GAW, HernandezPando R. Pathogenetic role, in human and murine tuberculosis, of changes in the peripheral metabolism of glucocorticoids and antiglucocorticoids. Psychoneuroendocrinology 1997; 22:S109–S113.

55. Walker BR, Williams BC. Corticosteroids and vascular tone: mapping the messenger maze. Clin Sci 1992; 82:597–605.

56. Walker BR, Best R. Clinical investigation of 11beta-hydroxysteroid dehydrogenase. Endocr Res 1995; 21:379–387.

57. Best R, Walker BR. Additional value of measurement of urinary cortisone and unconjugated cortisol metabolites in assessing the activity of 11 beta-hydroxysteroid dehydrogenase in vivo. Clin Endocrinol 1997; 47:231–236.

58. Walker BR, Best R, Noon JP, Watt GCM, Webb DJ. Seasonal variation in glucocorticoid activity in healthy men. J Clin Endocrinol Metab 1997; 82:4015–4019.

6   Androgens of Adrenal Origin

George Mastorakos and Anthony G. Doufas

CONTENTS

INTRODUCTION

The adrenal androgens (AAs), normally secreted by the fetal adrenal zone or the *zona reticularis*, are steroid hormones with weak androgen activity. Although AAs do not appear to play a major role in the fully androgenized adult man, they seem to play a role in the adult woman and in both sexes before puberty. Girls, women, and prepubertal boys may be negatively affected by AA hypersecretion in contrast to adult men. This chapter reviews the role and effects of AAs and analyzes the clinical significance of their hypersecretion during different stages of life in both sexes.

ANATOMY AND PHYSIOLOGY

Adrenal Anatomy

The adrenal glands, consisting of the cortex and medulla, are pyramidal in shape and juxtaposed to the upper poles of the kidneys. They receive their blood supply through the superior, middle, and inferior adrenal arteries, which, respectively, start from the phrenic arteries, aorta, and renal arteries and enter the adrenals through the cortices. Venus drainage takes place through a large central vein located in the medulla. The central vein of the left adrenal empties into the left renal vein and that of the right adrenal into the inferior vena cava. The adrenal cortex is divided into three histologic and functional zones: the outer, aldosterone-secreting *zona glomerulosa*; the intermediate, cortisol-secreting *zona fasciculata*; and the inner, androgen-secreting *zona reticularis*. Whereas the *zona glomerulosa* is primarily regulated by angiotensin II, both the *zona*

From: *Contemporary Endocrinology: Adrenal Disorders*
Edited by: A. N. Margioris and G. P. Chrousos © Humana Press, Totowa, NJ

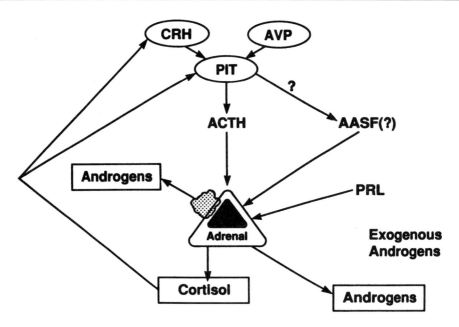

Fig. 1. Schematic description of the causes of adrenal androgen hypersecretion. Exposure to exogenous androgens is included.

fasciculata and the *zona reticularis* are regulated by corticotropin (Fig. 1) *(1)*. Indeed, both of these zones hypofunction and atrophy when corticotropin is deficient, whereas they hyperfunction and become hypertrophic and hyperplastic when corticotropin is in excess.

In the fetus, the adrenal cortices consist of the two adult adrenal *zonae glomerulosa* and *fasciculata* and an inner large fetal adrenal zone, which virtually disappears within weeks after birth *(2)*. Remaining cell foci from the fetal adrenal zone presumably give rise to the adrenal *zona reticularis* starting at the age of 4 to 5 yr in both sexes *(3)*. The growth of this zone continues until young adulthood (20 to 25 yr), remains at a plateau for 5 to 10 yr, and regresses gradually after the age of 35 yr. It seems that although there is no significant difference in the total width of the cortex in young compared to older men, aging results in alterations within the cortex of the adrenals in men. More specifically, there is a reduction in the size of the *zona reticularis* and a relative increase in the outer cortical zones *(4)*. These anatomical alterations are followed by a marked decline in circulating adrenal C19 steroids and their resulting androgen metabolites, which takes place mainly between the age groups of 20–30- and 50–60-yr olds, with smaller changes observed after age 60 *(5)*.

Adrenal Androgen Physiology

Regulation

Cotricotropin is a 39-amino-acid peptide synthesized and secreted by the anterior pituitary (Fig. 1). It is derived from proopiomelanocortin (POMC), a large precursor molecule from which β-lipotropic hormone and/or β-endorphin are also derived *(6,7)*. Corticotropin (1-39) is the predominant form of corticotropin in plasma and has a half-life of approx 10 min *(8)*. Corticotropin synthesis and secretion are primarily regulated

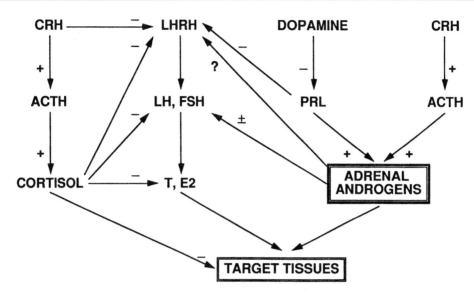

Fig. 2. Interactions among the hypothalamic-pituitary-adrenal axis, the PRL axis, and the reproductive axis. Abbreviations: LHRH, luteinizing hormone-releasing hormone; FSH, follicle-stimulating hormone; T, testosterone; E_2, estradiol-17β.

by corticotropin-releasing hormone (CRH) and arginine-vasopressin (AVP), both of which are produced by parvocellular neurons of the paraventricular nucleus of the hypothalamus and act in synergy with each other (Fig. 1) *(9,10)*. Corticotropin-stimulated cortisol exerts major feedback inhibitory influences at the level of both the hypothalamus and the anterior pituitary by suppressing CRH, AVP, and corticotropin synthesis and secretion. Because corticotropin is secreted in a pulsatile circadian and stress-responsive function, the AAs, like cortisol, generally have secretory patterns that follow those of corticotropin *(11,12)*. Rossi et al. showed that the canonic androgen receptor is present in human adrenocortical cells and that androgens may have a role in the adrenal cortex by reducing cell proliferation *(13)*. Furthermore, interleukin 6 (IL-6) and IL-6 receptor are expressed in adrenal cell cultures and IL-6 seems to regulate the adrenal synthesis of mineralocorticoids, glucocorticoids, and androgens. Thus, IL-6 exerts its acute action via the hypothalamus and the pituitary, being the major known stimulator of the HPA axis *(14,15)*. In the adrenal gland, it seems to be a long-term regulator of stress response, integrating the responses of all cortical zones to stimuli from the immune and endocrine system *(16)*. Interestingly, during acute psychological stress, stimulation of adrenal steroid release is accompanied by a shift toward DHEA. Augmentation of this effect by beta-adrenoceptor blockade indicates a beta-adrenoceptor-dependent mechanism affecting DHEA release *(17)*.

Both corticotropin and prolactin (PRL) stimulate AA secretion by the fetal adrenal zone (Fig. 2), but an as-yet-undefined placental factor appears to play a major role in sustaining this zone and in stimulating androgen secretion, together with corticotropin and/or PRL. Placental CRH production, which rises exponentially during human pregnancy, may play a key role in promoting dehydroepiandrosterone sulfate (DHEAS) production by the fetal adrenals, which could lead to increasing placental estrogen synthesis and contribute to the process of parturition in humans *(18)*. Glasow et al.

have found the PRL receptor in the human adrenal gland and suggested that PRL has a direct effect on adrenal steroidogenesis, thereby regulating adrenal function, which may be of particular relevance in clinical disorders with hyperprolactinemia *(19)*. Interestingly, adults with hyperprolactinemia have increased secretion of AAs by the *zona reticularis*, which is corrected by reduction of PRL secretion with bromocriptine *(20)*.

AAs are secreted in small amounts during infancy and early childhood, and their secretion gradually increases with age, paralleling the growth of the *zona reticularis*. The appearance of a slight amount of pubic hair as a result of AA rise has been called pubarche or adrenarche *(21)*. The mechanism(s) by which the *zona reticularis* develops with age and the regulation of adrenarche are not known. A programmed shift in production of intra-adrenal regulatory factors associated with differentiation of adrenal cells and changes in steroid biosynthesis might also take place independent of circulating factors. Recent findings by Gell et al. suggest that as children mature there is a decrease of 3β-hydroxysteroid dehydrogenase in the adrenal reticularis that may contribute to the increased production of DHEA and DHEAS seen during adrenarche by shifting pregnenolone through the 17α-hydroxylase/17, 20 lyase *(22)*. Recently, it has been shown that activation of the type 1 insulin-like growth factor (IGF) receptor increases ACTH responsiveness in fetal zone cells by modulating ACTH signal transduction. Also, locally produced IGF-2 modulates fetal adrenocortical cells function by increasing responsiveness to ACTH and possibly augmenting the potential for AA synthesis. Thus, the activation of type 1 IGF receptor on adrenal cortical cells may also play a pivotal role in AA production, both physiologically *in utero* and at adrenarche, and in pathophysiological conditions of hyperandrogenemia, such as the polycystic ovary syndrome *(23)*. The different steroidogenic potency of IGF-1 and IGF-2 might be explained by interaction of these ligands with locally produced IGF-binding proteins. These data indicate that the IGF system plays an important role in the regulation of the differential function of adult human adrenocortical cells *(24)*. During adrenarche, plasma concentrations of the AAs increase, whereas those of cortisol remain stable, suggesting that factors other than corticotropin are involved. However, recent findings imply a significant contribution of ACTH to the regulation of adrenarche in normal children either by having a priming effect on the adrenal gland or by acting in concert with other adrenal androgen stimulating factors *(25)*. Recent data suggest that the influence of sex and age is minor in the modulation of adrenal steroidogenesis and support the concept that extra-adrenal factors dominate the differential modulation of AAs and cortisol *(26)*. These may include POMC-derived peptides and an elusive adrenal androgen-stimulating factor (Fig. 1), *(27–32)*. Also, high-dose sex-steroid administration had marked effects on adrenal androgens levels, which decreased by 27–48% in males treated with ethinyloestradiol and increased by 23–70% in females treated with testosterone *(33)*. It is unlikely that the hypoestrogenism of menopause contributes to the decline of AAs noted with age. Furthermore, menopausal estrogen replacement, at least in physiological amounts administered transdermally, cannot be expected to reverse the suppressed production of these androgens *(34)*. It is worth noting that women who develop breast cancer in premenopausal years tend to have subnormal serum levels of AAs, whereas subjects who develop the disease in postmenopausal years have supranormal levels of these hormones. Androgens by acting via the androgen receptor, oppose estrogen-stimulated cell growth in premenopausal years. In postmenopausal women, elevated

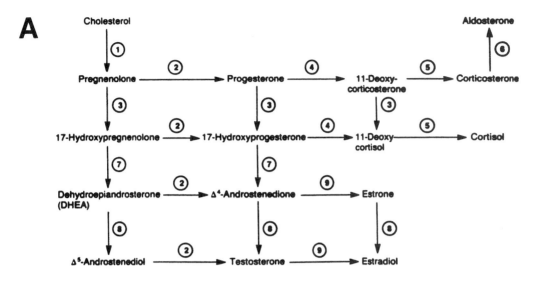

Fig. 3. (A) Adrenal androgen biosynthesis pathway. **(B)** The enzymes correspond to the numbers in the pathway.

AA levels stimulate cell growth by the action of the unique adrenal androgen 5-androstene-3β, 17β-diol, also termed ermaphrodiol, via its combination with the estrogen receptor in a hormone milieu lacking or having low concentrations of the classical estrogen 17 beta-estradiol *(35)*.

Biochemistry

Three 19-carbon compounds are the principal androgens secreted by the adrenals: dehydroepiandrosterone (DHEA) sulfate (DHEAS), DHEA, and Δ⁴-androstene-3, 17-dione (Δ⁴-androstenedione). Production of testosterone by these glands is minimal (Fig. 3). Although in quantity, DHEAS is the major product of the adrenal, this steroid *per se* is extremely weak as an androgen.

Peripheral Conversion and Excretion

Steroid precursors, and the AAs themselves, may be, respectively, converted to androgens or more potent androgens in peripheral tissues (Fig. 4). Major conversions

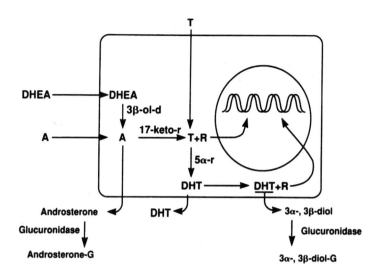

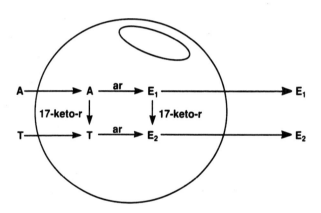

Fig. 4. Metabolism of the adrenal androgens in the pilosebaceous unit (**A**) and adipocyte tissue (**B**). Abbreviations: A, Δ^4-androstenedione; T, testosterone; DHT, dihydrotestosterone; R, receptor; 3β-ol-d, 3β-hydroxysteroid dehydrogenase; 17-keto-r, 17-ketosteroid reductase; 5α-r, 5α-reductase; 3α-, 3β-diol, 3α-androstenediol, 3β-androstenediol; 3α-, 3β-diol-G, 3α-diol-glucuronide, 3β-diol-glucuronide; androsterone-G, androsterone glucuronide; ar, aromatase; E_1, estrone; E_2, estradiol-17β.

are those of Δ^4-androstenedione to testosterone and testosterone to dihydrotestosterone. However, the peripheral biotransformation of DHEA, orally administered in 10 patients with complete panhypopituitarism, into potent androgens and estrogens may explain several of the reported beneficial actions of this steroid in aging people *(36)*. Major peripheral sites of androgen conversion are the hair follicles, the sebaceous glands, the prostate, and the external genitalia *(37,38)*.

Active uptake of androgens and *in situ* estrogen synthesis occur in peripheral adipose tissue (Fig. 4). Thus the enzymes aromatase and 17-ketosteroid reductase are highly active in fat cells *(39,40)*. The former is responsible for the transformation of Δ^4-androstenedione and testosterone, to estrone and estradiol, respectively. The latter transforms Δ^4-androstenedione to testosterone and estrone to estradiol. Aromatase activity is stimulated by glucocorticoids (41).

There is substantial evidence to suggest that different phenotypes of obesity are associated with different hormonal environments. Thus, although women with upper body obesity and those with lower body obesity have both increased aromatization of Δ^4-androstenedione to estrone and testosterone to estradiol, the former also have higher androgen production rates and elevated free testosterone levels, perhaps as a result of insulin resistance and functional ovarian hyperandrogenism (40). However, Vicennati et al. have shown recently that in premenopausal women there is no significant correlation between basal and stimulated androgen levels and body mass index, the waist-to-hip ratio, or basal and stimulated cortisol values (42).

The AAs and their metabolites are inactivated or degraded at various tissues, including the liver and kidneys (43). Major biochemical routes for inactivation and excretion are conjugations of these androgens, as well as estrogens to glucuronate or sulfate residues to produce hydrophilic glucuronides or sulfates that are excreted in the urine (Fig. 4).

Adrenal Androgen Effects

In adult men, the conversion of adrenal Δ^4-androstenedione to testosterone accounts for less than 5% of the production rate of the latter, making its participation in the physiologic androgenization of the male negligible. Excessive AA secretion appears to have no major clinical consequences in the adult man, although this may be debated. AA hypersecretion in prepubertal boys, on the other hand, has clearly been associated with isosexual precocious puberty.

In adult women, adrenal Δ^4-androstenedione and Δ^4-androstenedione generated from peripheral conversion of DHEA contribute substantially to total androgen production and effect. In the follicular phase of the menstrual cycle, adrenal precursors account for two-thirds of testosterone production and half of dihydrotestosterone production. In the midcycle, the ovarian contribution increases, and the adrenal precursors account for 40% of testosterone production. In women, increased AA production may be manifested as cystic acne, hirsutism, male-type baldness, menstrual irregularities, oligoovulation or anovulation, infertility, and/or frank virilization. Excessive adrenal androgen secretion in prepubertal or pubertal girls can cause heterosexual precocious puberty.

Both gonadal and AAs contribute to the positive impact of androgenic steroids on bone cell metabolism in vitro (44). Interestingly, a recent study found that the potential anabolic effect of androgens in bone may not be mediated at the level of the mature osteoblast, but at the level of fetal, less differentiated, osteoblastic cell lines (45).

ETIOLOGY OF ADRENAL ANDROGEN HYPERSECRETION

Primary Adrenal Causes

Benign Premature Adrenarche

Benign premature adrenarche is the isolated appearance of pubic and/or axillary hair before 8 yr in girls or 9 yr in boys without other signs of puberty or virilization and without an advanced bone age (46) (Table 1). It is characterized by increased production of AAs, is more common in girls than in boys, and usually occurs after 6 yr of age. Familial cases have been described, but are rare. In this nonprogressive disorder,

Table 1
Etiology of Adrenal Androgen Hypersecretion

Primary Adrenal
1. Benign premature adrenarche (adrenal androgen-stimulating factor?)
2. Adrenal tumors (adenomas, carcinomas)
3. ± Cushing syndrome
4. Hyperaldosteronism

Corticotropin hypersecretion
1. Congenital adrenal hyperplasia
2. Corticotropin-dependent Cushing's syndrome ± growth retardation
3. Glucocorticoid resistance ± hypermineralocorticoidism

Hyperprolactinemia
Exogenous
1. Androgens
2. Anabolic steroids

Other
Pregnancy
1. Placental sulfatase deficiency (no hyperandrogenism)
2. Placental aromatase deficiency (mother and female fetus virilization)

secondary sexual maturation occurs independently of gonadarche and is apparently caused by a factor other than corticotropin or is inherent to the adrenals. Benign premature adrenarche should be differentiated from late-onset forms of congenital adrenal hyperplasia that are clinically identical.

Adrenal Tumors

Primary adrenal tumors (adenomas and carcinomas) may autonomously hypersecrete androgens and/or other hormones *(47)*. Hormone-secreting adrenocortical adenomas and carcinomas are relatively rare. Adrenocortical adenomas typically present solely with clinical manifestations of hyperandrogenism because they usually secrete one type of hormone. In contrast, adrenocortical carcinomas may secrete androgens in conjunction with glucocorticoids and/or mineralocorticoids.

Corticotropin Hypersecretion

Congenital Adrenal Hyperplasia

Congenical adrenal hyperplasia is discussed in detail elsewhere in this volume.

Corticotropin-Dependent Cushing's Syndrome

Corticotropin-dependent Cushing's syndrome represents the most common cause of endogenous hypercortisolism, affecting approx 80–85% of the cases *(48)*. In 80% of these cases, it is caused by a pituitary adenoma (microadenoma or macroadenoma) secreting corticotropin or, rarely, by corticotroph cell hyperplasia (Fig. 5). In the remaining 20%, it is caused by corticotropin secreted ectopically from nonpituitary tumors, and occasionally it may be because of ectopic secretion of CRH by neoplasms. Corticotropin stimulates the adrenal cortex to hypersecrete both cortisol and AAs, causing combined hypercortisolism and hyperandrogenism. It seems that corticotropin alone does not control AA secretion and that the variability in the processing of POMC occurring in

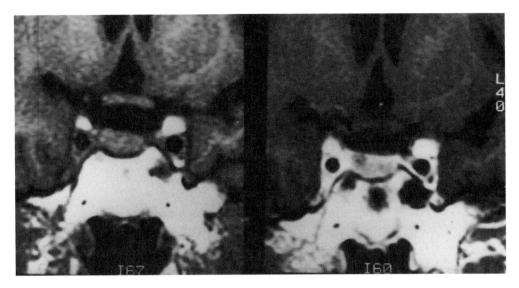

Fig. 5. Left: Coronal MR scan of the pituitary gland in a patient with Cushing's syndrome. MR-scan before administration of gadolinium shows normal pituitary. **Right:** MRI of the same pituitary gland after administration of gadolinium demonstrating a small adenoma *(white arrow)* in the right inferior part of the gland. (Courtesy of J. Doppman.)

Cushing's disease and ectopic ACTH syndrome may account for differences in the relation of cortisol to androgens observed between the disorders and when compared to that in normal subjects *(49)*. In severe cases, stimulation of steroid intermediates with mineralocorticoid activity, such as deoxycorticosterone and corticosterone, may result in excess of the steroids and cause severe hypertension and hypokalemic alkalosis.

Glucocorticoid Resistance

The syndrome of glucocorticoid resistance results from partial, albeit apparently generalized, inability of glucocorticoids to exert their effects on target tissues *(50,51)*. Because of resistance to the negative-feedback effects of cortisol, this syndrome is associated with compensatory elevation of circulating corticotropin and cortisol. Corticotropin causes excess secretion of adrenal steroids (cortisol, 11-deoxycorticosterone, and corticosterone) with salt-retaining activity and AAs. The manifestations of glucocorticoid resistance vary from asymptomatic, to chronic fatigue (perhaps reflecting glucocorticoid deficiency), to variable degrees of hypertension and/or hypokalemic alkalosis, and hyperandrogenism. The last of these can manifest in women as acne, hirsutism, male-type baldness, menstrual irregularities, oligoovulation or anovulation, and infertility; in men as infertility; and in children as precocious puberty. Different molecular defects of the highly-conserved glucocorticoid receptor gene, altering its functional characteristics, appear to cause glucocorticoid resistance.

Hyperprolactinemia

In the original description of the Forbes-Albright syndrome, urinary 17-ketosteroids were elevated in approximately half the patients *(52)*. Increased androgen secretion is indeed present in about 40% of hyperprolactinemic patients *(53–56)*. This could be caused either by concurrent ovarian hyperandrogenism or by stimulation of the *zona reticularis* by PRL. Interestingly, the increased levels of AAs in hyperprolactinemic patients with no stigmata of the polycystic ovary syndrome normalize during bromocriptine treatment *(20)*. Although hirsutism can be seen in women with hyperprolactinemia and elevated levels of androgens, only a small number show clear manifestations of hyperandrogenism. This may be explained by the generally mild elevation of AAs of low biological potency and by a decrease in peripheral target tissue 5α-reductase activity attributed to PRL-induced suppression of this enzyme *(57)*. The AAs that are elevated in hyperprolactinemia are mostly DHEAS and DHEA. The levels of the more potent testosterone and steroid metabolites resulting from peripheral 5α-reduction, such as dihydrotestosterone and androstenadiol, are, in fact, low or normal in these patients. The mechanisms by which inappropriate elevation of PRL stimulates AA secretion and inhibits 5α-reductase activity remain unclear.

Exogenous

All exogenous androgens can induce hyperandrogenism or frank virilization in women. Among the early manifestations are acne, development of hirsutism, coarsening of the voice, and oligomenorrhea or amenorrhea. Prolonged treatment can lead to irreversible changes. Exogenous androgens are prescribed therapeutically in several conditions, including aplastic anemia and hereditary angioneurotic edema *(58–61)*. Also, use of androgens as anabolic agents seems to be widespread among athletes of different sport disciplines. This abuse is because of the belief among athletes that these substances improve athletic performance. In fact, properly controlled studies have not shown changes in athletic performance, even when phenomenally high doses were employed *(62,63)*.

Other

Aromatization of fetal AAs and hydrolysis of the sulfate residue are essential for the placental production of estrogen. A placental defect in aromatization, desulfation, or both, results in low maternal urinary excretion of estrogens during pregnancy.

A number of cases of placental sulfatase deficiency, an X-linked disease, have been reported *(64)*. This enzyme is responsible for the hydrolysis of DHEAS, produced by the fetal adrenal, and of the 16α-hydroxy metabolite of DHEAS, produced by the fetal liver. This hydrolysis is followed by aromatization of these compounds to estradiol and estriol, respectively. Despite the defect in estriol production, infants of such pregnancies are usually normal at birth. Later in life, they may develop ichthyosis, potentially because of accumulation of cholesterol sulfate in the skin.

Placental aromatase deficiency can cause both maternal virilization during pregnancy and virilization of a female fetus (pseudohermaphroditism) *(65)*.

Over 50% of patients with the polycystic ovary syndrome (PCOS) demonstrate excess levels of AAs, particularly DHEAS. Nonetheless, the mechanism for this AAs excess remains unclear. Recent findings by Azziz et al. suggest that AA excess in PCOS patients is related to an exaggerated secretory response of the adrenal cortex for DHEAS and androstenedione, but not to an altered pituitary responsivity to CRH or to increased sensitivity of these AAs to ACTH stimulation. Whether the increased responsivity to ACTH for these steroids is secondary to increased *zonae reticularis* mass or to differences in P450c 17α-activity, particularly of the Δ^4 pathway, remains to be determined *(66)*.

In several species, including the human fetus, IGF-1 and -2 have been reported to modulate adrenal steroidogenesis, thus contributing to adrenal cortical differentiation *(23)*. L'Allemand et al. have shown that IGFs enhance the steroidogenesis and ACTH responsiveness of human cortical cells in culture and by this mechanism may contribute to clinical states with hyperandrogenemia *67*.

SIGNS AND SYMPTOMS OF ADRENAL ANDROGEN HYPERSECRETION

Prepubertal Clinical Presentation

Excess of AAs before puberty is responsible for clinical manifestations that vary with sex. In prepubertal boys, the excess of AAs leads to virilization manifested as penile enlargement, hair development in androgen-dependent areas of the skin, and development of other secondary sexual characteristics. This is defined as isosexual precocious puberty (peripheral isosexual precocity). In prepubertal girls, excess of androgens leads to inappropriate virilization manifested as acne, hirsutism, and clitoromegaly. This is defined as heterosexual precocious puberty (peripheral heterosexual precocity).

In both sexes, androgen excess increases height velocity and somatic development, as well as rate of skeletal maturation. Premature epiphyseal fusion in these children frequently leads to short adult height.

Pubertal Clinical Presentation

In boys, AA excess after the onset of puberty may lead to acceleration of the progression of puberty and possibly to premature epiphyseal fusion and compromised adult height. When the AA excess is in the context of Cushing's syndrome, however, arrest of puberty and growth may be observed because of the hypercortisolism. The latter exerts a profound inhibitory effect on the gonadal axis, resulting in suppression of testicular function, and on the growth axis, resulting in stunted growth. It should be noted, however, that even in the presence of hypercortisolism, AAs can accelerate bone maturation and cause premature epiphyseal fusion in the absence of substantial growth.

In girls, AA excess may result in virilization. Menstruation may be inhibited, and thus, primary or secondary amenorrhea or spanomenorrhea may occur. Acceleration of bone maturation takes place. Concurrent hypercortisolism may cause gonadal suppression and stunt the growth of these girls.

Adult Clinical Presentation

In adult men, AA excess may cause no apparent clinical symptomatology, but might also suppress luteinizing hormone (LH) and follicle-stimulating hormone, resulting in abnormal spermatogenesis and possibly infertility. In addition, AAs might potentiate the effects of testosterone on the skin and lead to acne or baldness. When AA excess is in the context of Cushing's syndrome, LH and testosterone secretion is suppressed. AA hypersecretion is insufficient to compensate for the decreased gonadal testosterone production, and the patient manifests signs of hypogonadism, such as decreased libido and impotence.

In adult women, AA excess is manifested as hyperandrogenism or frank virilization. Concurrent hypercortisolism may cause hypogonadism in these patients.

Table 2
Diagnosis of Adrenal Androgen Hypersecretion

Primary adrenal causes	
1. Benign premature adrenarche	Plasma steroid hormones, precocious puberty work-up, rule out late-onset congenital adrenal hyperplasia
2. Adrenal tumors	Plasma steroid hormones, dexamethasone suppression test, Cushing's syndrome work-up, 24-h urinary aldosterone excretion, adrenal ultrasound / computed tomography / MRI
Corticotropin hypersecretion	
1. Congenital adrenal hyperplasia	Plasma steroid precursors ± corticotropin stimulation
2. Corticotropin-dependent Cushing's syndrome	Dexamethasone suppression test, 24-hour UFC / 17-hydroxysteroid excretion, Cushing's syndrome work-up, plasma steroid hormones
3. Glucocorticoid resistance	Dexamethasone suppression test, 24-hour UFC / 17-hydroxysteroid excretion, hyperandrogenism work-up, precocious puberty work-up
Hyperprolactinemia	Hyperandrogenism work-up, serum PRL
Exogenous	History, plasma, and urinary measurements of synthetic androgens
Other	
Pregnancy	
1. Placental sulfatase deficiency	
2. Placental aromatase deficiency	

DIAGNOSIS OF ADRENAL ANDROGEN HYPERSECRETION

Primary Adrenal Causes

Benign Premature Adrenarche

The diagnosis of benign premature adrenarche (Table 2) is based on the exclusion of precocious puberty (Table 3) and late-onset congenital adrenal hyperplasia. The plasma concentrations of the AAs (DHEA, DHEAS, and Δ^4-androstenedione) as well as the levels of the 17-ketosteroids, their urinary metabolites, are increased for the age and are similar to those normally found in pubertal children with Tanner stage 2 pubic hair *(46, 68–70)*. Plasma levels of 17-hydroxyprogesterone, 11-deoxycortisol, and 17-hydroxy-pregnenolone in response to corticotropin do not increase to values diagnostic of mild or late-onset congenital adrenal hyperplasia caused, respectively, by 21-hydroxylase, 11-hydroxylase, or 3β-hydroxysteroid dehydrogenase-Δ^5, Δ^4-isomerase deficiency *(68)*. The AAs and their metabolites are suppressible by dexamethasone *(68,69)*. Gonadotropin levels are in the prepubertal normal range both at the basal state and after stimulation with gonadotropin-releasing hormone.

Table 3
Evaluation of Patients with Precocious Puberty

Laboratory evaluation
- 24-h urinary 17-ketosteroid, pregnanetriol, or 17-hydroxysteroid excretion
- Corticotropin stimulation test
- Plasma human chorionic gonadotropin
- Plasma LH and follicle-stimulating hormone (serial samples, LH-releasing hormone stimulation test)
- Plasma sex steroid concentration

Imaging evaluation
- Bone age
- Pelvic ultrasound
- Computed axial tomography (brain, abdomen)
- MRI (brain, abdomen)

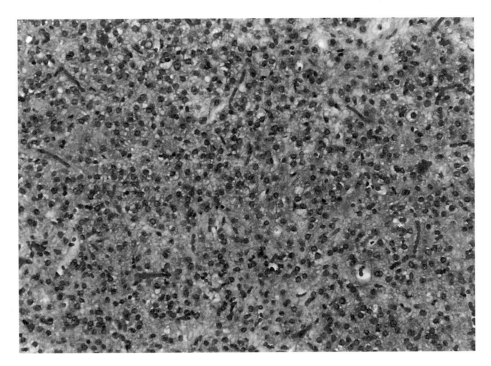

Fig. 6. Histology of a virilizing adrenocortical adenoma. (Courtesy of W. Travis.)

Adrenal Tumors

Benign virilizing adrenocortical adenomas can produce one or more of the AAs and/ or testosterone (Fig. 6). The plasma concentrations of these hormones are elevated, and usually they are not suppressed by dexamethasone *(48)*. These tumors are usually small (diameter <5 cm) and are not visible on ultrasound, but are visible on computed tomography (CT) or magnetic resonance imaging (MRI). These tumors do not show enhancement at the T2 relaxation time of MRI (Fig. 7).

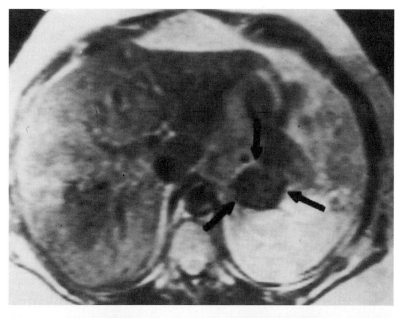

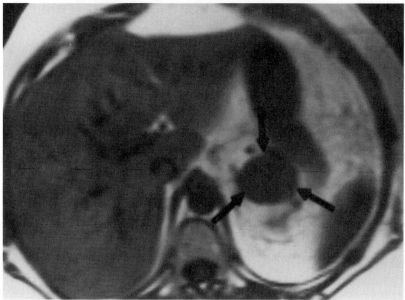

Fig. 7. MRI of a functioning adrenocortical adenoma. **Top:** T1-Weighted MR scan showing a left adrenal mass with low signal intensity similar of that of liver tissue. **Bottom:** The low signal intensity of this mass did not change during the T2-Weighted scan. (Courtesy of J. Doppman.)

Malignant virilizing adrenocortical carcinomas can produce several steroid intermediates, AAs, and/or testosterone, as well as compounds with glucocorticoid and mineralocorticoid activity *(47)* (Fig. 8). The elevated plasma levels of these steroids are usually not suppressible by dexamethasone, and the tumor is frequently palpable or visible on ultrasound. Generally, adrenocortical carcinomas are larger than 5 cm in diameter, and have already invaded the capsule of the gland or neighboring tissues by the time they

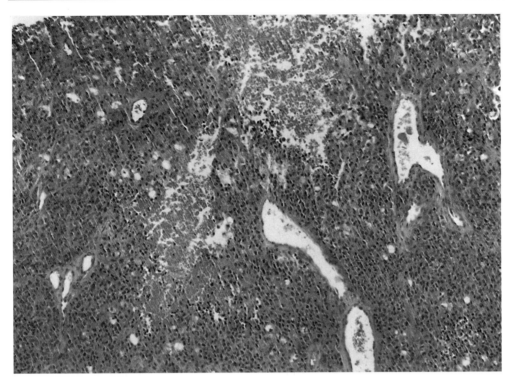

Fig. 8. Histology of an adrenocortical carcinoma. (Courtesy of W. Travis.)

are discovered. Unlike benign adenomas, MRI of these tumors shows enhancement at the T2 relaxation time (Fig. 9).

The diagnosis of Cushing's syndrome is made when 24-h urine-free cortisol (UFC) normalized for body surface area or 24-h urinary 17-hydroxysteroid normalized per gram of excreted creatinine is elevated *(48)*. The cicardian rhythm of plasma cortisol of these patients is frequently disrupted, and cortisol secretion is not suppressed properly by dexamethasone. If this is the case, the Cushing's syndrome evaluation should be pursued to confirm the differential diagnosis (Table 4). In patients with adrenal tumors causing Cushing's syndrome, AAs (DHEA, DHEAS, and Δ^4-androstenedione or testosterone) are frequently elevated. Circulating levels of plasma corticotropin, on the other hand, are persistently low or undetectable, contrary to the case for patients with Cushing's disease or an ectopic corticotropin-producing tumor, in whom the levels are normal or elevated. Presence of severe hypertension, hypokalemia, and alkalosis is usually caused by hyperproduction of steroid precursors with mineralocorticoid activity, such as deoxycorticosterone and corticosterone or aldosterone itself. These steroids can be measured in plasma, whereas aldosterone excretion can also be measured in the urine as total 24-h excretion.

Corticotropin Hypersecretion

Congenital Adrenal Hyperplasia

Congenital adrenal hyperplasia is discussed elsewhere in this volume.

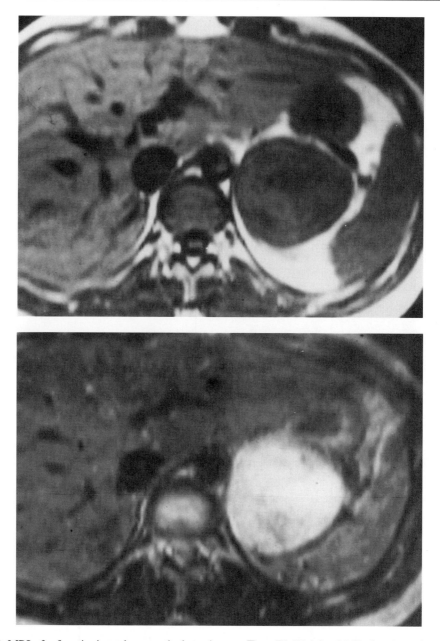

Fig. 9. MRI of a functioning adrenocortical carcinoma. **Top:** T1-Weighted MR showing a large left adrenal mass with low signal intensity similar to that of liver tissue. **Bottom:** T2-Weighted MR scan showing enhanced signal intensity of the same mass. (Courtesy of J. Doppman.)

Corticotropin-Dependent Cushing's Syndrome

When the diagnosis of Cushing's syndrome is established as aforementioned, the patient must be characterized as having or not having corticotropin-dependent Cushing's syndrome. If the former is true, further differentiation into pituitary vs ectopic Cushing's syndrome must be made (Table 4).

Table 4
Diagnostic Testing in Cushing's Syndrome and Pseudo-Cushing States[a]

Type	CRH	Liddle Test (Urinary 17-Hydroxysteroid)	Metyrapon E Tests (Urinary 17-Hydroxysteroid)	Computer Tomography/MRI	BIPSS[b]	Iodocholesterol Scan	ITT
Corticotropin-dependent Cushing's syndrome							
Pituitary	Corticotropin ↑ Cortisol ↑	Low dose − High dose ↓	↑	Pituitary ± Adrenal ↑ (macronodules)	Gradiant Lateralization	Bilateral uptake	Corticotropin − Cortisol −
Ectopic Corticotropin	Coricotropin − Cortisol −	Low dose − High dose −	−	Pituitary −	No gradient	Bilateral uptake	Corticotropin − Cortisol −
Ectopic CRH (rare)	High plasma CRH	Low dose − High dose −	?	Pituitary − Adrenal ↑	Gradiant[c]	Bilateral uptake[c]?	Corticotropin −[c] Cortisol −[c]
Corticotropin-independent Cushing's syndrome							
Adrenal adenoma	Corticotropin ↓ Cortisol−	Low dose− High dose −	−	+	Corticotropin↓	Uninlateral uptake	−
Adrenal carcinoma	Corticotropin ↓ Cortisol −	Low dose − High dose −	−	+	Corticotropin↓	−	−
Micronodular adrenal disease	Corticotropin ↓ Cortisol −	Low dose − High dose − paradoxic↑	−	±	Corticotropin↓	± Bilateral uptake	−
Pseudo-Cushing states (depression)							
	Corticotropin blunted Cortisol ↑	Low dose ±↓ High dose ↓	↑	?	?	Bilateral uptake[c]?	Corticotropin↑ Cortisol↑

From *ref. 48*, with permission.

[a]↑, elevation or enlargement; ↓, suppression; †, positive test; −, negative test or no change; ±, positive or negative.
[b]BIPSS, bilateral interior petrosal sinus sampling.
[c]Theoretically expected.

Glucocorticoid Resistance

In the glucocorticoid resistance syndrome, plasma cortisol is elevated, and 24-h UFC and 17-hydroxysteroid excretion is high *(51)*. Cortisol suppression by dexamethasone is compromised. Unlike what happens in Cushing's syndrome, plasma cortisol levels in glucocorticoid resistance retain a circardian rhythm and respond to stress tests, such as insulin-induced hypoglycemia.

Hyperprolactinemia

The hyperprolactinemia-related elevation of DHEA, DHEAS, and Δ^4-androstenedione rarely becomes clinically important. Elevated prolactin concentrations will lead to the diagnosis of the hyperprolactinemia in such patients.

Exogenous

Exogenous administration of androgens can be established as the cause of hyperandrogenism on the basis of the patient's history. Plasma and urinary measurements of the angiogenic substances and their metabolites are widely used in the identification of the synthetic compounds abused by athletes.

Other

In placental sulfatase or aromatase deficiency, the levels of estriol in the plasma and the urine of pregnant women are quite low *(65,72)*. The presence of pregnancy-related maternal hyperandrogenism or frank virilization will direct the diagnosis toward aromatase deficiency. A female fetus of such pregnancy may be virilized.

When a pregnant woman in the last trimester of pregnancy excretes inappropriately low levels of urinary estrogens for her gestational stage without evidence of fetal distress, one should consider fetal anencephaly, fetal adrenal hypoplasia, maternal use of certain drugs, and maternal renal disease *(73)*. When these causes are excluded, one must assess the placental capacity for estrogen synthesis. Loading the patient with DHEAS and DHEA may identify the enzyme deficiency *(74–76)*. Subjects with placental sulfatase deficiency will produce a normal increase in serum estradiol-17β levels in response to DHEA, but not DHEAS. Women with placental aromatase deficiency will show a response to neither DHEA or DHEAS.

Differential Diagnosis

Hypersecretion of androgens from the adrenal glands (Table 1) should be differentiated from clinical situations resulting from hypersecretion of androgens from the other sources, including androgen-producing gonads (polycystic ovary syndrome or gonadal tumors; these are discussed in detail elsewhere in this volume).

TREATMENT OF ADRENAL ANDROGEN HYPERSECRETION

Primary Adrenal Causes

Benign Premature Adrenarche

Once precocious puberty and late-onset congenital adrenal hyperplasia are excluded, no treatment is needed besides reassurance (Table 5). Gonadarche usually appears at a normal time.

Table 5
Treatment of Adrenal Androgen Hypersecretion

Primary adrenal causes

1. Benign premature adrenarche — No treatment
2. Adrenal tumors — Surgical resection, mitotane, steroid synthesis inhibitors

Corticotropin hypersecretion

1. Congenital adrenal hyperplasia — Hydrocortisone-Fludrocortisone
2. Corticotropin-dependent Cushing's syndrome — Excision of pituitary adenoma, X irradiation of pituitary, steroid synthesis inhibitors, excision of ectopic tumors, chemotherapy
3. Glucocorticoid resistance — Dexamethasone

Hyperprolactinemia — Dopaminergic agonists, excision of pituitary adenoma

Exogenous — Discontinuation of drugs

Other

Pregnancy

1. Placental sulfatase deficiency — No treatment
2. Placental aromatase deficiency — Dexamethasone

Adrenal Tumors

Surgical resection is the treatment of choice for all primary adrenal tumors *(47,48)*. Unilateral total adrenalectomy is recommended for the autonomous benign hormone-secreting adrenocortical adenomas. Complete resection of the tumor is also the treatment of choice for the adrenocortical carcinoma. Solitary local extensions, recurrences, or metastases of adrenocortical carcinomas should be removed surgically, if possible. Adrenocortical carcinomas are highly malignant neoplasms. Long-term remissions, however, have been reported after extensive resection, and long-term remissions have also followed surgical resection of hepatic, pulmonary, or cerebral metastases. Once it is known that the patient does not have a surgically curable disease, therapy with the adrenolytic agent mitotane is usually initiated. Mitotane given at maximally tolerated oral doses (up to 16 g/d) has some effectiveness in patients with metastatic adrenocortical carcinoma *(77)*. Tumor regression or arrest of growth has been observed in as many as one-third of the patients. The mean survival time of these patients, however, does not appear to be altered by the therapy. Occasionally for the correction of hyperandrogenism, hypercortisolism, and/or hypermineralocorticoidism, steroid synthesis inhibitors (ketoconazole, aminoglutethimide, metyrapone, trilostane, and etomidate) and androgen, glucocorticoid, or mineralocorticoid antagonists may be required. Radiation therapy is occasionally helpful for palliation of bone metastases.

Corticotropin Hypersecretion

Congenital Adrenal Hyperplasia

Congenital adrenal hyperplasia is discussed elsewhere in this volume.

Corticotropin-Dependent Cushing's Syndrome

The treatment of corticotropin-dependent Cushing's syndrome largely depends on the successful differential diagnosis and localization of the source of corticotropin *(47,48)*. If a corticotropin-producing pituitary adenoma is responsible for the syndrome, excision of the adenoma by transsphenoidal surgery is the therapy of choice. X irradiation of the pituitary can be recommended when complete removal of the pituitary adenoma cannot be attained or after two unsuccessful surgeries or recurrences. This is usually accompanied by treatment with low doses of mitotane (2–5 g/d). Patients who fail this therapy or who do not choose to pursue it in the first place always have the option of chronic medical therapy with steroid synthesis inhibitors (ketoconazole, aminoglutethimide, metyrapone, trilostane, and etomidate) or of bilateral adrenalectomy. When ectopic corticotropin- and/or CRH-producing tumors are responsible for the syndrome, they must be surgically excised and/or treated with therapy. If the source of corticotropin or CRH cannot be localized or if these tumors are inoperable, chronic medical therapy or bilateral adrenalectomy may be left as the only long-term alternative.

Glucocorticoid Resistance

Appropriate doses of a glucocorticoid with no intrinsic mineralocortcoid activity, such as dexamethasone, are recommended *(51,78)*. The goals of therapy are to eliminate the clinical manifestations of hyperandrogenisms and hypermineralocorticoidism and to normalize the production of AAs and their metabolites.

Hyperprolactinemia

The mild hyperandrogenism related to hyperprolactinemia is corrected with successful suppression of plasma PRL. The dopaminergic agonists bromocriptine and pergolide are quite efficient in suppressing PRL secretion regardless of whether a prolactinoma is present. Transsphenoidal adenomectomy of a nonresponsive prolactinoma that threatens vision may be rarely needed.

Exogenous

When exogenous androgens are administered for therapeutic purposes, other therapies should be sought or the cost–benefit ratio to the patient should be evaluated. Androgen-containing preparations taken to improve athletic performance should be discontinued.

Other

No particular measure should be taken in a pregnancy with placental sulfatase deficiency. Women with placental aromatase deficiency who are carrying a female fetus, however, may benefit from dexamethasone-replacement therapy. This compound crosses the placenta and suppresses the fetal adrenal zone.

PROGNOSIS OF ADRENAL ANDROGEN HYPERSECRETION

The prognosis of AA hypersecretion depends on the cause of the hyperandrogenism. Hyperandrogenism *per se* carries a good prognosis if treated properly and before it causes irreversible changes.

Primary Adrenal Causes

Benign Premature Adrenarche

This disorder has an excellent prognosis.

Adrenal Tumors

The prognosis of adrenocortical carcinomas is poor because the great majority of these tumors are diagnosed at an advanced stage. The 5-yr survival from the time of diagnosis is approx 22% after aggressive surgical therapy *(77)*. The prognosis of adrenocortical adenomas is excellent assuming proper diagnosis and surgery.

Corticotropin Hypersecretion

Congenital Adrenal Hyperplasia

The prognosis of congenital adrenal hyperplasia is discussed elsewhere in this volume.

Corticotropin-Dependent Cushing's Syndrome

If corticotropin-dependent Cushing's syndrome is caused by pituitary adenoma, its prognosis is excellent after proper surgical excision of the tumor. In the rare cases of corticotropin-dependent Cushing's syndrome caused by ectopic corticotropin and/or CRH secretion, the prognosis depends on the degree of malignancy of the original hormone-secreting neoplasm.

Glucocorticoid Resistance

The prognosis of glucocorticoid resistance is excellent assuming proper diagnosis and early therapy.

Hyperprolactinemia

The prognosis depends on the responsiveness of the PRL-secreting tumor to therapy. This is discussed elsewhere in the volume.

Exogenous

Hyperandrogenism caused by exogenous androgens has a good prognosis if the administration of these steroids is stopped promptly.

Other

No particular measure should be taken in a pregnancy with placental sulfatase deficiency. In theory, female fetuses carried by women with placental aromatase deficiency have a good prognosis when the mothers are treated with dexamethasone starting at gestation wk 5 or 6.

REFERENCES

1. Davis JO. Regulation of aldosterone secretion. In: Einstein AB, ed. *The adrenal cortex*. Little, Brown; Boston, 1967, pp. 203–247.
2. Bech K, Tygstrup I, Nerup J. The involution of the fetal adrenal cortex. A light microscopic study. Acta Pathol Microbial Scand 1969; 76: 391–400.
3. Dhom G. The prepubertal and pubertal growth of the adrenal (adrenarche). Beir Pathol 1973; 150:357–377.
4. Parker CR Jr, Mixon RL, Brissie RM, Grizzle WE. Aging alters zonation in the adrenals cortex of men. J Clin Endocrinol Metab 1997; 82: 3898–3901.

5. Labrie F, Belanger A, Cusan L, Gomez JL, Candas B. Marked decline in serum concentrations of adrenal C19 sex steroid precursors and conjugated androgen metabolites during aging. J Clin Endocrinol Metab 1997; 82: 2396–2402.

6. Brown JD, Doe RP. Pituitary pigmentary hormones: relationship of melanocyte-stimulating hormone to lipotropic hormone. JAMA 1978; 240: 1273–1278.

7. Krieger DT, Liotta LS, Suda T, et al. Human plasma immunoreactive lipotropin and adrenocorticotropin in normal subjects and in patients with pituitary adrenal disease. J Clin Endocrinol Metab 1979; 48: 566–571.

8. Nicolson WE, Liddle RA, Puett D, et al. Adrenocorticotropin hormone biotransformation, clearance and catabolism. Endocrinology 1978; 103: 1344–1351.

9. Vale W, Speiss J, Rivier C, et al. Characterization of a 41-residue ovine hypothalamic peptide that stimulates secretion of corticotropin and β-endorphin. Science 1981; 213: 1394–1397.

10. Lamberts SWJ, Verleun T, Oosterom R, et al. Corticotropin releasing factor and vasopressin exert a synergistic effect on adrenocorticotropin release in man. J Clin Endocrinol Metab 1984; 58: 298–303.

11. Rosenfeld RS, Rosenberg BJ, Fukushima DK, et al. 24-Hour secretory pattern of dehydroisoandrosterone sulfate. J Clin Endocrinol Metab 1975; 40: 850–855.

12. Feuillan P, Pang S, Avgerinos P, et al. Adaptation of the hypothalamic-pituitary-adrenal axis in patients with partial (late-onset) 21-hydroxylase deficiency. J Clin Endocrinol Metab 1988; 67: 154–160.

13. Rossi R, Zatelli MC, Valentini A, Cavazzini P, Fallo F, del Senno L, et al. Evidence for androgen receptor gene expression and growth inhibitory effect of dihydrotestosterone on human adrenocortical cells. J Clin Endocrinol Metab 1998; 159: 373–380.

14. Mastorakos G, Chrousos GP, Weber JS. Recombinant interleukin-6 activates the hypothalamic-pituitary-adrenal axis in humans. J Clin Endocrinol Metab 1993; 77: 1690–1694.

15. Mastorakos G, Weber JS, Magiakou MA, Gunn H, Chrousos GP. Hypothalamic-pituitary-adrenal axis activation and stimulation of systemic vasopressin secretion by recombinant interleukin-6 in humans: potential implications for the syndrome of inappropriate vasopressin secretion [ese comments]. J Clin Endocrinol Metab 1994; 79: 934–939.

16. Path G, Bornstein SR, Ehrhart-Bornstein M, Scherbaum WA. Interleukin-6 and the interleukin-6 receptor in the human adrenal gland: expression and effects on steroidogenesis. J Clin Endocrinol Metab 1997; 82: 2343–2349.

17. Oberbeck R, Benschop RJ, Jacobs R, Hosch W, Jetschmann JU, Schurmeyer TH, et al. Endocrine mechanisms of stress-induced DHEA-secretion. J Endocrinol Invest 1998; 21: 148–153.

18. Smith R, Mesiano R, Chan EC, Brown S, Jaffe RB. Corticotropin-releasing hormone directly and preferentially stimulates dehydroepiandrosterone sulfate secretion by human fetal adrenal cortical cells. J Clin Endocrinol Metab 1998; 83: 2916–2920.

19. Glasow A, Breidert M, Haidan A, Anderegg U, Kelly PA, Bornstein SR. Functional aspects of the effect of prolactin (PRL) on adrenal steroidogenesis and distribution of the PRL receptor in the human adrenal gland. J Clin Endocrinol Metab 1996; 81: 3103–3111.

20. Lobo RA, Kletzky OA, Kaptein EM, et al. Prolactin modulation of dehydroepiandrosterone sulfate secretion. Am J Obstet Gynecol 1980; 138: 632–636.

21. Smail PJ, Faiman C, Hobson WC, Fuller GB, Winter JS. Further studies on adrenarche in nonhuman primates. Endocrinology 1982; 111: 844–848.

22. Gell JS, Carr BR, Sasano H, Atkins B, Margraf L, Mason JI, et al. Adrenarche results from development of a 3beta-hydroxysteroid dehydrogenase-deficient adrenal reticularis. J Clin Endocrinol Metab 1998; 83: 3695–3701.

23. Mesiano S, Katz SL, Lee JY, Jaffe RB. Insulin-like growth factors augment steroid production and expression of steroidogenic enzymes in human fetal adrenal cortical cells: implications for adrenal androgen regulation. J Clin Endocrinol Metab 1997; 82: 1390–1396.

24. Fottner C, Engelhardt D, Weber MM. Regulation of steroidogenesis by insulin-like growth factors (IGFs) in adult human adrenocortical cells: IGF-I and, more potently, IGF-II preferentially enhance androgen biosynthesis through interaction with IGF-I receptor and IGF-binding proteins. J Endocrinol 1998; 158: 409–417.

25. Weber A, Clark AJ, Perry LA, Honour JW, Savage MO. Diminished adrenal androgen secretion in familial glucocorticoid deficiency implicates a significant role for ACTH in the induction of adrenarche. Clin Endocrinol (Oxf) 1997; 46: 431–437.

26. Fearon U, Clarke D, McKenna DJ, Cunningham SK. Intra-adrenal factors are not involved in the

differential control of cortisol and adrenal androgens in human adrenals. Eur J Endocrinol 1998; 138: 567–573.

27. Grumbach MM, Richards GE, Conte FA, et al. Clinical disorders of adrenal function and puberty: an assessment of the role of the adrenal cortex in normal and abnormal puberty in man and evidence for an ACTH-like pituitary adrenal androgen stimulating hormone. In: James VH, Serio M, eds. The endocrine function of the human adrenal cortex. Academic, London; 1978, pp. 583–612.
28. Parker LN, Lifrak ET, Odell WD. A 60,000 molecular weight human pituitary glycopeptide stimulates adrenal secretion. Endocrinology 1983; 113: 2092–2096.
29. Anderson DC. The adrenal androgen-stimulating hormone does not exist. Lancet 1980; 2:454–456.
30. Byrne GD, Perry YS, Winter JSD. Kinetic analysis of adrenal 3β-hydroxysteroid dehydrogenase activity during human development. J Clin Endocrinol Metab 1985; 60: 934–939.
31. McKenna TJ, Fearon U, Clarke D, Cunningham SK. A critical review of the origin and control of adrenal androgens. Baillieres Clin Obstet Gynaecol 1997; 11: 229–248.
32. Clarke D, Fearon U, Cunningham SK, McKenna TJ. The steroidogenic effects of beta-endorfin and joining peptide: a potential role in the modulation of adrenal androgen production. J Clin Endocrinol Metab 1996; 151: 301–307.
33. Polderman KH, Gooren LJ, van der Veen EA. Effects of gonadal androgens and oestrogens on adrenal androgens levels. Clin Endocrinol (Oxf) 1995; 43: 415–421.
34. Slayden SM, Crabbe L, Bae S, Potter HD, Azziz R, Parker CR Jr. The effect of 17 beta-estradiol on adrenocortical sensitivity, responsiveness, and steroidogenesis in postmenopausal women. J Clin Endocrinol Metab 1998; 83: 519–524.
35. Adams JB. Adrenal androgens and human breast cancer: a new appraisal. Breast Cancer Res Treat 1998; 51: 183–188.
36. Young J, Couzinet B, Nahoul K, Brailly S, Chanson P, Baulieu EE, et al. Panhypopituitarism as a model to study the metabolism of dehydroepiandrosterone (DHEA) in humans. J Clin Endocrinol Metab 1997; 82: 2578–2585.
37. Schweikert HU, Wilson JD. Regulation of human hair growth by steroid hormones: I. Testosterone metabolism in isolated hairs. J Clin Endocrinol Metab 1974; 38: 811–819.
38. Schweikert HU, Milewich L, Wilson JD. Aromatization of androstenedione by isolated human hairs. J Clin Endocrinol Metab 1975; 40: 413–417.
39. Deslypere JP, Verdonck L, Vermeulen A. Fat tissue: a steroid reservoir and site of steroid metabolism. J Clin Endocrinol Metab 1985; 61: 564–570.
40. Kirschner MA, Samojlik E, Drejka M, Szmal E, Schneider G, Ertel N. Androgen-estrogen metabolism in women with upper body versus lower body obesity. J Clin Endocrinol Metab 1990; 70: 473–479.
41. McNatty KP, Makris A, Reinhold VN, DeGrazia C, Osathanondh R, Ryan KJ. Metabolism of androstenedione by human ovarian tissues in vitro with particular reference to reductase and aromatase activity. Steroids 1979; 34: 429–443.
42. Vicennati V, Calzoni F, Gambineri A, Gagliardi L, Morselli Labate RM, Casimirri F, et al. Secretion of major adrenal androgens following ACTH administration in obese women with different body fat distribution. Horm Metab Res 1998; 30: 133–136.
43. Norman AW, Litwack G. Androgens. In: Norman and Litusassk, eds. Hormones. Academic, San Diego; 1987, pp. 483–513.
44. Kasperk CH, Wakley GK, Hierl T, Ziegler R. Gonadal and adrenal androgens are potent regulators of human bone cell metabolism in vitro. J Bone Miner Res 1997; 12: 464–471.
45. Hofbauer LC, Hicok KC, Khosla S. Effects of gonadal and adrenal androgens in a novel androgen-responsive human osteoblastic cell line. J Cell Biochem 1998; 71: 96–108.
46. Silverman SH, Migeon CJ, Rosenberg E, Wilkins L. Precocious growth of sexual hair without other secondary sexual development; "premature pubarche", a constitutional variation of adolescence. Pediatrics 1952; 10: 426–432.
47. Flack MR, Chrousos GP. Neoplasma of the adrenal cortex. In: Holland JF, Frei E III, Bast RC Jr, Kufe DW, Morton DL, Weichselbaum RR, eds. Cancer medicine. 3rd ed. Lea & Febiger, Philadelphia; 1993, pp. 1147–1153.
48. Kamilaris TC, Chrousos GP. Adrenal diseases. In: Moore WT, Eastman RC, eds. Diagnostic endocrinology. Decker, Philadelphia; 1990, pp. 79–109.
49. Cunningham SK, McKenna TJ. Dissociation of adrenal androgen and cortisol secretion in Cushing's syndrome. Clin Endocrinol (Oxf) 1994; 41: 795–800.

50. Chrousos GP, Karl M. The molecular mechanisms of glucocorticoid resistance. In: Saez JM, Brownie AC, Capponi A, Chambaz EM, Mantero F, eds. Cellular and molecular biology of the adrenal cortex. Colloque INSERM/John Libbey Eurotext, London; 1992, pp. 227–232.

51. Karl M, Chrousos GP. Familial glucocorticoid resistance: an overview. Exp Clin Endocrinol 1993; 101: 30–35.

52. Forbes A, Hanneman PH, Griswold GC, Albright F. Syndrome characterized by galactorrhea, amenorrhea, and low urinary FSH: comparison with acromegaly and normal lactation. J Clin Endocrinol Metab 1954; 14: 265–271.

53. Vermeulen A, Ando S. Prolactin and adrenal androgen secretion. Clin Endocrinol (Oxf) 1978; 8: 295–303.

54. Carter JN, Tyson JE, Warne GL, McNeilly AS, Fainman C, Friesen HG. Adrenocortical function in hyperprolactinemic women. J Clin Endocrinol Metab 1997; 45: 973–980.

55. Glickman SP, Rosenfield RL, Bergenstal RM, Helke J. Multiple androgenic abnormalities, including elevated free testosterone, in hyperprolactinemic women. J Clin Endocrinol Metab 1982; 55: 251–257.

56. Lobo RA, Kletzky OA. Normalization of androgen and sex hormone-binding globulin levels after treatment of hyperprolactinemia. J Clin Endocrinol Metab 1983; 56: 562–566.

57. Magrini G, Ebiner JR, Burckhardt P, Felber JP. Study of the relationship between plasma prolactin levels and androgen metabolism in man. J Clin Endocrinol Metab 1976; 43: 944–947.

58. Shahidi NT. Androgens and erythropoiesis. N Engl J Med 1973; 289: 72–80.

59. Evens RP, Amerson AB. Androgens and erythropoiesis. J Clin Pharmacol 1974; 14: 94–101.

60. Spaulding WB. Methyltestosterone therapy for hereditary episodic edema (hereditary angioneurotic edema). Ann Intern Med 1960; 53: 739–745.

61. Gould DJ, Cunliffe WJ, Smiddy FG. Anabolic steroids in hereditary angiooedema. Lancet 1978; 1: 770–771.

62. Rayn AJ. Anabolic steroids are fool's gold. Fed Proc 1981; 40: 2682–2688.

63. American College of Sports Medicine. Position statement on the use and abuse of anabolic-androgenic steroids in sports. Med Sci Sports Exerc 1977; 9: 11–13.

64. Tabei T, Heinrichs WL. Diagnosis of placental sulfatase deficiency. Am J Obstet Gynecol 1976; 124: 409–414.

65. Shozu M, Akasofu K, Harada T, Kubota Y. A new cause of female pseudohermaphroditism: placental aromatase deficiency. J Clin Endocrinol Metab 1991; 72: 560–566.

66. Azziz R, Black V, Hines GA, Fox LM, Boots LR. Adrenal androgen excess in the polycystic ovary syndrome: sensitivity and responsivity of the hypothalamic-pituitary-adrenal axis. J Clin Endocrinol Metab 1998; 83: 2317–2323.

67. L'Allemand D, Penhoat A, Lebrethon MC, Ardevol R, Baehr V, Oelkers W, et al. Insulin-like growth factors enhance steroidogenic enzyme and corticotropin receptor messenger ribonucleic acid levels and corticotropin steroidogenic responsiveness in cultured human adrenocortical cells. J Clin Endocrinol Metab 1996; 81: 3892–3897.

68. Korth-Schutz S, Levine LS, New MI. Serum androgens in normal prepubertal and pubertal children and in children with precocious puberty. J Clin Endocrinol Metab 1976; 42: 117–124.

69. Rosenfield RL. Plasma 17-ketosteroids and 17β-hydroxysteroid in girls with premature development of sexual hair. J Pediatr 1971; 79: 260–266.

70. Sizonenko PC, Paunier L. Correlation of plasma dehydroepiandrosterone, testosterone, FSH, and LH with stages of puberty and bone age in normal boys and girls and in patients with Addison's disease or hypogonadism or with premature or late adrenarche. J Clin Endocrinol Metab 1975; 41: 894–904.

71. Reiter EO, Kaplan SL, Conte FA, Grumbach MM. Responsivity of pituitary gonadotropes to luteinizing hormone-releasing factor in idiopathic precocious puberty, precocious thelarche, precocious adrenarche. Pediatr Res 1975; 9: 111–116.

72. Taylor NF. Review: placental sulphatase deficiency. J Inherti Metab Dis 1982; 5: 164–176.

73. Grant JK, Beastall GH. Clinical biochemistry of steroid hormones-methods and applications. Croom Helm, London; 1983.

74. Lauritzen C. Conversion of DHEA-sulfate to estrogens as a test of placental function. Horm Metab Res 1969; 1: 96.

75. France JT, Seddon RJ, Liggins GC. A study of a pregnancy with low estrogen production due to placental sulfatase deficiency. J Clin Endocrinol Metab 1973; 36: 1–9.

76. Klopper A, Varela-Torres R. Placental metabolism of dehydroepiandrosterone sulphate in normal pregnancy. Br J Obstet Gynaecol 1976; 83: 478–483.

77. Luton JP, Cerdas S, Billaud L, et al. Clinical features of adrenocortical carcinoma, prognostic factors, and the effect of mitotane therapy. N Engl J Med 1990; 322: 1195–1201.
78. Malchoff CD, Reardon G, Javier EC, Rogol AD, McDermott P, Loriaux DL, et al. Dexamethasone therapy for isosexual precocious pseudopuberty caused by generalized glucocorticoid resistance. J Clin Endocrinol Metab 1994; 79: 1632–1636.

7

Structure, Function, and Regulated Expression of the Steroidogenic Acute Regulatory (StAR) Protein

Molecular Insights Into the Acute Steroidogenic Response of the Adrenals and Gonads to Trophic Stimulation

Caleb B. Kallen, Futoshi Arakane, Teruo Sugawara, Marianthi Kiriakidou, Staci E. Pollack, Hidemichi Watari, Lane K. Christenson, Michiko Watari, and Jerome F. Strauss III

CONTENTS

ABSTRACT

Steroid hormones produced in the adrenals, gonads, and placenta are important regulators of tissue differentiation, development, and homeostasis. The first committed step in the synthesis of these hormones in all tissue types is the conversion of cholesterol into pregnenolone. This reaction is catalyzed by the cytochrome *P450* side-chain cleav-

From: *Contemporary Endocrinology: Adrenal Disorders*
Edited by: A. N. Margioris and G. P. Chrousos © Humana Press, Totowa, NJ

age enzyme ($P450_{scc}$), located on the matrix side of the inner mitochondrial membrane. This first step in steroidogenesis, which is highly regulated in a temporal and tissue-specific manner, is primarily controlled at the level of cholesterol availability to the inner-mitochondrial matrix rather than at the level of $P450_{scc}$ enzyme activity. It has been known for decades that the acute regulation of steroid-hormone synthesis in the adrenals and gonads is dependent upon the synthesis of a protein(s) in response to trophic hormones and that this protein is fast-acting (minutes) and functionally short-lived. The recently cloned Steroidogenic Acute Regulatory (StAR) protein appears to be the "labile protein" essential for the acute steroidogenic response. Absence of functional StAR protein causes congenital lipoid adrenal hyperplasia (lipoid CAH), a disease characterized by marked impairment of adrenal and gonadal steroid hormone synthesis. Recent data implicate cAMP-mediated pathways in the regulation of StAR mRNA expression via a mechanism that depends upon the orphan nuclear hormone receptor, steroidogenic factor-1 (SF-1). Additional data suggest that cAMP-mediated pathways stimulate StAR function at the posttranslational level by initiating protein kinase A (PKA)-mediated phosphorylation of StAR. Although StAR has been shown to be imported and processed by mitochondria, this event is not essential to StAR function. It appears that StAR acts on the outer mitochondrial membrane, stimulating sterol desorption from the sterol-rich outer membrane and its transfer to the relatively sterol-poor inner membrane.

SUBSTRATE AVAILABILITY IS A PRIMARY DETERMINANT OF STEROIDOGENESIS

The rate-limiting step in steroidogenesis is cholesterol delivery to the $P450_{scc}$ enzyme on the inner mitochondrial membrane *(1)*. This assertion is based on the observation that high-level steroidogenesis, comparable to that seen with stimulation by trophic hormones, can be produced by treating steroidogenic cells with freely diffusible cholesterol analogs, such as 22R-hydroxycholesterol or 20α-hydroxycholesterol *(2,3)*. These studies imply that the aqueous layer between the inner and outer mitochondrial membranes creates a barrier that impedes cholesterol transport to $P450_{scc}$, and that this barrier is breached upon acute stimulation of cells by trophic hormone. Cholesterol availability to $P450_{scc}$ can be conceived of as the sum of several coordinated events, some of which are constitutive and others that are acutely regulated: (1) uptake of extracellular cholesterol, derived largely from circulating lipoproteins; (2) intracellular trafficking of cholesterol from the plasma membranes, sites of *de novo* synthesis in the endoplasmic reticulum, lipid droplets, and the processed lipoprotein-carried cholesterol to the outer mitochondrial membrane; and (3) intramitochondrial transport of cholesterol from the outer to the inner mitochondrial membrane, where $P450_{scc}$ resides.

Briefly, uptake of circulating lipoproteins and their cargo of cholesterol is determined by the level of expression of lipoprotein receptors, which is upregulated in response to trophic hormones *(4)*. The transport of intracellular cholesterol from the plasma membrane and lipid droplets, as well as other organelles including lysosomes and endoplasmic reticulum to the mitochondrion, is poorly understood. Implicated in these processes are the activation of cholesterol ester hydrolase by trophic hormone *(5,6)*, the dynamic components of the cytoskeleton *(7,8)*, and the Nicmann-Pick C1 glycoprotein which governs movement of the cholesterol out of lysosomes *(8a)*. Whereas these cellular components are critical to the maintenance of the hormone-responsive steroidogenic cell, they appear to play a supporting role in the acute steroidogenic response. The rate-limiting step in steroidogenesis is the final step of cholesterol transport from the outer to the inner mitochondrial membrane.

IDENTIFICATION AND CLONING OF THE STEROIDOGENIC ACUTE REGULATORY PROTEIN

The potent effect of trophic hormones on steroidogenesis in the adrenals and gonads, resulting in a greater than 10-fold stimulation of steroid secretion occurs rapidly (within minutes). More chronic effects of trophic stimulation are well documented and include upregulation of the genes for the steroidogenic enzymes [for review, see *(9)*]. Seminal contributions by Ferguson *(10)* and Garren *(11)* demonstrated that the acute steroidogenic response depends upon protein synthesis, and is lost when cells are pretreated with inhibitors of protein synthesis (e.g., puromycin or cycloheximide). Further experiments demonstrated that pretreatment of cells with inhibitors of protein synthesis caused cholesterol to become increasingly localized to the outer mitochondrial membrane, where it is unavailable for metabolism by $P450_{scc}$ *(12)*. The emerging evidence supported a hypothesis that trophic hormone stimulates the synthesis of a "labile" or short-lived protein which functions to transport cholesterol from the outer to the inner mitochondrial membrane.

A number of candidate proteins for this labile factor were proposed, including sterol carrier protein 2, steroidogenesis activator peptide, and the peripheral benzodiazepine receptor [for review, see *(13)*]. In 1983, using two-dimensional gel electrophoresis, Orme-Johnson's laboratory *(14)* described a family of 37-, 32-, 30-kDa phosphoproteins that were rapidly induced in response to trophic hormone, and absent when cells were pretreated with cycloheximide. One of these proteins (pp30) was localized to the mitochondrion. The kinetics of appearance and the ACTH dose response of this phospho-protein correlated with ACTH-induced corticosteroid production by the adrenal cells under study. Further studies using pulse-chase radiolabeling demonstrated that the 37-kDa species represented short-lived (half lives 3–5 min) cytosolic precursors of the mitochondrial 30-kDa species, and that the proteins shared common proteolytic degradation profiles. The presence of phosphorylated residues on pp30 suggested that co- or posttranslational protein modification is correlated to protein function.

Important advances by Clark and colleagues enabled purification of murine pp30 *(16)*. Using peptide sequencing and degenerate oligonucleotide primers, they cloned the cDNA encoding a protein that they designated StAR protein from a MA-10 mouse Leydig tumor cell cDNA library. Expression of the StAR cDNA in MA-10 cells increased steroid production in the absence of trophic stimulation. Using an in vitro transcription/transplantation system, these investigators also demonstrated that the 37-kDa protein expressed by the StAR cDNA was imported and processed by isolated mitochondria, producing a 30-kDa protein.

Additional information regarding the expression, structure, and function of StAR, was gleaned in part from incisive experiments carried out using the human StAR cDNA *(16)*. The autosomal recessive disease known as congenital lipoid adrenal hyperplasia (lipoid CAH) was shown to result from mutations in the *StAR* gene [see this volume, and refs. (*17* and *18*)]. This disease is characterized by marked impairment of steroid hormone synthesis in the gonads and adrenals. The discovery of mutations in the *StAR* gene established a critical role of StAR in steroidogenesis. Confirmation of StAR's role in steroidogenesis was derived from the generation of a StAR knockout mouse that had a phenotype that parallels the human lipoid CAH (*19*).

StAR EXPRESSION AND StAR HOMOLOGS

The cloning of the human StAR cDNA and then the structural gene for StAR permitted extensive study of the gene's expression and insight into the protein's mechanism of action. The expression of StAR is directly correlated with steroidogenic activity in adrenal and gonadal cells (*13,20*). Human StAR mRNA is expressed in adult adrenal, ovary and testis as a major transcript of approx 1.6 kb, and lesser transcripts of 4.4 and 7.5 kb. The approx 1.6-kb transcript is expressed at low levels in the kidney (site of Vitamin D 1α hydroxylation) (*16*). No StAR mRNA was detected in human brain, liver, or placenta, the latter of which is consistent with the observation that placental steroidogenesis is StAR-independent. In accordance with this finding, pregnancies hosting fetuses affected with congenital lipoid CAH progress to term, demonstrating adequate placental progesterone production despite the fact that the placenta is an organ of fetal origin.

A possible explanation for StAR-independent steroidogenesis in the placenta is the existence of a StAR-like protein in this organ, which subserves StAR's function. *MLN64*, first identified as a gene highly expressed in certain breast cancers, is also expressed in placenta and brain, two tissues that produce steroid hormones, but do not contain detectable StAR mRNA (*21*). *MLN64* was found to have a carboxy terminus with strong homology to StAR (*21*). Moreover, *MLN64* sequences corresponding to essential domains in StAR were found to stimulate steroidogenesis in COS cells cotransfected with the cholesterol side-chain cleavage enzyme. Western blot analysis revealed that *MLN64* fragments representing domains of *MLN64* that are most similar to StAR and which displayed the greatest steroidogenic activity in COS cells were present in placenta and choriocarcinoma cells (*20*). Thus, a family of StAR-like proteins may exist that are expressed in a tissue-specific manner, and differentially regulated, promoting steroidogenesis in diverse cell types. Since other proteins sharing homology with the C-terminus of StAR have been identified, and the StAR motif has been named the START domain for StAR-related lipid transfer domains. Since those observations, the crystal structure of the "START domain" has been determined, demonstrating a hydrophobic tunnel structure capable of binding one molecule of cholesterol (*21a*).

TRANSCRIPTIONAL REGULATION

The human structural gene for StAR was mapped to chromosome 8p11.2 and spans 8 kb (*16,22*). The *StAR* structural gene consists of seven exons and six introns. A mutated *StAR* pseudogene, residing on chromosome 13, has been detected by reverse-transcribed polymerase chain reaction (RT-PCR) from testicular mRNA (*16*). The significance of this transcript is unknown, but it would not be expected to encode a functional StAR protein.

Cyclic AMP analogs stimulate *StAR* gene transcription by a process that can require ongoing protein synthesis *(20)*. The StAR promoter lacks cAMP-responsive elements (CRE) like several other steroidogenic enzyme gene promoters *(22,23)* and cyclic AMP-responsiveness of the StAR promoter was shown to be conferred by steroidogenic factor-1 (SF-1/AdBP4), an orphan member of the nuclear hormone receptor superfamily of transcription factors. SF-1 binding sites are present in the promoters of many of the genes encoding steroidogenic enzyme and they have been shown to confer cAMP-responsiveness to these promoters. SF-1 was shown to render the StAR promoter cAMP-responsive in the context of cells that do not express endogenous SF-1 (i.e., BeWo choriocarcinoma cells, HeLa cells, and SK-OV-3 cells).

Three SF-1 binding elements in the 5′-flanking region of the gene were identified *(24,25)*. These response elements were protected by SF-1 in DNase 1 footprint analysis and bound GST-SF-1 fusion protein in electrophoretic mobility-shift assays. The two proximal SF-1 response elements were shown to be critical for StAR promoter function in human granulosa-lutein cells, cells which express SF-1 and respond to cAMP with increased transcription of the endogenous *StAR* gene. Mutation of either element substantially reduced basal and forskolin-stimulated promoter activity. Mutation of the distal SF-1 binding site reduced basal, but not forskolin-stimulated, promoter activity in the granulosa-lutein cells. These findings demonstrated that multiple SF-1 response elements are required for maximal StAR promoter activity and for regulation by cAMP. The mechanism by which SF-1 confers cAMP-responsiveness at each of these sites, and the potential regulators of SF-1 function (i.e., ligands, other protein cofactors) are under investigation.

The *StAR* gene promoter also contains two *cis* elements that are responsive to CCAAT/enhanced-binding proteins (C/EBPs) *(27)*. One of these elements was shown to bind C/EBP β present in granulosa-lutein cell nuclear extracts. When this site was mutated, StAR promoter activity in granulosa-lutein cells was reduced, but the mutated promoter still showed a twofold increase in promoter activity in response to 8-Br-cAMP. 8-Br-cAMP treatment was shown to increase granulosa-lutein cell C/EBP β levels, explaining in part the requirement for ongoing protein synthesis for cAMP-induced *StAR* gene transcription in these cells. Therefore, part of the augmentation of *StAR* gene expression by trophic hormones encompasses signaling mediated by C/EBP β on top of the action of SF-1.

There is probably a role for Sp1 response elements in the StAR promoter in the transcriptional response to cAMP. Sp1 response elements are known to be important in conferring cAMP-responsiveness to other steroidogenic enzyme promoters *(26)*. It is noteworthy that Sp1 acts as a cofactor for the sterol regulatory element binding proteins (SREBPs) a family of ubiquitously expressed transcription factors essential for the regulation of many proteins important in the synthesis and metabolism of lipids. We have found that coexpression of SREBP1α increases in StAR promoter activity *(28)*.

Another member of the nuclear hormone receptor superfamily, *DAX*-1, has been implicated in the negative regulation of *StAR* gene expression. Mutations in the human *DAX*-1 gene cause X-linked adrenal hypoplasia congenita. *DAX*-1 was shown to repress both basal and cAMP-induced StAR promoter activity *(29)*. It has been suggested that *DAX*-1 inhibits *StAR* gene expression by binding to SF-1 or by directly binding to the StAR promoter.

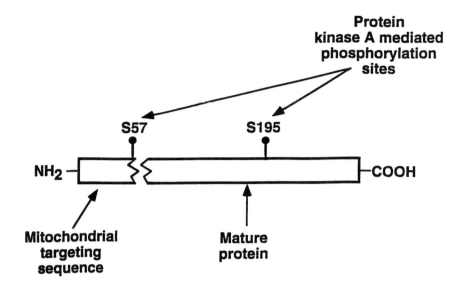

Fig. 1. Schematic of StAR protein structure. The 285 amino acid StAR protein has an amino acid terminal mitochondrial targeting sequence and two serine residues that serve as targets for protein kinase A (PKA-mediated phosphorylation. StAR phosphorylation is important for maximal steroidogenic activity. StAR import into mitochondria leads to cleavage of the targeting sequence.

StAR STRUCTURE AND FUNCTION

The human StAR cDNA encodes a 285 amino acid protein that migrates at approx 37 kDa on SDS polyacrylamide gels. The StAR protein sequence is highly conserved, exhibiting 85–88% identity and greater than 90% similarity among the species thus far compared (mouse, human, hamster, rat, cow, sheep, and pig). The protein contains putative phosphorylation sites for protein kinase A (PKA), CAM kinase, protein kinase C, creatine kinase, and P34CDC2 kinase. The amino terminal 33 amino acids of the predicted polypeptide possess a high-net positive charge and the potential to form an amphipathic helical structure typical of mitochondrial signal sequences (*see* Fig. 1). The murine protein contains an amino terminal R-X-Z-X-X-S sequence (where X is any amino acid and Z is a hydrophobic residue), characteristic of signal sequences cleaved by mitochondrial processing peptidase, although the serine residue at amino acid 43 is not conserved in the human. Both murine and human StAR proteins have been shown to be efficiently processed by mitochondria of steroidogenic and nonsteroidogenic tissues *(15,30)*. Whereas mitochondrial import and processing were formerly thought to be essential to StAR function, recent data suggest that mitochondrial importation may contribute to StAR inactivation and is unnecessary for cholesterol transport (Fig. 2). Physical studies on recombinant StAR protein suggests that it is a molten globule, a dynamic protein structure that lacks fixed interactions that would constrain the folded polypeptide chain organization *(31)*. The molten globule configuration appears at pH 3.5–4.0, a pH that may be generated in the immediate vicinity of mitochondria. The molten globule configuration may facilitate the unfolding of the protein in preparation for action on the mitochondria and the protein's subsequent movement through the import pore into the mitochondrial matrix.

Insight regarding StAR function has been provided from studies using a heterologous

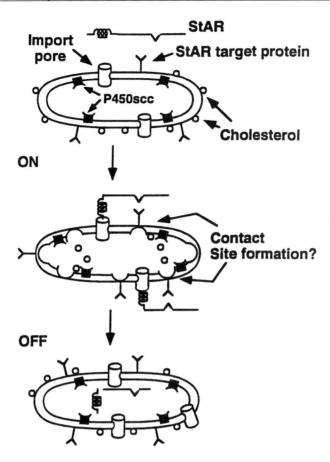

Fig. 2. Potential mechanisms of StAR function. StAR preprotein interacts with the outer mitochondrial membrane and transiently activates cholesterol transport to the inner mitochondrial membrane by promoting cholesterol desorption from the sterol-rich outer membrane to the sterol-poor inner membrane. Cholesterol may move through pre-existing contact sites or contact sites formed in response to StAR action. Cholesterol then serves as the substrate for P450scc, which catalyzes pregnenolone formation. The StAR protein is rapidly imported, and, therefore, rendered inactive for cholesterol transport. Cleavage of the StAR mitochondrial signal sequence following import into the mitochondria forms the mature 30-kDa protein.

cell-model system for steroidogenesis *(16)*. In this system, COS-1 cells (transformed monkey kidney cells) are transfected with a plasmid containing a fusion gene of cytochrome $P450_{scc}$, adrenodoxin, and adrenodoxin reductase establishing the mitochondrial enzyme system required for production of pregnenolone. These cells, which do not respond to trophic stimulation, can be cotransfected with a StAR expression plasmid, resulting in a fourfold or more increase in steroid production. This confirmation of StAR's role in steroid production was followed by experiments using truncation mutants of the *StAR* gene *(30,32)*. Surprisingly, these studies demonstrated that the amino terminus of StAR (up to N-62 amino acids and including the mitochondrial targeting sequence) were expendable for StAR function. Using the transfected cells, as well as in vitro import assays with isolated mitochondria, it was demonstrated that the amino terminal deletion, as predicted, abrogates StAR import without interfering with StAR's stimulatory effect on steroidogenesis. Moreover, certain patients with lipoid CAH have been shown to produce a mutant StAR protein that, although functionally inactive, is efficiently imported into mitochondria. This finding can be taken as further evidence that the process of StAR importation can be dissociated from StAR's steroidogenic action.

Carboxy terminal truncation mutants were also examined in the COS cell system. Removal of the terminal 28 amino acids inactivated StAR, and deletion of the C-terminal 10 amino acids reduced steroidogenic activity by approx 50%. These observations demonstrated the importance of the StAR C-terminal domains in the protein's action. The emerging picture of StAR structure and function is that the biological action of the protein is encoded in the C-terminus whereas the targeting function is encoded in the N-terminus.

How does StAR promote sterol translocation to the side-chain cleavage enzyme? Recombinant StAR protein lacking the first 62 amino acid residues encompassing the mitochondrial targeting sequence stimulated pregnenolone synthesis by isolated bovine corpus luteum mitochondria in a dose-dependent fashion *(30)*. A recombinant protein in which the A218V mutation was introduced that inactivates StAR function was unable to stimulate mitochondrial pregnenolone formation. These data suggest that StAR molecules, which are import incompetent, can stimulate steroidogenesis.

Using cholesterol-enriched phospatidylcholine vesicles as a donor and various organelles as acceptors, it was shown that N-62 recombinant StAR stimulates cholesterol transfer from sterol-rich donors to the sterol-poor acceptors, whereas the A218V mutant recombinant protein did not *(33)*. The StAR-mediated sterol movement could not be attributed to fusion of donor and acceptor membranes. The recombinant "wild-type" protein could not promote phospholipid transfer, revealing a selective lipid transfer activity. The interpretation of these findings is that StAR promotes cholesterol desorption from the sterol-rich membranes, driving it to sterol-poor acceptor membranes. This action of StAR evidently does not require a high-affinity StAR receptor because the protein can function in a vesicle-accceptor system. The organelle specificity of this lipid transfer activity of StAR is determined by the mitochondrial targeting sequence, which assures the efficient and rapid movement of the protein to its site of action.

StAR PHOSPHORYLATION

Comparison of the StAR protein sequences from multiple species has demonstrated two consensus motifs for protein kinase A (PKA) phosphorylation located at serine 57 and serine 195 in the human protein *(34)*. Cyclic AMP is a known activator of PKA, qualifying these sites as potential candidates for modulation of StAR activity via PKA-mediated phosphorylation. Alkaline phosphatase treatment of StAR-expressing COS-1 cell lysates resulted in loss on two acidic species noted by two-dimensional gel electrophoresis *(34)*. Moreover, ^{32}P was incorporated into StAR protein immunoprecipitated from COS-1 cell extracts, and treatment with 8-bromo-cAMP increased ^{32}P incorporation into the StAR preprotein. StAR protein generated by in vitro transcription/translation was phosphorylated by the protein kinase A catalytic subunit in the presence of $[\gamma\text{-}^{32}P]$ ATP. ^{32}P incorporation was diminished by mutation of these serine residues to alanines, both in COS-1 cell transfection experiments and using protein generated by in vitro transcription/translation incubated with the PKA catalytic subunit. These data are consistent with a role for PKA in StAR phosphorylation.

To assess the functional significance of StAR phosphorylation at these residues, the steroidogenic activity of the wild-type StAR and serine to alanine mutants was tested in COS-1 cells transfected with *P450*$_{scc}$. Mutation of the conserved PKA target site at serine 57 had no effect on pregnenolone synthesis, whereas mutation at residue 195 resulted in approx 50% reduction in steroid production. Mutation of serine 195 to an aspartic acid resulted in slightly increased StAR activity in the COS-1 cells, consistent with the notion that negative charge at this site, via phosphorylation or otherwise, enhances StAR function. These observations suggest that phosphorylation of serine 195 increases the biological activity of StAR and that this post- or cotranslational event accounts, in part, for the immediate effects of cAMP on steroid production.

CONCLUSION

The overwhelming evidence to date suggests that StAR is the "labile factor" produced in adrenal and gonadal cells in response to trophic stimulation that is responsible for cholesterol transport to the side-chain cleavage system. The StAR preprotein is synthesized in response to trophic hormones and to their downstream effector cAMP. The action of cAMP on StAR expression is mediated in part by SF-1 and augmented by other transcription factors including C/EBPβ. StAR has a short functional half-life, accounting for the rapid inhibitory effects of cycloheximide and other protein synthesis inhibitors on steroidogenesis. The StAR protein is phosphorylated by PKA, and possibly by other kinases, and PKA-mediated phosphorylation is essential for maximal steroidogenic activity. StAR acts on the mitochondrial outer membrane and is then imported and processed to the mature protein. The rapid mitochondrial import appears to account for the short functional half-life of StAR. The mechanisms by which StAR promotes cholesterol translocation appears to involve the ejection of sterol from the relatively sterol-rich outer mitochondrial membrane to the relatively sterol-poor inner membrane.

REFERENCES

1. Rennert H, Chang YJ, Strauss JF III. Intracellular cholesterol dynamics related to steroid hormone synthesis: a contemporary view. In: Adashi EY and Leung PCK, eds., The Ovary, New York. 1993, p. 147.
2. Toaff ME, Schleyer H, Strauss JF III. Presence of a low molecular weight inhibitor of succinate-supported cholesterol side chain cleavage in rat ovaries. Biochim Biophys Acta 1980; 617:291.
3. Tuckey RC, Atkinson HC. Pregnenolone synthesis from cholesterol and hydroxycholesterols by mitochondria from ovaries following the stimulation of immature rats with pregnant mare's serum gonadotropin and human choriogonadotropin. Eur J Biochem 1989; 186:255–259.
4. Gwynne JT, Strauss JF III. The role of lipoproteins in steroidogenesis and cholesterol metabolism in steroidogenic glands. Endocr Rev 1982; 3:299–329.
5. Tuckey RC, Stevenson PM. Cholesterol esterase and endogenous cholesterol ester pools in ovaries from maturing and superovulated immature rats. Biochim Biophys Acta 1980; 618:501–509.
6. Vahouny GV, Chanderbhan R, Noland BJ, Scallen TJ. Cholesterol ester hydrolase and sterol carrier proteins. Endocr Res 1984; 10:473–505.
7. Hall PF. The roles of calmodulin, actin, and vimentin in steroid synthesis by adrenal cells. Steroids 1997; 62:185–189.
8. Hall PF, Almahbobi G. Roles of microfilaments and intermediate filaments in adrenal steroidogenesis. Microsc Res Tech 1997; 36:463–479.
8a. Watari H, Blanchette-Mackie EJ, Dwyer NK, et al. NPCI-containing compartment of human granulosa-lutein cells: a role in the intracellular trafficking of cholesterol supporting steroidogenesis. Exp Cell Res 2000; 255:56–66.

9. Waterman MR, Simpson ER. Steroidogenic capacity in the adrenal cortex and its regulation. Prog Drug Res 1990; 34:359–381.

10. Ferguson JJ. Protein synthesis and adrenocorticotropin responsiveness. J Biol Chem 1963; 238:2754–2759.

11. Garren LD, Ney RL, Davis WW. Studies on the role of protein synthesis in the regulation of corticosterone production by adrenocorticotropic hormone in vivo. Proc Natl Acad Sci USA 1965; 53:1443–1450.

12. Privalle CT, Crivello JF, Jefcoate CR. Regulation of intramitochondrial cholesterol transfer to side-chain cleavage cytochrome P-450 in rat adrenal gland. Proc Natl Acad Sci USA 1983; 80:702–706.

13. Stocco DM, Clark BJ. Regulation of the acute production of steroids in steroidogenic cells. Endocr Rev 1996; 17:221–244.

14. Krueger RJ, Orme-Johnson NR. Acute adrenocorticotropic hormone stimulation of adrenal corticosteroidogenesis. Discovery of a rapidly induced protein. J Biol Chem 258; 1983; 10,159–10,167.

15. Clark BJ, Wells J, King SR, Stocco DM. The purification, cloning, and expression of a novel luteinizing hormone-induced mitochondrial protein in MA-10 mouse Leydig tumor cells. Characterization of the steroidogenic acute regulatory protein (StAR). J Biol Chem 1994; 269:28,314–28,322.

16. Sugawara T, Holt JA, Driscoll D, Strauss JF III, Lin D, Miller WL, et al. Human steroidogenic acute regulatory protein: functional activity in COS-1 cells, tissue-specific expression, and mapping of the structural gene to 8p11.2 and a pseudogene to chromosome 13. Proc Natl Acad Sci USA 1995; 92:4778–4782.

17. Lin D, Sugawara T, Strauss JF III, Clark BJ, Stocco DM, Saenger P, et al. Role of steroidogenic acute regulatory protein in adrenal and gonadal steroidogenesis. Science 1995; 267:1828–1831.

18. Bose H, Sugawara T, Strauss JF III, Miller WL. Genetics and pathophysiology of congenital lipoid adrenal hyperplasia. N Engl J Med 1996; 335:1870–1878.

19. Caron KM, Soo SC, Wetsel WC, Stocco DM, Clark BJ, Parker KL. Targeted disruption of the mouse gene encoding steroidogenic acute regulatory protein provides insights into congenital lipoid adrenal hyperplasia. Proc Natl Acad Sci USA 1997; 94:11,540–11,545.

20. Kiriakidou M, McAllister JM, Sugawara T, Strauss JF III. Expression of steroidogenic acute regulatory protein (StAR) in the human ovary. J Clin Endocrinol Metab 1996; 82:1776.

21. Watari H, Arakane F, Moog-Lutz C, Kallen CB, Tomasetto G, Gerton GL, et al. MLN64 contains a domain with homology to the steroidogenic acute regulatory protein (StAR) that stimulates steroidogenesis. Proc Natl Acad Sci USA 1997; 94:8462–8467.

21a. Tsujshita Y, Hurley JH. Structure and lipid transport mechanism of a StAR-related lipid transport domain. Nature Structure Biol 2000; 7:4080–414.

22. Sugawara T, Lin D, Holt JA, Martin KO, Javitt NB, Miller WL, Strauss JF III. Structure of the human steroidogenic acute regulatory protein (StAR) gene: StAR stimulates mitochondrial cholesterol 27-hydroxylase activity. Biochemistry 1995; 34:12506–12512.

23. Waterman MR. Biochemical diversity of the cAMP-dependent transcription of the steroid hydroxylase genes in the adrenal cortex. J Biol Chem 1994; 269:27783–27786.

24. Sugawara T, Holt JA, Kiriakidou M, Strauss JF III. Steroidogenic factor 1-dependent promoter activity of the human steroidogenic acute regulatory protein (StAR) gene. Biochemistry 1996; 35:9052–9059.

25. Sugawara T, Kiriakidou M, McAllister JM, Kallen CB, Strauss JF III. Multiple steroidogenic factor 1 binding elements in the human steroidogenic acute regulatory protein gene 5′-flanking region are required for maximal promoter activity and cyclic AMP responsiveness. Biochemistry 1997; 36:7249–7255.

26. Christenson LK, Johnson PF, McAllister JM, Strauss III JF. CCAAT/enhancer-binding proteins regulate expression of the human steroidogenic acute regulatory protein (StAR) gene. J Biol Chem 1999; 274:26591–26598.

27. Momoi K, Waterman MR, Simpson ER, Zanger UM. 3′,5′-cyclic adenosine monophosphate-dependent transcription of the CYP11A (cholesterol side chain cleavage cytochrome P450) gene involves a DNA response element containing a putative binding site for transcription factor Spl. Mol Endocrinol 1992; 6:1682–1690.

28. Christenson LK, McAllister JM, Martin K, Javitt NB, Osborne TF, Strauss JF III. Oxysterol regulation of steroidogenic acute regulatory protein (StAR) gene expression: structural specificity, transcriptional and post-transcriptional actions. J Biol Chem 1998; 273:30,729–30,735.

29. Zazopoulos E, Lalli E, Stocco DM, Sassone-Corsi P. DNA binding and transcriptional repression by DAX-1 blocks steroidogenesis. Nature 1997; 390:311–315.

30. Arakane F, Kallen CB, Watari H, Foster JA, Sepuri NBV, Pain D, et al. The mechanism of action of steroidogenic acute regulatory protein (StAR): StAR acts on the outside of mitochondria to stimulate steroidogenesis. J Biol Chem 1998; 273:16,339–16,345.

31. Bose HS, Whittal RM, Baldwin MA, Miller WL. The active form of the steroidogenic acute regulatory protein, StAR, appears to be a molten globule. Proc Natl Acad Sci USA 1999; 96:7250–7255.

32. Arakane F, Sugawara T, Nishino H, Liu Z, Holt JA, Pain D, et al. Steroidogenic acute regulatory protein (StAR) retains activity in the absence of its mitochondrial import sequence: implications for the mechanism of StAR action. Proc Natl Acad Sci USA 1996; 93:13,731–13,736.

33. Kallen CB, Billheimer JT, Summers SA, Stayrook S, Lewis M, Strauss JF III. Steroidogenic acute regulatory protein (StAR) is a sterol transfer protein. J Biol Chem 1998; 273:16,339–16,943.

34. Arakane F, King SR, Du Y, Kallen CB, Walsh LP, Watari H, et al. Phosphorylation of steroidogenic acute regulatory protein (StAR) modulates its steroidogenic activity. J Biol Chem 1997; 272:32,656–32,662.

8 Regulation of Adrenocortical Function by the Sympathoadrenal System

Physiology and Pathology

Monika Ehrhart-Bornstein and Stefan R. Bornstein

CONTENTS

INTRODUCTION

In the first complete description of the adrenal gland in 1852, von Kölliker described the adrenal as composed of two different tissues, with the cortex belonging to the "blood-vascular glands" and the medulla, a part of the nervous system, resembling a ganglion *(1)*. The astonishing arrangement of these two tissues justifies the question: What is a ganglion doing inside a gland *(2)?*

It is now generally accepted that adrenocortical steroids influence the differentiation of adrenomedullary cells from norepinephrine-producing neuronal precursor cells toward epinephrine-producing adrenomedullary chromaffin cells. Steroids not only induce the production of epinephrine [for review, *(3)*], they also direct the phenotypic development of adrenal chromaffin cells ([for review, *(4)*]. Therefore, the location of the adrenal medulla within a steroid-producing endocrine gland appears to be essential for the development and function of chromaffin cells. However, multiple lines of evidence in recent years suggest that the interaction between the two parts of the adrenal is not a

From: *Contemporary Endocrinology: Adrenal Disorders*
Edited by: A. N. Margioris and G. P. Chrousos © Humana Press, Totowa, NJ

one-way street, but rather, bidirectional *(5)*. Indeed, the influence of the sympathoadre-nomedullary system on the adrenal cortex includes its diurnal variations of steroidogene-sis, which depends on the integrity of the sympathetic innervation *(6–8)*. Neural input also appears to mediate the compensatory growth of the remaining adrenal following unilateral adrenalectomy [for review, *(9)*]. These effects of the adrenal medulla on the cortex may be associated to alterations of the sensitivity of the latter to adrenocortico-tropin (ACTH) because splanchnic nerve stimulation has been shown to enhance the production of glucocorticoids in response to ACTH *(10)*. Indeed, sections of both splanchnic nerves, in lambs, decreases adrenocortical sensitivity to ACTH *(11)*. In addition, it now appears that splanchnic innervation may be also able to stimulate adrenocortical steroidogenesis in the absence of pituitary ACTH. Thus, in isolated perfused porcine, adrenal glands with intact splanchnic innervation steroidogenesis could be stimulated independently of the hypothalamus-pituitary-adrenal (HPA) axis through electrical activation of the sympathoadrenal system *(12–15)*, indicating an ACTH-independent effect of sympathetic innervation on adrenocortical function. Thus, the "ganglion" in the middle of a steroid-producing endocrine gland appears to be an important local regulator of its function.

INNERVATION OF THE ADRENAL CORTEX

Neuroendocrine regulation of this type may depend on neurotransmitters released from nerve endings on the adrenal cortex. Indeed, the adrenal cortex receives innerv-ations from two different sources *(16)*. Some nerves have their cell bodies located outside the adrenal and reach the cortex with the blood vessels. These are regulated independently from the splanchnic innervation of the gland. Other neurons originate in cell bodies located within the adrenal medulla *(16,17)* and may be regulated by splanchnic nerve activity. These adrenal nerves are mainly catecholaminergic, as well as peptidergic storing catecholamines (dopamine, epinephrine, and norepinephrine) and a wide variety of neuropeptides including opioids, calcitonin-gene-related peptide (CGRP), neuropeptide Y (NPY), vasoactive intestinal polypeptide (VIP), corticotropin-releasing hormone (CRH), and substance P in the same secretory granules [for review *(5)*]. All these neurotransmitters and neuropeptides have been shown to modulate adrenocortical function.

INVOLVEMENT OF THE ADRENAL MEDULLA

The adrenomedullary chromaffin cells synthesize and secrete neurotransmitters and neuropeptides under splanchnic control. It has been shown that the main adrenomedul-lary secretory products, the catecholamines epinephrine and norepinephrine, stimulate mammalian adrenocortical function in perfused adrenals *(12,14)* and of adrenocortical cells in primary culture, via transcriptional regulation of steroid-producing enzymes *(18,19)*. In isolated cells, the possibility of intra–adrenal interactions and effects of epinephrine on adrenal vasculature have been excluded. Thus, it appears that catechola-mines released from the adrenal medulla stimulate adrenocortical steroidogenesis in a direct mode of action being responsible for the observed activation of the mammalian adrenal cortex following stimulation of the sympathoadrenal system.

Serotonin (5-HT), a neurotransmitter also produced in the adrenal medulla of several species, influences the activity of the adrenal cortex *(20–23)*. Indeed, 5-HT stimulates corticosteroid production at the adrenocortical level in several animal models [for review, *(24)*], as well as that of humans *(25,26)*.

As aforementioned, adrenomedullary chromaffin cells also produce, store, and secrete a whole series of neuropeptides, including enkephalins, CGRP, NPY, neurotensin, galanin, substance P, vasopressin, oxytocin, VIP, somatostatin, PACAP, and POMC [for review, *(5)*]. Several of these peptides influence adrenocortical steroid production in many species. The effect of adrenomedullary neuropeptides on steroidogenesis varies from stimulation to inhibition. Some neuropeptides synthesized in chromaffin cells influence predominantly the release of mineralocorticoids in the zona glomerulosa. This correlates well with morphological observations confirming the presence of chromaffin cell accumulations in the subcapsular area of *zona glomerulosa (27–30)*. Some peptides appear to exert different effects on adrenal cortex depending on the system used, i.e., if it is in vivo or in vitro. The action of these peptides most probably depends on intact adrenal architecture. Indeed, increasing evidence exists for an indirect influence of several peptides, such as PACAP *(31)* and VIP *(32,33)* on adrenocortical function via the release of catecholamines from the medulla.

Coculture of bovine adrenomedullary chromaffin cells with bovine adrenocortical cells have supplied direct evidence for a paracrine influence of chromaffin cells on adrenocortical cells. In these systems, adrenocortical and medullary cells are separated by semipermeable membranes. We could show that secretory products released from chromaffin cells under basal conditions are potent stimulators of adrenocortical steroidogenesis. This stimulatory effect is independent of a direct cell–cell contact *(34)*.

It is now well established that catecholamines and neuropeptides are costored and coreleased from the same secretory granules [for review, *(35,36)*]. If adrenomedullary secretory products are able to differentially stimulate or inhibit adrenocortical function, mechanisms should exist that differentially regulate the synthesis and the release of each of these peptides. In fact, it now appears that multiple populations of chromaffin cells exist within the adrenal medulla each different on its peptide composition *(37,38)*. The differential expression of adrenomedullary proteins and peptides seems to be the result of a concerted action of neurogenic and humoral factors of different origin. Indeed, each stressor stimulates certain subtypes of adrenomedullary cells *(39)*. The neurotransmitters released from splanchnic nerves could be involved in the regulation of this differential biosynthesis *(40–42)*. In reciprocity, it is the adrenal cortex that influences the differentiation of adrenomedullary cells. Glucocorticoids not only promote differentiation of adrenomedullary cells with respect to their catecholamine content, but also with respect to the formation of peptides and proteins like enkephalins, and chromogranins *(40,43,44)*. A third set of potential regulators of adrenomedullary differentiation are immune factors like interleukin 1 (IL-1) and tumor necrosis factor (TNF)-alpha *(45)*. Interestingly, IL-1 alpha and TNF-alpha that differentially regulate Met-enkephalin, VIP, neurotensin, and substance P biosynthesis in chromaffin cells *(45)* are locally produced by adrenocortical cells, as well as by resident immune cells *(46–48)*. In the human adrenal, these cytokines are mainly produced by cells of the adrenocortical zone, which are in direct contact with the adrenal medulla, i.e., the *zona reticularis (46,47)*. Thus, a regulatory circuit seems to exist within the adrenal. In addition to the influence of adrenocortical steroids on the differentiation of adrenomedullary cells, the adrenal cortex may also influence the peptide composition of chromaffin granules by releasing cytokines. Adrenomedullary secretory products, in turn, are able to differentially stimulate or inhibit adrenocortical function.

HOW DO ADRENOMEDULLARY SECRETORY PRODUCTS REACH THE ADRENAL CORTEX?

The accepted "text book" view, based on routine histological investigations in the adult mammalian adrenal, holds that the two different endocrine tissues are clearly separated in an outer steroid-producing cortex and a central medulla (49–51). However, this concept of adrenal gland anatomy is not supported by morphological characteristics. In fact, the cells of the adrenal medulla and the adrenal cortex are significantly interwoven in many mammals, including humans. Indeed, adrenomedullary chromaffin cells can be found in all zones of the adult adrenal cortex. Some form ray-like structures stretching from the adrenal medulla through the entire cortex (27,28,52,53). There are also chromaffin cells appearing as islets or even single cells located in the zona fasciculata and reticularis, as identified by immunohistochemical staining, surrounded by steroid-producing cells. In the zona glomerulosa, chromaffin cells spread frequently into the subcapsular region, forming nests of cells (27–30). The occurrence of these adreno-medullary chromaffin cells in the adrenal cortex may be caused by the embryologic development of the adrenal. In humans, chromaffin precursor cells start to invade the adrenal at week 6 GA [(54,55) and references therein]. Chromaffin cells located in the cortex probably derive from cells whose migration to the medulla has stopped prematurely. On the other hand, cortical cells are present within the adrenal medulla. A rime of cortical cells is present around the bigger vessels, as well as isolated accumulations of cells embedded in the surrounding chromaffin tissue some connected to the adrenal cortex. In fact, the adrenal medulla appears, in part, to be peppered with cortical cells (29,56). Within the human adrenal, these cortical islets are composed of cells from all three cortical zones (Fig. 1). Ultrastructural analyses of the contact zones in all three zones of the adrenal cortex revealed that cortical and chromaffin cells are opposed to each other without separation by connective tissue or interstitium (29,56,57). This intimate intermingling of the two cell types allows extensive contact zones for paracrine interaction.

In addition to a direct paracrine action, some adrenomedullary secretory products may reach the adrenal cortex via interstitial fluid and lymphatics. Small molecules such as catecholamines appear to enter the blood vessels directly and, therefore, can only influence adrenocortical cells, which are in direct contact to a chromaffin cell. Larger molecules, such as proteins and neuropeptides appear to pass via the interstitial space into the lymph and may, via this route, reach adrenocortical cells (58).

SYMPATHOADRENAL REGULATION OF ADRENAL BLOOD FLOW

In addition to the direct effect of chromaffin cells on adrenocortical cells, adrenocortical innervation and adrenomedullary secretory products may be involved in the regulation of adrenal blood flow and, thus, influence the adrenocortical cells in an indirect manner. Indeed, the mammalian adrenal cortex is a highly vascularized organ and it has been shown that adrenal blood flow is affected by splanchnic nerves (59,60). In the rat adrenal gland, glucocorticoid secretion is closely linked to blood flow (61,62).

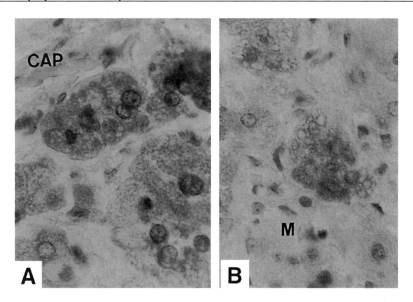

Fig. 1. Paraffin section of human adrenal immunostained for angiotensin II type 1 receptor (Ang II R1). **(A)** Cells of the *zona glomerulosa* located in the subcapsular area and **(B)** *zona glomerulosa* cells located in the adrenal medulla are stained. CAP: adrenal capsule, M: adrenal medulla.

Neurons containing vasoactive factors like catecholamines, VIP and NPY *(16,63)* and adrenomedullary cells *(27,28,30,53)* that are able to produce vasoactive substances are concentrated in the area of the subcapsular arteriolar plexus. This plexus may be responsible for the regulation of blood flow through the adrenal gland *(64)* and evidence exists that the adrenal blood flow rate may be regulated in part by several neuropeptides including VIP, substance P, NPY, neurotensin, and enkephalins released from the capsular region of the adrenal gland in response to splanchnic nerve stimulation *(65)*. In conclusion, neurotransmitters and neuropeptides appear to regulate adrenocortical cell function via two distinct mechanisms: a direct action on adrenocortical cells and indirectly by regulation of blood flow.

CLINICAL IMPLICATIONS

Is a neuroadrenocortical interaction within the adrenal gland relevant to human physiology and pathophysiology? It is well-established that the adrenal cortex is mainly regulated by pituitary ACTH, and hypophysectomy leads to atrophy of the adrenal cortex. On the other hand, it has been known for many years that individuals given dexamethasone in doses large enough to suppress pituitary function are able to respond to major stresses by increasing their endogenous glucocorticoid production *(66)*. Furthermore, in patients with proven pituitary ACTH deficiency, CRH induced a significant increase in plasma cortisol, preceded by a rise in plasma ACTH *(67)*, indicating the involvement of an extrapituitary, perhaps intraadrenal CRH/ACTH-system. It is also of interest, that the mechanism of adrenal stimulation in diabetic patients may be not mediated entirely by the pituitary, because there is a diminished pituitary response to metapyrone *(68)*. Therefore, in some extreme instances the production of adrenal steroids may be regulated not by the hypothalamus-pituitary axis, but by local factors. In

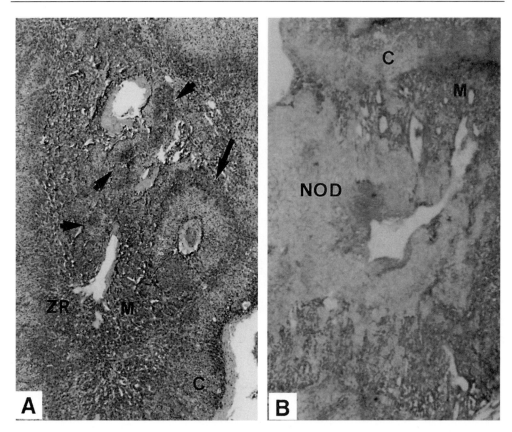

Fig. 2. (A) Paraffin section of human adrenal. The *zona reticularis* (ZR) was immunostained for MHC class II, which is specifically expressed by *reticularis* cells in the human adrenal *(84,85).* Besides adrenocortical tissue around large blood vessels (large arrow), the adrenal medulla (M) is interspersed with small adrenocortical islets (small arrows). **(B)** Human adrenal from a patient with an adrenocortical nodule. Adrenomedullary chromaffin tissue is immunostained for chromogranin A. The adrenocortical nodule was originating from cortical cells located in the medulla. C: normal cortex, M: adrenal medulla, immunostained for chromogranin A, NOD: adrenocortical nodule (reproduced from ref *86).*

addition, a clear discrepancy between pituitary ACTH production and adrenal-steroid release also occurs in several physiological situations *(69–71),* during the development of the adrenal gland and in puberty *(72)* suggesting the existence of additional regulatory mechanisms.

As aforementioned, in human adrenals, adrenomedullary and adrenocortical tissues are extensively intermingled *(56).* This provides the anatomical basis for a close cell-to-cell interaction allowing for a close coordination of the two stress systems. Interestingly, cells of all three zones of the cortex are present in the human adrenal medulla (Fig. 1). The occurrence of adrenocortical cells within the medulla has direct consequences during isolation of adrenomedullary tissue for autologous transplantation to the caudate nucleus as a treatment in patients suffering from Parkinson's disease. As pointed out by Carmichael et al. *(73),* it is especially important to minimize the percentage of cortical cells and to remove these islets in the surgical preparations because

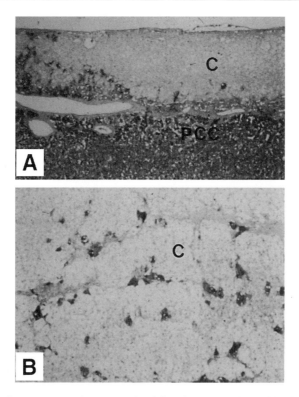

Fig. 3. Human pheochromocytoma immunostained for chromogranin A. (**A,B**) The remnant cortex is infiltrated by pheochromocytoma tumor cells with close cellular interaction of pheochromocytes with adrenocortical cells. PCC: pheochromocytoma, C: adrenal cortex.

cortical steroids may stimulate the conversion of dopamine to epinephrine and, thus, compromise the beneficial effect of the implantation.

Another important observation is the apparently frequent origination of adrenal nodules and adenoma from cortical islets in the medulla (Fig. 2). It therefore seems that these islets being under the direct influence of the surrounding adrenomedullary tissue may be at a higher risk to develop pathological characteristics compared to cortical cells located in the adrenal cortex.

Some recent observations have suggested that the intraadrenal interactions may be responsible for the pathology of the adrenal cortex in addition to the regulation of adrenocortical function in different physiological situations. Clinical case reports describe patients presenting clinically with adrenocortical hyperfunction where the histopathological investigation reveals a pheochromocytoma (74–76). Indeed, some Cushing's syndromes may be caused by ectopic production of ACTH in pre-existing pheochromocytoma [(77) and literature herein]). However, also non-ACTH-mediated Cushing's syndromes may exist in patients with pheochromocytoma (78). In these cases, adrenocortical hyperfunction probably is caused by the stimulatory effect of an adrenomedullary secretory product not related to ACTH. In the adrenals of patients with controversial clinical and pathological features, the adrenal cortex often is invaded by pheochromocytes (Fig. 3). The stimulation of adrenocortical function in these cases could be due to the stimulatory influence of secretagogs released from the pheochromo-cytoma. On the other hand, corticotropin-independent Cushing's syndrome may be the result of an aberrant expression or an overresponsiveness of receptors for secretagogs released from the adrenal medulla, such as β-receptors *(79)*, vasopressin receptors *(80)*, or IL-1 receptors *(81)*. In addition a case has been described where Cushing's syndrome was caused by a member of the glucagon/VIP peptide family, gastric inhibitory polypeptide *(82)*.

CONCLUSIONS

The adrenal medulla appears to exert important paracrine regulatory effects on the adrenal cortex. It is thus possible that a cortical–chromaffin cell interaction is crucial in the response of the adrenal gland to stress and the overall adaptive mechanisms [reviewed in *(83)*], as well as in the pathophysiology of the adrenal gland.

ACKNOWLEDGMENT

Work done in the author's laboratory was supported by the Willhelm Sander-Stiftung (Grant 95.033.1 to M.E.-B.), by the Deutsche Forschungsgemeinschaft (DFG Grant Bo 1141/2-2 to S.R.B.), and by the Bundesministerium für Bildung, Forschung und Technologie (BMBF), Interdisciplinary Center for Clinical Research at the University of Leipzig (IZKF Project B1).

REFERENCES

1. von Kölliker A. Handbuch der Gewebelehre des Menschen. Leipzig, 1852.
2. Carmichael SW. What is a ganglion doing inside a gland? IBRO News 1989; 17:6.
3. Axelrod J, Reisine TD. Stress hormones: their interaction and regulation. Science 1984; 224:452–459.
4. Hofmann HD, Seidl K, Unsicker K. Development and plasticity of adrenal chromaffin cells: clues based on in vitro studies. J Electron Microsc Tech 1989; 12:397–407.
5. Ehrhart-Bornstein M, Hinson JP, Bornstein SR, Scherbaum WA, Vinson GP. Intraadrenal interactions in the regulation of adrenocortical steroidogenesis. Endocr Rev 1998; 19:101–143.
6. Ottenweller JE, Meier AH. Adrenal innervation may be an extrapituitary mechanism able to regulate adrenocortical rhythmicity in rats. Endocrinology 1982; 111:1334–1338.
7. Dijkstra I, Binnekade R, Tilders FJH. Diurnal variation in resting levels of corticosterone is not mediated by variation in adrenal responsiveness to adrenocorticotropin but involves splanchnic nerve integrity. Endocrinology 1996; 137:540–547.
8. Jasper MS, Engeland WC. Splanchnic neural activity modulates ultradian and circadian rhythms in adrenocortical secretion in awake rats. Neuroendocrinology 1994; 59:97–109.
9. Dallman MF. Control of adrenocortical growth in vivo. Endocr Res 1984; 10:213–242.
10. Edwards AV, Jones CV. The effect of splanchnic nerve stimulation on adrenocortical activity in conscious calves. J Physiol 1987; 382:385–396.
11. Edwards AV, Jones CT, Bloom SR. Reduced adrenal cortical sensitivity to ACTH in lambs with cut splanchnic nerves. J Endocrinol 1986; 110:81–85.
12. Bornstein SR, Ehrhart-Bornstein M, Scherbaum WA, Pfeiffer EF, Holst JJ. Effects of splanchnic nerve stimulation on the adrenal cortex may be mediated by chromaffin cells in a paracrine manner. Endocrinology 1990; 127:900–906.
13. Ehrhart-Bornstein M, Bornstein SR, Scherbaum WA, Pfeiffer EF, Holst JJ. The role of the vasoactive intestinal peptide in a neuroendocrine regulation of the adrenal cortex. Neuroendocrinology 1991; 54:623–628.
14. Ehrhart-Bornstein M, Bornstein SR, Güse-Behling H, Stromeyer H, Scherbaum WA, Adler G, Holst JJ. Sympathoadrenal regulation of adrenal androstenedione release. Neuroendocrinology 1994; 59:406–412.

15. Ehrhart-Bornstein M, Bornstein SR, González-Hernández JA, Holst JJ, Waterman MR, Scherbaum WA. Sympathoadrenal regulation of adrenocortical steroidogenesis. Endocr Res 1995; 21:13–24.

16. Holzwarth MA, Cunningham LA, Kleitman N. The role of adrenal nerves in the regulation of adrenocortical functions. Ann NY Acad Sci 1987; 512:442–464.

17. Kesse WK, Parker TL, Coupland RE. The innervation of the adrenal gland: I. The source of pre- and postganglionic nerve fibers to the rat adrenal gland. J Anat 1988; 157:33–41.

18. Ehrhart-Bornstein M, Bornstein SR, Trzeciak WH, Usadel H, Güse-Behling H, Waterman MR, Scherbaum WA. Adrenaline stimulates cholesterol side chain cleavage cytochrome P450 mRNA accumulation in bovine adrenocortical cells. J Endocrinol 1991; 131:R5–R8.

19. Güse-Behling H, Ehrhart-Bornstein M, Bornstein SR, Waterman MR, Scherbaum WA, Adler G. Regulation of adrenal steroidogenesis by adrenaline: Expression of cytochrome P450 genes. J Endocrinol 1992; 135:229–237.

20. Ritzén M, Hammerström L, Ullberg S. Autoradiographic distribution of 5-hydroxytryptamine and 5-hydroxytryptophan in the mouse. Biochem Pharmacol 1965; 14:313–383.

21. Holzwarth MA, Brownfield MS. Serotonin coexists with epinephrine in rat adrenal medulla. Neuroendocrinology 1985; 41:230–236.

22. Verhofstad AAJ, Jonsson G. Immunohistochemical and neurochemical evidence for the presence of serotonin in the adrenal medulla of the rat. Neuroscience 1983; 10:1443–1453.

23. Delarue C, Leboulenger F, Morra M, Héry F, Verhofstad AAJ, Bérod A, et al. Immunohistochemical and biochemical evidence for the presence of serotinin in amphibian adrenal chromaffin cells. Brain Res 1988; 459:17–26.

24. Contesse V, Delarue C, Leboulenger F, Lefebvre H, Héry F, Vaudry H. Serotonin produced in the adrenal gland regulates corticosteroid secretion through a paracrine mode of communication. In: Facchinetti F, Henderson IW, Pieratoni R, Polzonetti-Magni A, eds. Cellular Communication in Reproduction. J Endocrinol Ltd. Bristol, 1993, pp. 187–198.

25. Lefebvre H, Contesse V, Delarue C, Feuilloley M, Hery F, Grise P, et al. Serotonin-induced stimulation of cortisol secretion from human adrenocortical tissue is mediated through activation of a serotonin-4 receptor subtype. Neuroscience 1992; 47:999–1007.

26. Lefebvre H, Contesse V, Delarue C, Soubrane C, Legrand A, Kuhn J, et al. Effect of the serotonin-4 receptor agonist zacopride on aldosterone secretion from human adrenal cortex: in vivo and in vitro studies. J Clin Endocrinol Metab 1993; 77:1662–1666.

27. Fortak W, Kmiec B. [About occurrence of the chromophilic cells in the adrenal cortex of white rats]. Endokrynol Pol 1968; 19:117–128.

28. Gallo-Payet N, Pothier P, Isler H. On the presence of chromaffin cells in the adrenal cortex: their possible role in adrenocortical function. Biochem Cell Biol 1987; 65:588–592.

29. Bornstein SR, Ehrhart-Bornstein M, Usadel H, Böckmann M, Scherbaum WA. Morphological evidence for a close interaction of chromaffin cells with cortical cells within the adrenal gland. Cell Tissue Res 1991; 265:1–9.

30. Berka JL, Kelly DJ, Robinson DB, Alcorn D, Marley PD, Fernley RT, Skinner SL. Adrenaline cells of the rat adrenal cortex and medulla contain renin and prorenin. Mol Cell Endocrinol 1996; 119:175–184.

31. Neri G, Andreis PG, Prayer-Galetti T, Rossi GP, Malendowicz LK, Nussdorfer GG. Pituitary adenylate-cyclase activating peptide enhances aldosterone secretion of human adrenal gland: evidence for an indirect mechanism, probably involving the local release of catecholamines. J Clin Endocrinol Metab 1996; 81:169–173.

32. Hinson JP, Kapas S, Orford CD, Vinson GP. Vasoactive intestinal peptide stimulation of aldosterone secretion by the rat adrenal cortex may be mediated by the local release of catecholamines. J Endocrinol 1992; 133:253–258.

33. Bornstein SR, Haidan A, Ehrhart-Bornstein M. Cellular communication in the neuroadrenocortical axis: role of vasoactive intestinal polypeptide (VIP). Endocr Res 1996; 22:819–829.

34. Haidan A, Bornstein SR, Glasow A, Uhlmann K, Lübke C, Ehrhart-Bornstein M. Basal steroidogenic activity of adrenocortical cells is increased tenfold by co-culture with chromaffin cells. Endocrinology 1998; 139:772–780.

35. Winkler H, Apps DK, Fischer-Colbrie R. The molecular function of adrenal chromaffin granules: established facts and unresolved topics. Neuroscience 1986; 18:261–290.

36. Carmichael SW. Cytochemistry of the adrenal medulla. In: Ogawa K and Barka T, eds. Electron Microscopic Cytochemistry and Immunocytochemistry in Biomedicine. CRC Press, Boca Raton, FL, 1993, pp. 562–583.

37. Siegel RE, Eiden LE, Pruss RM. Multiple populations of neuropeptide-containing cells in cultures of the bovine adrenal medulla. Brain Res 1985; 349:267–270.

38. Linnoila RI, Diaugustine RP, Hervonen A, Miller RJ. Distribution of [Met^5]- and [Leu^5]-enkephalin-, vasoactive intestinal polypeptide- and substance P-like immunoreactivities in human adrenal glands. Neuroscience 1980; 5:2247–2259.

39. Vaupel R, Jarry H, Schlomer HT, Wuttke W. Differential response of substance P-containing subtypes of adrenomedullary cells to different stressors. Endocrinology 1988; 123:2140–2145.

40. Fischer-Colbrie R, Iacangelo A, Eiden LE. Neural and humoral factors separately regulate neuropeptide Y, enkephalin, and chromogranin A and B mRNA levels in rat adrenal medulla. Proc Natl Acad Sci USA 1988; 85:3240–3244.

41. Pruss RM, Mezey E, Forman DS, Eiden LE, Hotchkiss AJ, Di Maggio DA, et al. Enkephalin and neuropeptide Y: two colocalized neuropeptides are independently regulated in primary cultures of bovine chromaffin cells. Neuropeptides 1986; 7:315–327.

42. Tschernitz C, Laslop A, Eiter C, Kroesen S, Winkler H. Biosynthesis of large dense-core vesicles in PC12 cells: effects of depolarization and second messengers on the mRNA levels of their constituents. Brain Res Mol Brain Res 1995; 31:131–140.

43. Sietzen M, Schober M, Fischer-Colbrie R, Scherman D, Sperk G, Winkler H. Rat adrenal medulla: levels of chromogranins, enkephalins, dopamine beta-hydroxylase and of the amine transporter are changed by nervous activity and hypophysectomy. Neuroscience 1987; 22:131–139.

44. Inturrisi CE, Branch AD, Robertson HD, Howells RD, Franklin SO, Shapiro JR, et al. Glucocorticoid regulation of enkephalins in cultured rat adrenal medulla. Mol Endocrinol 1988; 2:633–640.

45. Eskay RL, Eiden LE. Interleukin-1α and tumor necrosis factor-α differentially regulate enkephalin, vasoactive intestinal polypeptide, neurotensin, and substance P biosynthesis in chromaffin cells. Endocrinology 1992; 130:2252–2258.

46. González-Hernández JA, Bornstein SR, Ehrhart-Bornstein M, Geschwend JE, Gwosdow AR, Jirikowski GF, et al. Interleukin 1 is expressed in human adrenal gland in vivo. Possible role in a local immune-adrenal axis. Clin Exp Immunol 1995; 99:137–141.

47. González-Hernández JA, Ehrhart-Bornstein M, Späth-Schwalbe E, Scherbaum WA, Bornstein SR. Human adrenal cells express TNFα-mRNA: evidence for a paracrine control of adrenal function. J Clin Endocrinol Metab 1996; 81:807–813.

48. Judd AM, Mac Leod RM. Differential release of tumor necrosis factor and II-6 from adrenal zona glomerulosa cells in vitro. Am J Physiol 1995; 268:E114–20.

49. Landsberg L, Young JB. Williams Textbook of Endocrinology. Saunders, Philadelphia, PA, 1992, p. 624.

50. Orth DN, Kovacs WJ, DeBold CR. The adrenal cortex. In: Wilson JD and Foster DW, eds. Williams Textbook of Endocrinology. Saunders, Philadelphia, PA, 1992; pp. 489–619.

51. Rittmaster RS, Cutler GBJ. Morphology of the adrenal cortex and medulla. In: Becker KL, ed. Principles and Practice of Endocrinology and Metabolism. Lippincott, Philadelphia, PA; 1990, pp. 572–579.

52. Kmiec B. Histologic and histochemical observations on regeneration of the adrenal medulla after enucleation in white rats. Folia Morphol (Warsz) 1968; 27:238–245.

53. Nussdorfer GG. Cytophysiology of the adrenal cortex. Int Rev Cytol 1986; 98:1–395.

54. Ehrhart-Bornstein M, Breidert M, Guadanucci P, Wozniak W, Bocian-Sobkowska J, Malendowicz LK, et al. 17α-Hydroxylase and chromogranin A in 6th week human fetal adrenals. Horm Metab Res 1997; 29:30–32.

55. Molenaar WM, Lee V-M, Trojanowski JQ. Early fetal acquisition of the chromaffin and neuronal immunophenotype by human adrenal medulary cells. An immunohistological study using monoclonal antibodies to chromogranin A, synaptophysin, tyrosin hydroxilase and neuronal cytoskeletal proteins. Exp Neurol 1990; 108:1–9.

56. Bornstein SR, González-Hernández JA, Ehrhart-Bornstein M, Adler G, Scherbaum WA. Intimate contact of chromaffin and cortical cells within the human adrenal gland forms the cellular basis for important intraadrenal interactions. J Clin Endocrinol Metab 1994; 78:225–232.

57. Bornstein SR, Ehrhart-Bornstein M. Ultrastructural evidence for a paracrine regulation of the rat adrenal cortex mediated by the local release of catecholamines from chromaffin cells. Endocrinology 1992; 131:3126–3128.

58. Carmichael SW, Stoddard SL, O'Connor DT, Yaksh TL, Tyce GM. The secretion of catecholamines, chromogranin A and neuropeptide Y from the adrenal medulla of the cat via the adrenolumbar vein and thoracic duct: different anatomic routes based on size. Neuroscience 1990; 34:433–440.

59. Engeland WC, Gann DS. Splanchnic nerve stimulation modulates steroid secretion in hypophysecto-mized dogs. Neuroendocrinology 1989; 50:124–131.

60. Engeland WC, Lilly MP, Gann DS. Sympathetic adrenal denervation decreases adrenal blood flow without altering the cortisol response to hemorrhage. Endocrinology 1985; 117:1000–1010.

61. Hinson JP, Vinson GP, Whitehouse BJ. The relationship between perfusion medium flow rate and steroid secretion in the isolated perfused rat adrenal gland. J Endocrinol 1986; 111:391–396.

62. Vinson GP, Hinson JP. Blood flow and hormone secretion in the adrenal gland. In: James VHT, ed. The Adrenal Gland. Raven, New York, 1992; pp. 71–86.

63. Vizi ES, Toth IE, Szalay KS, Windisch K, Orso E, Szabo D, et al. Catecholamines released from local adrenergic axon terminals are possibly involved in fine-tuning of steroid secretion from zona glomerulosa cells: functional and morphological evidence. J Endocrinol 1992; 135:551–561.

64. Vinson GP, Pudney JA, Whitehouse BJ. The mammalian adrenal circulation and the relationship between adrenal blood flow and steroidogenesis. J Endocrinol 1985; 105:285–294.

65. Hinson JP, Cameron LA, Purbrick A, Kapas S. The role of neuropeptides in the regulation of adrenal vascular tone: effects of vasoactive intestinal polypeptide, substance P, neuropeptide Y, neurotensin, Met-enkephalin, and Leu-enkephalin on perfusion medium flow rate in the intact perfused rat adrenal. Regul Peptides 1994; 51:55–61.

66. Liddle GW, Estep HL, Kendall Jr JW, Williams Jr WC, Townes AW. Clinical application of a new test of pituitary reserve. J Clin Endocrinol 1959; 19:875–894.

67. Fehm HL, Holl R, Späth-Schwalbe E, Born J, Voigt KH. Ability of corticotropin releasing hormone to simulate cortisol secretion independent from pituitary adrenocorticotropin. Life Sci 1988; 42:679–686.

68. Lentle BC, Thomas JP. Adrenal function and the complications of diabetes mellitus. Lancet II; 1964; 544–549.

69. Krieger DT. Plasma ACTH and corticosteroids. In: Groot LJ, Cahill GF, Martini L, Nelson DH, Odell WD, Potts JT, et al., eds. Endocrinology, vol. 2. Grune and Stratton, New York, 1979; pp. 1139–1156.

70. Fehm HL, Klein E, Holl R, Voigt KH. Evidence for extrapituitary mechanisms mediating the morning peak of plasma cortisol in man. J Clin Endocrinol Metab 1984; 58:410–414.

71. Fehm HL, Steiner K, Klein E, Voigt KH. Evidence for ACTH-unrelated mechanisms in the regulation of cortisol secretion in man. Klin Wochenschr 1984; 62:19–24.

72. Parker LN, Odell WD. Control of adrenal androgen secretion. Endocr Rev 1980; 1:392–410.

73. Carmichael SW, Stoddard SL, Kelly PJ. Technical aspects of transplantation of the adrenal medulla to the caudate nucleus as a treatment for Parkinson's disease. Meth Neurosci 1994; 21:272–277.

74. LeCompte PM. Cushing's syndrome with possible pheochromocytoma: report of a case. Am J Pathol 1944; 20:689–707.

75. Mathison DA, Waterhouse CA. Cushing's syndrome with hypertensive crisis and mixed adrenal cortical adenoma-pheochromocytoma (cortico-medullary adenoma). Am J Med 1969; 47:635–641.

76. Kovacs K, Horvath E. Ultrastructural features of corticomedullary cells in a human adrenal cortical adenoma and in rat adrenal cortex. Anat Anz 1973; 134:387–389.

77. Wajchenberg BL, Mendonca BB, Liberman B, Pereira MAA, Kirschner MA. Ectopic ACTH syndrome. J Steroid Biochem Mol Biol 1995; 53:139–151.

78. Khoo DHC, Fok ACK, Tan L, Cheng C, Wong KS. Non-ACTH mediated Cushing's syndrome in a patient with phaechromocytoma. 10th Int. Congress Endocrinology, San FranciscoP3-582 (Abstract).

79. Lacroix A, Tremblay J, Rousseau G, Bouvier M, Hamet P. Propranolol therapy for ectopic β-adrenergic receptors in adrenal Cushing's syndrome. N Engl J Med 1997; 337:1429–1434.

80. Perraudin V, Delarue C, De Keyzer Y, Bertagna X, Kuhn J-M, Contesse V, et al. Vasopressin-responsive adrenocortical tumor in a mild Cushing's syndrome: in vivo and in vitro studies. J Clin Endocrinol Metab 1995; 80:2661–2667.

81. Willenberg HS, Stratakis CA, Marx C, Ehrhart-Bornstein M, Chrousos GP, Bornstein SR. Aberrant interleukin-1 receptor in a cortisol-secreting adrenal adenoma causing Cushing's syndrome. N Engl J Med 1998; 339:27–31.

82. Lacroix A, Bolté E, Tremblay J, Dupré J, Poitras P, Fournier H, et al. Gastric inhibitory polypeptide-dependent cortisol hypersecretion—a new cause of Cushing's syndrome. N Engl J Med 1992; 327:974–980.

83. Chrousos GP. Organization and integration of the endocrine system. In: Sperling M, ed. Pediatric Endocrinology. Saunders, Philadelphia, PA 1996, pp. 1–14.

84. Khoury EL, Greenspan JS, Greenspan FS. Adrenocortical cells of the zona reticularis normally express HLA-DR antigenic determinants. Am J Pathol 1987; 127:580–591.

85. Marx C, Wolkersdörfer GW, Brown J, Scherbaum WA, Bornstein SR. MHC class II expression—A new tool to assess dignity in adrenocortical tumours. J Clin Endocrinol Metab 1996; 81:4488–4491.
86. Bornstein SR, Stratakis CA, Chrousos GP. Adrenocortical tumors: recent advances in basic concepts and clinical management. Ann Intern Med 1999; 130:757–765.

9

Interleukin (IL)-1 Family of Cytokines and Corticotropin-Releasing Hormone (CRH) in the Adrenal Gland

Andrew N. Margioris, Erene Dermitzaki, Maria Venihaki, and Achille Gravanis

CONTENTS

INTRODUCTION

It is now well-established that the interleukin (IL)-1 family of cytokines initiates the acute immune response and, at the same time and in order to adapt the organism to the stress of inflammation, activates the two stress axes, i.e., the hypothalamus-pituitary-adrenal (HPA) and the sympathetic. The initiation of the stress response by the IL-1 cytokines takes place centrally, at the central nervous system. There, the IL-1 cytokines stimulate the production of corticotropin-releasing hormone (CRH) in the parvocellular part of the paraventricular hypothalamic nucleus and the production of norepinephrine in hypothalamus and locus ceruleus.

Based on multiple lines of data, it now appears that the interaction between the IL-1

From: *Contemporary Endocrinology: Adrenal Disorders*
Edited by: A. N. Margioris and G. P. Chrousos © Humana Press, Totowa, NJ

cytokines and the stress axes also takes place at a more peripheral level. At this level, the effect of IL-1 cytokines does not aim in the adaptation of the whole organism to the inflammatory response, but rather in the participation of local regulatory networks for a tissue-specific "fine-tuning." A second characteristic of the immune–stress systems interaction, at this level, is the bidirectional character of this interaction, i.e., the latter can modify the production and/or the release of local cytokines. The adrenal gland can be viewed as an example of this peripheral interaction. Thus, the IL-1 cytokines and CRH, which have been shown to be produced within the adrenals by several types of parenchymal cells and resident macrophages, form a complex paracrine network within the gland also composed by other cytokines, catecholamines, locally produced neuropeptides (adrenocorticotropic hormone (ACTH), endogenous opioids, substance P, and so on), corticoids, and prostaglandins. This paracrine network takes the role of a local microregulator of the production and secretion of glucocorticoids and adrenal catecholamines (1–3).

THE IL-1 FAMILY OF CYTOKINES

The IL-1 family of cytokines is produced by activated monocytes/macrophages during the acute phase of inflammatory response. The IL-1 cytokines are also produced by a variety of other cells including neutrophils, keratinocytes, epithelial cells, fibroblasts, and adrenal cortical and medullary cells. The cytokines interleukin (IL)-1α and IL-1β have a 25% homology in amino acids. The biological action of IL-1 cytokines is the result of their binding to the IL-1 receptor-type 1 (Rt1). A second IL-1 receptor, the IL-1Rt2 does not produce any biological effect and most probably represents a "decoy receptor." A third member of the IL-1 family of cytokines is the IL-1 receptor antagonist (ra), which exhibits the same affinity toward both types of IL-1 receptors, but lacks any agonistic activity (4,5). By alternative splicing of its immature transcript, two forms of IL-1ra are obtained, the sIL-1ra, which is secretable and thus biologically active, and icIL-1ra, which is confined within the intracellular space because it lacks a signal sequence for secretion (5,6). Coexpression of the two forms of IL-1ra has been demonstrated only in human fibroblasts and glioblastoma cells (7,8). As it is expected, the inhibitory effect of IL-1ra is accomplished via its binding to the type 1 IL-1R.

In addition to their role in initiating inflammation, the IL-1 cytokines also activate the two stress axes at the level of the central nervous system in order to adapt the organism to the arising inflammatory response. Indeed, the IL-1 cytokines stimulate the synthesis and secretion of hypothalamic CRH (9–13) and the production of norepinephrine, dopamine, and serotonin from anterior hypothalamus (14) and locus ceruleus. Finally, the IL-1 cytokines exert a wide variety of other noninflammatory effects on the peripheral components of the two stress systems including effects on adrenal cortex and medulla and the peripheral sympathetic system.

THE ADRENAL GLAND PRODUCES IL-1 CYTOKINES

The IL-1 cytokines are produced by several types of cells within the adrenal gland:

IL-1 in the Cortex

In humans, the combination of *in situ* hybridization and immunostaining have shown that IL-1β is mainly localized in the cortical 17α-hydroxylase positive steroid-producing cells of the *zona reticularis* surrounding the adrenomedullary cells *(15,16)*. To our knowledge, there is no localization study regarding the IL-1α and IL-1ra in the adrenal cortex.

IL-1 in the Medulla

The production of IL-1 cytokines from adrenomedullary chromaffin cells is cell-specific, meaning that each type of IL-1 cytokine is produced by a distinct type of chromaffin cell. It should be mentioned here that chromaffin cells can be distinguished into adrenaline- and noradrenaline-producing. *In situ* hybridization analysis of bovine and ovine adrenals with probes complementary to the coding region of bovine phenylethanolamine N-methyltransferase (PNMT) proenkephalin A mRNA shows that the adrenaline producing cells are localized in the outer cell layer of the adrenal medulla and that these cells also produce proenkephalin A, precursor of the delta type of endogenous opioids *(17)*. The noradrenaline (i.e., PNMT-negative) cells are concentrated at the center of the gland and most probably produce prodynorphin, the precursor of the endogenous kappa type of opioids *(18)*. The two types of chromaffin cells also differ in several other characteristics. Thus, tetraethylammonium chloride is more effective in stimulating catecholamine synthesis and secretion from primary cultures of noradrenaline-rich (noradrenergic, i.e., PNMT-negative) cells compared to adrenaline-rich (adrenergic) bovine chromaffin cells *(19)*.

As far as adrenal IL-1 cytokines are concerned, the following pattern has emerged: the IL-1α cytokine is present only in adrenergic PNMT-positive chromaffin cells; its synthesis is induced by cholinergic stimulation *(20)*. On the other hand, the IL-1β mRNA and protein, although detectable in adrenal chromaffin cells *(16,21)*, are mainly confined in the noradrenergic (i.e., PNMT-negative) chromaffin cells, at least in rodents *(9,19,22)*. *In situ* hybridization experiments have demonstrated that the IL-1β-producing cells, concentrated as it was described in the inner-medullary zone can be stimulated by bacterial lipopolysacharides (LPS). They respond by increasing their synthesis of IL-1β *(21)*. The strongest hybridization signal is seen after 1.5 h of exposure decreasing to basal at 3 h. By comparison, the production of preproenkephalin A mRNA peaks later suggesting that the IL-1 cytokines act as mediators of the LPS effect on this opioid precursor. Finally, the IL-1ra cytokine is detectable mainly in the adrenergic PNMT-positive chromaffin cells and to a lesser degree in the noradrenergic (PNMT-negative) cells *(23)*.

IL-1 in Resident Macrophages

Most of the adrenal CD68+ macrophages are located in the cortex close to the adrenal medulla. As expected, they produce large quantities of all IL-1 cytokines *(15,16)*.

IL-1 in Pheochromocytomas

Immunoreactive IL-1α and its transcript are present in the PC12 rat pheochromocytoma cell line; their production is induced by NGF *(11)*. The IL-1 transcripts and proteins are also present in human pheochromocytoma cells *(24,25)*. NGF induces the expression of the IL-1a gene in PC12 cells via the TrkA receptor pathway *(26)*. It is suggested that the ability of factors like NGF to affect IL-1 synthesis signifies the importance of the latter as growth factors. Indeed, the IL-1 cytokines promote glial cell proliferation and induce the expression of NGF at the sites of peripheral nerve injury.

THE ADRENAL GLAND PRODUCES CRH

CRH is the principal stimulator of the HPA stress axis, the final product of which is the synthesis and secretion of glucocorticoids from the adrenal cortex. CRH is a 41-amino acid neuropeptide produced by the parvocellular cells of the paraventricular hypothalamic nucleus. It is stored into secretory vesicles in the median eminence from where it is secreted in the portal circulation, reaches the anterior pituitary corticotrophs, binds to its receptors, and stimulates the synthesis of proopiomelanocortin (POMC) and the secretion of ACTH. The synthesis of hypothalamic CRH is regulated negatively by glucocorticoids and positively by several neuropeptides and neurotransmitters. The expression of the *CRH* gene is regulated by a variety of second messengers, the most important of which is cAMP. Indeed, a cAMP-responsive element has been localized in the promoter region of the *CRH* gene.

In addition to its effects on the HPA axis, CRH exerts a host of other effects within the central nervous system including stimulation of the catecholaminergic stress axis, inhibition of hypothalamic GnRH production (and thus suppression of the hypothalamus-pituitary-gonadal axis), and multiple behavioral effects including regulation of appetite.

Regarding the catecholaminergic system, CRH activates it, but it is also activated by catecholamines in a self-potentiating loop, which is interrupted by glucocorticoids. More specifically, in microdialysate experiments using catheterized conscious and freely moving rats, it has been demonstrated that CRH stimulates the release of catecholamines from the anterior and medial hypothalamus, medial prefrontal cortex, hippocampal dentate gyrus, and locus ceruleus *(27–30)*. The CRH antagonist ahCRH blocks this effect, suggesting the mediation of CRH receptors *(30)*. In addition to its effect on catecholamine release, CRH also affects their synthesis because it has been shown that it stimulates the transcription of tyrosine hydroxylase, the principal enzyme of catecholamine synthesis *(31–33)*. Indeed, it now appears that the effect of CRH on catecholamine synthesis is much more biologically important than its effect on catechol-amine secretion. The stimulatory effect of CRH on catecholamine production appears to be exerted via paracrine pathways because there is a very close anatomical proximity between CRH and noradrenergic neurons in the locus ceruleus *(34–37)*. CRH also affects the synthesis of dopamine in the central nervous system. Indeed, CRH stimulates the synthesis of synaptosomal dopamine in rat and mouse striatum in vitro, via the activation of tyrosine hydroxylase *(31–32)*. Similarly, the administration of CRH to humans in vivo causes a delayed increase of the plasma levels of homovanillinic acid, the major dopamine metabolite *(33)*.

CRH is also produced by the adrenal chromaffin cells of most species. Indeed, production of CRH has been documented in normal human adrenal medulla *(38–41)*, the adrenal medulla of rodents *(2,10,42–44)*, cows *(45–47)*, and dogs *(48,49)*. The production of CRH by the adrenals of such a wide variety of species suggests that it most probably plays an important role within the gland. The identification of specific CRH-binding sites within the adrenal gland supports this hypothesis *(50,51)*. Indeed, CRH induces the synthesis of epinephrine from normal primate and rodent adrenal chromaffin cells *(44,50)*. This effect of CRH is most probably mediated by a CRH receptor because the CRH antagonist ahCRH blocks it.

The ability of chromaffin cells to synthesize CRH is retained following their transfor-mation to pheochromocytomas *(39–41, 52–55)*. Indeed, the presence of the CRH transcript and its peptide product have been documented in primary cultures of human pheochromocytomas *(56)*, the PC12 rat pheochromocytoma cell line *(44)*, and the human pheochromocytoma KAT45 cell line *(57)*. CRH stimulates the synthesis of dopamine from the PC12 rat pheochromocytoma cells, and norepinephrine from KAT45 human pheochromocytoma cells.

IL-1 CYTOKINES STIMULATE HYPOTHALAMIC CRH

One of the major leaps in our understanding of the interaction between the immune system and the stress axes took place in the late 80s when it was proven that the IL-1 cytokines exert a direct stimulatory effect on the synthesis and secretion of hypothalamic CRH *(58,59)*. As it will be mentioned later, this effect of IL-1 cytokines is retained in several peripheral neural and no-neural sites including the adrenal gland. The IL-1 cytokines also affect the production of other neuropeptides from the adrenal medulla including vasoactive intestinal polypeptide (VIP), the delta endogenous opioid agonist met-enkephalin *(60)*, the kappa opioid agonist dynorphin, and POMC-derived peptides such as is the ACTH *(57)*. The production of neurotensin and substance P appears not to be affected by the IL-1 cytokines.

IL-1 CYTOKINES STIMULATE THE ADRENAL CORTEX

The IL-1 cytokines directly stimulate adrenal steroidogenesis. Thus, in rats, IL-1 stimulates adrenal production of corticosterone *(61)* without inducing any significant increase of the level of circulating ACTH suggesting a direct effect on adrenal cells or the existence of an alternative ACTH-independent pathway through which the IL-1 cytokines accomplish their stimulatory effect on glucocorticoid production *(62)*. Indeed, it now appears that the IL-1 cytokines stimulate the production of epinephrine from the PNMT-positive adrenal chromaffin cells located in the outer-medullary layer in the vicinity of adrenal cortical cells. Subsequently, epinephrine stimulates the production of glucocorticoids from cortical cells via α-adrenergic receptors on the surface of the steroid-producing. Indeed, the presence of the α-adrenergic antagonist phentolamine inhibits the IL-1-stimulated release of corticosterone *(61,63)*, whereas propranolol (β-adrenergic antagonist) does not have any effect. As it could be expected from the fact that the IL-1 cytokines exert a direct effect on adrenal medulla, phentolamine and propranolol have no effect on ACTH stimulated corticosterone release *(64)*. To make matters more complicated, the stimulatory effect of IL-1 on corticosterone production is completely blocked by αhCRF suggesting that the direct effect of IL-1 on the adrenal gland involves activation of the intra-adrenal CRH system *(62)*. Indeed, rat adrenal medullary cells respond to IL-1 by increasing their release of ACTH and CRH, in addition to catecholamines *(2)*. The IL-1 cytokines also stimulate the synthesis of CRH and ACTH from PC12 rat pheochromocytoma *(44)* and from KAT45 human pheochromocytoma cells *(57)* suggesting that this sequence of events is preserved in pheochromocytomas. However, hypercortisolemia in adrenaline-producing human pheochromocytomas is not so widespread as these data might suggest *(57)*. In conclusion, the following hypothetical sequence of events may take place within the adrenal gland following exposure to IL-1 cytokines: the latter stimulate the production of norepineph-rine and CRH from the inner-medullary chromaffin cells. CRH, and/or other neuropeptides (ACTH ?) stimulate the production of epinephrine from the outer-zone chromaffin cells which, in turn, via α-adrenergic receptors on the surface of cortical cells in the *zona fasciculata* induces the production of glucocorticoids.

The IL-1 cytokines also stimulate the production of prostaglandins from primary cultures of rat adrenal cells *(61)*. However, the stimulatory effect of IL-1 cytokines on corticosterone is independent of prostaglandin production *(61)*. The significance of IL-1-induced prostaglandin production, in the adrenal gland, is currently unknown.

General conclusion: it now appears that the IL-1 cytokines can stimulate the production of glucocorticoids by at least three pathways: through the stimulation of hypothalamic CRH and the resulting activation of the HPA axis, through the direct activation of the intra-adrenal CRH-ACTH axis, and through the stimulation of a catecholamine-dependent and prostaglandin-independent pathway.

IL-1 CYTOKINES STIMULATE THE CENTRAL CATECHOLAMINERGIC SYSTEM

The IL-1 cytokines enhance norepinephrine turnover in hypothalamus and hippocampus, serotonin turnover in hippocampus and prefrontal cortex, and dopamine utilization in the prefrontal cortex *(65)*. The IL-1-mediated activation of the noradrenergic innervation of the paraventricular nucleus represents part of the mechanism by which the IL-1 cytokines stimulate hypothalamic CRH *(66)*. The augmented norepinephrine turnover following exposure to IL-1 is demonstrable only in whole hypothalami and in several specific hypothalamic nuclei and not in other central nervous system areas such as is the medulla oblongata and cerebral cortex suggesting that the effect of IL-1 cytokines is site-specific and, thus, physiologically relevant. The IL-1-induced increase in hypothalamic norepinephrine is blocked by pretreatment with either indomethacin (cyclooxygenase inhibitor) or anticorticotropin-releasing hormone antibody, but not by naloxone indicating the involvement of prostaglandins and CRH, but not opioids. Indeed, it appears that IL-1 activates noradrenergic neurons projecting to the hypothalamus and that CRH and eicosanoid-cyclooxygenase products within the brain are involved in this process *(67,68)*.

IL-1 CYTOKINES STIMULATE THE PERIPHERAL CATECHOLAMINERGIC SYSTEM

Multiple lines of evidence suggest that the IL-1 cytokines stimulate the peripheral part of the catecholaminergic system, although some authors report the opposite *(69)*. Indeed, the IL-1 cytokines accelerate norepinephrine turnover in the spleen, lung, diaphragm, and pancreas *(67,68)*. The sympathetic outflow to the spleen is an interesting model. More specifically, norepinephrine recovered in splenic dialysates is mainly derived from terminals of splenic sympathetic nerves. Intraperitoneal injection of IL-1β produces an immediate increase in the recovered norepinephrine *(70,71)*. The CRF antagonist αhCRF attenuates the IL-1β-induced norepinephrine recovery suggesting the mediation of CRH *(71)*. In similarity to the central catecholaminergic system, some of the effects of IL-1 cytokines on the peripheral catecholaminergic system are mediated by prostaglandins *(72)*. Thus, it now becomes clear that the stimulatory effects of IL-1 cytokines in both central and peripheral catecholaminergic systems involves CRH and prostaglandins.

IL-1 CYTOKINES STIMULATE THE PRODUCTION OF ADRENAL CATECHOLAMINES

Multiple lines of evidence indicate that the functional type of IL-1 receptors, the IL-1t1, is present in the adrenal gland of several species localized mainly in the medulla, suggesting that IL-1 cytokines exert local effects. However, *in situ* hybridization of mouse adrenals with an antisense cRNA probe for the IL-1t1 receptor has been reported as negative *(73)*. As mentioned above, in similarity to the central and peripheral catecholaminergic systems, the IL-1 cytokines also stimulate the production of catecholamines from the adrenal gland. Thus, in bovine adrenals, both IL-1α and IL-1β increase the production of epinephrine following a 24-h exposure *(13,64)*. This effect involves stimulation of catecholamine synthesis because the IL-1 cytokines induce the production of aromatic L-amino acid decarboxylase mRNA, an essential step in their synthetic pathway *(12)*. Furthermore, in vivo experiments have shown that IL-1β (given intravenously) results in an increase of catecholamine levels in systemic circulation *(72)*, an effect attributed to a direct action on the adrenal medulla because the IL-1 crossing of the blood brain barrier is limited and the intracerebroventricular injection of IL-1β produces mainly fever and minimal, if any, elevation of systemic catecholamines *(72)*. Interestingly, it has been recently reported that human mononuclear cells produce factors that stimulate the production of catecholamines from primary cultures of porcine adrenomedullary chromaffin cells quite independent of the IL-1 cytokines, which appear to be ineffective in this animal model, suggesting a species-specific adrenal response to immune system *(74)*. However, in PC12 rat pheochromocytoma cells, the IL-1 cytokines do induce the expression of aromatic L-amino acid decarboxylase suggesting the preservation of this pathway in pheochromocytomas *(12)*.

BIDIRECTIONAL IL-1–CRH INTERACTION

Multiple lines of evidence suggest that, in the periphery, the interaction between immune system and CRH is a bidirectional process, i.e. CRH modulates several local parameters of the immune system. Thus, CRH increases lymphocyte proliferation and natural killer cytotoxicity *(75)*. Furthermore, treatment of murine leukocytes with CRH enhances natural killer cell activity *(76,77)*. CRH inhibits vascular leakage in experimental models of tissue injury *(78)*. Regarding the IL-1 cytokines, it has been shown that following exposure to CRH the production of IL-1β and IL-1ra transcripts and peptide products increase in human peripheral monocytes in culture. This CRH effect is blocked by its antagonist ahCRH *(70)*. In addition, intraperitoneal injection of CRH increases the number of IL-1 binding sites in mouse pituitary without affecting its binding to hippocampus, spleen, or testis *(80)*. In AtT-20 cell cultures, CRH increases Bmax (concentration) of IL-1 receptors without altering KD (affinity); this CRF effect appears to be mediated through specific CRH-binding sites because ahCRF blocks it *(81)*. CRH stimulates the proliferation of human blood lymphocytes in culture in the absence and presence of T-cell mitogens, such as concanavalin A and phytohemaglutinin. The stimulation of concanavalin A response is augmented by CRH and blocked by ahCRF *(82)*. However, CRF has no effect on TNF, IL-1, and IL-6 production from murine-adherent peritoneal exudate cells, whereas hydrocortisone exerts a dramatic inhibitory effect on these cytokines *(83)*. It has been hypothesized that CRH may be affecting the production of cytokines via "POMC-regulated transcription factors" *(84)*.

REFERENCES

1. Bartfai T, Schultzberg M. Cytokines in neuronal cell types. Neurochem Int 1993; 22:435–444.
2. Mazzocchi G, Malendowicz LK, Markowska A, Nussdorfer GG. Effect of hypophysectomy on cortico-tropin-releasing hormone and adrenocorticotropin immunoreactivities in the rat adrenal gland. Mol Cell Neurosci 1994; 5:345–349.
3. Nussdorfer GG, Mazzocchi G. Immune-endocrine interactions in the mammalian adrenal gland: facts and hypotheses. Int Rev Cytol 1998; 183:143–184.
4. Carter DB, Deibel MR, Dunn CJ, Tomich C-S, Laborte AL, Slighton JL, et al. Purification, cloning, expression and biological characterization of an interleukin-1 receptor antagonist protein. Nature 1990; 344:633–638.
5. Eisenberg SP, Evans RJ, Arend WP, Verderber E, Brewer T, Hannum CH, et al. Primary structure and functional expression from complementary DNA of a human interleukin-1 receptor antagonist. Nature 1990; 343:341–346.
6. Haskill S, Martin G, Van Le L, Morris J, Peace A, Bigler CF, et al. cDNA cloning of an intracellular form of the human interleukin-1 receptor antagonist associated with epithelium. Proc Natl Acad Sci USA 1991; 88:3681–3685.
7. Krzesicki RF, Hatfield CA, Bienkowski MJ, Mcguide JC, Winterrowd GE, Chapman DL, et al. Regulation of expression of IL-1 receptor antagonist protein in human synovial and dermal fibroblasts. J Immunol 1993; 150:4008–4018.
8. Tada M, Dierens A-C, Desbaillets I, Jaufeerlly R, Hamou M-F, De Tribolet N. Production of interleukin-1 receptor antagonist by human glioblastoma cells in vitro and in vivo. J Neuroimmunol 50:187–194.
9. Schultzberg M, Andersson C, Unden A, Troye-Blomberg M, Svenson SB, Bartfai T. Interleukin-1 in adrenal chromaffin cells. Neuroscience 1989; 30:805–810.
10. Naito Y, Fukata J, Nakaishi S, Nakai Y, Hirai Y, Tamai S, et al. Chronic effects of interleukin-1 on hypothalamus, pituitary, and adrenal glands in rat. Neuroendocrinology 1990; 51:637–641.
11. Alheim K, Andersson C, Tingsborg S, Ziolkowska M, Schultzberg M, Bartfai T. Interleukin 1 expression is inducible by nerve growth factor in PC12 pheochromocytoma cells. Proc Natl Acad Sci USA 1991; 88:9301–9306.
12. Li XM, Jourio AV, Boulton AA. Induction of aromatic L-amino acid decarboxylase mRNA by interleukin-1beta and prostaglandin E2 in PC12 cells. Neurochem Res 1994; 19:591–595.
13. Yanagihara N, Minami K, Shirakawa F, Uezono Y, Kobayashi H, Eto S, et al. Stimulatory effect of IL-1b on catecholamine secretion from cultured bovine adrenal medullary cells. Biochem Biophys Res Com 1994; 198:81–87.
14. Shintani F, Kanba S, Nakaki T, Nibuya M, Kinoshita N, Suzuki E, et al. Interleukin-1 beta augments release of norepinephrine, dopamine, and serotonin in the rat anterior hypothalamus. J Neurosci 1993; 13:3574–3581.
15. Gonzalez-Hernandez JA, Bornstein M, Geschwend JE, Adler G, Scherbaum WA. Macrophages within the human adrenal gland. Morphological data for a possible local immune-neuroendocrine interaction. Cell Tissue Res 1994; 278:201–205.
16. Gonzalez-Hernandez JA, Bornstein SR, Ehrhart-Bornstein M, Gschwend JE, Gwosdow A, Jirikowski G, et al. IL-1 is expressed in human adrenal gland in vivo. Possible role in a local immune-adrenal axis. Clin Exp Immunol 1995; 99:137–141.
17. Wan DC, Scanlon D, Choi CL, Bunn SJ, Howe PR, Livett BG. Co-localization of RNAs coding for phenylethanolamine N-methyltransferase and proenkephalin A in bovine and ovine adrenals. J Auton Nerv Syst 1989; 26:231–240.
18. Margioris AN. Opioids in neural and non-neural tissues. Trends Endocrinol Metab 1993; 4:163–168.
19. Cahill AL, Eertmoed AL, Mangoura D, Perlman RL. Differential regulation of phenylethanolamine N-methyltransferase expression in two distinct subpopulations of bovine chromaffin cells. J Neurochem 1996; 67:1217–1224.
20. Andersson C, Svenson SB, Van Deventer S, Cerami A, Bartfai T. Interleukin-1alpha expression is inducible by cholinergic stimulation in the rat adrenal gland. Neuroscience 1992; 47:481–485.
21. Nobel CS, Schultzberg M. Induction of interleukin-1 beta mRNA and enkephalin mRNA in the rat adrenal gland by lipopolysaccharides studied by in situ hybridization histochemistry. Neuroimmuno-modulation 1995; 2:61–73.

22. Schultzberg M, Svenson SB, Unden A, Bartfai T. Interleukin-1-like immunoreactivity in peripheral tissues. J Neuroscience Res 1987; 18:184–189.

23. Schultzberg M, Tingsboro S, Nobel S, Lundkvist J, Svenson SB, Simoncsits A, et al. Interleukin-1 receptor antagonist protein and mRNA in the rat adrenal gland. J Interf Cytokine Res 1995; 15:721–729.

24. Bornstein SR, Erhrart-Bornstein M, Gonzalez-Hernandez JA, Schroder S, Scherbaum WA. Expression of interleukin-1 in human pheochromocytoma. J Endocrinol Invest 1996; 19:693–698.

25. Venihaki M, Gravanis A, Margioris AN. KAT45 human pheochromocytoma cell line. A new model for the in vitro study of neuro-immunohormonal interactions. Ann NY Acad Sci 1998; 840:425–433.

26. Alheim K, McDowell TL, Symons JA, Duff GW, Bartfai T. An AP-1 site is involved in the NGF induction of IL-1 alpha in PC12 cells. Neurochem Int 1996; 29:487–496.

27. Emoto H, Yokoo H, Yoshida M, Tanaka M. Corticotropin-releasing factor enhances noradrenaline release in the rat hypothalamus assessed by intracerebral microdialysis. Brain Research 1993; 601:286–289.

28. Lavicky J, Dunn AJ. Corticotropin-releasing factor stimulates catecholamine release in hypothalamus and prefrontal cortex in freely moving rats as assessed by microdialysis. J Neurochem 1993; 60:602–612.

29. Lee EHY, Chang SY, Chen AYJ. CRH facilitates NE release from the hippocampus: a microdialysis study. Neuroscience Res 1994; 19:327–330.

30. Smagin GN, Swirgiel AH, Dunn AJ. Corticotropin-releasing factor administered into the locus coeruleus, but not the parabrachial nucleus, stimulates norepinephrine release in the prefrontal cortex. Brain Res Bull 1995; 36:71–76.

31. Olianas MC, Onali P. Corticotropin-releasing factor activates tyrosine hydroxylase in rat and mouse striatal homogenates. Eur J Pharmacol 1998; 150:389–392.

32. Olianas MC, Onali P. Stimulation of synaptosomal dopamine synthesis by corticotropin-releasing factor in rat striatum: role of Ca^{2+}-dependent mechanisms. Europ J Pharmacol 1989; 166:165–174.

33. Posener JA, Schidkraut JJ, Williams GH, Gleason RE, Salomon MS, Mecheri G, et al. Acute and delayed effects of corticotropin-releasing hormone on dopamine activity in man. Biol Psychiatry 1994; 36:616–621.

34. Valentino RJ, Foote SL, Aston-Jones G. Corticotropin-releasing factor activates noradrenergic neurons in the locus coeruleus. Brain Res 1983; 270:363–367.

35. Valentino RJ, Wehby RG. Corticotropin-releasing factor: Evidence for a neurotransmitter role in the locus coeruleus during hemodynamic stress. Neuroendocrinology 1988; 48:674–677.

36. Valentino RJ, Page ME, Curtis AL. Activation of noradrenergic locus coeruleus neurons by hemodynamic stress is due to local release of corticotropin-releasing factor. Brain Res 1991; 555:25–34.

37. Valentino RJ, Page ME, Van Bockstaele E, Aston-Jones G. Corticotropin-releasing factor innervation of the locus-coeruleus region: distribution of fibers and source of input. Neuroscience 1992; 48:689–705.

38. Suda T, Tomori N, Tozawa F, Mouri T, Demura H, Schizume K. Distribution and characterization of immunoreactive corticotropin-releasing factor in human tissues. J Clin Endocrinol Metab 1984; 59:861–867.

39. Suda T, Tomori N, Yajima F, Odagiri E, Demura H, Shizume K. Characterization of immunoreactive corticotropin and corticotropin-releasing factor in human adrenal and ovarian tumors. Act Endocrinol (Copenh) 1986; 111:546–552.

40. Nicholson WE, DeCherney GS, Jackson RV, Orth DN. Pituitary and hypothalamic hormones in normal and neoplastic adrenal medulla: biologically active corticotropin-releasing hormone and corticotropin. Regul Pep 1987; 18:173–188.

41. Usui T, Nakai Y, Tsukada T, Jingami H, Takahashi H, Fukata J, et al. Expression of the adrenocorticotropin-releasing hormone precursor gene in placenta and other nonhypothalamic tissues in man. Mol Endocrinol 1988; 2:871–875.

42. Merchenthaler I. Corticotropin-releasing factor (CRF)-like immunoreactivity in the rat central nervous system. Extrahypothalamic distribution. Peptides 1984; 5:53–69.

43. Bagdy G, Calogero AE, Szemeredi K, Chrousos GP, Gold PW. Effects of cortisol treatment on brain and adrenal corticotropin-releasing hormone (CRH) content and other parameters regulated by CRH. Regul Pept 1990; 31:83–92.

44. Venihaki M, Gravanis A, Margioris AN. Comparative study between normal rat chromaffin and PC12 ratpheochromocytoma cells: production and effects of corticotropin-releasing hormone. Endocrinology 1997; 138:698–704.

45. Hashimoto K, Murakami K, Hattori T, Niimi M, Fujimo K, Ota Z. Corticotropin-releasing factor (CRF)-like immunoreactivity in the adrenal medulla. Peptides 1984; 5:707–712.

46. Edwards AV, Jones CT. Secretion of corticotropin releasing factor from the adrenal during splachnic nerve stimulation in conscious calves. J Physiol (London) 1988; 40:89–100.

47. Minamino N, Uehara A, Arimura A. Biological and immunological characterization of corticotropin-releasing activity in bovine adrenal medulla. Peptides 1988; 9:37–45.

48. Bruhn TO, Engeland WC, Anthony ELP, Gann DS, Jackson IDM. Corticotropin-releasing factor in the dog adrenal medulla is secreted in response to hemorrhage. Endocrinology 1987a; 120:25–33.

49. Bruhn TO, Engeland WC, Anthony ELP, Gann DS, Jackson IDM. Corticotropin-releasing factor in the adrenal medulla. Ann NY Acad Sci 1987b; 512:115–128.

50. Udelsman R, Harwood JP, Millan MA, Chrousos GP, Golstein DS, Zimlichman R, et al. Functional corticotropin-releasing factor receptors in the primate peripheral sympathetic nervous system. Nature 1986; 6049:147–150.

51. Aguilera G, Millan MA, Hauger RL, Catt KJ. Corticotropin-releasing factor receptors: distribution and regulation in brain, pituitary and peripheral tissues. Ann NY Acad Sci 1987; 512:48–66.

52. Sasaki A, Yumita S, Kimura S, Miura Y, Yoshinaga K. Immunoreactive corticotropin-releasing hormone, somatostatin, and peptide histidine methionine are present in adrenal pheochromocytomas, but not in extra-adrenal pheochromocytoma. J Clin Endocrinol Metab 1990; 70:996–999.

53. O'Brien T, Young WF, Davila DG, Scheithauer BW, Kovacs K, Hovath E, et al. Cushing's syndrome associated with ectopic production of corticotropin-releasing hormone, corticotropin and vasopressin by pheochromocytoma. Clin Endocrinol Oxf 1992; 37:460–467.

54. Tsuchihashi T, Yamaguchi K, Abe K, Yanihara N, Saito S. Production of immunoreactive corticotropin-releasing hormone in various neuroendocrine tumors. Jpn J Clin Oncol 1992; 22:232–237.

55. Saeger W, Reincke M, Scholz GH, Ludecke DK. Ectopic ACTH- or CRH-secreting tumors in Cushing's syndrome. Zentralbl Pathol 1993; 139:157–163.

56. Liu J, Heikkila P, Voutilainen R, Karonen SL, Kahri AI. Pheochromocytoma expressing adrenocorticotropin and corticotropin-releasing hormone; regulation by glucocorticoids and nerve growth factor. Eur J Endocrinol 1994; 131:221–228.

57. Venihaki M, Ain K, Dermitzaki E, Gravanis A, Margioris AN. KAT45, a noradrenergic human pheochromocytoma cell line producing corticotropin-releasing hormone. Endocrinology 1998; 139:713–722.

58. Berkenbosch F, Van Oers J, Del Rey A, Tilders F, Besedovsky H. Corticotropin-releasing factor-producing neurons in the rat activated by interleukin-1. Science 1987; 238:524–526.

59. Sapolsky R, Rivier C, Yamamoto G, Plotsky P, Vale W. Interleukin-1 stimulates the secretion of hypothalamic corticotropin-releasing factor. Science 1987; 238:522–524.

60. Eskay RL, Eiden LE. Interleukin-1 alpha and tumor necrosis factor-alpha differentially regulate enkephalin, vasoactive intestinal polypeptide, neurotensin, and substance P biosynthesis in chromaffin cells. Endocrinology 1992; 130:2252–2258.

61. O'Konnel NA, Kumar A, Chatzipanteli K, Mohan A, Agarwal RK, Head C, et al. Interleukin-1 regulates corticosterone secretion from the rat adrenal gland through a catecholamine-dependent and prostaglandin E2-independent mechanism. Endocrinology 1994; 135:460–467.

62. Andreis PG, Neri G, Belloni AS, Mazzocchi G, Kasprzak A, Nussdorfer GG. Interleukin-1 beta enhances corticosterone secretion by acting directly on the rat adrenal gland. Endocrinology 1991; 129:53–57.

63. Gwosdow AR, O'Connell NA, Spencer JA, Kumar MS, Agarwal RK, Bode HH, et al. Interleukin-1-induced corticosterone release occurs by an adrenergic mechanism from rat adrenal gland. Am J Physiol 1992; 263:E461–466.

64. Gwosdow AR. Mechanisms of interleukin-1-induced hormone secretion from the rat adrenal gland. Endocr Res 1995; 21:25–37.

65. Zalcman S, Green-Johnson JM, Murray L, Nance DM, Dyck D, Anisman H, et al. Cytokine-specific central monoamine alterations induced by interleukin-1, -2 and -6. Brain Res 1994; 643:40–49.

66. MohanKumar PS, Quadri SK. Systemic administration of interleukin-1 stimulates norepinephrine release in the paraventricular nucleus. Life Sci 1993; 52:1961–1967.

67. Terao A, Oikawa M, Saito M. Cytokine-induced change in hypothalamic norepinephrine turnover: involvement of corticotropin-releasing hormone and prostaglandins. Brain Res 1993; 622:257–261.

68. Terao A, Oikawa M, Saito M. Tissue-specific increase in norepinephrine turnover by central interleukin-1 but not by interleukin-6, in rats. Am J Physiol 1994; 266:R400–R404.

69. Hurst S, Collins SM. Interleukin-1 beta modulation of norepinephrine release from rat myenteric nerves. Am J Physiol 1993; 264:G30–G35.

70. Vriend CY, Zuo L, Dyck DG, Nance DM, Greenberg AH. Central administration of interleukin-1 beta increases norepinephrine turnover in the spleen. Brain Res Bull 1993; 31:39–42.

71. Shimizu N, Hori T, Nakane H. An interleukin-1 beta-induced noradrenaline release in the spleen is mediated by brain corticotropin-releasing factor: an in vivo microdialysis study in conscious rats. Brain Behav Immun 1994; 8:14–23.

72. Sakata Y, Morimoto A, Murakami N. Changes in plasma catecholamines during fever induced by bacterial endotoxin and interleukin-1 beta. Jpn J Physiol 1994; 44:693–703.

73. Cunningham Jr ET, Wada E, Carter DB, Tracey DE, Battey JF, DeSouza EB. *In situ* histochemical localization of type 1 interleukin-1 receptor messenger RNA in the central nervous system, pituitary, and adrenal gland of the mouse. Neurosci 1992; 12:1101–1114.

74. Lujan HJ, Mathews HL, Gamelli RL, Jones SB. Human immune cells mediate catecholamine secretion from adrenal chromaffin cells. Crit Care Med 1998; 26:1218–1224.

75. Jain R, Zwickler D, Hollander CS, Brand H, Saperstein A, Hutchinson B, et al. Corticotropin-releasing factor modulates the immune response to stress in the rat. Endocrinology 1991; 128:1329–1336.

76. Carr DJ, Weigent DA, Blalock JE. Hormones common to the neuroendocrine and immune systems. Drug Des Deliv 1989; 4:187–195.

77. Carr DJ, DeCosta BR, Jacobson AE, Rice KC, Blalock JE. Corticotropin-releasing hormone augments natural killer cell activity through a naloxone-sensitive pathway. J Neuroimmunol 1990; 28:53–61.

78. Thomas HA, Ling N, Wei ET. CRF and related peptides as antiinflammatory agonists. Ann NY Acad Sci 1993; 697:219–228.

79. Paez Pereda M, Sauer J, Perez Castro C, Finkielman S, Stalla GK, Holsboer F, et al. Corticotropin-releasing hormone differentially modulates the interleukin-1 system according to the level of monocyte activation by endotoxin. Endocrinology 1995; 136:5504–5510.

80. Takao T, Tojo C, Nishioka T, Hashimoto K, De Souza EB. Corticotropin-releasing factor treatment upregulates interleukin-1 receptors in the mouse pituitary: reversal by dexamethasone. Brain Res 1995; 688:219–222.

81. Webster EL, Tracey DE, De Souza EB. Upregulation of interleukin-1 receptors in mouse AtT-20 pituitary tumor cells following treatment with corticotropin-releasing factor. Endocrinology 1991; 129:2796–2798.

82. Singh VK. Stimulatory effect of corticotropin-releasing neurohormone on human lymphocyte proliferation and interleukin-2 receptor expression. J Neuroimmunol 1989; 23:257–262.

83. Doherty GM, Jensen JC, Buresh CM, Norton JA. Hormonal regulation of inflammatory cell cytokine transcript and bioactivity production in response to endotoxin. Cytokine 1992; 4:55–62.

84. Lininio J, Gold PW, Wong ML. A molecular mechanism for stress-induced alterations in susceptibility to disease. Lancet 1995; 346:104–106.

II THE ADRENAL GLAND: *PATHOPHYSIOLOGY*

10 Overview of Hyper- and Hypocortisolism

W.W. de Herder and S.W.J. Lamberts

CONTENTS

HYPERCORTISOLISM

Cushing's Syndrome and Pseudo-Cushing States

A spectrum of physiological and pathological conditions is accompanied by prolonged activation of the hypothalamus-pituitary-adrenocortical (HPA) axis (*see* Table 1) *(1)*. Part of the patients with these conditions are likely to develop features of Cushing's syndrome. In this respect, the term "preclinical Cushing's syndrome" refers to a disorder in which the hypercortisolism has escaped from the normal feedback control mechanisms, but yet insufficiently to cause clinically recognizable Cushing's syndrome. It is generally easy to recognize overt Cushing's syndrome from the classical clinical features. However, in the conditions listed in Table 1, the clinical picture and laboratory findings may be conflicting. It is obvious, that making a correct diagnosis is crucial for subsequent therapy.

Of particular importance is the clinical differentiation between patients with spontaneous Cushing's syndrome and patients with "cushingoid" obesity. Some of the classic clinical features, like truncal obesity, hirsutism, hypertension, and abnormal glucose tolerance are not helpful distinguishing between these two patient groups. However, osteoporosis, muscle weakness, bruising, and hypokalemia are helpful differential diagnostic features (Table 2) *(2–4)*.

Pregnancy is rare in overt Cushing's syndrome because increased circulating cortisol and adrenal androgen levels suppress the activity of the female reproductive system. In pregnant patients with Cushing's syndrome, adrenocorticotropin (ACTH)-dependent (mostly Cushing's disease) and ACTH independent (mostly benign adrenocortical tumors) Cushing's syndrome are equally represented *(5)*. In normal pregnancy, increased levels of unbound corticotropin releasing-hormone (CRH) in the circulation, which is of placental origin, stimulates the maternal pituitary-adrenocortical axis. In a subgroup

From: *Contemporary Endocrinology: Adrenal Disorders*
Edited by: A. N. Margioris and G. P. Chrousos © Humana Press, Totowa, NJ

Table 1
Classification of Hypercortisolism (Adapted from Tsigos, et al. [1])

Chronic stress
Chronic exercise
Chronic disease
Psychiatric disorders
    Melancholic depression
    Anorexia nervosa
    Obsessive-compulsive disorder
    Panic disorder
    Chronic alcoholism
    Alcohol and narcotic withdrawal
Cushing's syndrome (endogenous/factitious)
Diabetes mellitus with neuropathy
Truncal obesity
Pregnancy
Malnutrition
Glucocorticoid resistance
Cortisol hyperreactive syndrome (AERD)

Table 2
Clinical and Laboratory Features of Cushing's Syndrome vs Cushingoid Obesity (Adapted from Kreisberg [2] et al. [3] and Ross and Linch [4])

Feature	Likelihood ratio[a]
Generalized obesity	0.05
Abnormal glucose tolerance	1.14
Oligomemorrhea	1.41
Hirsutism	1.72
Hypertension	2.29
Truncal obesity	3.10
Hypokalemia	6.25
Bruising	8.83
Muscle weakness	9.29
Osteoporosis	21.33

[a]The probability that a feature will appear in Cushing's syndrome (prevalence), as compared with the probability that it will appear in cushingoid obesity.

of patients with pregnancy-related Cushing's syndrome, placental CRH has been identified as a mediator of disease activity (6,7).

In the context of the Von Munchausen syndrome, exogenous Cushing's syndrome, caused by factitious administration of glucocorticoids is uncommon. In these patients, the clinical features may vary, making the differentiation from cyclic Cushing's syndrome difficult (see later). However, the medical history of these patients can provide important clues. Striking alterations in the urinary glucocorticoid excretion, discrepancies between plasma and urine glucocorticoid levels and evidence of adrenal atrophy on imaging

Table 3
Causes of Cushing's Syndrome

ACTH-dependent Cushing's syndrome
    Cushing's disease
        corticotrope microadenoma (diameter <10 mm)
        corticotrope macroadenoma (diameter >10 mm)
        corticotrope hyperplasia/multiple corticotrope microadenomas
    Ectopic ACTH syndrome
    Ectopic CRH syndrome

ACTH-independent Cushing's syndrome
    Adrenocortical adenoma (some patients with adrenal incidentalomas)
    Adrenocortical carcinoma
    ACTH-independent bilateral adrenocortical disease (*see* Table 4)

Pregnancy-induced Cushing's syndrome
Factitious Cushing's syndrome

studies should also rise suspicion. In these patients, high-pressure liquid chromatography (HPLC) analysis of urine for the detection of synthetic glucocorticoids is the most sensitive test *(8,9)*.

Another diagnostic pitfall can be caused by variable cortisol excretion in a subset of patients with Cushing's syndrome. An extreme variety of this is the so-called "cyclic," "episodic," "periodic," or "fluctuating Cushing's syndrome," also called "variable hormonogenesis." In these patients basal cortisol secretion may intermittently fall in the normal, or subnormal range, obscuring the laboratory evidence of hypercortisolism. Variability may also occur in the results of standard dynamic tests, used for determination of the etiology of hypercortisolism. This implies that in case of inconsistent diagnostic tests, testing should be repeated after fixed time intervals, in the hope that the diagnosis might become clearer in time. Fluctuating hypercortisolism can confound diagnosis in all etiologies of Cushing's syndrome *(10,11)*.

In patients presenting with incidentally detected adrenal tumors (adrenal incidentalomas), hypertension, noninsulin-dependent diabetes mellitus and obesity can be hallmarks of preclinical Cushing's syndrome. Although the natural course of these tumors still remains obscure, secondary adrenocortical insufficiency may follow surgical removal of the incidentaloma in these patients *(12–15)*.

Historically, spontaneous Cushing syndrome is divided into ACTH-dependent and ACTH-independent (Table 3). In the first category are Cushing's disease, ectopic ACTH syndrome and ectopic CRH syndrome. These conditions generally, but not always, result in bilateral adrenal enlargement. In some of these patients, bilateral adrenal nodular hyperplasia, or solitary adrenal macro-, or microadenomas may develop as anatomical variants. In the second category, one finds autonomous cortisol producing adenomas and carcinomas.

In recent years, the ACTH-independent bilateral adrenal micro- and macronodular hyperplasias (AIMIH and AIMAH) have been added to the spectrum of ACTH-independent Cushing's syndrome (Table 4) *(16)*. A still growing number of etiologies resulting in either spontaneous, and/or familial forms have been postulated and/or identified. Derangements in ligand-receptor interactions are common etiologies in these subgroups.

Table 4
The Spectrum of ACTH-Independent Bilateral Adrenocortical Disease

Primary pigmented nodular adrenocortical disease
  Isolated
  Familial
  Hereditary Carney complex (*see* Chapter 21)
ACTH-independent bilateral micronodular and macronodular adrenal hyperplasia
Isolated
    Via transition from Cushing's disease to ACTH-independent bilateral micro-, or
      macronodular adrenal hyperplasia
    Via activating mutation(s) of the $G_s$alpha subunit of the stimulatory G protein that
      activates adenylate cyclase (McCune-Albright syndrome)
    Via overexpression of GIP receptors (Food-dependent Cushing's syndrome)
    Via overexpression of beta-adrenergic receptors (Catecholamine-dependent Cushing's
      syndrome)
    Via overexpression of estrogen receptors (pregnancy)
    Via overexpression of LH receptors (pregnancy)
    Via overexpression of serotonin 5HT–4 receptors
    Via increased expression or response of V_1AVP receptors
    Via overexpression IL-1 receptors?
  Familial

Prolonged ACTH stimulation in ACTH-dependent Cushing's syndrome (mostly Cushing's disease) may result in the development of ACTH-independent autonomous adrenocortical hyperfunction *(17,18)*. The ACTH receptor interacts with the alpha subunit of the stimulatory G protein ($G_s$alpha), which activates adenylate cyclase. In the McCune–Albright syndrome, activating mutations in the $G_s$alpha protein result in constitutive activation of the signal transduction pathway generating cAMP. Apart from ACTH-independent bilateral adrenal nodular hyperplasia, this condition is characterized by polyostotic fibrous dysplasia, hypophosphatemic osteomalacia, café au lait pigmentations of the skin, growth hormone- or prolactin or TSH-secreting pituitary adenomas, primary hyperthyroidism, and sexual precocity *(19)*. Adrenocortical pathology and histology of these patients show a typical mosaic pattern of nodules, which carry the mutation and zones of atrophy consisting of cells that do not carry the mutation and are not stimulated by ACTH in the presence of hypercortisolism *(19)*.

Carney complex is an autosomal-dominant transmitted multisystem tumor syndrome. These patients can develop ACTH-independent autonomous adrenocortical hyperfunction, myxomas, pigmented skin lesions (lentigines, blue nevi), peripheral nerve tumors (schwannomas), testicular tumors (Sertoli cell tumor, Leydig cell tumor, adrenocortical rest tumor), mammary myxoid fibromas, and pituitary somatotroph adenomas *(20)*. The pathology and histology of the adrenal glands in these patients show a unique architecture of multiple pigmented nodules that are composed of large cells that contain lipofuscin and adrenocortical atrophy between these nodules. This syndrome has been linked to a yet unknown gene on the short arm of chromosome 2 *(21)*. Carney complex will be further discussed in Chapter 21. Primary pigmented nodular adrenocortical disease has also been reported as a spontaneous disorder and as an isolated familial disorder without association with the other clinical abnormalities of Carney complex.

In food-dependent Cushing's syndrome, overexpression of the receptor for gastric inhibitory polypeptide (= glucose-dependent insulinotropic polypeptide [GIP]) on adrenocortical cells (22), leads to either bilateral adrenal macronodular hyperplasia (23–26), or to an adrenocortical adenoma (27–31). In some cases, administration of the somatostatin receptor-analog, octreotide, has caused a short-term inhibition of the postprandial GIP release and subsequently has resulted in clinical and biochemical amelioration (24,28).

Caticha and colleagues have studied a patient with ACTH-independent bilateral adrenal nodular hyperplasia, who developed features of Cushing's syndrome during pregnancy and during estrogen–progestin treatment. In cultured adrenocortical cells of this patient, cortisol production was directly stimulated by estradiol (32). In a postmenopausal patient with ACTH-independent macronodular hyperplasia and Cushing's syndrome, Lacroix and colleagues have demonstrated that cortisol production could be stimulated by the administration of human chorionic gonadotropin (hCG), luteinizing hormone releasing-hormone (GnRH), and luteinizing hormone (LH). These findings were suggestive for the ectopic expression of LH/hCG receptors. The administration of the long-acting LH analog, Leuprolide acetate resulted in control of hypercortisolism (33). In the same patient, cortisol production could also be stimulated by the oral administration of cisapride and metoclopramide, which was suggestive for the additional expression of serotonin 5HT-4 receptors on the adrenals (33).

In another patient with ACTH-independent macronodular hyperplasia, Lacroix and colleagues have demonstrated that the Cushing's syndrome was secondary to the abnormal adrenocortical expression of beta-adrenergic receptors. In this patient, treatment with propranolol resulted in a reduction of hypercortisolism (34).

In vasopressin-responsive Cushing's syndrome, there is abnormal hyperresponsiveness of an eutopic V1 vasopressin receptor in either cortisol-producing adenomas (35), or bilateral macronodular adrenocortical hyperplasias (36,37). In a case of ACTH-independent Cushing's syndrome, aberrant expression of the interleukin 1 (IL-1) receptor, which is not a G-protein-linked receptor, in an adrenocortical adenoma was held responsible for the aberrant stimulation of cortisol production by interleukin 1. In this adenoma, high local interleukin levels, produced by a massive mononuclear infiltrate of CD45- and CD68-containing leukocytes and macrophages could have caused Cushing's syndrome (38). Until now, this condition has not been reported in association with ACTH-independent bilateral adrenocortical hyperplasias.

Glucocorticoid Resistance

A variety of molecular defects in the glucocorticoid receptor gene can cause changes in the functional characteristics, or number of intracellular glucocorticoid receptors. In these situations, the complex negative feedback system of the HPA axis is also activated, which results in the clinical syndromes of generalized (familial) primary (partial) glucocorticoid receptor resistance. In these syndromes, increased circulating levels of cortisol, adrenocortical androgens, and mineralocorticoids can be found. The clinical features of glucocorticoid resistance vary from hypertension and/or hypokalemic alkalosis and/or features of hyperandrogenism (hirsuitism, acne, menstrual irregularities, oligoanovulation, and infertility in females, infertility in men) to chronic fatigue. Most of the classical clinical features of Cushing's syndrome are absent (39).

AERD

Recently, a new syndrome named apparent E (=cortisone) reductase deficiency (AERD) has been described. In two sisters with AERD, there were biochemical evidence of increased cortisol production, but absence of clinical symptoms of Cushing's syndrome. Symptoms of hyperandrogenism were related to increased adrenocortical production of androgens and cortisol metabolites. The putative biochemical mechanism in these patients is an alteration in the cortisol metabolism, resulting in the increased urinary excretion of corticosteroid metabolites with 11-carbonyl groups and the diminished urinary excretion of 11β-hydroxylated steroids. The exact nature of this alteration has not been further characterized yet (40).

HYPOCORTISOLISM

Primary Bilateral Adrenocortical Failure

Because the first description of the syndrome of primary adrenocortical failure by Thomas Addison in 1855, the spectrum of etiologies of this syndrome has changed. In the early years, tuberculosis accounted for most cases of primary adrenocortical failure. This number gradually decreased from 70% in 1930 to 31% in 1968 (East coast region of the United Kingdom [41]), to 17% in 1974 (Denmark [42]), and finally to 0–7% in 1994 (Dutch survey of Addison's patients [43], Nottingham, U.K. [44]). Currently, autoimmune adrenalitis is the most common cause of primary adrenocortical failure. About 55% of these patients have circulating antibodies against the steroidogenic enzyme 21-hydroxylase (45). In Table 5, the etiologies of primary and secondary adrenocortical insufficiency are given.

Patients with autoimmune polyglandular syndromes and circulating antibodies against the steroidogenic enzyme 21-hydroxylase are at a high risk for developing Addison's disease and, therefore, should be carefully followed up. In these patients, repeated CRH and/or ACTH testing may lead to early recognition of primary adrenocortical failure. Alternatively, adult patients presenting with clinically manifested Addison's disease should be screened for other autoimmune diseases associated with type II polyglandular autoimmune syndrome (46,47).

X-linked adrenoleukodystrophy (ALD) is characterized by primary adrenocortical failure and demyelinization with the central and peripheral nervous system. In these patients, the oxidation of very long chain fatty acids (VLCFAs), particularly, hexacosanoic acid, pentacosaic acid, and tetracosanoic acid, is impaired. This results in the accumulation of these VLCFAs in tissues and body fluids. At least seven clinical subtypes have been described. Primary adrenocortical failure may be the only clinical presentation of ALD. Although it was initially believed that most, if not all, patients presented before the age of 15, Laureti and colleagues have shown that ALD-associated adrenocortical failure can first occur in young adult males. Therefore, young adult males with primary adrenocortical failure, and in whom antibodies against the steroidogenic enzyme 21-hydroxylase are absent, should be screened by determination of the plasma VLCFA concentration to exclude ALD (48,49). Hereditary ACTH insensitivity syndromes are characterized by hypocortisolism in the presence of high plasma ACTH levels generally occurring early in childhood (50). The renin–angiotensin–aldosterone axis is normal, with an unaltered aldosterone response to angiotensin II. It has been reported as a spontaneous disorder, as an isolated familial disorder and in association

Table 5
Etiologies of Primary and Secondary Adrenocortical Insufficiency

Primary Adrenocortical Failure

from birth
  Congenital adrenal hypoplasia (familial or isolated)
  Hereditary syndrome of glucocorticoid deficiency

in youth/young adults
  Autoimmune (isolated or as a part of the type 1 polyglandular syndrome)
  X-linked adrenoleukodystrophy (only in males)
  Tuberculosis

mostly in adulthood
  Autoimmune (isolated or as a part of the type II polyglandular
syndrome)
  Tuberculosis
  Systemic fungal infections
  AIDS
  Bilateral adrenal metastases
  Bilateral adrenal hemorrhage and/or necrosis
  Drugs (ketoconazole, metyrapone, etomidate, o,p′-DDD)

Secondary Adrenocortical Failure

Pituitary
      macroadenoma
      necrosis or bleeding into macroadenoma
      postpartum necrosis (Sheehan's syndrome)
      metastasis
      surgery and/or radiation
      empty sella syndrome
      hypophysitis
      infection (in AIDS)
  Isolated ACTH deficiency (congenital, acquired)
  Head (or pituitary) trauma
  Suprasellar tumors
  Sarcoidosis
  Histiocytosis X
  Withdrawal of long-term glucocorticoid therapy, or megestrol acetate

with achalasia, absence of lacrimation and autonomic and motor neuropathy as well as other associated features. The latter complex of symptoms is also known as the triple A syndrome, or Allgrove syndrome *(50,51)*. A variety of mutations in the ACTH receptor gene underlie the ACTH resistance syndromes *(50,52,53)*.

In patients infected with the human immunodeficiency virus (HIV), adrenocortical insufficiency is a well-known complication *(54,55)*. Multiple etiological factors have been recognized. Evidence of opportunistic infections (with cytomegalovirus (CMV), *Mycobacterium avium, Toxoplasma gondii*) of the adrenals has been frequently found in postmortem studies of patients having died from AIDS. Some cases of CMV-induced adrenocortical necrosis, resulting in primary adrenocortical failure *(56),* and CMV-induced hypothalamic destruction, resulting in secondary adrenocortical insufficiency *(57)* have been reported. Certain antimycotic drugs, like ketoconazole and fluconazole interfere with adrenocortical steroidogenesis and can cause primary adrenocortical insufficiency in patients with limited adrenocortical reserve (58). The drugs rifampicin and phenytoin are frequently administered to AIDS patients and increase cortisol metabolism (59,60). Megestrol acetate, a drug with intrinsic glucocorticoid activity, is frequently used for AIDS-related anorexia. After prolonged administration of megestrol acetate, acute withdrawal can, therefore, result in secondary adrenocortical insufficiency (61). Adrenal destruction by neoplasms like Kaposi's sarcoma and bilateral adrenal bleeding are less frequent causes of primary adrenocortical failure in AIDS patients. Furthermore, acquired glucocorticoid resistance has been demonstrated in HIV-infected patients (59,62,63).

Secondary Adrenocortical Failure

Glucocorticoid-induced ACTH deficiency is the most common cause of secondary adrenocortical failure. In these circumstances, supraphysiological doses of glucocorticoids have been given long enough to result in suppression of the hypothalamic CRH production and a blunted ACTH response to CRH.

Secondary adrenocortical failure caused by acquired ACTH deficiency may also result from intrinsic pituitary diseases, or from CRH deficiency caused by hypothalamic pathology. Most frequently, pituitary hormone-hypersecreting macroadenomas (tumor diameter >10 mm), clinically nonfunctioning pituitary macroadenomas, or suprasellar tumors are found. In these patients, features of hyposecretion of other anterior pituitary hormones, as well as accompanying neurologic or opthalmologic defects are common. Anterior pituitary hormonal deficiency may either directly result from pituitary infiltration by the tumor, or indirectly from compression of the hypothalamic-pituitary axis by the tumor, or as a consequence of surgical hypophysectomy, or radiotherapy directed at the tumor (64).

Congenital isolated ACTH deficiency is a rare disorder, which may occur as an isolated, or familial variant. Abnormal cleavage patterns of proopiomelanocortin (POMC) (65) or POMC mutations are involved in the pathogenesis of these syndromes (66). Acquired isolated ACTH deficiency is most probably caused by primary failure of the pituitary corticotropes. Most patients are between the ages of 30 and 50 years of age. In these patients, no other pituitary or suprasellar pathologies (apart from lymphocytic hypophysitis) have been recognized. Acquired isolated ACTH deficiency has been reported in combination with type I diabetes mellitus, primary autoimmune hypothyroidism, and lymphocytic hypophysitis, which suggests that autoimmunity may play a role in its pathogenesis (67,68).

The Paradox of Clinical Hypercortisolism and Biochemical Hypocortisolism: Cortisol Hyperreactive Syndrome

Until now, one patient with the combination of clinical features of Cushing's syndrome and paradoxical hypocortisolism has been reported (69). In cultured fibroblasts from this patient, the administration of glucocorticoids resulted in a supernormal induction of aromatase activity and a stronger than normal inhibition of the incorporation of [³H]thymidine by these cells. It was concluded that this patient was hyperreactive to glucocorticoids, although the mechanism of this hyperreactivity still remains to be elucidated.

REFERENCES

1. Tsigos C, Papanicolaou DA, Chrousos GP. Advances in the diagnosis and treatment of Cushing's syndrome. Baill Clin Endocrinol Metab 1995; 9:315–336.
2. Kreisberg R. Clinical problem-solving. Half a loaf. Engl J Med 1994; 330:1295–1299.
3. Nugent CA, Warner HRDJT, Tyler FH. Probability theory in the diagnosis of Cushing's syndrome. J Clin Endocrinol 1963; 24:621–627.
4. Ross EJ, Linch DC. Cushing's syndrome—killing disease: discriminatory value of signs and symptoms aiding early diagnosis. Lancet 1982; 2:646–649.
5. Sheeler LR. Cushing's syndrome and pregnancy. Endocrinol Metab Clin N Am 1994; 23:619–627.
6. Aron DC, Schnall AM, Sheeler LR. Spontaneous resolution of Cushing's syndrome after pregnancy. Am J Obstet Gynecol 1990; 162:472–474.
7. Wallace C, Toth EL, Lewanczuk RZ, Siminoski K. Pregnancy-induced Cushing's syndrome in multiple pregnancies. J Clin Endocrinol Metab 1996; 81:15–21.
8. Cizza G, Nieman LK, Doppman JL, Passaro MD, Czerwiec FS, Chrousos GP et al. Factitious Cushing syndrome. J Clin Endocrinol Metab 1996; 81:3573–3577.
9. Lin CL, Wu TJ, Machacek DA, Jiang NS, Kao PC. Urinary free cortisol and cortisone determined by high performance liquid chromatography in the diagnosis of Cushing's syndrome. J Clin Endocrinol Metab 1997; 82:151–155.
10. Atkinson AB, Kennedy AL, Carson DJ, Hadden DR, Weaver JA, Sheridan B. Five cases of cyclical Cushing's syndrome. Br Med J (Clin Res Ed) 1985; 291:1453–1457.
11. Shapiro MS, Shenkman L. Variable hormonogenesis in Cushing's syndrome. Q J Med 1991; 79:351–363.
12. Reincke M, Nieke J, Krestin GP, Saeger W, Allolio Winkelmann W. Preclinical Cushing's syndrome in adrenal "incidentalomas": comparison with adrenal Cushing's syndrome. J Clin Endocrinol Metab 1992; 75:826–832.
13. Newell-Price J, Grossman A. Adrenal incidentaloma: subclinical Cushing's syndrome. Postgrad Med J 1996; 72:207–210.
14. Terzolo M, Osella G, Ali A, Borretta G, Cesario F, Paccotti P, et al. Subclinical Cushing's syndrome in adrenal incidentaloma. Clin Endocrinol (Oxf) 1998; 48:89–97.
15. Aron DC. Adrenal incidentalomas and glucocorticoid autonomy. Clin Endocrinol (Oxf) 1998; 49:157–158.
16. Malchoff CD, MacGillivray D, Malchoff DM. Adrenocorticotropic hormone-independent adrenal hyperplasia. Endocrinologist 1996; 6:79–85.
17. Hocher B, Bahr V, Dorfmuller S, Oelkers W. Hypercortisolism with non-pigmented micronodular adrenal hyperplasia: transition from pituitary-dependent to adrenal-dependent Cushing's syndrome. Acta Endocrinol (Copenh) 1993; 128:120–125.
18. Hermus AR, Pieters GF, Smals AG, Pesman GJ, Lamberts SW, Benraad TJ et al. Transition from pituitary-dependent to adrenal-dependent Cushing's syndrome. N Engl J Med 1988; 318:966–970.
19. Weinstein LS, Shenker A, Gejman PV, Merino MJ, Friedman E, Spiegel AM. Activating mutations of the stimulatory G protein in the McCune-Albright syndrome. N Engl J Med 1991; 325:1688–1695.
20. Young WF Jr, Carney JA, Musa BU, Wulffraat NM, Lens JW, Drexhage HA. Familial Cushing's syndrome due to primary pigmented nodular adrenocortical disease. Reinvestigation 50 years later. N Engl J Med 1989; 321:1659–1664.
21. Stratakis CA, Jenkins RB, Pras E, Mitsiadis CS, Ra SB, Stalboerger PG et al. Cytogenetic and microsatellite alterations in tumors from patients with the syndrome of myxomas, spotty skin pigmentation, and endocrine overactivity (Carney complex). J Clin Endocrinol Metab 1996; 81:3607–3614.
22. N'Diaye N, Tremblay J, Hamet P, de Herder WW, Lacroix A. Adrenocortical overexpression of gastric inhibitory polypeptide receptor underlies food-dependent Cushing's syndrome. J Clin Endocrinol Metab 1998; 83:2781–2785.
23. Lacroix A, Bolte E, Tremblay J, Dupre J, Poitras P, Fournier H, et al. Gastric inhibitory polypeptide-dependent cortisol hypersecretion—a new cause of Cushing's syndrome. N Engl J Med 1992; 327:974–980.
24. Reznik Y, Allali-Zerah V, Chayvialle JA, Leroyer R, Leymarie P, Travert G, et al. Food-dependent Cushing's syndrome mediated by aberrant adrenal sensitivity to gastric inhibitory polypeptide. N Engl J Med 1992; 327:981–986.

25. Lebrethon MC, Avallet O, Reznik Y, Archambeaud F, Combes J, Usdin TB, et al. Food-dependent Cushing's syndrome: characterization and functional role of gastric inhibitory polypeptide receptor in the adrenals of three patients. J Clin Endocrinol Metab 1998; 83:4514–4519.

26. N'Diaye N, Hamet P, Tremblay J, Boutin JM, Gaboury L, Lacroix A. Asynchronous development of bilateral nodular adrenal hyperplasia in gastric inhibitory polypeptide-dependent Cushing's syndrome. J Clin Endocrinol Metab 1999; 84:2616–2622.

27. Hamet P, Larochelle P, Franks DJ, Cartier P, Bolte. Cushing syndrome with food-dependent periodic hormonogenesis. Clin Invest Med 1987; 10:530–533.

28. de Herder WW, Hofland LJ, Usdin TB, de Jong FH, Uitterlinden P, van Koetsveld P, et al. Food-dependent Cushing's syndrome resulting from abundant expression of gastric inhibitory polypeptide receptors in adrenal adenoma cells. J Clin Endocrinol Metab 1996; 81:3168–3172.

29. Chabre O, Liakos P, Vivier J, Chaffanjon P, Labat-Moleur F, Martinie M, et al. Cushing's syndrome due to a gastric inhibitory polypeptide-dependent adrenal adenoma: insights into hormonal control of adrenocortical tumorigenesis. J Clin Endocrinol Metab 1998; 83:3134–3143.

30. Lebrethon MC, Avallet O, Reznik Y, Archambeaud F, Combes J, Usdin TB, et al. Food-dependent Cushing's syndrome: characterization and functional role of gastric inhibitory polypeptide receptor in the adrenals of three patients. J Clin Endocrinol Metab 1998; 83:4514–4519.

31. Luton JP, Bertherat J, Kuhn JM, Bertagna X. Expression aberrante du récepteur du GIP (gastric inhibitory polypeptide) dans un adenome de la cortico-surrénale responsable d'un syndrome de Cushing dépendant d'alimentation. Bull Acad Natl Med 1998; 182:1839–1849.

32. Caticha O, Odell WD, Wilson DE, Dowdell LA, Noth RH, Swislocki AL, et al. Estradiol stimulates cortisol production by adrenal cells in estrogen-dependent primary adrenocortical nodular dysplasia. J Clin Endocrinol Metab 1993; 77:494–497.

33. Lacroix A, N'Diaye N, Hamet P, Tremblay J, Boutin J, Sairam MR. LH-dependent Cushing's syndrome (CS) in a woman with bilateral macronodular adrenal hyperplasia: control of hypercortisolism with leuprolide. 80th Annual Meeting of the Endocrine Society, June 24–27, Abstract P2-398, 1998.

34. Lacroix A, Tremblay J, Rousseau G, Bouvier M, Hamet P. Propranolol therapy for ectopic beta-adrenergic receptors in adrenal Cushing's syndrome. N Engl J Med 1997; 337:1429–1434.

35. Perraudin V, Delarue C, de Keyzer Y, Bertagna X, Kuhn JM, Contesse V, et al. Vasopressin-responsive adrenocortical tumor in a mild Cushing's syndrome: in vivo and in vitro studies. J Clin Endocrinol Metab 1995; 80:2661–2667.

36. Horiba N, Suda T, Aiba M, Naruse M, Nomura K, Imamura M, et al. Lysine vasopressin stimulation of cortisol secretion in patients with adrenocorticotropin-independent macronodular adrenal hyperplasia. J Clin Endocrinol Metab 1995; 80:2336–2341.

37. Lacroix A, Tremblay J, Touyz RM, Deng LY, Lariviere R, Cusson JR, et al. Abnormal adrenal and vascular responses to vasopressin mediated by a V1-vasopressin receptor in a patient with adrenocorticotropin-independent macronodular adrenal hyperplasia, Cushing's syndrome, and orthostatic hypotension. J Clin Endocrinol Metab 1997; 82:2414–2422.

38. Willenberg HS, Stratakis CA, Marx C, Ehrhart-Bornstein M, Chrousos GP, Bornstein SR. Aberrant interleukin-1 receptors in a cortisol-secreting adrenal adenoma causing Cushing's syndrome. N Engl J Med 1998; 339:27–31.

39. Chrousos GP, Detera-Wadleigh SD, Karl M. Syndromes of glucocorticoid resistance. Ann Intern Med 1993; 119:1113–1124.

40. Phillipov G, Palermo M, Shackleton CH. Apparent cortisone reductase deficiency: a unique form of hypercortisolism. J Clin Endocrinol Metab 1996; 81:3855–3860.

41. Stuart Mason A, Meade TW, Morris JN. Epidemiological and clinical picture of Addinson's disease. Lancet 1968; ii:744–747.

42. Nerup J. Addison's disease—clinical studies. A repo of 108 cases. Acta Endocrinol (Copenh) 1974; 76:127–141.

43. Zelissen PMJ. Addison patiënten in Nederland. Den Haag: Nederlandse Vereniging voor Addison Patiënten, 1994.

44. Kong M-F, Jeffcoate W. Eighty-six cases of Addison's disease. Clin Endocrinol (Oxf) 1994; 41:757–761.

45. Chen S, Sawicka J, Betterle C, Powell M, Prentice L, Volpato M, et al. Autoantibodies to steroidogenic enzymes in autoimmune polyglandular syndrome, Addison's disease, and premature ovarian failure. J Clin Endocrinol Metab 1996; 81:1871–1876.

46. Baker JR Jr. Autoimmune endocrine disease. JAMA 1997; 278:1931–1937.

47. Riley WJ. Autoimmune polyglandular syndromes. Horm Res 1992; 38 Suppl 2:9–15.
48. Laureti S, Casucci G, Santeusanio F, Angeletti G, Aubourg P, Brunetti P. X-linked adrenoleukodystrophy is a frequent cause of idiopathic Addison's disease in young adult male patients. J Clin Endocrinol Metab 1996; 81:470–474.
49. Laureti S, Aubourg P, Calcinaro F, Rocchiccioli F, Casucci G, Angeletti G, et al. Etiological diagnosis of primary adrenal insufficiency using an original flowchart of immune and biochemical markers. J Clin Endocrinol Metab 1998; 83:3163–3168.
50. Clark AJ, Weber A. Adrenocorticotropin insensitivity syndromes. Endocr Rev 1998; 19:828–843.
51. Stuckey BG, Mastaglia FL, Reed WD, Pullan PT. Glucocorticoid insufficiency, achalasia, alacrima with autonomic motor neuropathy. Ann Intern Med 1987; 106:61–63.
52. Tsigos C, Arai K, Latronico AC, DiGeorge AM, Rapaport R, Chrousos GP. A novel mutation of the adrenocorticotropin receptor (ACTH-R) gene in a family with the syndrome of isolated glucocorticoid deficiency, but no ACTH-R abnormalities in two families with the triple A syndrome. J Clin Endocrinol Metab 1995; 80:2186–2189.
53. Naville D, Barjhoux L, Jaillard C, Faury D, Despert Esteva B, et al. Demonstration by transfection studies that mutations in the adrenocorticotropin receptor gene are one cause of the hereditary syndrome of glucocorticoid deficiency. J Clin Endocrinol Metab 1996; 81:1442–1448.
54. Aron DC. Endocrine complications of the acquired immunodeficiency syndrome. Arch Intern Med 1989; 149:330–333.
55. Sellmeyer DE, Grunfeld C. Endocrine and metabolic disturbances in human immunodeficiency virus infection and the acquired immune deficiency syndrome. Endocr Rev 1996; 17:518–532.
56. Piedrola G, Casado JL, Lopez E, Moreno A, Perez-Elias MJ, Garcia-Robles R. Clinical features of adrenal insufficiency in patients with acquired immunodeficiency syndrome. Clin Endocrinol 1996; 45:97–101.
57. Sullivan WM, Kelley GG, O'Connor PG, Dickey PS, Kim JH, Robbins R, et al. Hypopituitarism associated with a hypothalamic CMV infection in a patient with AIDS. Am J Med 1992; 92:221–223.
58. Gradon JD, Sepkowitz DV. Fluconazole-associated acute adrenal insufficiency. Postgrad Med J 1991; 67:1084–1085.
59. Grinspoon SK, Donovan DS, Jr, Bilezikian JP. Aetiology and pathogenesis of hormonal and metabolic disorders in HIV infection. Baillieres Clin Endocrinol Metab 1994; 8:735–755.
60. Grinspoon SK, Bilezikian JP. HIV disease and the endocrine system. N Engl J Med 1992; 327:1360–1365.
61. Leinung MC, Liporace R, Miller CH. Induction of adrenal suppression by megestrol acetate in patients with AIDS. Ann Intern Med 1995; 122:843–845.
62. Vago T, Clerici M, Norbiato G. Glucocorticoids and t immune system in AIDS. Baill Clin Endocrinol Metab 1994; 8:789–802.
63. Norbiato G, Bevilacqua M, Vago T, Baldi G, Chebat E, Bertora P, et al. Cortisol resistance in acquired immunodeficiency syndrome. J Clin Endocrinol Metab 1992; 74:608–613.
64. Lamberts SW, de Herder WW, van der Lely AJ. Pituitary insufficiency. Lancet 1998; 352:127–134.
65. Nussey SS, Soo SC, Gibson S, Gout I, White A, Bain M, et al. Isolated congenital ACTH deficiency: a cleavage enzyme defect? Clin Endocrinol (Oxf) 1993; 39:381–385.
66. Krude H, Biebermann H, Luck W, Horn R, Brabant G, Gruters A. Severe early-onset obesity, adrenal insufficiency and red hair pigmentation caused by POMC mutations in humans. Nat Genet 1998; 19:155–157.
67. Koide Y, Kimura S, Inoue S, Ikeda M, Uchida K, Ando, et al. Responsiveness of hypophyseal-adrenocortical axis to repetitive administration of synthetic ovine corticotropin-releasing hormone in patients with isolated adrenocorticotropin deficiency. J Clin Endocrinol Metab 1986; 63:329–335.

11 ACTH Resistance

Constantine Tsigos, MD, PhD

The recent cloning of the adrenocorticotropic hormone (ACTH) receptor gene has greatly increased our understanding of the molecular basis of ACTH action and, hence, of the normal and pathologic functioning of its principal target organ, the adrenal cortex. This chapter will focus on the clinical forms of hereditary ACTH-resistance syndromes and their association with abnormalities of the ACTH receptor gene.

THE ACTH RECEPTOR

Biology of the ACTH Receptor

The ACTH receptor (melanocortin receptor 2, MC2), together with the other melano-cortin receptors, form a distinct subfamily of the G-protein-coupled receptors *(1)*. As such, they consist of seven hydrophobic membrane-spanning α-elices connected by hydrophilic loops exposed on either side of the plasma membrane. They share, however, a number of unique structural characteristics *(2)*. Thus, they lack several amino acid residues present in most of the other members of this superfamily, such as the proline residues in the fourth and fifth transmembrane domains, which introduce bents in the α-helical structure, and one or both cysteine residues thought to form bisulfide bonds between the first and second extracellular loops. Three-dimensional modeling of the skin melanocortin receptor (MC1), suggested that the binding pocket for the ligand is located between the second, third, and sixth transmembrane domains, with several points of interaction between receptor and ligand *(3)*. Each of the melanocortin receptors, including the ACTH receptor, couples to Gs and adenylyl cyclase, but displays a unique pharmacological profile for activation by the different melanocortin peptides. The ACTH receptor exhibits an absolute specificity for ACTH, requiring two peptide domains for recognition and activation, the core H-F-R-W sequence present in all the melanocortin peptides and a highly basic motif found in the midportion of ACTH *(4)*. The core H-F-R-W pharmacophore is a full agonist, albeit at low affinity, of the other four melanocortin receptors.

From: *Contemporary Endocrinology: Adrenal Disorders*
Edited by: A. N. Margioris and G. P. Chrousos © Humana Press, Totowa, NJ

The chromosomal localization of the intronless human ACTH receptor gene has been determined in the distal end of chromosome 18 (18p11.2) *(5)*. Northern blot analysis has revealed ACTH receptor mRNA only in the adrenal cortex and not in a variety of other human tissues *(1)*. *In situ* hybridization has actually demonstrated that the receptor is expressed in all three adrenocortical *zonae (1)*. More recently, reverse-transcriptase polymerase chain reaction (RT-PCR) has identified expression of the ACTH receptor in the adipose tissue *(6)*. There is, however, a spectrum of other extra-adrenal tissues that bind ACTH without detectable expression of the receptor, most notably, mononuclear leukocytes *(7)*, the skin *(8)*, and the brain *(9,10)*. Thus, the ACTH actions in these tissues are probably mediated by other melanocortin receptors that bind ACTH, e.g., the skin MSH receptor (MC1) in the skin, MC3 and MC4 melanocortin receptors in the brain, and so on *(1,8,11)*.

The ACTH receptor is the smallest member of the G-protein-coupled-receptor super-family, consisting of 297 amino acids. It has a molecular weight in its unmodified form of 33. There are two potential sites for N-linked glycosylation in the extracellular N-terminal region, so that the molecular weight of the mature form of the receptor might be 43 *(12)*.

Recently, the 5′-untranslated region of the ACTH receptor mRNA was determined and a major transcription start site is located in an upstream exon separated by more than 1.8 kb of an intronic sequence *(13)*. In addition, 1 kb of the 5′ flanking promoter region of the ACTH receptor gene was cloned and shown to have several cAMP responsive element (CRE)-like sequences *(14)*. This might explain why, in contrast to the commonly observed homologous downregulation of target tissue receptors by their own hormone ligands, ACTH apparently upregulates its own receptors and increases their numbers in the cells of the *zonae fasciculata* and *reticularis (15,16)*. In addition, ACTH produces dose- and time-dependent increases in the transcription rate of the ACTH receptor and, in the ACTH receptor, mRNA longevity. It appears, therefore, that ACTH receptor regulation is a significant component of hypothalamic-pituitary-adrenal (HPA) axis control. Teleologically, this may represent an advantage for this axis, one of the two principal effector limbs of the stress system *(17)*.

Dose-dependent increases in the transcription of the ACTH receptor mRNA in the *zonae fasciculata* and *reticularis* are also induced by angiotensin II *(15,16)*, which acts primarily by causing elevations of Ca^{2+} and diacylglycerol. Thus, it is likely that the ACTH receptor gene is regulated by multiple-signal transduction pathways, including those of kinase A and C.

Signaling Through the ACTH Receptor

ACTH, a 39 amino acid peptide, is the major circulating proteolytic product of proopiomelanocortin (POMC) and the principal regulator of adrenocortical steroidogenesis *(17)*. The biologic activity of ACTH resides in the N-terminal portion of its molecule with the first 24 amino acids being necessary for maximal activity.

ACTH regulates glucocorticoid and adrenal androgen secretion by the *zonae fasciculata* and *reticularis,* respectively, and participates in the control of aldosterone secretion by the *zona glomerulosa (18)*. Specific ACTH receptors mediate all actions of ACTH. Upon binding with ACTH, the receptors are activated, and, in turn, activate the hetero-trimeric G-protein complex, which subsequently activates adenylase cyclase *(11)*. This enzyme catalyzes cyclic AMP generation, which results in stimulation of protein kinase

A and the release of the activated catalytic subunit. This, in turn, stimulates cholesterol ester hydrolase, the enzyme responsible for the conversion of cholesterol esters to cholesterol. Cholesterol is then transported inside the mitochondria for side-chain cleavage and the subsequent steroidogenesis steps.

In addition to the direct effect on steroidogenesis, ACTH also has an important trophic effect on the adrenal cortices *(19)*. Thus, ACTH excess produces adrenal hyperplasia, and, conversely, ACTH deficiency causes atrophy. Adrenocortical dysfunction might also result from abnormalities of the ACTH receptor or downstream the signaling cascade. However, unlike the case of the TSH receptor in hyperfunctioning thyroid adenomas, the ACTH receptor does not appear to function as a protooncogene in adrenocortical tumors *(20)*.

CLINICAL SYNDROMES OF ACTH RESISTANCE

Hereditary Isolated Glucocorticoid Deficiency

Clinical Presentation

Hereditary isolated glucocorticoid deficiency, first described in 1959 by Shepherd et al. *(21)*, is a rare autosomal recessive disorder that manifests as primary adrenal insufficiency, usually without mineralocorticoid deficiency *(22–26)*. If unsuspected, the disease can be lethal. Indeed, among over 50 published cases, 18 have died as a result of the disease. Affected children commonly present within the first two to three yr of life with hyperpigmentation, recurrent hypoglycemia that can lead to convulsions or coma, chronic asthenia, and failure to thrive. Typically, plasma cortisol levels are undetectable and do not respond to exogenous ACTH, whereas endogenous plasma ACTH concentrations are very high, consistent with resistance to ACTH action. Aldosterone and adrenal androgen responses to ACTH are also lost in these patients. However, renin and aldosterone levels are usually normal and responds appropriately to activation of the renin–angiotensin axis (e.g., by salt restriction, orthostasis, and furosemide-induced diuresis).

Histological examination of the adrenal glands from patients who died from the disease has revealed that the ACTH-dependent *zonae fasciculata* and *reticularis* are extremely atrophic, reduced to a narrow band of fibrous tissue, whereas the angiotensin II-dependent *zona glomerulosa* is relatively well-preserved *(21–23)*. This has led to suggestions that the disorder might reflect a defect in the membrane ACTH receptor, in the intracellular ACTH signaling pathway, or in adrenocortical development.

Molecular Pathophysiology

The cloning of the ACTH receptor gene in 1992 has permitted a test of the hypothesis that it might be the disease locus. This was the most likely possibility, given the isolated nature of the defect and its characteristic limitation to the two inner ACTH-dependent adrenocortical *zonae*. Indeed, in our initial patient with isolated glucocorticoid deficiency, an African American boy, DNA sequencing revealed two different point mutations in the ACTH receptor gene *(27)*. The maternal allele contained a stop codon at amino acid 201 of the third cytosolic loop (Fig. 1), resulting in a truncated receptor protein, which lacked a major part of the third cytosolic loop, the sixth and seventh transmembrane domains, the third extracellular loop, and the cytosolic carboxy-tail. In the paternal allele, neutral Ser[120] within the apolar third transmembrane domain was

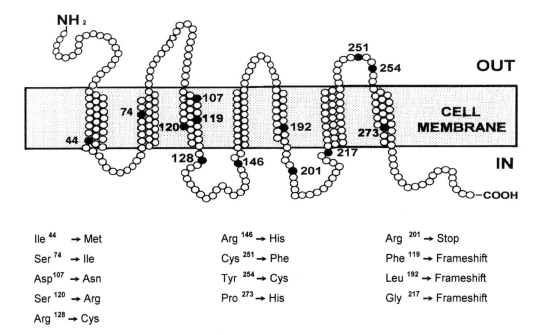

Fig. 1. Schematic representation of the ACTH receptor with the characteristic seven transmembrane domain structure, indicating the position of amino acid substitutions thus far identified to be associated with hereditary isolated glucocorticoid deficiency.

replaced by the basic Arg, most probably disrupting receptor structure and ligand binding, as this domain is important for the formation of the binding pocket of the receptor. Interestingly, the heterozygote parents and grandparents of the proband, carrying either mutation, showed exaggerated and prolonged ACTH responses to ovine CRH, suggestive of subclinical resistance to ACTH *(27)*. The Ser[120] to Arg substitution has also been identified in another African American family with isolated glucocorticoid deficiency (C. Tsigos, unpublished observations).

In a different African American kindred with isolated glucocorticoid deficiency, we found a homozygote point mutation, changing Tyr[254] to Cys in the third extracellular loop of the receptor protein. This mutation probably interferes with bisulfide bond formation and, hence, with the tertiary structure of the receptor *(28)*. Similar point mutations introducing extra cysteines in the extracellular loops of the V2 vasopressin receptor in kindreds with nephrogenic diabetes insipidus also result in a dysfunctional receptor *(29)*.

Ten additional point mutations and frameshift mutations have been reported as homozygote or compound heterozygote mutations in different pedigrees with isolated glucocorticoid deficiency. These mutations are scattered throughout the ACTH receptor molecule and affect all aspects of receptor function as outlined in Table 1 and Fig. 1. Clark et al. *(30)* reported a homozygous point mutation that converted Ser[74] to Ile. This mutation is in the second transmembrane domain of the ACTH receptor, where two independent mutations that profoundly affect the function of the homologous skin MSH receptor have also been found *(31)*. The Ser[74] to Ile mutation was later identified in four additional kindreds and appears to be the most frequent alteration in this disorder.

Table 1
Mutations of the ACTH Receptor Gene so far Identified in Patients with Hereditary
Isolated Glucocorticoid Deficiency

Mutation	Probable effect of mutation	Reference
S120R	Possible structural disruption	Tsigos et al. (1993)
S741	Possible loss of ligand affinity	Clark et al. (1993)
I44M	Possible loss of ligand affinity	Weber et al. (1995)
Y254C	Possible structural disruption	Tsigos et al. (1995)
R146H	Loss of signal transduction	Weber et al. (1995)
R128C	Loss of signal transduction	Weber et al. (1995)
D107N	Possible loss of ligand affinity	Naville et al. (1996)
C251F	Possible structural disruption	Naville et al. (1996)
P272H	Possible structural disruption	Stratakis et al. (1997)
R201X	Truncated receptor	Tsigos et al. (1993)
L192fs	Truncated receptor	Weber et al. (1995)
G217fs	Truncated receptor	Naville et al. (1996)
F119fs	Truncated receptor	Elias et al. (1997)

In one of the families, the S741 mutation was in compound heterozygote form, with a point mutation converting Arg^{128} into a cysteine *(32)*. Arg^{128} is a highly conserved residue on the C-terminal side of the third transmembrane domain of the receptor (Fig. 1), a very important region for interacting with and activating Gs-protein. In another family, the S741 mutation was combined with a deletion of a single C residue in codon 119 in the other allele, resulting in a frameshift of the coding sequence and, after a short length of four nonsense residues, in a premature stop codon *(33)*. In a third family, the S741 mutation was in compound heterozygote form with a Pro-to-His substitution at position 273 of the protein (P273H) *(34)*. This mutation, the closest one to the carboxyl terminus of the protein, may affect the intramolecular structure of the receptor and may, hence, disrupt its function.

Weber et al. *(32)* reported a Finnish pedigree that combined a frameshift mutation (caused by a 2-bp deletion) after Leu^{192} in the fifth transmembrane domain with a point mutation substituting Iso^{44} by methionine in the other allele. The former mutation results in major disruption of the structure of the ACTH receptor and, most probably, complete loss of its function. In contrast, it is not clear how the 144M mutation alters, if at all, receptor function, as the hydrophobic Iso^{44} in the first transmembrane domain is not a conserved residue. Weber et al. *(32)* also reported two independent families, one of Pakistani and one of African American ancestry, which were both homozygote for a mutation changing Arg^{146} to His. Arg^{146} is located in the C-terminal end of the second intracellular loop, and might be expected to have an important role in signal transduction.

Naville et al. *(35)* reported a patient with isolated glucocorticoid deficiency with a homozygote mutation, converting the negatively charged Asp^{107} in the third transmembrane domain to an uncharged Asn residue *(32)*. They also described a compound-heterozygote patient, in whom the paternal allele contained a 1-nucleotide insertion at the junction of the third intracellular loop and the sixth transmembrane domain, which modified the reading frame after residue Gly^{217}, eventually leading to a stop codon. The maternal allele of the same patient contained a point mutation converting Cys^{251} to Phe, also in the third extracellular loop. All three mutations were expressed in the

M3 cell line, in which no response to physiological ACTH concentrations was detected for the mutant receptors. It would, indeed, be expected that the G217fs mutation would lead to the production of a truncated receptor protein unable to transduce the signal. The D107N and C251F mutations must affect amino acids that are important for ligand binding and/or signal transduction. These two residues are conserved in all members of the melanocortin receptor family. Interestingly, the ACTH receptor has two more Cys residues, other than C^{251}, in its short third extracellular loop, all conserved among the melanocortin receptor family.

Unfortunately, expression studies of the mutant ACTH receptors have been hampered by problems with low-transfection efficiency and/or the presence of endogenous ACTH receptor-like activity in the various cell lines tried. The recent report of a subclone of the mouse-adrenocortical Y1 cell line that lacks endogenous receptor expression may lead the way for further studies of cloned ACTH receptors. ACTH ligand-binding studies are also quite difficult, further complicating the investigation of the structure/ function relationships of the ACTH receptor. Undoubtedly, greater understanding of the relevance of the mutations for ACTH receptor function will have to await further expression and binding studies. It is also hoped that development of antibodies against the ACTH receptor will soon be successful, as this would also greatly facilitate these studies.

Not all clinically defined cases of hereditary-isolated glucocorticoid deficiency, however, are associated with mutations within the coding region of the ACTH receptor gene. Weber et al. *(36)* and Naville et al. *(35)* have actually described 4 and 13 such families, respectively, which were clinically indistinguishable from those, in whom mutations were identified. Abnormalities in the promoter region of the ACTH receptor could be responsible in these cases. However, Weber et al. *(36),* using a pair of polymorphic dinucleotide repeats that is localized in the same region of chromosome 18, to which the human ACTH receptor has been mapped (18p11.2) *(5),* demonstrated no apparent linkage between the disease and the ACTH receptor gene in four families. These findings suggest that the etiology of isolated glucocorticoid deficiency might be heterogenous and that gene(s) other than that of the ACTH receptor might produce the same phenotype.

Triple A Syndrome

Clinical Presentation

A subset of the patients with hereditary unresponsiveness to ACTH, in addition to hypocortisolism, develops alacrima (lack of tears) and achalasia of the esophagus (leading to difficulty in swallowing) *(37–40).* This constellation of symptoms is referred to as triple A syndrome, first described in 1978 by Allgrove et al. *(37).* Low tear production, usually present from early infancy, may be confirmed with the Shirmer's test, whereas esophageal dysmotility can be demonstrated by barium swallow and/or endoscopic examination. In some cases, the diagnosis of achalasia may precede the diagnosis of cortisol deficiency. Occasional patients may also develop variable degrees of mineralocorticoid deficiency. Histologic postmortem examination of the adrenals reveals atrophic inner zones of the cortex, an appearance very similar to that in isolated glucocorticoid deficiency. More recently, it has become apparent that progressive and variable neurologic impairment that involves both central and peripheral neurons is

Table 2
Clinical Features of the Triple A Syndrome in a
Survey of 20 Cases[a]

Clinical Feature	Frequency (%)
Glucocorticoid deficiency	100
Alacrima	95
Achalasia	75
Mineralocorticoid deficiency	15
Neurological deficits (85%)	
Motor dysfunction	85
Autonomic dysfunction	70
Sensory impairment	25
Mental retardation/learning disabilities	55

[a]Obtained from ref. *40*.

also frequently associated with the triple A syndrome. Neurological defects may include autonomic and peripheral neuropathy, ataxia, and mental retardation and may thus result in a severely disabling disease *(39,40)*. Table 2 summarizes the clinical features in one recent survey of 20 triple A cases.

Treatment for both ACTH resistance syndromes, the isolated glucocorticoid deficiency and the triple A syndrome, consists of glucocorticoid replacement therapy and, when appropriate, additional mineralocorticoid replacement. Patients with isolated glucocorticoid deficiency achieve normal growth and development with steroid replacement and live an otherwise normal life. For the patients with the triple A syndrome, however, the quality of life depends on the severity and course of esophageal dysmotility and neurological impairment that may develop. The former can effectively be treated with surgical intervention (Heller's myotomy), but there is no known means to prevent or influence the latter.

Molecular Pathophysiology

It had been originally proposed that the ACTH receptor may also be defective in the triple A syndrome, but we had been unable to find mutations in the entire coding region of this gene in several families with the triple A syndrome *(28,41)*. Thus, a developmental defect might be implicated in the pathogenesis of this syndrome or an abnormality in the intracellular signaling of ACTH. Alternatively, a defect in a transcription factor for genes regulating the neuroendocrine system could be underlying the complex phenotype of the syndrome. The first big step toward resolving this question was recently made by the chromosomal localization by linkage analysis of the gene responsible for the triple A syndrome to a 6cM area in chromosome 12 *(42)*. There are several known genes already mapped to this critical region on 12q13, none of which are strong candidates, however, to explain the entire triple A phenotype. Preliminary cytogenetic analysis focusing on the cosegregating segment on chromosome 12q13 did not reveal any visible rearrangements in several patients from different pedigrees *(42)*. Thus, a positional candidate gene approach appears to be the most feasible and attractive strategy for the eventual identification of the causative gene. Understanding the molecular defect of the triple A syndrome would be very important as it may allow presymptomatic testing in neonates in affected families and may raise the prospect of rational design of therapies for this condition.

REFERENCES

1. Mountjoy KG, Robbins LS, Mortrud MT, Cone RD. The cloning of a family of genes that encode the melanocortin receptors. Science 1992; 257:1248–1251.
2. Cone RD, Lu D, Koppula S, et al. The melanocortin receptors: agonists, antagonists, and the hormonal control of pigmentation. Recent Prog Horm Res 1996; 51:287–317.
3. Prusis P, Frandberg P-A, Muceniece R, Kalvinsh I, Wikberg JES. A three dimensional model for the interaction of MSH with the melanocortin-1 receptor. Bioch Biophys Res Comm 1995; 210:205–210.
4. Kepas S, Cammas FM, Hinson JP, Clark AJL. Agonist and receptor binding properties of adrenocortico-tropin peptides using the cloned mouse adrenocorticotropin receptor expressed in a stably transfected HeLa cell line. Endocrinology 1996; 137:3291–3294.
5. Vamvakopoulos NC, Durkin S, Nierman W, Chrousos GP. Mapping of the human adrenocorticotropin hormone receptor (ACTH-R) gene to the small arm of chromosome 18 (18p. 11.21-pter). Genomics 1993; 18:454–455.
6. Boston BA, Cone RD. Characterization of melanocortin receptor subtype expression in murine adipose tissues and in the 3T3-L1 cell line. Endocrinology 1996; 137:2043–2050.
7. Smith EM, Brosnan P, Meyer WH, Blalock JE. An ACTH receptor on human mononuclear lympho-cytes. N Engl J Med 1987; 317:1266–1269.
8. Suzuki I, Cone RD, Sungbin IM, Nordlung J, Abdel-Malek ZA. Binding of melanotropic hormones to the melanocortin receptor MC1R on human melanocytes stimulates proliferation and melanogenesis. Endocrinology 1996; 137:1627–1633.
9. Low MJ, Simerly RB, Cone RD. Receptors for the melanocortin peptides in the central nervous system. Curr Opin Endocrinol Diab 1994; 1:79–88.
10. Cone RD, Mountjoy KG, Robbins LS, Nadeau JH, Johnson KR, Roselli-Rehfus L, et al. Cloning and functional characterization of a family of receptors for the melanotropin peptides. Ann NY Acad Sci 1993; 680:342–363.
11. Tsigos C, Arai K, Latronico AC, Weber E, Chrousos GP. Receptors for melanocortin peptides in the hypothalamic-pituitary-adrenal axis and skin. Ann NY Acad Sci 1995; 771:352–363.
12. Penhoat A, Jaillard C, Saez JM. Identification and characterization of corticotropin receptors in bovine and human adrenals. J Steroid Bioch Mol Biol 1993; 44:21–27.
13. Naville D, Barjhoux L, Jaillard C, Lebrethon MC, Saez JM, Begeot M. Characterization of the transcription start site of the ACTH receptor gene: presence of an intronic sequence in the 5′-flanking region. Mol Cell Endocrinol 1994; 106:131–135.
14. Naville D, Jaillard C, Barjhoux L, Durand P, Begeot M. Genomic structure and promoter characteriza-tion of the human ACTH receptor gene. Bioch Biophys Res Comm 1997; 230:7–12.
15. Lebrethon MC, Naville D, Begeot M, Saez JM. Regulation of corticotropin receptor number and messenger RNA in cultured human adrenocortical cells by corticotropin and angiotensin II. J Clin Invest 1994; 93:1828–1833.
16. Mountjoy KG, Bird IM, Rainey WE, Cone RD. ACTH induces upregulation of ACTH receptor mRNA in mouse and human adrenocortical cell lines. Mol Cell Endocrinol 1994; 99:R17–R20.
17. Tsigos C, Chrousos GP. Physiology of the hypothalamic-pituitary adrenal axis in health and dysregula-tion in psychiatric and autoimmune disorders. Endocrinol Metab Clin N Am 1994; 23:451–466.
18. Aguilera G. Factors controlling steroid biosynthesis in the zona glomerulosa of the adrenal. J Biochem Molec Biol 1993; 45:147–152.
19. Kimura T. Effects of hypophysectomy and ACTH administration on the level of adrenal cholesterol side chain desmolase. Endocrinology 1969; 85:492–499.
20. Latronico AC, Reinke M, Mendonca BB, Arai K, Chrousos GP, Tsigos C. No evidence for oncogenic mutations in the adrenocorticotropin receptor gene in human adrenocortical neoplasms. J Clin Endocri-nol Metab 1995; 80:875–877.
21. Sheppard TH, Landing BE, Mason DG. Familial Addison's disease. Case report of two sisters with corticoid deficiency unassociated with hypoaldosteronism. J Dis Child 1959; 97:154–162.
22. Migeon CJ, Kenny FM, Kowarski, Snipes CA, Spaulding JS, Finkelstein JW, et al. The syndrome of congenital unresponsiveness to ACTH. Report of six cases. Pediat Res 1968; 2:501–513.

23. Kelch RP, Kaplan SL, Biglieri EG, Daniels GH, Epstein CJ, Grumbach MM. Hereditary adrenocortical unresponsiveness to adrenocorticotropin hormone. J Pediatr 1972; 81:726–736.
24. Thistletwaite D, Darling JAB, Fraser R, Mason PA, Rees LH, Harkness RA. Familial glucocorticoid deficiency. Studies of diagnosis and pathogenesis. Arch Dis Child 1975; 50:291–297.
25. Spark RF, Etzkorn JR. Absent aldosterone response to ACTH in familial glucocorticoid deficiency. N Engl J Med 1977; 297:917–920.
26. Yamaoka T, Kudo T, Takuwa Y, Kawakami Y, Itakura M, Yamashita K. Hereditary adrenocortical unresponsiveness to adrenocorticotropin with a postreceptor defect. J Clin Endocrinol Metab 1992; 75:270–274.
27. Tsigos C, Arai K, Hung W, Chrousos GP. Hereditary isolated glucocorticoid deficiency associated with abnormalities of the adrenocorticotropin receptor gene. J Clin Invest 1993; 92:2458–2461.
28. Tsigos C, Arai K, Latronico AC, DiGeorge AM, Rapaport R, Chrousos GP. A novel mutation of the adrenocorticotropin receptor (ACTH-R) gene in a family with the syndrome of isolated glucocorticoid deficiency, but no ACTH-R abnormalities in two families with the triple A syndrome. J Clin Endocrinol Metab 1995; 80:875–877.
29. Pan Y, Metzenberg A, Das S, Jing B, Gitschier J. Mutations in the V2 vasopressin receptor gene are associated with X-linked nephrogenic diabetes insipidus. Nature Genet 1992; 2:103–106.
30. Clark AJL, McLoughlin L, Grossman A. Familial glucocorticoid deficiency associated with point mutation in the adrenocorticotropin receptor. Lancet 1993; 341:461–462.
31. Robbins LS, Nadeau JH, Johnson XR, Kelly MA, Roselli-Rehfuss L, Baack E, et al. Pigmentation phenotypes of variant extension locus alleles result from point mutations that alter MSH receptor function. Cell 1993; 72:827–834.
32. Weber A, Toppari J, Harvey RD, Klann RC, Shaw NJ, Ricker AT, et al. Adrenocorticotropin receptor gene mutations in familial glucocorticoid deficiency: relationships with clinical features in four families. J Clin Endocrinol Metab 1995; 80:65–71.
33. Elias LLK, Klann R, Prarasam G, Pullinger G, Canas TA, Clark AJL. Severe ACTH insensitivity results from a novel compound heterozygote mutation of the ACTH receptor. 79th Ann Meet Endocrine Soc, Minneapolis, MN, (Abstract) 1997; P2–506.
34. Stratakis CA, Wu SM, Bourdony CJ, Cohen D, Rennert OM, Chan WY. Hereditary isolated glucocorticoid deficiency: description of a kindred with adrenocorticotropin (ACTH) unresponsiveness and identification of a novel mutation (P273H) of the ACTH-receptor (MC2R). 79th Ann Endocrine Soc, Minneapolis, MN, 1997; (Abstract):P3–483.
35. Naville D, Barjhoux L, Jaillard C, Fauty D, Despert F, Esteva B, et al. Demonstration by transfection studies that mutations in the adrenocorticotropin receptor gene are one cause of the hereditary syndrome of glucocorticoid deficiency. J Clin Endocrinol Metab 1996; 81:1442–1448.
36. Weber A, Clark AJL. Mutations of the ACTH receptor gene are only one cause of familial glucocorticoid deficiency. Hum Mol Genet 1993; 58:5–588.
37. Allgrove J, Clayden GS, Grant BD, Macaulay JC. Familial glucocorticoid deficiency with achalasia of the cardia and deficient tear production. Lancet 1978; 1:1284–1286.
38. Geffner ME, Lippe BM, Kaplan SA, Berquist WE, Bateman JB, Paterno VI, et al. Selective ACTH insensitivity, achalasia, and alacrima: a multi-system disorder presenting in childhood. Pediatr Res 1983; 17:532–536.
39. Moore PSJ, Couch RM, Perry YS, Shuckett EP, Winter JSD. Allgrove syndrome: an autosomal recessive syndrome of ACTH insensitivity, achalasia and alacrima. Clin Endocrinol 1991; 34:107–114.
40. Grant DB, Barnes ND, Dumic M, Ginalska-Malinowska M, Milla PJ, Petrykowski W, et al. Neurological and adrenal dysfunction in the adrenal insufficiency/alacrima/achalasia (3A) syndrome. Arch Dis Child 1993; 68:779–782.
41. Heinrichs C, Tsigos C, Deschepper J, Dugardeyn C, Goyens P, Ganem G, et al. Clinical and physiological heterogeneity in two siblings with hereditary resistance to adrenocorticotropin: biochemical and molecular studies. Eur J Paed 1995; 154:191–196.
42. Weber A, Wienker TF, Jung M, et al. Linkage of the gene for the triple A syndrome to chromosome 12q13 near the type II keratin gene cluster. Hum Mol Gen 1996; 12:2061–2066.

12 Syndromes of Ectopic ACTH Secretion

Recent Pathophysiological Aspects

Yves de Keyzer, Marie Laure Raffin-Sanson, Agnès Picon, and Xavier Bertagna

CONTENTS

HISTORICALLY
HOW ACTH IS PRODUCED BY NONPITUITARY TUMORS
REFERENCES

HISTORICALLY

Cushing's syndrome refers to the manifestations of chronic glucocorticoid excess and may result from various causes that are all associated with tumors. The most common one being that which was first recognized by Harvey Cushing, and therefore called Cushing's disease, is caused by adrenocorticotropic hormone (ACTH) hypersecretion by a pituitary corticotroph adenoma. The ectopic ACTH syndrome is another, much rarer (approx 5–10%), cause owing to a variety of so-called ACTH-secreting nonpituitary tumors. Finally, approx 30% of Cushing's syndrome patients are ACTH nondependent because of primary adrenocortical tumors, most often unilateral, either benign or malignant.

The first case of ectopic ACTH syndrome probably was reported by Brown in 1928, who described a bearded woman with diabetes who had an oat-cell carcinoma of the lung *(1)*. The discovery of ACTH, the development of an ACTH bioassay, and the pioneering work of Liddle's group *(2)* subsequently identified cases of patients with Cushing's syndrome in whom ACTH was produced by "nonendocrine" tumors. In the initial paper by Meador et al. *(3)*, most of these patients had lung tumors, the extracts of which contained bioactive ACTH. The concept of "ectopic hormone secretion" was then born, and its fine pathophysiological mechanism still remains highly intriguing today with the continuation of remarkable progress being made, essentially through the recent advances in molecular endocrinology and the unraveling of the details of ACTH biosynthesis.

From: *Contemporary Endocrinology: Adrenal Disorders*
Edited by: A. N. Margioris and G. P. Chrousos © Humana Press, Totowa, NJ

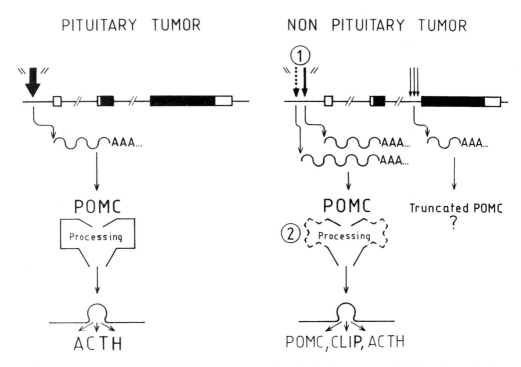

Fig. 1. A schematic view of POMC gene expression in pituitary tumors (left) and nonpituitary tumors (right).

HOW ACTH IS PRODUCED BY NONPITUITARY TUMORS

Altered Proopiomelanocortin (POMC) Processing in ACTH-Secreting Nonpituitary Tumors (Figs. 1 and 2)

... Is Frequent ...

When the ectopic ACTH syndrome was first described it was thought to originate from nonendocrine tumors as stated in the title of the original paper of Meador et al. *(3)*. Today we know that almost all of these tumors, including those found in the lung, such as bronchial carcinoids or small-cell carcinomas of the lung (SCCLs), are genuine endocrine tumors. Their neuroendocrine phenotype is ascertained not only on a morphological basis with the presence of neurosecretory granules, but also biochemically by the presence of granins *(4)*. Other markers of neuroendocrine differentiation have been found more recently with the two specific PCs (prohormone convertases) PC1 and PC2, which participate in the processing of polypeptide precursors to bioactive peptide and/or neuropeptide hormones and transmitters *(5,6)*.

In nonpituitary tumors, various maturation processes—presumably under the action of local PCs *(5)*—operate that are appropriate for the resident hormone precursor of the given tissue (procalcitonin in a medullary thyroid carcinoma, progastrin-releasing peptide in a bronchial tumor) and are more or less efficient for an ectopic precursor like POMC. Hence, an abnormal maturation pattern of POMC is a classic feature of the ectopic ACTH syndrome. POMC may be poorly processed *(7–10)* or, in the contrary, abnormal fragments, such as corticotrophin-like intermediary lobe peptide (CLIP) and hβMSH5-22 may be generated *(11–14)*. Recent studies have shown that PC2 was

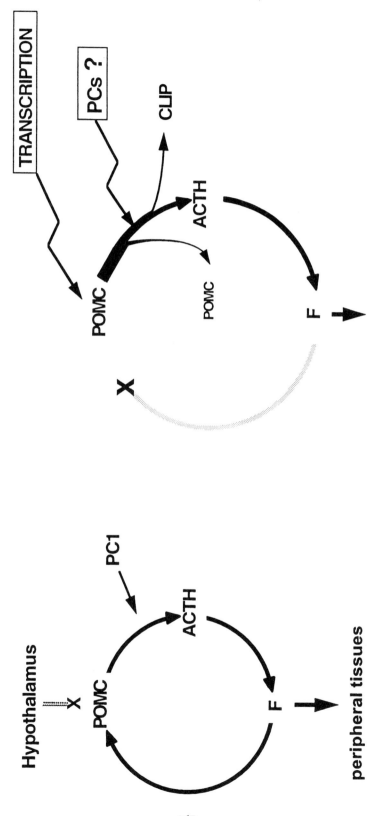

Fig. 2. A schematic view of the pathophysiological determinants for ACTH oversecretion in pituitary tumors (Cushing's disease, left) and in nonpituitary tumors (ectopic ACTH secretion, right).

specifically present in tumors that contained CLIP and not in those that contained predominantly ACTH *(15)*. These processing abnormalities diminish the tissue's ability to secrete authentic ACTH—the sole bioactive peptide in terms of steroidogenesis— and somehow protect the patients from the consequences of the tumor production. They also provide the investigator with subtle molecular clues that an ACTH-dependent Cushing's syndrome may originate from a nonpituitary source (Fig. 1).

A frequent feature of the ectopic ACTH syndrome is a discrepant lipotropin (LPH) ACTH ratio in blood that is unexpectedly high *(16)*. Recent studies have shown that this feature is associated with tumors that have a high content of CLIP. Each molecule of ACTH that is further processed to CLIP is indeed lost for the ACTH RIA and/ or IRMA.

In many cases, intact POMC, or biosynthetic intermediate to ACTH, may be the predominant molecular weight (MW) forms secreted. Several groups have developed specific IRMAs for POMC or other partially processed precursors. These elegant approaches take advantage of various monoclonal, or polyclonal, antibodies to develop a variety of "sandwich" recognition on different locations of the precursor molecule *(17–19)*. Recent studies on large series demonstrated that aggressive tumors, like SCCL, preferentially release intact POMC, whereas carcinoids rather overprocess the precursor, releasing ACTH and smaller peptides like CLIP. It was proposed that the ratio of circulating POMC/ACTH was positively correlated with the aggressivity of the tumor *(19)*.

... But Not Specific

Abnormal processing of POMC is not specific to nonpituitary tumors and is found occasionally in rare pituitary macroadenomas and in some exceptional pituitary cancers. High-molecular-weight immunoreactive ACTH-like materials have been identified by gel exclusion chromatography *(20–22)* in the plasma of such patients. In some cases, a direct POMC IRMA in blood suggests that unprocessed precursor may be directly secreted by the pituitary tumor *(19, 23)*. In other tumors, abnormal POMC fragments, such as CLIP, have been found. Although so far no one has been able to examine, at the same time, the presence of POMC and CLIP in such tumors. This situation recalls that which is physiologically observed in the early postnatal days in the rat: at that period of life, anterior pituitary corticotrophs contain, at the same time, POMC, CLIP, and ACTH *(24)*. Thus, further studies are needed to establish a complete pattern of POMC processing in these rare tumors and to confirm whether their POMC profiles more or less mimic that of a nonmature corticotroph cell of the anterior pituitary. It is highly likely that these processing abnormalities contribute to the relative "silence" of these tumors.

How (and Why) the POMC Gene is Transcribed in ACTH-Secreting Nonpituitary Tumors

Some POMC Gene Transcription Occurs Normally in Nonpituitary Tissues

POMC mRNA is present in many normal nonpituitary tissues, in animal, and in humans *(25)*. In most of these tissues, POMC gene expression is quantitatively and qualitatively different from that in the pituitary. The tissue concentration of POMC mRNA is low and the mRNAs are essentially made of short, truncated, transcripts of ca. 800 nucleotides (nt). These transcripts result from heterogeneous transcription initiations at the 5' end of exon 3 (25); they are nonfunctional and cannot be efficiently translated into POMC peptides (26).

Abnormal POMC Transcripts in ACTH-Secreting Nonpituitary Tumors (Fig. 1)

When ACTH-secreting nonpituitary tumors were examined by the classic Northern blot approach to estimate the molecular size of POMC transcripts, it was found that several had a high-molecular-weight POMC mRNA of about 1450 nt, which was always associated with a normal-sized (pituitary-like) 1200 nt POMC mRNA (27). Using a genomic probe corresponding to sequences upstream of the pituitary cap site, it was shown that this mRNA species was 5' extended (27).

S1 mapping studies with different probes derived from a large DNA fragment encompassing 3.0 kb upstream from the usual (pituitary) cap site (referred as + 1), revealed that the 5' extended POMC mRNA corresponded to a population of three transcripts with 5' ends located at −108 and −217 for the two major ones, and −369 for the third one.

The 5' extended POMC mRNAs thus included longer, 5' noncoding sequences of 215, 324, and 476 nt, respectively. Only one initiation codon was present in the additional sequence, at position −367. Its use would not disrupt the POMC reading frame, the only consequence would be the translation of a larger prePOMC molecule with an N-terminal region extended by 158 amino acids. This additional peptide fragment would not contain the high proportion of hydrophobic residues required for a classical signal peptide and probably could not engage this protein into the secretory pathway. Such a protein has not been detected so far.

Analysis of the human genomic sequence (28) revealed the following motifs preceding the initiation sites of −369 and −217 : ATATTTA at −396, CCCGCCCG at −275, and ATAATTTA at −241. It is tempting to speculate that, like TATAA and GC boxes, these sequences are involved in the transcription of at least some of the 5' extended POMC mRNAs. No characteristic feature could be identified within the 100 nt upstream from position −108. However, this region was GC-rich (72%) and could contain unknown or cryptic promoter sequences.

S1 mapping with 5' extended probes has assessed the relative ratio of the pituitary-like and 5' extended mRNAs. They show that in the majority of ACTH-secreting nonpituitary tumors, the pituitary-sized (1200 nt) mRNA is predominant, although in some instances, the 5' extended transcript accounts for up to approx 50% of POMC mRNA. Further studies should test the hypothesis that this 5' extended mRNA is associated with less-differentiated and more-aggressive neuroendocrine tumors, such as SCCLs, by contrast with highly differentiated, rather indolent tumors like bronchial carcinoids, which most often contain the pituitary-like 1200 nt POMC mRNA as the highly predominant, if not sole, transcript of the POMC gene.

Pheochromocytoma is a rare, but classical, cause of the ectopic ACTH syndrome. For this reason a systematic screening of POMC mRNA was performed in a series of 11 such tumors. All contained the short (approx 800 nt) POMC mRNA, identical to that in the normal human adrenal. Unexpectedly, in two tumors that were not associated with the ectopic ACTH syndrome, equivalent amounts of the 1200 nt POMC mRNA and of the 1450 nt POMC mRNA were detected (29). When a similar search was performed in a variety of bronchial tumors, it confirmed that small (800 nt) POMC mRNAs were present in normal lungs and in all types of bronchial tumors. When neuroendocrine lung tumors (carcinoids) were specifically examined a 1200 nt, POMC mRNA was present in addition to the small mRNAs in many patients without the ectopic ACTH syndrome. In patients with the ectopic ACTH syndrome, the 1200 nt POMC mRNA was always present in large amounts and was the highly predominant, if not sole, POMC transcript *(30)*.

Thus, most nonpituitary tissues and tumors normally express a small POMC mRNA that most likely has no functional significance. In an occasional tumor, a shift of transcription initiation triggers the generation of a 1200 nt (or pituitary-like) POMC mRNA. This latter event only can then be considered as ectopic. It is suggested that it is the necessary condition for the production of ACTH by a nonpituitary tumor. Ectopic ACTH secretion by a nonpituitary tumor is obligatorily triggered by activation of DNA sequences located upstream of the pituitary transcription initiation site and thus generating a POMC mRNA that contains exon 1. Studies in corticotroph cells have shown that these sequences are responsive to cAMP *(31)*. This hypothesis was used to suppress ectopic ACTH secretion by a metastatic pancreatic tumor using a somatostatin analog that presumably reduced intratumoral cAMP content *(32)*. It may also explain the apparently aberrant suppression of POMC gene expression by dopamine agonists in some SCCL that presumably express a functional dopamine receptor.

What Triggers POMC Gene Transcription in ACTH-Secreting Nonpituitary Tumors?

Until recently, few studies have addressed the basic question of POMC transcription in nonpituitary tumor cells because of the lack of convenient models. However, several POMC-producing SCCL cell lines are now available. Southern blot analyses have found no evidence for POMC gene rearrangements *(34)*, in contrast with a case of ectopic parathyroid hormone secretion by an ovarian tumor *(35)*, and as recently demonstrated with the PRAD gene in several parathyroid adenomas *(36)*. Using transient expression of human POMC-luciferase fusion genes in one such cell line, DMS-79, it was shown that the normal human POMC gene promoter was functional in these tumoral bronchial cells. Transcription requires the same 417 nt promoter fragment as in AtT-20 cells, but the respective contribution of definite regions vary between each cell line. For example, the DE-2 element of the rat POMC gene promoter, which induced a 20-fold increase in the transcription rate of a minimal rat POMC gene in AtT-20, is totally inactive in DMS-79 cells *(34)*. Thus, POMC gene transcription is achieved through a different set of transacting factors.

In most, but not all, patients with the ectopic ACTH syndrome, ACTH and cortisol are unresponsive to the high-dose dexamethasone suppression test. This is used as a diagnostic tool to distinguish them from patients with Cushing's disease. The mechanism of the glucocorticoid resistance has been examined in SCCL *(37)* cell lines and seems to be heterogeneous. In some cases, the resistance is only relative and can be overcome with high levels of glucocorticoids *(38)*. Other cell lines apparently contain few, if any, GRs as judged by binding studies; expression of wild-type GR in an unresponsive cell line that already contained GR restored glucocorticoid signaling as measured with cotransfected glucocorticoid-responsive reporter genes. It is not clear, however, if the primary resistance resulted from structural abnormality of the native GR *(39)*, a low level of expression, or some intrinsic property of the cell line *(40)*. It has also been claimed that overexpression of 11β-hydroxysteroid dehydrogenase, an enzyme-converting cortisol into its inactive metabolite cortisone, might diminish the biological effects of endogenous glucocorticoids *(40)*.

These results raise the question of whether POMC is merely expressed by a set of nonspecific factors that also pick up the POMC gene by virtue of some permissive chromatin structure in the vicinity of the gene. Thus, SCCL lines that derive from highly malignant, poorly differentiated bronchial cancers may represent a specific and unusual situation that is far from that in a normal pituitary. Bronchial carcinoids, in contrast, are highly differentiated and rather indolent neuroendocrine tumors that can also express the POMC gene and induce the ectopic ACTH syndrome. The mechanism of POMC gene transcription in these tumors might be different and perhaps more related to that classic pituitary mechanism.

The Ectopic ACTH Syndrome: Two Different Entities

Classically

The first description of the ectopic ACTH syndrome was in patients who bore obvious and aggressive tumors, mainly SCCLs *(3)*, most often leading to a rapid fatal outcome. The clinical features were dominated by muscle wasting, weight loss, and hyperpigmentation, thereby being quite different from the usual manifestations of the Cushing's disease *(2)*. High levels of circulating cortisol and mineralocorticoids induced severe hypokalemia. Hormonal investigations revealed highly elevated ACTH plasma levels and classical dynamic tests, such as the high-dose dexamethasone suppression test, the metyrapone test, the vasopressin test, and, lastly, the corticotrophin-releasing hormone (CRH) test, are typically unresponsive, stressing the autonomous character of ACTH secretion by such tumors *(41)*.

More Recently

This rather unique presentation of the ectopic ACTH syndrome is contradicted by features observed in another set of tumors responsible for what has been recently denominated "the occult" ectopic ACTH syndrome *(42–44)* or the chronic ectopic corticotropin syndrome *(45)*. These patients bear a small tumor that escapes usual detection means. Further to this diagnostic difficulty, they often behave in a "pituitary-like" manner and have led many endocrinologists to the erroneous diagnosis of Cushing's disease and eventually to unwarranted and inefficient pituitary-directed therapies. The clinical features resemble that of Cushing's disease with a mild and slowly progressive hypercortisolism, and, what is most intriguing, some of these tumors respond to the classic dynamic tests in a fashion similar to that of a pituitary corticotroph tumor. Almost one-third suppress cortisol secretion under the high-dose dexamethasone suppression test *(41,43,44,46–48)*, and some well-documented cases show ACTH response to metyrapone and/or CRH stimulation *(49,50)*.

Carcinoid tumors, especially in the bronchial tree, constitute the vast majority of these ACTH-secreting nonpituitary tumors responsible for the occult ectopic ACTH syndrome *(41,43,45)*. They are uniformly small tumoral lesions with a high degree of neuroendocrine differentiation as assessed by the presence of secretory granules at the electron microscopy and their biochemical correlates, the secretogranins *(4,51)*. Also, they are characterized by their high content in the two PCs that are specifically associated with the neuroendocrine cells (PC1 and PC2) and whose function is to process polypeptide precursors to their bioactive peptide hormones *(6,15,52)*.

Such tumors may be an endocrinologist's nightmare *(42)*. They have led to the development of an aggressive investigation procedure, bilateral inferior petrosal sinus sampling, as the best diagnostic approach to recognize the nonpituitary origin of an ACTH secretion, if not to locate its precise site *(53,54)*.

Basically, these tumors are the targets of researchers to help find out the reasons for their strange (or unanticipated) behaviors. Recently, it has been shown that they may contain glucocorticoid receptors *(48,50)*, thus offering a tentative explanation for their pituitary-like behavior, although it does not help to understand why they occasionally express the POMC gene. It was inescapable to explore the possibility that they also express other genes, specifically associated with the corticotroph phenotype. A special interest has evidently been brought by the recent cloning of the V3 vasopressin receptor *(55–58)*. This long-sought receptor, believed to be intimately linked with the corticotroph phenotype, offered a privileged molecular tool to shed new light on the pathophysiology of ACTH-secreting nonpituitary tumors.

The V3 Vasopressin Receptor and the Ectopic ACTH Syndrome

Expression of V3 receptor, CRH receptor, and POMC genes, was examined simultaneously in various types of ACTH-secreting tumors using a comparative RT-PCR approach. Six of eight bronchial carcinoids responsible for the ectopic ACTH syndrome had both POMC- and V3-receptor signals as high as those in pituitary corticotroph adenomas. In contrast, no POMC signal and only a very faint V3-receptor signal were detected in six of eight nonsecreting bronchial carcinoids. Northern blot analysis showed V3-receptor mRNA of identical size in ACTH-secreting bronchial carcinoids and pituitary tumors. Other types of aggressive nonpituitary tumors responsible for ectopic ACTH syndrome (two metastases of neuroendocrine tumors of unknown origin, one metastatic medullary thyroid carcinoma, one malignant and one benign pheochromocytoma) presented much lower levels of both POMC- and V3-receptor gene expression than those found in ACTH-secreting bronchial carcinoids. In contrast with the V3 receptor, CRH-receptor mRNA was detected in many neuroendocrine tumors irrespective of their POMC status.

Assessment of V3-receptor gene expression in ACTH-producing nonpituitary tumors characterized bronchial carcinoids as a particular subset of tumors where both V3 receptor- and POMC genes may be expressed in a pattern indistinguishable from that in pituitary corticotroph adenomas. They can use the normal promoter generating only the pituitary-like, 1200 nt, POMC mRNA *(27)*; produce equal, if not higher, levels of POMC mRNA and POMC peptides *(30,59)*; and process the precursor to release large amounts of bioactive ACTH *(60)*. The apparent coordinate expression of two different genes (coding for the V3 receptor and for POMC), which characterize the pituitary corticotroph cell, strengthens the idea that a broad process of corticotroph differentiation is achieved in these nonpituitary tumors *(61)*.

The classical dogma states that, in contrast with pituitary tumors, ACTH-secreting nonpituitary tumors do not respond to vasopressin stimulation. Yet, some exceptional cases had been reported where vasopressin had induced ACTH rise in vivo *(62)*, and in vitro studies on bronchial carcinoids have also showed a stimulatory effect of vasopressin on ACTH release *(50,63)*.

The functional or causal role for the V3 receptor in ACTH-secreting nonpituitary tumors is not known. If it contributes to an increase in POMC gene expression and/

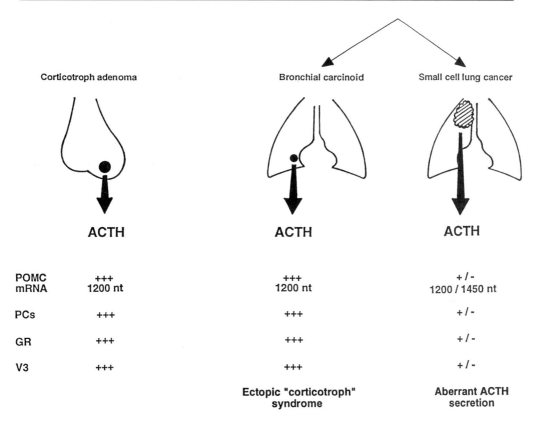

	Corticotroph adenoma	Bronchial carcinoid	Small cell lung cancer
	ACTH	ACTH	ACTH
POMC mRNA	+++ 1200 nt	+++ 1200 nt	+ / - 1200 / 1450 nt
PCs	+++	+++	+ / -
GR	+++	+++	+ / -
V3	+++	+++	+ / -
		Ectopic "corticotroph" syndrome	Aberrant ACTH secretion

Fig. 3. Ectopic ACTH syndrome: two different entities? GR: glucocorticoid receptor; V3: vasopressin receptor V3.

or ACTH secretion, it may act through simple overexpression of a wild-type receptor, as recently shown in experimental models for adrenergic receptors in the heart *(64)*, through expression of a constitutively activated receptor as shown in human pathological states with LH- and TSH receptors *(65)*, or through chronic receptor stimulation under the auto- or paracrine action of locally produced vasopressin *(66,67)*. Alternatively, expression of a common transactivating factor(s) involved in the tissue-specific expression of both the V3- and the POMC genes in pituitary corticotroph cells, may cause ectopic ACTH secretion, at least in this newly characterized subset of nonpituitary tumors. Two factors have recently been identified that seem to be involved in POMC gene expression in the pituitary, Cute *(68)*, and Ptx1 *(69)*. Further studies will examine their possible role in ectopic ACTH syndrome.

Two Different Entities: Ectopic Corticotroph Syndrome or Aberrant ACTH Secretion (Fig. 3)

The intimate mechanism that triggers POMC gene transcription in a nonpituitary tumor causing ectopic ACTH syndrome remains mysterious. Is it because of the fortuitous result of a wide and nonspecific genetic turbulence, which also picks up the POMC gene or, alternatively, to the faithful transposition of a more or less complete corticotroph phenotype out of pituitary limits?

The SCCLs and the bronchial carcinoid tumor are two contrasted examples. The former are highly malignant, display few biochemical markers of neuroendocrine differentiation *(70)*, produce low levels and altered molecular forms of POMC mRNA *(27)* and POMC peptides *(60,71)*, and, rarely and barely express the V3-receptor gene. The latter, in contrast, are rather indolent tumors, have high contents of biochemical neuroendocrine markers, produce large amounts of normal (pituitary-like) POMC mRNA, and express high levels of the corticotroph-specific V3 receptor, thus, the ectopic ACTH syndrome appears to be made of two different entities. When it is because of indolent and highly differentiated tumors, with the highest levels of V3 receptor, like bronchial carcinoids, it might be best called ectopic corticotroph syndrome. In contrast, when it is caused by aggressive, poorly differentiated tumors with much lower V3 receptor, it might be best called aberrant ACTH secretion syndrome (Fig. 3).

REFERENCES

1. Brown WH. A case of pluriglandular syndrome: Diabetes of bearded women. Lancet 1928; 2:1022–1023.
2. Liddle GW, Nicholson WE, Island DP, Orth DN, Abe L, Lowder SC. Clinical and laboratory studies of ectopic humoral syndromes. Rec Prog Horm Res 1969; 25:283–314.
3. Meador CK, Liddle GW, Island DP, Nicholson WE, Lucas CP, Nuckton JG, et al. Cause of Cushing's syndrome in patients with tumors arising from "nonendocrine" tissue. J Clin Endocrinol Metab 1962; 22:6893–6703.
4. Vieau D, Linard CG, Mbikay M, Lenne F, Chretien M, Luton J-P, et al. Expression of the neuroendocrine cell marker 7B2 in human ACTH secreting tumors. Clin Endocrinol 1992; 36:597–603.
5. Seidah NG, Chrétien M. Proprotein and prohormone convertases: a family of subtilases generating diverse bioactive polypeptides. Brain Res 1999; 848:45–62.
6. Scopsi L, Gullo M, Rilke F, Martin S, Steiner DF. Proprotein convertases (PC1/PC3 and PC2) in normal and neoplastic human tissues: their use as markers of neuroendocrine differenciation. J Clin Endocrinol Metab 1995; 80:294–301.
7. Bertagna X, Nicholson WE, Sorenson GD, Pettengill OS, Mount CD, Orth DN. Corticotropin, lipotropin, and β-endorphin production by a human nonpituitary tumor in tissue culture: evidence for a common precursor. Proc Natl Acad Sci USA 1978; 75:5160–5164.
8. Ratter SJ, Gillies G, Hope H, Hale AC, Grossman A, Gaillard R, et al. Pro-opiocortin related peptides in human pituitary and ectopic ACTH secreting tumors. Clin Endocrinol 1983; 18:211–218.
9. Ratter SJ, Lowry PJ, Besser GM, Rees LH. Chromatographic characterization of ACTH in human plasma. J Endocrinol 1980; 85:359–364.
10. Yalow RS, Berson SA. Size heterogeneity of immunoreactive human ACTH in plasma and in extracts of pituitary glands and ACTH-producing thymoma. Biochem Biophys Res Commun 1971; 44:439–445.
11. Bertagna X, Lenne F, Comar D, Massias JF, Wajcman H, Baudin V, et al. . Human beta-melanocyte stimulating hormone revisited. Proc Natl Acad Sci USA 1986; 83:9719–9723.
12. Orth DN, Nicholson WE, Mitchell WM, Island DP, Liddle GW. Biologic and immunologic characterization and physical separation of ACTH and ACTH fragments in the ectopic ACTH syndrome. J Clin Invest 1973; 52:1756–1769.
13. Ratcliffe JG, Scott AP, Bennett HPJ, Lowry PJ, McMartin C, Strong JA, et al. Production of a corticotrophin-like intermediate lobe peptide and of corticotrophin by a bronchial carcinoid tumour. Clin Endocrinol 1973; 2:51–55.
14. Vieau D, Massias JF, Girard F, Luton J-P, Bertagna X. Corticotrophin-like intermediary lobe peptide as a marker of alternate proopiomelanocortin processing in ACTH-producing non-pituitary tumours. Clin Endocrinol 1989; 31:691–700.
15. Vieau D, Seidah NG, Chrétien M, Bertagna X. Expression of the prohormone convertase PC2 correlates with the presence of CLIP in human ACTH secreting tumors. J Clin Endocrinol Metab 1994; 79:1503–1509.
16. Kuhn JM, Proeschel MF, Seurin D, Bertagna X, Luton J-P, Girard F. Comparative assessment of ACTH and lipotropin plasma levels in the diagnosis and follow-up of patients with Cushing's syndrome: a study of 210 cases. Am J Med 1989. 86:678–684.

17. Crosby SR, Stewart MF, Ratcliffe JG, White A. Direct measurement of the precursors of adrenocortico-tropin in human plasma by two-site immunoradiometric assay. J Clin Endocrinol Metab 1988; 67:1272–1277.
18. Lowry PJ, Linton EA, Hodgkinson SC. Analysis of peptide hormones of the hypothalamic pituitary adrenal axis using "two-site" immunoradiometric assays. Horm Res 1989; 32:25–29.
19. Raffin-Sanson M-L, Massias JF, Dumont C, Raux-Demay MC, Proeschel MF, Luton JP, et al. High plasma proopiomelanocortin in aggressive ACTH-secreting tumors. J Clin Endocrinol Metab 1996; 81:4272–4277.
20. Fuller PJ, Lim ATW, Barlow JW, White EL, Khalid BA, Copolov DL, et al. A pituitary tumor producing high molecular weight adrenocorticotropin-related peptides: clinical and cell culture studies. J Clin Endocrinol Metab 1984; 58:134–142.
21. Hale AC, Millar JB, Ratter SJ, Pickard JD, Doniach I, Rees LH. A case of pituitary dependent Cushing's disease with clinical and biochemical features of the ectopic ACTH syndrome. Clin Endocrinol 1985; 22:479–488.
22. Reincke M, Allolio B, Saeger W, Kaulen D, Winkelmann W. A pituitary adenoma secreting high molecular weight adrenocorticotropin without evidence of Cushing's disease. J Clin Endocrinol Metab 1987; 65:1296–1300.
23. Gibson S, Ray DW, Crosby SR, Dornan TL, Jennings AM, Bevan JS, et al. Impaired processing of Proopiomelanocortin in corticotroph macroadenomas. J Clin Endocrinol Metab 1996; 81:497–502.
24. Noel G, Mains RE. Plasticity of peptide biosynthesis in corticotropes: independent regulation of different steps in processing. Endocrinology 1991; 129:1317–1325.
25. Lacaze-Masmonteil T, de Keyzer Y, Luton J-P, Kahn A, Bertagna X. Characterization of proopiomela-nocortin transcripts in human non-pituitary tissues. Proc Natl Acad Sci USA 1987; 84:7261–7265.
26. Clark AJL, Lavender PM, Coates P, Johnson MR, Rees LH. In vitro and in vivo analysis of the processing and fate of the peptide products of the short proopiomelanocortin mRNA. Mol Endocrinol 1990; 4:1737–1743.
27. de Keyzer Y, Bertagna X, Luton J-P, Kahn A. Variable modes of Proopiomelanocortin gene transcrip-tion in human tumors. Mol Endocrinol 1989; 3:215–223.
28. Takahashi H, Hakamata Y, Watanabe Y, Kikuno R, Miyata T, Numa S. Complete nucleotide sequence of the human corticotropin-β-lipotropin precursor gene. Nucleic Acids Res 1983; 11:6847–6858.
29. de Keyzer Y, Rousseau-Merck MF, Luton J-P, Girard F, Kahn A, Bertagna X. Proopiomelanocortin gene expression in human phaechromocytomas. J Mol Endocrinol 1989; 2:175–181.
30. Texier PL, de Keyzer Y, Lacave R, Vieau D, Lenne F, Rojas-Miranda A, et al. Proopiomelanocortin gene expression in normal and tumoral human lung. J Clin Endocrinol Metab 1991; 73:414–420.
31. Boutillier AL, Monnier D, Lorang D, Lundblad JR, Roberts JL, Loeffler JP. Corticotrophin releasing hormone stimulates proopiomelanocortin transcription by cFos-dependent and -independent pathways: characterization of an AP1 site in exon 1. Mol Endocrinol 1995; 9:745–755.
32. Bertagna X, Favrod-Coune C, Escourolle H, Beuzeboc P, Christoforov B, Girard F, et al. Suppression of ectopic ACTH secretion by the long-acting somatostatin analog SMS 201-995. J Clin Endocrinol Metab 1989; 68:988–991.
33. Farrel WE, Clark AJL, Stewart MF, Crosby SR, White A. Bromocriptine inhibits Pro-opiomelanocortin mRNA and ACTH precursor secretion in small cell lung cancer cell lines. J Clin Invest 1992; 90:705–710.
34. Picon A, Leblond-Francillard M, Raffin-Sanson M-L, Lenne F, Bertagna X, de Keyzer Y. Functional analysis of the human proopiomelanocortin promoter in the small cell lung carcinoma cell line DMS 79. J Mol Endocrinol 1995; 15:187–194.
35. Nussbaum SR, Gaz RD, Arnold A. Hypercalcemia and ectopic secretion of parathyroid hormone by an ovarian carcinoma with rearrangement of the gene for parathyroid hormone. N Engl J Med 1990; 323:1324–1328.
36. Arnold A. Molecular genetics of a parathyroid gland neoplasia. J Clin Endocrinol Metab 1993; 77:1108–1112.
37. Clark AJL, Stewart MF, Lavender PM, Farrel W, Crosby SR, Rees LH, et al. Defective glucocorticoid regulation of proopiomelanocortin gene expression and peptide secretion in a small cell lung cancer cell line. J Clin Endocrinol Metab 1990; 70:485–490.
38. Farrel WE, Stewart MF, Clark AJL, Crosby SR, Davis JRE, White A. Glucocorticoid inhibition of ACTH peptides: small cell lung cancer cell lines are more resistant than pituitary corticotroph adenoma cells. J Mol Endocrinol 1993; 10:25–32.

39. Gaitan D, DeBold CR, Turney MK, Zhou PH, Orth DN, Kovacs WJ. Glucocorticoid receptor structure and function in an adrenocorticotropin-secreting small lung cancer. Mol Endocrinol 1995; 9:1193–1201.

40. Picon A, Bertagua X, de Keyzer Y. Analysis of the human proopiomelanocortin gene promoter in a small cell lung carcinoma cell line reveals an unusual role for E_2F transcription factors. Oncogene 1999; 18:2627–2633.

41. Wajchenberg BL, Mendonca BB, Liberman B, Pereira MA, Carneiro PC, Wakamatsu A, et al. Ectopic adrenocorticotropic hormone syndrome. Endocr Rev 1994; 15:752–787.

42. Findling JW, Tyrrel JB. Occult ectopic secretion of corticotropin. Arch Intern Med 1986; 146:929–933.

43. Mason AMS, Ratcliffe JG, Buckle RM, Mason AS. ACTH secretion by bronchial carcinoid tumours. Clin Endocrinol 1972; 1:3–25.

44. Howlett TA, Drury PL, Perry L, Doniach I, Rees LH, Besser GM. Diagnosis and management of ACTH-dependent Cushing's syndrome: comparison of the features in ectopic and pituitary ACTH production. Clin Endocrinol 1986; 24:699–713.

45. Orth DN. Cushing's syndrome. N Engl J Med 1995; 332:791–803.

46. Nieman LK, Chrousos GP, Oldfield EH, Avgerinos PC, Cutler GB, Loriaux DL. The ovine corticotropin-releasing hormone stimulation test and the dexamethasone suppression test in the differential diagnosis of Cushing's syndrome. Ann Intern Med 1986; 105:862–867.

47. Strott CA, Nugent CA, Tyler FH. Cushing's syndrome caused by bronchial adenoma. Am J Med 1968; 44:97–104.

48. Florkowski CM, Wittert GA, Lewis JG, Donald RA, Espiner EA. Glucocorticoid responsive ACTH secreting bronchial carcinoid tumors contain high concentrations of glucocorticoid receptors. Clin Endocrinol 1994; 40:269–274.

49. Malchoff CD, Orth DN, Abboud C, Carney JA, Pairolero PC, Carey RM. Ectopic ACTH syndrome caused by a bronchial carcinoid tumor responsive to dexamethasone, metyrapone, and corticotropin-releasing factor. Am J Med 1988; 84:760–764.

50. Suda T, Tozawa F, Dobashi I, Horiba N, Ohmori N, Yamakado M. Corticotropin-releasing hormone, proopiomelanocortin, and glucocorticoid receptor gene expression in adrenocorticotropin-producing tumors in vitro. J Clin Invest 1993; 92:2790–2795.

51. Vieau D, Rojas-Miranda A, Verley JM, Lenne F, Bertagna X. The secretory granule peptides 7B2 and CCB are sensitive biochemical markers of neuroendocrine bronchial tumors in man. Clin Endocrinol 1991; 35:319–325.

52. Creemers J, Roebroek A, Van de Ven W. Expression in human lung tumor cells of the proprotein processing enzyme PC1/PC3: cloning and primary sequence of a 5Kb cDNA. FEBS Lett 1992; 300:82–88.

53. Oldfield EH, Doppman JL, Nieman LK, Chrousos GP, Miller DL, Katz DA, et al. Petrosal sinus sampling with and without corticotropin-releasing hormone for the differential diagnosis of Cushing's syndrome. N Engl J Med 1991; 325:897–905.

54. Findling JW, Kehoe ME, Shaker JL, Raff H. Routine inferior petrosal sinus sampling in the differential diagnosis of adrenocorticotropin (ACTH)-dependent Cushing's syndrome: early recognition of the occult ectopic ACTH syndrome. J Clin Endocrinol Metab 1991; 73:408–413.

55. de Keyzer Y, Auzan C, Lenne F, Beldjord C, Thibonnier M, Bertagna X, et al. Cloning and characterization of the human V3 pituitary vasopressin receptor. FEBS Lett 1994; 356:215–220.

56. Sugimoto T, Saito M, Mochizuki S, Watanabe Y, Hashimoto S, Kawashima H. Molecular cloning and functional expression of a cDNA encoding the human V1b vasopressin receptor. J Biol Chem 1994; 269:27088–27092.

57. Saito M, Sugimoto T, Tahara A, Kawashima H. Molecular cloning and characterization of rat V1b vasopressin receptor: evidence for its expression in extra-pituitary tissues. Biochem Biophys Res Commun 1995; 212:751–757.

58. Lolait SJ, O'Carroll A-M, Mahan LC, Felder CC, Button DC, Young W Scott III, et al. Extrapituitary expression of the rat V1b vasopressin receptor gene. Proc Natl Acad Sci USA 1995; 92:6783–6787.

59. de Keyzer Y, Bertagna X, Lenne F, Girard F, Luton J-P, Kahn A. Altered proopiomelanocortin gene expression in ACTH-producing non-pituitary tumors. J Clin Invest 1985; 76:1892–1898.

60. Bertagna X. Proopiomelanocortin-derived peptides. In: Aron DC, Tyrrell JB, eds. Endocrinology and Metabolism Clinics of North America: Cushing's Syndrome. W.B. Saunders, Philadelphia. 1994, pp. 467–485.

61. de Keyzer Y, Clauser E, Bertagna X. The pituitary V3 vasopressin receptor and the ectopic ACTH syndrome. Curr Opin Endocrinol Diab 1996; 3:125–131.

62. Raux MC, Binoux M, Luton J-P, Gourmelen M, Girard F. Studies of ACTH secretion control in 116 cases of Cushing's syndrome. J Clin Endocrinol Metab 1975; 40:186–197.

63. Hirata Y, Yamamoto H, Matsukura S, Imura H. In vitro release and biosynthesis of tumor ACTH in ectopic ACTH-producing tumors. J Clin Endocrinol Metab 1975; 41:106–114.

64. Milano CA, Allen LF, Rockman HA, Dolber PC, McMinn TR, Chien KR, et al. Enhanced myocardial function in transgenic mice overexpressing the Béta2-adrenergic receptor. Science 1994; 264:582–586.

65. Parma J, Duprez L, Van Sande J, Cochaux P, Gervy C, Mockel J, et al. Somatic mutations in the thyrotropin receptor gene cause hyperfunctioning thyroid adenomas. Nature 1993; 365:649–651.

66. Utiger RD. Inappropriate antidiuresis and carcinoma of the lung: detection of arginine vasopressin in tumor extracts by immunoassay. J Clin Endocrinol Metab 1966; 26:970–974.

67. Becker KL. Historical perspective on the pulmonary endocrine cell. In: Becker KL, Gazdar AF, eds., The Endocrine Lung in Health and Disease. W.B. Saunders Company, Philadelphia 1984, pp. 156–161.

68. Therrien M, Drouin J. Cell-specific helix-loop-helix factor required for pituitary expression of the proopiomelanocortin gene. Mol Cell Biol 1993; 13:2342–2353.

69. Tremblay J, Lammonerie T, Lanctot C, Therrien M, Drouin J. A novel homeobox transcription factor is expressed in early pituitary development and is a major determinant for cell-specific transcription of the proopiomelanocortin gene. Am Endocr Soc 1995; Washington: (Abstr.).

70. Warren WH, Gould VE, Faber LP, Kittle CF, Memoli VA. Neuroendocrine neoplasms of the broncho-pulmonary tract. A classification of the spectrum of carcinoid to small cell carcinoma and intervening variants. J Thorac Cardiovasc Surg 1985; 89:819–825.

71. Stewart PM, Gibson S, Crosby SR, Penn R, Holder R, Ferry D, et al. ACTH precursors characterize the ectopic ACTH syndrome. Clin Endocrinol 1994; 40:199–204.

13 Clinical Presentation and Diagnosis of Cushing's Syndrome

Andrew N. Margioris
and George P. Chrousos

CONTENTS

DEFINITION AND HISTORICAL DATA

Prolonged exposure to high levels of glucocorticoids results in a syndrome first described by Cushing. Harvey Williams Cushing (1869–1939) reported the clinical syndrome of amenorrhea, bruising, cutaneous striae, facial plethora, high blood pressure, hirsutism, and myopathy and attributed it to "pituitary basophilism" *(1)*. Bishop and Close were the first to name the new syndrome after Cushing in a case recognized as such the year Cushing published his paper *(2)*. Albright was the first to recognize the role of glucocorticoids in this syndrome *(3)*. A few years later, excessive secretion of corticotropin (ACTH) from pituitary was shown to be the cause of Cushing's disease *(4)*. The ectopic ACTH syndrome was described by the same person who later established the dexamethasone suppression test, the long-standing golden standard for the differential diagnosis of Cushing's syndrome *(5)*.

ETIOLOGY

The source of glucocorticoids can be exogenous or endogenous. The former may be iatrogenic or factitious *(6)* whereas the latter is caused by increased adrenal cortisol production, which may be ACTH-dependent or ACTH-independent.

ACTH-dependent Cushing's syndrome may be caused by (1) overproduction of ACTH (from corticotroph cell tumors, corticotropinomas) of the anterior pituitary gland; (2) as a result of excessive production of ACTH from ectopic sources *(7)*, or (3) rarely, from ectopic corticotropin-releasing hormone (CRH) secretion.

From: *Contemporary Endocrinology: Adrenal Disorders*
Edited by: A. N. Margioris and G. P. Chrousos © Humana Press, Totowa, NJ

Corticotropinomas cause approx 65% of endogenous Cushing's syndrome, which has been traditionally referred to as Cushing's disease. The overwhelming majority of corticotropinomas (microadenomas and macroadenomas) are unencapsulated benign tumors. The macroadenomas are characterized by a greater and more autonomous ACTH secretion, inducing more pronounced biological signs of hypercorticism, and are more often accompanied by visual field defects and impairment of other pituitary hormonal secretion *(8)*. The typical patient with pituitary Cushing's disease presents with a history of gradually increasing symptomatology. In a significant proportion of patients, Cushing's disease is associated with bilateral macronodular adrenal hyperplasia, with nodules visible on CT and MRI. Some of these macronodules rarely become autonomous, i.e., produce cortisol independently of ACTH. This has been called transitional Cushing's syndrome. Aberrant interleukin 1 (IL-1) receptors have been recently described in such nodules *(9)*.

The ACTH-independent Cushing's syndrome results from adrenals that have become autonomous from either benign or malignant adrenocortical tumors or from other autonomous processes. Primary bilateral adrenocortical diseases are rare entities that have recently been appreciated as important causes of Cushing's syndrome *(10)*. They include (1) primary pigmented adrenocortical disease (PPNAD), also known as "micronodular adrenal disease," which is a genetic disorder that is often associated with Carney complex, and (2) massive macronodular adrenocortical disease (MMAD), a rare disorder of unknown etiology that affects older adults.

Carney complex is a multiple endocrine neoplasia (MEN) syndrome that affects the adrenal cortex, the pituitary, thyroid, and gonads. It is associated with pigmentation abnormalities, myxomas, and other mesenchymal and neural crest neoplasms. The inheritance of the complex is autosomal dominant, and genetic mapping has shown that at least two loci are involved in its pathogenesis *(11)*. MMAD appears to be an isolated finding in most cases, and a genetic defect has not yet been defined. Ectopic expression of hormone receptors has been implicated in several cases of MMAD, but an underlying deficit has not been detected.

Bilateral adrenocortical hyperplasia has also been described in McCune-Albright syndrome and MEN type-1, but this finding is not always associated with hypercortisolism.

The melancholic phase of primary affective disorders can cause reactive hypercortisolism (Pseudo-Cushing's) most probably from an overactive hypothalamus causing a CRH-mediated overstimulation of anterior pituitary corticotrophs *(12,13)*. An association between human immunodeficiency virus infection and pseudo-Cushing's syndrome has been recently described *(14,15)*. New antiretroviral therapies have been implicated.

Chronic active alcoholism also causes pseudo-Cushing's syndrome although the clinical and laboratory findings subside within days following discontinuation of alcohol.

Finally, recurrent Cushing's syndrome may be the result of ectopic adrenal tissue or tumor fragmentation during surgical manipulations *(16)*.

CLINICAL PRESENTATION

Types of Clinical Presentation

The clinical presentation of hypercortisolism can be influenced heavily from the etiology of the disease. Thus, patients with ACTH-dependent Cushing's syndrome form cortisol-secreting pituitary adenomas present with a mild clinical picture and gradual progress. On the other hand, patients with ACTH-independent Cushing's syndrome from adrenocortical carcinoma present with a dramatic clinical picture, which worsens rapidly and is accompanied by signs of virilization or feminization from the overproduction of adrenal androgens or estrogens. These patients may also have hypermineralocorticoidism with hypertension and hypokalemic alcalosis, from the overproduction of aldosterone, deoxy-corticosterone, or corticosterone, which possess sodium-retaining activity.

The clinical presentation of patients with ectopic ACTH production depends on the degree of hypercortisolism and the severity of the illness. In general, three clinical forms of the ectopic ACTH syndrome are recognized: the plethoric, the cachectic, and the pigmentary forms. Patients with the most benign nonpituitary ACTH-producing tumors, such as bronchial carcinoids, medullary thyroid carcinomas, or pheochromocytomas, develop the typical plethoric form which, on clinical grounds, is indistinguishable from pituitary-dependent Cushing's syndrome.

Patients with the most malignant forms of nonpituitary ACTH-producing tumors, such as lung cancer, exhibit a rapidly progressing catabolic picture dominated by cachexia, darkening of the skin, hypokalemic alkalosis, and hyperglycemia. Darkening of the skin becomes the dominant feature accompanied by varying degrees of plethora.

In a few patients with Cushing's syndrome, the elevated secretion of cortisol may exhibit cyclical periodicity, the duration of each cycle ranging from few days to several months. Discrepancies between the clinical findings and the biochemical profile are suggestive of the diagnosis.

Finally, hypercortisolism has been observed in several psychiatric diseases. Of these, chronic alcoholism and melancholic depression may be difficult to differentiate from mild Cushing's disease when accompanied by obesity, hirsutism, and menstrual irregularities. Chronic active alcoholism may mimic the clinical and hormonal characteristics of Cushing's syndrome and, in this case, the condition has been referred to as alcoholic Pseudo-Cushing's. As aforementioned, the clinical and laboratory findings subside within days following the discontinuation of alcohol. The melancholic phase of primary affective disorders is frequently associated with sustained hypercortisolism. It is theorized that endogenous depression may result in an overactive hypothalamus causing a CRH-mediated overstimulation of anterior pituitary corticotrophs. Clinically, these patients may have several symptoms of true Cushing's disease including generalized obesity, hypertension, hirsutism, and menstrual irregularities. Some of these patients may have incomplete suppression of plasma cortisol after dexamethasone (dex) administration and mildly elevated 24-h UFC excretion. In approx 70% of patients with endogenous depression there is an ACTH and cortisol response to insulin-induced hypoglycemia. In contrast, approx 80% of all patients with Cushing's syndrome fail to do so. In addition, 75% of all patients with depression have a blunted response of ACTH to CRH, probably as a result of appropriate suppression of their pituitary glands by the elevated plasma cortisol levels, whereas most patients with Cushing's disease have "normal" or exaggerated ACTH responses. The recently described combined dex/oCRH test can distinguish almost 100% of the patients, because patients with depression have no response to CRH after dex, whereas patients with Cushing's disease do *(12)*. It has been suggested that suppression of endogenous glucocorticoids may be beneficial in some severe cases of major depression resistant to antidepressant therapy.

Fat Deposition and Body Habitus

Obesity is present in over 90% of patients with Cushing's syndrome. It can be generalized or, in about 50% of the cases, trunkal, and combined with thin extremities (centripedal obesity). Redistribution of fat deposition to unusual sites is characteristic of Cushing's syndrome. Fat may be deposited on the face "moon facies," the dorsal aspect of the neck (buffalo hump), the supraclavicular fossae, the visceral and retroperitoneal spaces, and the mediastinum. The latter is characterized by large amounts of mature adipose tissue within the mediastinum that may simulate mass lesions leading to diagnostic error *(17)*.

Skin

High-circulating glucocorticoids inhibit the synthesis of collagen and other ground substances in the skin, causing a thin, "paper-like" skin, red or violaceous striae, increased bruisability caused by capillary fragility, facial acne, hirsutism, acanthosis nigricans, fungal infections, and hyperpigmentation.

In children and adolescents with Cushing's syndrome, the skin manifestations of hypercortisolism were extremely common. Thus, almost 80% of them exhibited purple subcutaneous striae, 60% steroid-induced acne, 60% hirsutism, 30% acanthosis nigricans, 30% ecchymoses, 20% hyperpigmentation, and 10% fungal infections *(18)*. These symptoms decreased dramatically within the three postoperative months and progressively disappeared within the first year of the follow-up period with the exception of light-colored striae.

Muscles

Chronic hypercortisolism causes generalized myopathy, which is more severe in the proximal muscles. Muscles that exercise are usually spared.

Sodium and Water Homeostasis, Blood Pressure

Moderate increase of systemic blood pressure is almost always present in Cushing's syndrome. It has been shown that cortisol increases blood pressure, in a dose-dependent manner, accompanied by sodium retention. This effect of cortisol is not prevented by the coadministration of the type 1-mineralocorticoid receptor antagonist spironolactone suggesting that sodium retention is not the primary mechanism of cortisol-induced hypertension. Because sympathetic activity is also unaffected, it has been proposed that nitric oxide may play a role in cortisol-induced hypertension *(19)*.

Severe hypertension with hypokalemic alkalosis is dominant in ectopic ACTH production or in adrenocortical carcinomas. Similarly, hypertension and hypokalemic alkalosis may characterize the ACTH-independent bilateral macronodular adrenocortical hyperplasia secondary to excessive secretion of mineralocorticoids rather than because of a mineralocorticoid effect of cortisol *(20)*.

Occult hypermineralocorticoidism in patients with Cushing's syndrome is responsible for the greater-than-normal Na+/H+ exchange (NHE), which results in peripheral edema, high diastolic blood pressure, and hypokalemia. The enhanced NHE is normalized by treatment with spironolactone. This effect of hypercortisolism is most probably caused by functional hypermineralocorticoidism from the incomplete peripheral conversion of cortisol (which binds to mineralocorticoid receptors) into the metabolically inactive cortisone, because these patients exhibit high urine tetrahydrocortisol plus 5-alpha-tetrahydrocortisol to tetrahydrocortisone ratio *(21)*.

Carbohydrate Metabolism

Glucocorticoids antagonize the hypoglycemic effects of insulin. Thus, increased concentrations of serum cortisol result in glucose intolerance. Indeed, fasting hyperglycemia is present in at least 15% of patients with Cushing's syndrome. Genetically predisposed patients may develop frank diabetes mellitus.

Bone Metabolism

Glucocorticoids inhibit the formation of bone matrix by suppressing the production of extracellular collagen *(22)*. They also suppress gastrointestinal absorption of calcium and stimulate its urinary secretion. It has been shown that patients with Cushing's syndrome have reduced osteoblastic function, increased bone resorption, reduced bone mineral density, and that the severity of these abnormalities is statistically related to the severity of disease activity, as indicated by urinary free cortisol *(23)*. Indeed, in Cushing's syndrome patients, serum bone Gla protein, a marker of osteoblastic function, is reduced, whereas bone resorption is increased as indicated by increased urinary hydroxyproline and urinary deoxypyridinoline. Their bone mineral density is reduced at all sites with the spinal trabecular the most severely affected. In long-standing hypercortisolism, the worsening bone demineralization and osteoporosis leads to pathologic bone fractures in over 50% of patients.

Aseptic avascular necrosis of the femoral and humeral heads appears to be less frequent in patients with the endogenous syndrome than in patients treated with pharmacologic doses of glucocorticoids.

Growth

Glucocorticoids inhibit the production of growth hormone and somatomedin C, as well as their biological effects. Indeed, new bone formation is severely suppressed in patients with Cushing's syndrome. During childhood, hypercortisolism can present as growth retardation.

Gonadal Axis

The hypothalamic-pituitary-adrenal and the hypothalamic-pituitary-gonadal axes interact at multiple levels. Thus, CRH is responsible for the "hypothalamic" amenorrhea of stress, which is also seen in melancholic depression, malnutrition, eating disorders, chronic active alcoholism, chronic excessive exercise, and the hypogonadism of Cushing's syndrome. Indeed, CRH and the proopiomelanocortin (POMC) product beta-endorphin inhibit the production of LHRH, whereas the ovarian estrogens stimulate the expression of the CRH gene, as well as the other stress axis, the noradrenergic system. These interactions may explain adult women's slight hypercortisolism and the preponderance of affective, anxiety and eating disorders, the mood cycles, and their slightly higher vulnerability to autoimmune and inflammatory diseases *(24)*.

High levels of glucocorticoids suppress the hypothalamic-pituitary-gonadal axis at multiple levels. They inhibit the production of LHRH, LH, and FSH, and that of ovarian estrogen and progesterone and, at the same time, render their target tissues resistant to them. Approx 80% of patients with Cushing's syndrome have menstrual irregularities or amenorrhea, which appear to be the result of hypercortisolemic inhibition of gonado-tropin release acting at a hypothalamic level, rather than raised circulating androgen levels *(25)*.

During adolescence, hypercortisolism can present as delayed or arrested puberty.

Thyroid Function

Hypercortisolemia inhibits the secretion of thyroid stimulating hormone (TSH) and the conversion of the relatively inactive tetra-iodo-thyronine (T_4) to the more active tri-iodo-thyronine (T_3).

Nervous System

The presence of hypercortisolism affects the nervous system in many ways: (1) It can cause pseudotumor cerebri (mainly in male children, but also in adults of both sexes); (2) it can cause generalized proximal myopathy, which may result in severe muscle atrophy. The patients complain of muscle weakness and, on examination, they are unable to rise from the squatting position; (3) hypercortisolism can also cause spinal lipomatosis, which may result in spinal cord or nerve-root compression; and (4) hypercortisolism-induced perineural lipomatosis can cause nerve entrapment syndromes *(26)*.

It should be noted that hypercortisolism may alter the electrical activity of the brain, causing changes in the electroencephalogram.

Behavior

Hypercortisolism affects behavioral and cognitive functions. Approx 70% of patients with Cushing's syndrome have some psychiatric manifestations that may predate all other symptoms in at least 50% of the cases *(27)*. They range from mild mood changes to severe psychosis.

About half of the adult patients with Cushing's syndrome meet the strict criteria for a major affective disorder. The earliest symptoms are euphoria or hypomania and mild irritability and later emotional lability, fatigue, and depression. It should be noted here that depression from other etiologies might result in the activation of the hypothalamic-pituitary-adrenal axis at the level of hypothalamus *(28)*. However, hypercortisolism-induced depression is distinctive in that it is usually intermittent than constant, lasting a few days in contrast to most patients suffering from depression of other etiologies. In some cases, the depression can be severe enough to become the dominant feature of Cushing's syndrome. Recently, major depression (according to DSM-IV criteria) has been found in 54% of patients with pituitary-dependent Cushing's disease *(29)*. It was significantly associated with older age, females, higher pretreatment urinary cortisol levels, relatively more severe clinical condition, and absence of pituitary adenoma. Patients with Cushing's disease and depression appear to suffer from a more severe form of illness, both in terms of cortisol production and clinical presentation, compared to those who were not depressed. Because of these connections, the presence of depression is an important clinical feature that should not be neglected *(26)*.

High levels of glucocorticoids also impair several cognitive functions including memory and attention span. In children, "compulsive diligence" in performing their homework may indicate the development of a cognition defect.

Sleep is affected with typically decreased REM latency and stage 4 (deep) sleep and increased daytime sleepiness. Impotence and decreased libido are very common phenomena.

DIAGNOSIS

The tests to diagnose Cushing's syndrome are divided into screening, confirmatory, and tests to make the differential diagnosis and localize the cause of hypercortisolemia. The main purpose of the screening tests is to identify the few patients with Cushing's syndrome from the large population of patients with similar clinical presentation (i.e., having obesity, hypertension, hyperglycemia, and so on) but do not suffer from hypercortisolism. It should be noted that the diagnosis and differential diagnosis of Cushing's syndrome can be extremely difficult *(30)*.

Routine Clinical Chemistry

The routine clinical chemistry profile may show hyperglycemia, hypokalemic alkalosis, and hypercalcemia, whereas the blood count shows neutrophilia, lymphopenia, and eosinopenia. Hypokalemic alkalosis is more common in patients with the ectopic ACTH syndrome and in patients with Cushing's disease from macroadenomas *(8)*.

Plasma Cortisol

Random, single determinations of plasma cortisol are of no real diagnostic value because the normal secretion of cortisol is episodic and its plasma concentrations frequently overlap with that of patients with Cushing's syndrome. Lack of diurnal variation in the levels of plasma cortisol can only be suggestive of Cushing's syndrome.

The Overnight 1-mg Dexamethasone Suppression Test

Most patients with Cushing's syndrome will have an 8:00 AM plasma cortisol of more than 5 µg/dL, after the administration of 1 mg of dexamethasone (15 µg/Kg body weight) at 11:00 PM the night before. Normals will show suppression to levels below 5 µg/dL. Patients with alcoholic or psychiatric hypercortisolism may fail to show suppression. Patients on estrogen treatment or with liver disease may also fail to show suppression because of increased levels of cortisol binding globulin (false-positive test). In such patients, the 24-h urine-free cortisol excretion is usually normal. False-positive tests may also be caused by several drugs, such as phenytoin and phenobarbital, that accelerate the metabolism of dexamethasone. Poor absorption of dex may also cause false-positive responses and should be kept in mind.

Urinary-Free Cortisol

The 24-h urinary-free cortisol (UFC) excretion test is the golden standard for the diagnosis of Cushing's syndrome. This test appears to be the most reliable initial test for the diagnosis of Cushing's syndrome, provided that the urine collection is complete. UFC of less than 100 µg/d excludes the diagnosis of Cushing's disease in the majority of subjects. False-negative tests can be observed on patients with periodic Cushing's syndrome and in patients with severe renal failure. False-positive tests can occur on patients with alcoholic or psychiatric hypercortisolism or glucocorticoid resistance.

Because a complete collection of urine for UFC determination is not easy to achieve, an overnight UFC determination has been proposed. It appears that the overnight

UFC to urine creatinine ratio exhibits almost 100% sensitivity and more than 90% specificity *(31)*.

Urine 17-Hydroxysteroids

The 24-h urinary excretion of 17-hydroxysteroids (17OHS) corrected for the amount of excreted creatinine can be used as an alternative of the UFC. Indeed, this test is accurate only if the excretion of 17OHS is corrected for the amount of excreted creatinine (17OHS/gm creatinine) because this correction significantly decreases the percentage of false-positive values in obese patients.

Late-Night Salivary Cortisol

The concentration of cortisol in saliva is in equilibrium with free-serum cortisol. Measurement of late-night salivary cortisol appears to be a simple and reliable screening test for Cushing's syndrome and complements the UFC test. Indeed, patients with proven Cushing's syndrome have significantly elevated 2300-h salivary cortisol compared to normal subjects. The combination of an elevated 2300-h salivary cortisol and an elevated UFC has been shown to identify all patients with proven Cushing's syndrome (100% sensitivity) *(32)*. The concentration of morning salivary cortisol of patients with Cushing's syndrome overlaps with that of normal subjects.

Midnight Serum Cortisol

A midnight cortisol value greater than 7.5 µg/dL correctly distinguishes Cushing's syndrome from pseudo-Cushing states. The sensitivity of the test is high (96%) compared to that obtained for any other test including urinary cortisol (45%), 17OHCS (22%), any other individual cortisol time-point (10–92%), the morning (23%) or the evening (93%) cortisol mean, and the ratio (11%) of morning to evening values *(33)*.

The Liddle Dexamethasone Suppression Test

This test was first described by Grant Liddle. It has since been used as the golden standard for the differential diagnosis of hypercortisolism. It consists of six sequential 24-h urinary collections for measurement of 17OHS or UFC: 2 d prior to the administration of dexamethasone (designated as days 1 and 2 of the test), during the administration of 0.5 mg dexamethasone × 4/d × 2 d (days 3 and 4) (low-dose dexamethasone), and 2 mg dexamethasone × 4/d × 2 d (days 5 and 6) (high-dose dexamethasone). The low-dose dexamethasone suppression test is used to confirm the diagnosis of Cushing's syndrome irrespectively of the etiology. The high-dose dexamethasone suppression test differentiates between the various etiologies of Cushing's syndrome. Urinary 17OHS usually decrease to below 3.5 mg/g of creatinine, on the second day of the low-dose dexamethasone test (day 4) in normal subjects, whereas in patients with Cushing's syndrome (of any etiology), it is higher than 3.5 mg/g creatinine. More than 85% of the patients with pituitary-dependent Cushing's syndrome demonstrate a decrease of their 17OHS excretion to values less than 50% of the baseline, and of UFC excretion to values less than 90% of the baseline (days 1 and 2), on the sixth day of the test (high dexamethasone), whereas less than 15% of all patients with ectopic ACTH secretion or the ACTH-independent form of Cushing's syndrome respond in this manner.

The Overnight 8-mg Dexamethasone Suppression Test

This is an alternative to the standard, but rather cumbersome, Liddle's test. However, few patients with ACTH-producing pituitary adenoma show no suppression of plasma cortisol after the administration of 8 mg of dexamethasone. In a recently published paper, two patients with Cushing's disease did not respond to this test *(34)*. The authors also found decreased expression of the glucocorticoid receptor alpha in their pituitary adenomas that could explain the insensitivity to the 8-mg dexamethasone suppression test.

Metyrapone Test

This compound blocks the conversion of 11alpha-deoxycortisol to cortisol. In more than 80% of patients with pituitary-dependent Cushing's syndrome, an oral dose of 750 mg every 4 h for six doses will cause a decrease of plasma cortisol levels and a compensatory increase of plasma 11alpha-deoxycortisol to levels above 10 μg/dL. As 11alpha-deoxycortisol is metabolized to 17OHS, patients with pituitary-dependent Cushing's syndrome have increased 17OHS excretion that exceeds the baseline by 50% on the day of the test or the ensuing day. Patients with the ectopic ACTH syndrome or with adrenal adenomas or carcinomas do not increase their plasma 11alpha-deoxy-cortisol or their 24-h urinary 17OHS excretion, because the production of their ACTH and/or cortisol does not respond to glucocorticoid negative feedback.

Plasma ACTH

The concentration of plasma ACTH on patients with pituitary-dependent Cushing's syndrome is normal or mildly elevated. In patients with the ectopic ACTH syndrome, it is usually higher than in pituitary-dependent Cushing's, although there is a large area of overlap between the two conditions. ACTH is usually undetectable or very low on patients with ACTH-independent Cushing's. High-molecular-weight forms of immuno-reactive ACTH are observed in 25% of patients with the ectopic ACTH syndrome. The ACTH precursor proopiomelanocortin is also elevated in the majority of these patients.

CRH Test and Combined CRH/Dexamethasone Test

The intravenous administration of synthetic ovine CRH to healthy subjects results in a dose-dependent increase of plasma ACTH and cortisol. The same dose of human CRH elicits a similar response in magnitude, but shorter in duration. Some degree of flushing (mainly facial), metallic taste, increased respiratory rate, and hypotension have been reported to occur in 10 to 20% of all subjects receiving intravenous ovine CRH. The frequency of these side effects appears to be dose-dependent. A CRH response is defined as an increase of plasma ACTH or cortisol to more than four times the intraassay coefficient of variation above the baseline, which is usually around 20%. Most patients with Cushing's disease respond with elevations of ACTH and cortisol, whereas most patients with the ectopic ACTH syndrome do not respond. Patients with ACTH-independent Cushing's syndrome show no response of ACTH or cortisol to CRH. The diagnostic accuracy of the ovine CRH-stimulation and the dexamethasone-suppression tests are similar. A combined strategy using both the dexamethasone-suppression and the CRH-stimulation tests usually yields superior sensitivity and diagnostic accuracy in the differential diagnosis of Cushing's disease from Pseudo-Cushing states *(35,36)*.

Recently, the combined Dex-CRH test was found to be of value in the differential diagnosis between patients with mild Cushing's syndrome vs normal *(37)*.

Simultaneous Bilateral Inferior Petrosal Sinus Sampling (SBIPSS)

The differential diagnosis of ACTH-dependent Cushing's syndromes can be quite difficult because the pituitary microadenomas and the ectopic ACTH-secreting tumors are frequently very small to be localized by imaging techniques. SBIPSS is one of the most specific methods to determine the source of ACTH *(38)*. During SBIPSS, catheters are led into each inferior petrosal sinus via the ipsilateral femoral vein. Venous blood from the anterior pituitary drains into the cavernous sinus and from there into the superior and inferior petrosal sinuses. The location of the catheters is confirmed by the injection of radiopaque solution. Samples for plasma ACTH are collected simultaneously from each inferior petrosal sinus and from a peripheral vein, before and 3, 5, and 10 min after the intravenous injection of 1 µg/kg of ovine CRH. Patients with the ectopic ACTH syndrome have no ACTH concentration gradient between either inferior petrosal sinus and the peripheral blood. The presence of plasma ACTH concentration gradient between either site and the peripheral vein (baseline gradient >1.6, post CRH gradient >3.2) is highly suggestive of Cushing's disease. It should be mentioned that unilateral, or nonsimultaneous sampling, may provide false-negative results because inferior petrosal vein ACTH levels contralateral to pituitary adenomas, are often no different from those in peripheral plasma. SBIPSS can also be useful, in the localization of a microadenoma within the pituitary. Indeed, a gradient of plasma ACTH concentrations, between the two petrosal sinuses (ratio >1.6), suggests correctly the location of the adenoma in about 70% of the cases. This is particularly important in cases in which the neurosurgeon fails to visualize the tumor during the operation. In these cases, hemipituitectomy can be performed, at an attempt to cure Cushing's disease without causing permanent pituitary-hormone deficiencies.

Measurement of immunoreactive CRH in the inferior petrosal sinus plasma has been shown to have no diagnostic significance because it does not differ between patients with Cushing's disease, pseudo-Cushing's states and normals *(39)*.

Single Sequential Inferior Petrosal Sinus Sampling

Recently, a simplified method of inferior petrosal sinus sampling has been described using a single sequential sampling from each of the inferior petrosal sinuses, following initial hCRH stimulation. It was shown to be as accurate as the more complex test using multiple bilateral simultaneous inferior petrosal sinus samples. In addition, the use of indwelling cerebral venous catheters is avoided preventing the possible damage of the brain stem *(40)*.

Cavernous Sinus Sampling

An alternative method to inferior petrosal sinus sampling is the selective venous sampling from the cavernous sinus *(41)*. It has been shown that cavernous sinus sampling, without CRH administration, can demonstrate hypersecretion of ACTH from the pituitary gland with a high diagnostic accuracy, whereas the intercavernous gradients indicate the correct lateralization in laterally localized microadenomas. However, it was found that the best results were obtained from sampling the posterior portion of the cavernous sinus.

Imaging

Most patients with ACTH-dependent Cushing's syndrome have ACTH-secreting microadenomas with a diameter of less than 5 mm. Thus, plain sella X-rays and sella tomographies are normal in the majority of cases. High-resolution gadolinium MRI identifies pituitary ACTH-producing tumors in more than 50% of the cases although this number has been recently disputed *(42)*. CT or MRI of the adrenals are useful for the diagnosis of Cushing's syndrome from cortisol-secreting adrenal adenomas or carcinomas. Adrenocortical carcinomas are usually quite large at the time of diagnosis and enhance on the T_2 relaxation time, whereas most adrenocortical adenomas are usually less than 5 cm in diameter and do not enhance on T_2. The differential diagnosis of the ACTH-dependent Cushing's syndrome can be quite difficult, because frequently, the pituitary microadenomas and the ectopic ACTH-secreting tumors are not localizable by imaging techniques.

The [111In-DTPA-D-Phe1]octreotide scintigraphy scan can locate ACTH-producing carcinoids containing somatostatin receptors *(43)*.

REFERENCES

1. Cushing HW. The basophil adenomas of the pituitary body and their clinical manifestations (pituitary basophilism). Bull Johns Hopkins Hosp 1932; 50:137–195.
2. Bishop PMF, Close HG. A case of basophil adenoma of the anterior lobe of the pituitary. "Cushing's Syndrome". Guy's Hosp Rep 1932; 82:143–153.
3. Albright F. Cushing's syndrome. Harvey Lecture Ser 1942–1943; 38:123–186.
4. Kepler EJ, Sprague RG, Claegt OT, Ower MP, Mason H, Rodgers HM. Adrenocortical tumor associated with Cushing's syndrome. J Clin Endocrinol 1948; 8:499–531.
5. Liddle GW. Tests of pituitary-adrenal supressibility in the diagnosis of Cushing's syndrome. J Clin Endocrinol Met 1960; 20:1539.
6. Quddusi S, Browne P, Toivola B, Hirsch IB. Cushing's syndrome due to surreptitious glucocorticoid administration. Arch Intern Med 1998; 158:294–296.
7. Arioglu E, Doppman J, Gomes M, Kleiner D, Mauro D, Barlow C, et al. Cushing's syndrome caused by corticotropin secretion by pulmonary tumorlets. N Engl J Med 1998; 339:883–886.
8. Selvais P, Donckier J, Buysschaert M, Maiter D. Cushing's disease: a comparison of pituitary corticotroph microadenomas and macroadenomas. Eur J Endocrinol 1998; 138:153–159.
9. Willenberg HS, Stratakis CA, Marx C, Ehrhart-Bornstein M, Chrousos GP, Bornstein SR. Aberrant interleukin-1 receptors in a cortisol-secreting adrenal adenoma causing Cushing's syndrome. N Engl J Med 1998; 339:27–31.
10. Stratakis CA, Kirschner LS. Clinical and genetic analysis of primary bilateral adrenal diseases (micro- and macronodular disease) leading to Cushing's syndrome. Horm Metab Res 1998; 30:456–463.
11. Stratakis CA, Carney JA, Lin JP, Papanicolaou DA, Karl M, Kastner DL, et al. Carney complex, a familial multiple neoplasia and lentiginosis syndrome. Analysis of 11 kindreds and linkage to the short arm of chromosome 2. J Clin Invest 1996; 97:699–705.
12. Yanovski JA, Cutler GB Jr, Chrousos GP, Nieman LK. The corticotropin-releasing hormone stimulation test following dexamethasone administration (dex/CRH test): a new test to distinguish Cushing's syndrome from pseudo-Cushing's states. J Am Med Assoc 1993; 269:2232–2238.
13. Newell-Price J, Trainer P, Besser M, Grossman A. The diagnosis and differential diagnosis of Cushing's syndrome and pseudo-Cushing's states. Endocr Rev 1998; 19:647–672.
14. Miller KK, Daly PA, Sentochnik D, Doweiko J, Samore M, Basgoz NO, et al. Pseudo-Cushing's syndrome in human immunodeficiency virus-infected patients. Clin Infect Dis 1998; 27:68–72.
15. Lo JC, Mulligan K, Tai VW, Algren H, Schambelan M. "Buffalo hump" in men with HIV-1 infection. Lancet 1998; 351:867–870.
16. Leibowitz J, Pertsemilidis D, Gabrilove JL. Recurrent Cushing's syndrome due to recurrent adrenocortical tumor—fragmentation of tumor in ectopic adrenal tissue? J Clin Endocrinol Metab 1998; 83:3786–3789.

17. Nguyen KQ, Hoeffel C, Le LH, Phan HT. Mediastinal lipomatosis. South Med J 1998; 91:1169–1172.

18. Stratakis CA, Mastorakos G, Mitsiades NS, Mitsiades CS, Chrousos GP. Skin manifestations of Cushing's disease in children and adolescents before and after the resolution of hypercortisolemia. Pediatr Dermatol 1998; 15:253–258.

19. Kelly JJ, Mangos G, Williamson PM, Whitworth JA. Cortisol and hypertension. Clin Exp Pharmacol Physiol 1998; 25:S51–56.

20. Hayashi Y, Takeda Y, Kaneko K, Koyama H, Aiba M, Ideka U, et al. A case of Cushing's syndrome due to ACTH-independent bilateral macronodular hyperplasia associated with excessive secretion of mineralocorticoids. Endocr J 1998; 45:485–491.

21. Koren W, Grienspuhn A, Kuznetsov SR, Berezin M, Rosenthal T, Postnov YV. Enhanced Na+/H+ exchange in Cushing's syndrome reflects functional hypermineralocorticoidism. J Hypertens 1998; 16:1187–1191.

22. Sartorio A, Conti A, Ambrosi B. Bone and collagen turnover in patients with active and preclinical Cushing's syndrome and in subjects with adrenal incidentaloma. J Clin Endocrinol Metab 1998; 83:2605–2606.

23. Chiodini I, Carnevale V, Torlontano M, Fusilli S, Guglielmi G, Pileri M, et al. Alterations of bone turnover and bone mass at different skeletal sites due to pure glucocorticoid excess: study in eumenorrheic patients with Cushing's syndrome. J Clin Endocrinol Metab 1998; 83:1863–1867.

24. Chrousos GP, Torpy DJ, Gold PW. Interactions between the hypothalamic-pituitary-adrenal axis and the female reproductive system: clinical implications. Ann Intern Med 1998; 129:229–240.

25. Lado-Abeal J, Rodriguez-Arnao J, Newell-Price JD, Perry LA, Grossman AB, et al. Menstrual abnormalities in women with Cushing's disease are correlated with hypercortisolemia rather than raised circulating androgen levels. J Clin Endocrinol Metab 1998; 83:3083–3088.

26. Margioris AN, Chrousos GP. Adrenal disorders. In: Vinken PJ, Bruyn GW, (Ser. eds.); Goetz CG, Aminoff MJ, (Vol eds), Systemic Diseases. Part II. Handbook of Clinical Neurologyl. Vol 70 (Rev. Ser. 26), 1998; Elsevier Science, New York.

27. Dorn LD, Burgess ES, Dubbert B, Simpson SE, Friedman T, Kling M, et al. Psychopathology in patients with endogenous Cushing's syndrome: 'atypical' or melancholic features. Clin Endocrinol 1995; 43:433–442.

28. Michelson D, Gold PW. Pathophysiologic and somatic investigations of hypothalamic-pituitary-adrenal axis activation in patients with depression. Ann N Y Acad Sci 1998; 840:717–722.

29. Sonino N, Fava GA, Raffi AR, Boscaro M, Fallo F. Clinical correlates of major depression in Cushing's disease. Psychopathology 1998; 31:302–306.

30. Loh KC, Fitzgerald PA, Miller TR, Tyrrell JB. Perils and pitfalls in the diagnosis of Cushing's syndrome. West J Med 1998; 169:46–50.

31. Corcuff JB, Tabarin A, Rashedi M, Duclos M, Roger P, Ducassou D. Overnight urinary-free cortisol determination: a screening test for the diagnosis of Cushing's syndrome. Clin Endocrinol (Oxf) 1998; 48:503–508.

32. Raff H, Raff JL, Findling JW. Late-night salivary cortisol as a screening test for Cushing's syndrome. J Clin Endocrinol Metab 1998; 83:2681–2686.

33. Papanicolaou DA, Yanovski JA, Cutler GB Jr, Chrousos GP, Nieman LK. A single midnight serum cortisol measurement distinguishes Cushing's syndrome from pseudo-Cushing states. J Clin Endocrinol Metab 1998; 83:1163–1167.

34. Mu YM, Takayanagi R, Imasaki K, Ohe K, Ikuyama S, Yanase T, et al. Low level of glucocorticoid receptor messenger ribonucleic acid in pituitary adenomas manifesting Cushing's disease with resistance to a high dose-dexamethasone suppression test. Clin Endocrinol (Oxf) 1998; 49:301–306.

35. Tsigos C, Kamilaris TC, Chrousos GP. Adrenal diseases. In: Moore WT, Eastman RC, eds., Diagnostic Endocrinology. Second ed. Mosby, St Louis, MO, 1996, pp 125–156.

36. Tsigos C, Chrousos GP. Differential diagnosis and management of Cushing's syndrome. Annu Rev Med 1996; 47:443–461.

37. Yanovski JA, Cutler GB Jr, Chrousos GP, Nieman LK. The dexamethasone-suppressed corticotropin-releasing hormone stimulation test differentiates mild Cushing's disease from normal physiology. J Clin Endocrinol Metab 1998; 83:348–352.

38. Oldfield EH, Doppman JL. Petrosal versus cavernous sinus sampling. J Neurosurg 1998; 89:890–893.

39. Yanovski JA, Nieman LK, Doppman JL, Chrousos GP, Wilder RL, Gold PW, et al. Plasma levels of corticotropin-releasing hormone in the inferior petrosal sinuses of healthy volunteers, patients with

Cushing's syndrome, and patients with pseudo-Cushing states. J Clin Endocrinol Metab 1998; 83:1485–1488.

40. Padayatty SJ, Orme SM, Nelson M, Lamb JT, Belchetz PE. Bilateral sequential inferior petrosal sinus sampling with corticotrophin-releasing hormone stimulation in the diagnosis of Cushing's disease. Eur J Endocrinol 1998; 139:161–166.

41. Tabarin A, Laurent F, Catargi B, Olivier-Puel F, Lescene R, Berge J, et al. Comparative evaluation of conventional and dynamic magnetic resonance imaging of the pituitary gland for the diagnosis of Cushing's disease. Clin Endocrinol (Oxf) 1998; 49:293–300.

42. Matte J, Roufosse F, Rocmans P, Schoutens A, Jacobovitz D, Mockel J. Ectopic Cushing's syndrome and pulmonary carcinoid tumour identified by [111In-DTPA-D-Phe1]octreotide. Postgrad Med J 1998; 74:108–110.

43. Teramoto A, Yoshida Y, Sanno N, Nemoto S. Cavernous sinus sampling in patients with adrenocorticotrophic hormone-dependent Cushing's syndrome with emphasis on inter- and intracavernous adrenocorticotrophic hormone gradients. J Neurosurg 1998; 89:762–768.

14

The Desmopressin Test

A New Tool in the Functional Evaluation of the Pituitary-Adrenal Axis in Patients with Cushing's Syndrome?

S. Tsagarakis and N. Thalassinos

CONTENTS

INTRODUCTION

Noniatrogenic Cushing's syndrome is a rare clinical entity that is caused by an inappropriately elevated endogenous cortisol production and results in significant morbidity and mortality in affected patients. Despite its rarity, Cushing's syndrome represents one of the most challenging diseases in clinical endocrinology because, despite the use of a variety of tests, its diagnosis and/or differential diagnosis often remains uncertain *(1)*. It has long been known that vasopressin contributes to the regulation of the hypothalamo-pituitary-adrenal (HPA) axis: although it is a weak ACTH-releasing secretagog, vasopressin has a significant synergistic effect with CRH that grossly potentiates pituitary ACTH secretion *(2)*. This action is thought to occur via the specific corticotroph vasopressin receptor also known as V3 (or V1b) receptor *(3)*. In the past, several investigators have used the administration of vasopressin analog (LVP or AVP) to differentiate between the ACTH-dependent forms of Cushing's syndrome *(4)*. Thus, positive ACTH and cortisol responses to vasopressin analogs have been observed in the majority of patients with pituitary-dependent Cushing's syndrome, whereas no such

From: *Contemporary Endocrinology: Adrenal Disorders*
Edited by: A. N. Margioris and G. P. Chrousos © Humana Press, Totowa, NJ

responses were observed in most patients with ectopic ACTH secretion. However, these vasopressin tests had a lower diagnostic accuracy compared to the more widely used CRH test *(5)*. Moreover, because of its smooth-muscle constricting actions, administration of vasopressin analogs is commonly associated with several side effects. For these reasons, these tests have not gained wide acceptance for their use in the investigation of patients with Cushing's syndrome. Desmopressin, a long-acting analog of vasopressin, appears to be free of the V1 receptor-mediated pressor side effects, and a desmopressin test has been recently introduced in clinical practice as an adjunctive tool in the diagnosis and differential diagnosis of Cushing's syndrome *(6)*. In the present chapter, we will review current knowledge on the diagnostic value of this test in the work-up of patients with proven or suspected Cushing's syndrome.

DESMOPRESSIN ACTIONS ON THE NORMAL AND ABNORMAL PITUITARY-ADRENAL AXIS

There exist three types of vasopressin receptors: the V1a (or V1), V2, and V1b (or V3) receptors *(7–9)*. They are all members of the G-protein-coupled receptor family, structurally characterized by a single polypeptide chain with seven intramembrane domains. The V1 (or V1a) receptor, which acts by activating phospholipase C, is mainly present in the liver, vascular smooth muscle, brain, mesangial cells, and platelets. The V2 receptor, which acts by activating adenylate cyclase, is mainly expressed in the kidney. The V3 (or V1b) subtype receptor, which is also linked to phospholipase C, is found almost exclusively on pituitary corticotrops. Desmopressin is a long-acting vasopressin analog *(10)*, which has a high relative affinity for the renal V2 receptors with little V1-mediated activity. In contrast to other vasopressin analogs (LVP or AVP) desmopressin has no ACTH-releasing activity when given in normal human volunteers under basal conditions *(11)*. However, although ineffective on basal ACTH levels, it has been shown in a recent report to potentiate CRH-induced ACTH secretion in normal human volunteers *(12)*. This finding indicates the presence of desmopressin responding receptors in the normal corticotrophs. The vasopressin-receptor subtypes of normal corticotrophs activated by desmopressin are not well-established, but they may involve both the V2 or V3 subtypes. The V2 receptors, although thought to be specific for the kidney, have also been found to be expressed in low levels in other tissues including normal corticotrophs *(13)*. The V3 receptors are normally found in pituitary corticotrophs and, it cannot be excluded that desmopressin, a V2 agonist, is completely devoid of crossreaction with this type of receptor. It is also of note that both of these subtypes of receptors are upregulated in the majority of corticotroph adenomas studied by a quantitative PCR-based method *(13)*. This finding may be responsible for the high incidence of responsiveness to desmopressin in patients with such tumors. However, the V3 receptors are also frequently found in many ectopic tumors capable of ectopically secreting ACTH *(14)*.

EFFECTS OF DESMOPRESSIN ADMINISTRATION IN PATIENTS WITH VARIOUS FORMS OF CUSHING'S SYNDROME

Malebri et al. *(15)* were the first who administered desmopressin (5 or 10 μg iv bolus) in patients with various forms of Cushing's syndrome. Despite its known lack of responsiveness in normal subjects, desmopressin administration produced a signifi-

Table 1
The Desmopressin Test in the Differential Diagnosis of Cushing's Syndrome

Reference	Cortisol response		ACTH response	
	CD	EAS	CD	EAS
Malebri et al. *(15)*	15/16	0/3	4/5	0/1
Newell-Price et al. *(17)*	14/17	1/5	12/17	2/5
Colombo et al. *(16)*	14/17	0/1	14/17	0/1
Tsagarakis et al. *(19)*	21/25	0/3	23/25	0/3
TOTAL	64/75	1/14	53/64	2/12
Sensitivity		**85%**		**82%**
Specificity		**92%**		**83%**

CD = Cushing's disease, EAS = Ectopic ACTH syndrome.

cant rise of cortisol secretion in 15/16 patients with Cushing's disease. Patients with other forms of Cushing's syndrome, including eight patients with cortisol-producing adrenal adenomas and three patients with proven or suspected ectopic ACTH secretion, were unresponsive. Similar results were also presented in subsequent studies *(16,17)*: thus, by using the response criteria for CRH testing as defined by Kaye and Crapo *(18)*, Newell-Price et al. demonstrated a positive response of cortisol in 14/17 and ACTH levels in 12/17, whereas Colombo et al. demonstrated a positive cortisol and ACTH response in 14/17 of patients with Cushing's disease. More recently, we evaluated our results on the use of desmopressin tests in patients with Cushing's disease, and we found a positive cortisol in 21/25 and ACTH response in 23/25 of patients studied *(19)*. The combined data from all these series are shown in Table 1. Responsiveness to desmopressin administration, however, has only been studied in an overall limited number of patients with ocult ectopic ACTH secretion. Only 1/14 and 2/12 patients with proven or suspected ectopic ACTH secretion had a positive cortisol or ACTH, respectively, following desmopressin administration. No patient with cortisol-producing adrenal adenoma had a positive response to desmopressin. Thus, the prevalence of subjects who met the criteria adopted to define positive cortisol, and ACTH responses to the desmopressin test was significantly higher in the group of patients with Cushing's disease than in the group of patients with other forms of Cushing's syndrome.

On the basis of the aforementioned findings, it has been suggested that the desmopressin test may be occasionally useful in the differentiation between the various forms of ACTH-dependent Cushing's syndrome. On the basis of published series, the overall calculated sensitivity and specificity of cortisol responsiveness to the desmopressin test, in differentiating among the causes of ACTH-dependent Cushing's syndrome, are 85% and 92%, respectively. A slightly lower sensitivity of 82% and specificity of 83% is obtained for positive ACTH responses. Therefore, as a test, the desmopressin test has a comparable sensitivity and specificity with those reported for the most commonly used high-dose dexamethasone suppression test and CRH test. Interestingly, there are several patients with Cushing's disease that do not respond to CRH, but they respond to desmopressin *(16)*. Therefore, its routine use may provide some evidence in favor of Cushing's disease in those CRH unresponsive patients. However, caution is required regarding the specificity of positive cortisol or ACTH responses to desmopressin, because in view of the small number of patients with ectopic ACTH syndrome studied so far, the actual frequency of positive responses cannot be stated with confidence. In fact, Arlt et al. recently reported a patient with an ACTH-producing bronchial carcinoid tumor with a positive cortisol and ACTH response to desmopressin testing (20). We also noted a positive desmopressin response in a patient with ectopic ACTH secretion originating from a medullary thyroid carcinoma in a patient with the MEN2A syndrome.

Combined Stimulation with Desmopressin and CRH

Dickstein et al. reported that a combined test using CRH plus AVP had a better sensitivity than the CRH test in patients with Cushing's disease (4). Based on these findings, Newell-Price et al. recently reported their experience of a combined test using CRH and desmopressin in differentiating between the two forms of ACTH-dependent Cushing's syndrome (17). In this study, all 17 patients with histologically confirmed Cushing's disease had a positive cortisol or ACTH response following the combined adminstration of CRH and desmopressin. Interestingly, the combined administration resulted in nonoverlapping cortisol and ACTH responses between the 17 patients with Cushing's disease and the five patients with the ectopic ACTH syndrome included in this study, enabling thus a complete discrimination between these entities. It is of note, that a higher percent rise has been adopted as the cutoff point for the differentiation among these conditions. However, although the combined test may offer a better differentiation, its specificity requires further assessment by studying a larger number of patients with ectopic ACTH secretion. Recently, we have observed a significant ACTH and cortisol response (114% and 228%, respectively) in a patient with an histologically confirmed bronchial carcinoid tumor.

The Use of the Combined Stimulation with CRH and Desmopressin During Bilateral Inferior Petrosal Sampling

In view of the difficulties in arriving to a confident diagnosis in many patients with ACTH-dependent Cushing's syndrome, bilateral inferior petrosal sinus sampling (BIPSS) for ACTH measurements is now widely used in many centers with a special interest to Cushing's syndrome (21). Compared to the noninvasive tests, BIPSS is the most useful investigative tool in the differential diagnosis of ACTH-dependent Cushing's syndrome (5). The diagnostic accuracy of this procedure is improved by the assessment of the central to peripheral ACTH gradients obtained following the administration of CRH to stimulate ACTH secretion (21,22). However, as shown in several series, few patients with Cushing's disease respond to CRH and some of them do not demonstrate diagnostic ACTH gradients following petrosal sinus sampling with CRH stimulation alone (23). As it has recently been reported, the combined administration of CRH and desmopressin is a more-potent stimulus for pituitary-derived ACTH release in patients with Cushing's disease, we examined whether the diagnostic accuracy of this procedure could be improved by the use of the combined stimulation with CRH and desmopressin. We studied 37 patients with ACTH-dependent Cushing's syndrome: 33 with Cushing's disease and four with occult ectopic ACTH syndrome. In the patients with CD, stimulation with CRH alone (100 μg iv) during BIPSS was performed in 16, and with CRH (100 μg iv) plus desmopressin (10 μg iv) in the remaining 17 patients. In the patients with ectopic ACTH secretion, petrosal sinus sampling was performed with CRH stimulation in three and CRH plus desmopressin in one patient. As shown in Fig. 1, in patients with Cushing's disease the mean peak ACTH levels were signifi-

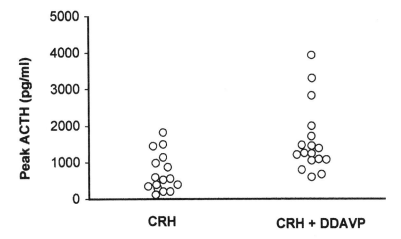

Fig. 1. Peak ACTH levels from the dominant site during bilateral inferior petrosal sinus sampling in patients with Cushing's disease. As a group, patients undergoing stimulation with a combined stimulus of CRH and DDAVP had mean peak ACTH levels higher than those observed in a group of patients who had stimulation with CRH alone ($p<0.01$) (S. Tsagarakis and N. Thalassinos, unpublished observations).

cantly higher in the group given a combined stimulus than in the group who had only CRH stimulation. Dominant central to peripheral ACTH ratios greater than two were observed in 13/16 patients undergoing stimulation with CRH alone. However, all 17 patients following the combined stimulation with CRH and desmopressin had C:P ratios greater than 2. None of the patients with the ectopic ACTH syndrome had a C:P ratio greater than 2. It is of note that the single patient with an occult bronchial carcinoid who was studied following a combined stimulation during petrosal sinus sampling had a C:P ratio of less than 2, despite a significant peripheral ACTH and cortisol response. It may thus be concluded that as the combined use of CRH and desmopressin induces a higher ACTH output from pituitary corticotroph adenomas, the use of a combined stimulus may improve the diagnostic accuracy of this procedure.

The Desmopressin Test in the Postoperative Assessment of Patients Undergoing Transsphenoidal Surgery for Cushing's Disease

As most patients with Cushing's disease demonstrate an abnormal response to desmo-pressin, it could be argued that the complete removal of a corticotroph adenoma would be associated with a disappearance of such an aberrant response. In fact, Colombo et al. demonstrated the lack in desmopressin responsiveness in a limited number of patients with Cushing's disease cured by transsphenoidal surgery *(16)*: postoperatively, there was no response to desmopressin at either 1 or 12 mo in six and five cured patients, respectively. In contrast, they observed positive responses in three noncured patients tested at 1 mo following surgery. It is of note that in all five cured patients studied 12 mo postoperatively, administration of CRH caused a marked release of ACTH and cortisol. It may thus be suggested that a lack of response to desmopressin may be used as an additional test during the immediate period following surgery or in subsequent years to ascertain cure of Cushing's disease.

THE USE OF THE DESMOPRESSIN TEST IN THE DIFFERENTIATION OF CUSHING'S SYNDROME FROM "PSEUDO-CUSHING'S STATES"

As aforementioned, the desmopressin test, either alone or given in combination with CRH, may be of some value as an adjunctive tool in the differential diagnosis of the various causes of ACTH-dependent Cushing's syndrome. Furthermore, as normal subjects do not respond to desmopressin *(11,12)*, another possible application of this test could be to differentiate patients with Cushing's disease from those individuals suspected to have this disease. This is of particular importance in certain clinical conditions, such as depression, stress, renal failure, alcoholism, and obesity, (frequently encountered as "pseudo-Cushing's states"), in which the correct differentiation by means of the routinely used diagnostic tests often remains uncertain *(24)*. Because, among the various causes of Cushing's syndrome, it is Cushing's disease that is most commonly confused with these "pseudo-Cushing's states," a test such as the desmopressin test with a high probability to reflect a neoplastic pituitary phenotype may be of some value, in order to increase diagnostic confidence in difficult cases. So far, the diagnostic value of the desmopressin in differentiating between depression and obesity has been reported and will be briefly discussed.

The Desmopressin Test in Depression

Recently, Malebri et al. studied the ability of desmopressin administration to differentiate depression from Cushing's disease *(25)*. They studied the prevalence of positive desmopressin responses in a small number of 11 depressed women, 14 patients with Cushing's disease, and 20 normal volunteers. A positive cortisol response to desmopressin (defined as a rise greater than 36% over baseline) was observed with the following frequencies: 100% in patients with Cushing's disease, 36% of depressed patients and in only 10% of normal volunteers. Thus the desmopressin test had a 100% sensitivity, but a 64% specificity in differentiating between Cushing's disease and depression.

The Desmopressin Test in Obesity

Obesity, is another condition commonly seen in endocrine practice that may raise the possibility of Cushing's syndrome and may thus require exclusion *(26)*. Previous reports have described a hyperresponsive HPA axis in obese subjects, particularly those with central obesity, after different stimulation tests *(27–29)*. We recently studied the responsiveness of the HPA axis to desmopressin in a group of obese subjects and furthermore, we investigated the ability of desmopressin administration to differentiate between patients with obesity and Cushing's disease *(19)*. Using a response criterion of at least a 20% rise in the circulating plasma cortisol level over baseline, 21/25 of patients with Cushing's disease responded to desmopressin, whereas only 3/20 of the obese patients showed a positive response (Fig. 2a). Regarding ACTH, using the response criterion of at least a 50% rise in the circulating plasma ACTH level over baseline, 23/25 of patients with Cushing's disease responded to desmopressin, whereas only 3/20 of the obese patients showed a positive response (Fig. 2b). Thus, the prevalence of subjects who met the criteria adopted to define positive cortisol and ACTH responses to desmopressin was significantly higher in the group of patients with Cushing's disease than in the group of patients with obesity, with cortisol responses leading to a 84%

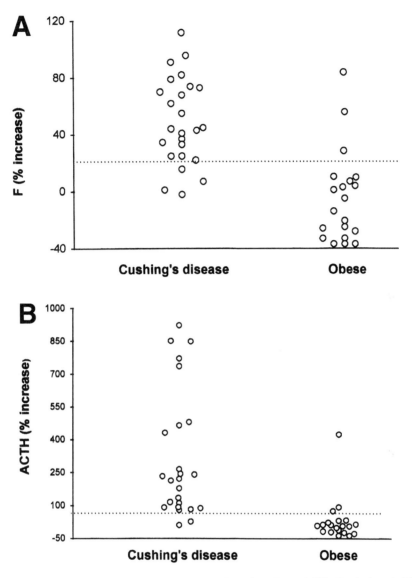

Fig. 2. Individual data showing the percent change from baseline of **(A)** Cortisol and **(B)** ACTH following desmopressin administration in patients with CD and obese subjects. Dotted lines cross the Y axes at 20% **(A)** and 50% **(B)**. Despite a substantial overlap the frequency of positive responses was significantly higher in patients with CD than in obese subjects (from S. Tsagarakis, et al. *ref. (19)*, in press).

sensitivity and a 85% specificity, and ACTH responses to a 92% sensitivity and 85% specificity for the diagnosis of Cushing's disease.

CONCLUSIONS AND RECOMMENDATIONS FOR THE USE OF THE DESMOPRESSIN TEST IN CLINICAL PRACTICE

Based on the data presented in this chapter, there is some evidence that the desmopressin test may be occasionally useful in the investigation of patients with suspected or proven Cushing's syndrome. The major challenge in the differential diagnosis of Cushing's syndrome is to identify the site of the ACTH-secreting tumor. In the majority of cases, the tumor is a pituitary corticotroph microadenoma, whereas in the remaining patients, ACTH hypersecretion originates from small, and thus radiologically unidentified, ectopic sites *(30)*. Accurate diagnosis is of paramount importance in order to effectively remove such tumors by surgery. The long used high-dose dexamethasone suppression test has recently been criticized for its low efficacy in differentiating among the causes of ACTH-dependent Cushing's syndrome *(31)*. The CRH test seems superior, but varying numbers of false positive (5–10%) or negative (7–14%) results have been reported *(5,30)*. Even the most invasive method of bilateral inferior petrosal sinus sampling has failed to yield a 100% diagnostic accuracy.

Despite some initial enthusiasm that the desmopressin test may be a good alternative in the differential diagnosis of ACTH-dependent Cushing's syndrome, its value has now been limited by an increasing number of false-positive responses. However, as the current policy by many investigators is to use more, rather than fewer, tests in an effort to increase diagnostic confidence, the addition of the desmopressin test, which uncovers an independent property manifested by the majority of pituitary corticotroph adenomas, may provide further ground in favor of Cushing's disease. In fact, desmopressin is inexpensive, widely available worldwide, and its administration is not associated with noxious side effects. In future, as the combined administration of CRH and desmopressin represents the most sensitive way to stimulate ACTH secretion in patients with Cushing's disease, it seems most likely, that the combined test may well replace separate testing by CRH and desmopressin. However, it remains yet unclear as to what extent such an increase in sensitivity of the combined test affects its specificity, but this requires further study in a larger group of patients with the ectopic ACTH secretion syndrome. Moreover, the combined use of CRH and desmopressin may also become the stimulus of choice in patients undergoing BIPSS, particularly those patients that do not respond to the administration of CRH.

The use of desmopressin in the postoperative assessment of patients following the removal of a corticotroph adenoma represents a promising and attractive advance in the follow-up of such patients. It is now increasingly recognized that the best long-term results of transspenoidal surgery appear to be in those patients with unmeasurable serum cortisol levels in the immediate postoperative period *(32)*. However, long-term clinical remissions have been obtained in patients with postoperatively measurable serum cortisol levels caused by partial removal of a pituitary ACTH-secreting tumor. Such patients may present with suppressible cortisol levels to exogenous dexamethasone and they may also present with varying types of responses to CRH testing. A positive desmopressin response may thus represent a more sensitive test for the existence of a pituitary tumor remnant, and may thus be of enormous value for deciding whether to administer additional therapy. However, more data are required before the inclusion of the desmopressin test as a criterion for additional treatment in such patients.

There is also some preliminary evidence that the desmopressin test may help in the occasionally difficult differentiation between Cushing's disease, (but not other forms of Cushing's syndrome), and "pseudo-Cushing's states." Although Cushing's syndrome may be excluded on clinical grounds in most cases, laboratory differentiation may often be confusing because of the varying degrees of the diagnostic accuracies of the currently used confirmatory tests (overnight and standard low-dose dexamethasone suppression, urinary-free cortisol measurements). To our experience, standard 2-d low-dose dexa-methasone suppression is the test of choice *(33),* but its specificity may be affected by concomitant stress or certain conditions that affect the absorption and metabolism of oral dexamethasone (e.g., renal failure, antiepileptics). Moreover, a false-negative rate of 2% has recently been reported *(34),* which may be even higher in patients with mild CD *(35).* Therefore, as none of the aforementioned commonly used tests cannot be taken alone as definitive, it is suggested that the desmopressin test may well add useful information in differentiating Cushing's disease from pseudo-Cushing states, in those occasional patients with equivocal results. Most of the former will respond to the standard low-dose dexamethasone suppression test, which is very rarely seen in Cushing's disease. However, for those few false-positive and/or -negative patients to dexamethasone suppression, desmopressin test may add useful diagnostic information.

REFERENCES

1. Jeffcoate W. Probability in practice in the diagnosis of Cushing's syndrome. Clin Endocrinol 1997; 47:271–272.
2. Gillies GE, Linton EA, Lowry PJ. Corticotrophin releasing activity of the new CRF is potentiated several times by vasopressin. Nature 1982; 299:355–357.
3. Antoni FA. Novel ligand specificity of pituitary vasopressin receptors in the rat. Neuroendocrinology 1984; 39:186–188.
4. Dickstein G, DeBold CR, Gaitan D, DeCherney GS, Jackson RV, Sheldon WR, et al. Plasma corticotropin and cortisol responses to ovine corticotropin-releasing hormone (CRH), arginine vasopressin (AVP), CRH plus AVP, and CRH plus metyrapone in patients with Cushing's disease. J Clin Endocrinol Metab 1996; 81:2934–2941
5. Newell-Price J, Trainer P, Besser M, Grssman A. The diagnosis and differential diagnosis of Cushing's syndrome and pseudo-Cushing's states. Endocrine Rev 1998; 19:647–672.
6. Newell-Price J. The desmopressin test and Cushing's syndrome: current state of play. Clin Endocrinol 1997; 47:173–174.
7. Thibonnier M, Auzan C, Madhun Z, Wilkins P, Berti-Mattera L, Clauser E. Molecular cloning, sequencing and functional expression of a cDNA encoding the human V1a vasopressin receptor. J Biol Chem 1994; 269:3304–3310.
8. Sugimoto T, Sato M, Mochizuki S, et al. Molecular cloning and functional expression of a cDNA encoding the human V1b vasopressin receptor. J Biol Chem 1994; 269:27,088–27,092.
9. De Keyzer Y, Auzan C, Lenne F, et al. Cloning and characterisation of the human V3 pituitary vasopressin receptor. FEBS Lett 1994; 356:215–220.
10. Sawyer WH, Acosta M, Manning M. Structural changes in the arginine vasopressin molecule that prolong its antidiuretic action. Endocrinology 1974; 95:140–149.
11. Gaillard RC, Riondel AM, Ling N, Muller AF. Corticotropin releasing factor activity of CRF 41 in normal man is potentiated by angiotensin II and vasopressin but not desmopressin. Life Sci 1988; 43:1935–1944.
12. Ceresini G, Freddi M, Paccotti P, Valenti G, Merchenthaler I. Effects of ovine corticotropin-releasing hormone injection and desmopressin coadministration on galanin and adrenocorticotropin plasma levels in normal women. J Clin Endocrinol Metab 1997; 82:607–610.
13. Dahia PLM, Ahmed-Shuaib A, Jacobs RA, Chew SL, Honegger J, Fahlbusch R. Vasopressin receptor expression and mutation analysis in corticotropin-secreting tumors. J Clin Endocrinol Metab 1996; 81:1768–1771.
14. De Keyzer, Lenne F, Auzan C, Jegou S, Rene P, Vaudry H, et al. The pituitary V3 vasopressin receptor and the corticotroph phenotype in ectopic ACTH syndrome. J Clin Invest 1996; 97:1311–1318.
15. Malebri DA, Mendonca BB, Liberman B, Toledo SPA, Corradini MCM, Cunha-Neto MB, et al. The desmopressin stimulation test in the differential diagnosis of Cushing's syndrome. Clin Endocrinol 1993; 38:463–472.
16. Colombo P, Passini E, Re T, Faglia G, Ambrosi B. Effect of desmopressin on ACTH and cortisol secretion in states of ACTH excess. Clin Endocrinol 1997; 46:661–668.

17. Newell-Price J, Perry L, Medbak S, Monson J, Savage M, Besser M, et al. A combined test using desmopressin and corticotropin-releasing hormone in the differential diagnosis of Cushing's syndrome. J Clin Endocrinol Metab 1997; 82:176–181.
18. Kaye TB, Crapo L. The Cushing's syndrome: an update on diagnostic tests. Ann Intern Med 1990; 112:432–444.
19. Tsagarakis S, Vasiliou V, Kokkoris P, Stavropoulos G, Thalassinos N. Comparison of cortisol and ACTH responses to the desmopressin test between patients with Cushing's syndrome and simple obesity. Clin Endocrinol, 1999; 51:473–479.
20. Arlt W, Dahia PLM, Callies F, Nordmeyer JP, Allolio B, Grossman AB, et al. Ectopic ACTH production by a bronchial carcinoid tumour responsive to desmopressin *in vivo* and *in vitro*. Clin Endocrinol 1997; 47:623–627.
21. Oldfield EH, Doppman JL, Nieman LK, Chrousos GP, Miller DL, Katz DA, et al. Petrosal sinus sampling with and without corticotropin-releasing hormone for the differential diagnosis of Cushing's syndrome. N Engl J Med 1991; 325:897–905.
22. Kaltsas G, Giannulis MG, Newell-Price JDC, Dacie JE, Thakkar C, Afshar F, et al. A critical analysis of the value of simultaneous inferior petrosal sinus sampling in Cushing's disease and the occult ectopic adrenocorticotropin syndrome. J Clin Endocrinol 1999; 84:487–492.
23. Lopez J, Barcelo B, Lucas T, Salame F, Alameda C, Boronat M, et al. Petrosal sinus sampling for the diagnosis of Cushing's disease: evidence of false negative results. Clin Endocrinol 1996; 45:147–156.
24. Yanovski JA, Cutler GB, Chrousos GP, Nieman LK. Corticotropin-releasing hormone stimulation following low-dose dexamethasone suppression. J Am Med Assoc 1993; 269:2232–2238.
25. Malebri DA, Candida M, Fragoso BV, Vieira Filho AHG, Brenhla EML, Mendonca BB. Cortisol and adrenocorticotropin response to desmopressin in women with Cushing's disease compared with depressive illness. J Clin Endocrinol Metab 1996; 81:2233–2237.
26. Kopelman PG. Investigation of obesity. Clin Endocrinol 1994; 41:703–708.
27. Bjorntorp P. Visceral obesity: a "civilization syndrome". Obesity Res 1993; 1:206–222.
28. Pasquali R, Contobelli S, Casimiri F, Capelli M, Bortoluzzi L, Flamia R, et al. The hypothalamic-pituitary-adrenal axis in obese women with different patterns of body fat distribution. J Clin Endocrinol Metab 1993; 77:341–346.
29. Weaver JU, Kopelman PG, McLoughlin L, Forsling M, Grossman A. Hyperactivity of the hypothalamo-pituitary adrenal axis in obesity: a study of ACTH, β-lipotropin and cortisol responses to insulin-induced hypoglycaemia. Clin Endocrinol 1993; 39:345–350.
30. Trainer PJ, Grossman A. The diagnosis and differential diagnosis of Cushing's syndrome. Clin Endocrinol 1991; 34:317–330.
31. Aron DC, Raff H, Findling JW. Effectiveness versus efficacy: the limited value in clinical practice of high dose dexamethasone suppression testing in the differential diagnosis of adrenocortiotropin-dependent Cushing's syndrome. J Clin Endocrinol Metab 1997; 82:1780–1785.
32. McCance DR, Besser M, Atkinson AB. Assessment of cure after transsphenoidal surgery for Cushing's disease. Clin Endocrinol 1996; 44:1–6.
33. Tsagarakis S, Kokkoris P, Roboti C, Malagari C, Kaskarelis J, Vlassopoulou V, et al. The low-dose dexamethasone suppression test in patients with adrenal incidentalomas: comparisons with clinically euadrenal subjects and patients with Cushing's syndrome. Clin Endocrinol 1998; 48:627–634.
34. Newell-Price J, Trainer P, Perry L, Wass J, Grossman A, Besser M. A single midnight cortisol has 100% sensitivity for the diagnosis of Cushing's syndrome. Clin Endocrinol 1995; 43:545–550.
35. Yanovski JA, Cutler GB, Chrousos GP, Nieman LK. The dexamethasone-suppressed corticotropin-releasing hormone stimulation test differentiates mild Cushing's disease from normal physiology. J Clin Endocrinol Metab 1998; 83:348–352.

15 Pseudo-Cushing Syndrome

Theodore Friedman

CONTENTS

WHAT IS PSEUDO-CUSHING'S?

Cushing's syndrome is a rare disorder that can severely affect the patient. It is the result of prolonged exposure to high levels of exogenous or endogenous glucocorticoids. Symptoms of patients with Cushing's syndrome include weight gain, easy bruising, menstrual irregularities, increased appetite, trouble sleeping, depression or mood swings, anxiety, fatigue and altered mentation (trouble concentrating or decreased memory) *(1–3)*. Physical abnormalities include new onset obesity (primarily in the abdominal and buttock regions), buffalo hump, filling in of the regions above the collarbone, thinning of the extremities, rounding and reddening of the face, thin skin, decreased muscle strength, high blood pressure, stretch marks, and excess hair growth in women. Although some patients may have most or all of these signs and symptoms so that the diagnosis of Cushing's syndrome may be easy to make, other patients may have mild Cushing's syndrome and go to their health care providers at an early stage of the disease. This is especially true as Cushing's syndrome has been publicized in the lay literature, *(4)* and with the proliferation of Internet-related information sites and Cushing's support groups, more patients are aware that Cushing's syndrome may explain their medical problems. Thus, patients are seeking medical attention earlier. However, other medical conditions may also result in some of the signs, symptoms, and laboratory abnormalities seen in patients with Cushing's syndrome, without the patient actually having Cushing's syndrome. These conditions are called pseudo-Cushing's states and

From: *Contemporary Endocrinology: Adrenal Disorders*
Edited by: A. N. Margioris and G. P. Chrousos © Humana Press, Totowa, NJ

include conditions such as severe stresses (illness or emotional stress), alcoholism or alcohol withdrawal, and psychiatric conditions such as depression, panic disorders, and psychotic conditions. The pathophysiology leading to increased cortisol production in alcoholism and depression is discussed later. Pseudo-Cushing's states are classically defined as those conditions associated with increased cortisol production [usually measured by urinary-free cortisol (UFC) measurements], but with less clinical signs and symptoms than true Cushing's syndrome. Resolution of the underlying primary condition leads to disappearance of the signs and symptoms of Cushing's syndrome. In this chapter, we will also discuss conditions that mimic the clinical stigmata of Cushing's syndrome, but lack elevated cortisol production.

It should be noted that the psychiatric conditions causing pseudo-Cushing's states, such as depression, are quite common and a patient with one of these conditions may appear similar to the rarer patient with Cushing's syndrome. Thus, it is quite important to determine if the patient has Cushing's syndrome or a pseudo-Cushing's state in a time- and cost-effective manner, because if a patient with a pseudo-Cushing's state is misdiagnosed as having Cushing's syndrome, that patient could undergo needless, and potentially harmful, testing and unnecessary invasive procedures or even surgery. On the other hand, if a patient truly has Cushing's syndrome, it would be important to confirm the diagnosis and eliminate the possibility of a pseudo-Cushing's state, so that the etiology of the Cushing's syndrome can be determined and the patient can receive the appropriate surgery. It is important to make the diagnosis of Cushing's syndrome before investigating the type of Cushing's syndrome (differential diagnosis), as the tests employed in the latter require the patient to be hypercortisolemic.

CONDITIONS LEADING TO PSEUDO-CUSHING'S STATES

Both physiological and nonphysiological conditions can lead to elevated cortisol production, leading to some signs and symptoms of hypercortisolism (Table 1). The physiological conditions include stress associated with surgery and severe illness, and emotional, caloric, and aerobic stress. Rosmond et al. *(5)* found that stress-related cortisol secretion was associated with lack of diurnal variation of cortisol, high cortisol levels after dexamethasone suppression, central obesity, hypertension, hyperlipidemia, and insulin-resistance. The pathophysiological conditions include both alcoholism *(6,7)* and psychiatric disorders *(8,9)*. Poorly controled diabetes is also associated with hypercortisolism *(10,11)*. The hypercortisolism of alcoholism has been described much more frequently in Europe *(6,12–14);* it may be rarer in the United States. Wand and Dobs *(15)* estimated that 5% of the alcoholic population in the Baltimore area had clinical signs of hypercortisolism. The psychiatric disorders leading to a pseudo-Cushing's states commonly confused with Cushing's syndrome include depression and anxiety disorders. Depression leading to increased cortisol production is quite common and is discussed later. Anorexia nervosa and bulimia usually do not present with symptoms of Cushing's syndrome. Renal failure leading to high cortisol production, although rare, poses significant diagnostic and therapeutic problems *(16–18)*. Severe obesity may lead to mild elevations in cortisol production, however, in both obesity and renal failure, most of the other stigmata of Cushing's syndrome are lacking.

Primary glucocorticoid-receptor resistance *(19–21)* leads to elevated cortisol levels and may also be confused with Cushing's syndrome. The diminished feedback by

Table 1
Pseudo-Cushing States

High Cortisol Secretion Rate without Convincing Clinical Features
of Cushing Syndrome

Stress
   Surgery
   Severe illness
   Emotional
   Caloric
   Aerobic
Alcoholism
   Long-term active alcoholism
   Ethanol withdrawal
Psychiatric Disorders
   Depression (particularly melancholic depression)
   Anorexia nervosa
   Bulimia
   Psychoses
   Panic Disorders
Renal Failure
Severe Obesity
Primary Glucocorticoid Receptor Resistance
Excessive Fluid Intake (Psychogenic Polydipsia or Diabetes Insipidus)
Factitious Glucocorticoid Intake
Uncontrolled Diabetes

Conditions with Eucortisolemia That May Mimic Cushing's Syndrome

Obesity
Metabolic Syndrome
Polycystic Ovary Syndrome
Growth Hormone Deficiency
HIV Infection
Glucocorticoid Hyperresponsivity
Impaired Cortisol Catabolism

glucocorticoids leads to high levels of ACTH and cortisol. Because hypertension and hyperandrogenism leading to hirsutism, acne, and oligomenorrhea exist, the patients may present with some symptoms of Cushing's syndrome. However, the classic end-organ effects of hypercortisolism including easy bruising, thin skin, and proximal muscle weakness, are absent.

Excessive fluid intake because of psychogenic polydipsia or diabetes insipidus has recently been described to cause an elevation in urinary cortisol excretion *(22)*. In these conditions, it is hypothesized that high urinary volumes result in a loss of the renal medullary gradient and the inability to reabsorb cortisol.

Finally, a common and often difficult to diagnose cause of increased cortisol levels associated with the stigmata of Cushing's syndrome is factitious glucocorticoid intake *(23)*. The patient may be taking hydrocortisone, prednisone, dexamethasone or other synthetic glucocorticoid or rarely, ACTH. Cortisol levels may be high (in the case of hydrocortisone) or low (in case of prednisone or dexamethasone), depending on whether the glucocorticoid crossreacts with the cortisol assay. In exogenous glucocorticoid intake. ACTH levels are low and imaging may show atrophic adrenal glands. The patient is frequently in the medical profession, presents with severe symptoms of a rapid onset, and is often quite impatient in demanding a rapid work-up. A high degree of suspicion is needed to uncover this disorder, which is associated with a high morbidity and mortality.

The normal circadian rhythm of cortisol is maintained in renal failure, excessive fluid intake, glucocorticoid resistance, renal failure, and most psychiatric conditions, allowing these conditions to be distinguished from Cushing's syndrome.

OTHER CONDITIONS THAT MAY MIMIC CUSHING'S SYNDROME

In addition to pseudo-Cushing's states in which cortisol production is increased, there exists other states, with normal cortisol production that nevertheless may mimic Cushing's syndrome (Table 1). The most common of these conditions is obesity and particularly the central obesity associated with the metabolic syndrome *(24)* [previously called syndrome X *(25)*]. Although cortisol production may be mildly increased *(26–29)* in some obese patients, direct evidence of hypercortisolism is usually absent and the cortisol levels are only mildly elevated. Similarly, polycystic ovary syndrome (PCOS), although associated with some signs and symptoms of hypercortisolism such as hirsutism, central obesity, and oligomenorrhea, is characterized by eucortisolemia. Usually, a careful history and physical can separate patients with obesity or PCOS from those with true Cushing's syndrome.

Patients with adult pituitary growth hormone (GH) deficiency may present with symptoms similar to those of Cushing's syndrome. These include weight gain accompanied by central obesity, low energy and fatigue, reduced muscle strength, altered lipid composition, and impaired psychological sense of well-being *(30)*. GH deficiency should be suspected in patients with previous insults to their pituitary including surgery, radiation, and presence of a pituitary tumor. Idiopathic adult GH deficiency is infrequently reported, but may be a common disorder. Patients with a history of pituitary damage should be evaluated by either two GH stimulation tests (arginine, L-dopa, GHRH, clonidine or exercise) or with an insulin-tolerance test. In patients without a history of pituitary damage, the paradigm for evaluation is less clear. A prudent approach in patients with symptoms of GH deficiency would be to initially measure a serum IGF-1 level. If the value is in the lower 25% for the patient's age and sex, we then perform either the two GH stimulation tests or the insulin tolerance test. It should be mentioned, however, that patients with GH deficiency are eucortisolemic.

Recently, it was noted that human immunodeficiency virus-1 (HIV)-positive patients, especially those on retroviral protease inhibitors have many of the signs and symptoms of Cushing's syndrome, including new onset central obesity, dorsocervical fat accumulation (buffalo hump), hyperlipemia, and abnormal glucose homeostasis *(31–34)*. These abnormalities have been called protease inhibitor-associated lipodystrophy (PIAL) *(35)*. In a study of HIV-positive patients on protease inhibitors, decreased UFC, but increased 17-hydroxysteroid (17-OHS), excretion was found *(35)*. Serum and urine cortisol were found to suppress normally to dexamethasone. The authors concluded that altered cortisol production was unlikely to explain the central obesity *(35)*. Although it was thought that the altered fat distribution was caused by the protease inhibitors, a recent report in HIV-infected women suggests that the body fat changes occur regardless of protease inhibitor use *(36)*. Thus, the HIV-induced malnutrition of patients not on protease inhibitors may mask the central obesity, which would be further exacerbated by weight gain and increased adiposity after protease inhibitor treatment *(36)*. Although this condition is quite interesting, it is unlikely that these patients will be mistaken for patients with true Cushing's syndrome.

On the other hand, there are two conditions that, although rarely described in the literature, may completely mimic Cushing's syndrome, but are also not associated with systemic hypercortisolism. These include hyperresponsivity of the glucocorticoid receptor and impaired catabolism of cortisol at the level of the tissue. One patient has been studied with symptoms of hypercortisolemia, but low UFC levels *(37–39)*. The patient's fibroblasts were isolated and found to be hyperresponsive to glucocorticoids. Although only one patient with this condition has been described in the literature, others may exist but have eluded being diagnosed, as screening tests (UFCs or dexamethasone suppression) would likely be normal in patients with this condition and the patient would probably not be further evaluated. Interestingly, a polymorphism at the glucocorticoid receptor was found in 6% of normal Dutch men and was consistent with cortisol hyperresponsivity associated with significantly greater cortisol suppression by dexamethasone, higher body mass index, and lower bone density than noncarriers *(40)*.

Glucocorticoid action at the prereceptor level is regulated, in part, by 11β-hydroxysteroid dehydrogenase (11β-HSD), an enzyme that interconverts bioactive cortisol and bioinactive cortisone *(41)*. There are two isoforms of this enzyme, 11β-HSD1, a low-affinity enzyme present in omental fat, hepatic, gonadal, and neural tissues and 11β-HSD2, a high affinity enzyme present in the colon and kidney. In omental fat cells, 11β-HSD1 predominately converts cortisone to cortisol *(42,43)*, whereas in the kidney, 11β-HSD2 predominantly inactivates cortisol, protecting the nonselective mineralocorticoid receptor from cortisol excess. Because patients with Cushing's syndrome have central obesity, Stewart and colleagues *(42,44)* proposed that enhanced conversion of cortisone to cortisol by 11β-HSD1 in the omentum may lead to similar symptoms of hypercortisolism in patients without true Cushing's syndrome. Patients with excess 11β-HSD1 would have normal plasma and urine levels of cortisol, but have symptoms of hypercortisolism. There are no specific inhibitors of 11β-HSD1 currently available; licorice and carbenoxolone inhibit both 11β-HSD1 and 11β-HSD2 and may cause mineralocorticoid hypertension. This condition, although not yet documented, may explain the findings of eucortisolemic individuals with the stigmata of Cushing's syndrome.

PATHOPHYSIOLOGY OF PSEUDO-CUSHING'S STATES

Explanations for the hypercortisolemia in the pseudo-Cushing's states of depression and alcoholism have been proposed. Patients with depression, particularly melancholic depression *(45)*, have hypercortisolemia and it is thought that the primary defect is at or above the level of the hypothalamus *(45–48)*. This hypothesis is based on the following evidence: (1) The ACTH response to exogenous corticotrophin-releasing hormone (CRH) is attenuated, indicating that the pituitary corticotroph is appropriately restrained by the negative feedback of the elevated levels of glucocorticoids. (2) Baseline evening plasma cortisol levels are elevated in depressed patients, but the cortisol response to CRH is similar as normals. (3) Depressed patients have an increased response to exogenous ACTH compared to controls. (4) Normal controls receiving a continuous infusion of CRH have a similar degree of hypercortisolism as those with depression. (5) Cerebrospinal levels of CRH are elevated in patients with depression. To integrate these findings, it is hypothesized that endogenous CRH is elevated in depression, with this being the earliest abnormality. The adrenal glands would then hypertrophy leading to the increased response of cortisol to ACTH. Cortisol feedback to the corticotroph would remain present [although also blunted as depressed patients have reduced suppression to dexamethasone *(49–51)*], so that exogenous CRH causes a blunted ACTH response, but a normal cortisol response. This theory is supported by the finding of adrenal enlargement in depressed patients *(52)*. In conclusion, depression is likely a state of CRH excess, whereas true Cushing's syndrome is a state of CRH deficiency. This difference is exploited in many of the tests designed to distinguish Cushing's syndrome from pseudo-Cushing's states.

In experimental animals given alcohol, there is a hypersecretion of CRH along with a partial reduction in the pituitary to both suppression by glucocorticoid and stimulation by CRH *(53,54)*. The increased CRH secretion may be at the hypothalamic or suprahypothalamic level (i.e., limbic cortex) *(55)*. It is further postulated that in alcohol abusers, the decreased responsiveness to CRH is caused by either downregulation of the CRH receptors in the pituitary, or alcohol's influence on transmembrane signal transduction *(56–58)*. Moreover, in alcoholism, there appears to be impaired binding of cortisol to cortisol-binding globulin (CBG), leading to elevated levels of free cortisol *(59)*. Another possible explanation for pseudo-Cushing's syndrome in patients with alcohol abuse is impaired hepatic metabolism of cortisol *(60)*. Finally, genetic influences may determine why only some alcoholics develop pseudo-Cushing's syndrome *(61,62)*.

INITIAL WORKUP OF PATIENTS WITH POSSIBLE HYPERCORTISOLISM

What should an endocrinologist do if a patient has some of the signs and symptoms of Cushing's syndrome? Patients should have a careful history and physical, looking for findings specific for Cushing's syndrome. Attention should be directed to the time-course of the symptoms (new, sudden onset of weight gain and other symptoms suggest Cushing's syndrome, whereas long-standing, nonprogressing symptoms suggest pseudo-Cushing's states). Comparison with old pictures is often very helpful. New onset sleep disturbances, including frequent awakening with associated daytime fatigue are constant in Cushing's syndrome. Typically, but not always, the obesity of Cushing's syndrome is centripetal, with a wasting of the arms and legs, distinct from the generalized weight gain seen in idiopathic obesity. Rounding of the face (moon facies) and a dorsocervical fat pad ("buffalo hump") occurs in non-Cushing's syndrome-related obesity, whereas facial plethora and supraclavicular and temporal filling are more specific for Cushing's syndrome. Thinning of the skin on the top of the hands is a very specific sign in younger adults with Cushing's syndrome and should always be examined. Once a careful history and physical is performed, patients suspected of having hypercortisolemia should begin their laboratory investigation to distinguish between true Cushing's syndrome and other states. It is recommended that UFC measurement should be the initial screening test for patients suspected of hypercortisolemia as this test has a high degree

Table 2
Tests to Distinguish Pseudo-Cushing's States from Early Cushing's Syndrome

Recommended	Possibly Recommended	Not Recommended
Urinary-Free Cortisol	Low-Dose Dexamethasone	Morning Plasma Cortisol
Dexamethasone-CRH Test	Test	Levels
Diurnal Plasma Cortisol Tests	Loperamide Test	Petrosasl Sinus Sampling
Diurnal Salivary Cortisol	Naloxone Stimulation Test	Pituitary MRI
Tests	IL-6 Test	

of sensitivity and is easy to perform. Low-dose dexamethasone screening has many disadvantages compared to UFC measurement and although capable of providing useful information, cannot be recommended over UFC determinations.

The author recommends measurements of three 24-h urine samples for UFC. An elevated UFC on at least one occasion was found in 184/194 (95%) with Cushing's syndrome *(63)*. This test is a good screen to help determine if the patient has Cushing's syndrome, is completely normal, or has an intermediate value and requires further testing to distinguish between pseudo-Cushing's states and Cushing's syndrome. Patients need to be instructed to discard the first morning void and then collect all urine until the next morning void. If all the UFCs are in the normal range (usually less than 50 or 90 µg/d (138 or 248 nmol/L), depending on the assay), it is unlikely that the patient has Cushing's syndrome. If some of the UFCs are more than 3.5 times the upper limit of normal (usually more than 175 or 315 µg/d, 491 or 870 nmol/L, depending on the assay), the patient probably has Cushing's syndrome and should have a work-up to determine the etiology of the Cushing's syndrome. If the patient's UFCs fall in the range between the upper limit of normal and 3.5 times the upper limit of normal, the patient needs to have further tests to distinguish between Cushing's syndrome and pseudo-Cushing's states. Once the initial screen (UFC) has determined that the patient has hypercortisolism, more sophisticated tests are needed to make the diagnosis of Cushing's syndrome.

TESTS TO DISTINGUISH PSEUDO-CUSHING'S STATES FROM CUSHING'S SYNDROME

There are many tests that can be done to distinguish between mild Cushing's syndrome and pseudo-Cushing's states (Table 2). The distinction between these two groups is the consideration of importance, as patients with severe Cushing's syndrome can probably be easily identified and normal patients can also be easily excluded. For this reason, the diagnostic accuracy for older tests that were based on separating normal volunteers from those with severe Cushing's syndrome are probably not relevant. The two very good, relatively new tests to help the endocrinologist distinguish between mild Cushing's syndrome and pseudo-Cushing's states in those patients with a mildly elevated UFC, are the diurnal plasma cortisol test and the dexamethasone-CRH test. Salivary nighttime cortisol tests are also promising. Other tests including the low-dose dexamethasone test, loperamide test, insulin-tolerance test, CRH test, morning plasma free cortisol, and pituitary imaging, although capable of providing additional information for the evaluation of Cushing's syndrome, exhibit an overlap between mild Cushing's syndrome and pseudo-Cushing's states and are probably inferior to the diurnal plasma cortisol and the dexamethasone-CRH test. There is no role for morning plasma total cortisol levels or petrosal sinus sampling.

Diurnal Cortisol Tests

The disruption of the circadian rhythm of cortisol (and ACTH) is a distinguishing characteristic of Cushing's syndrome. Normally, cortisol reaches a peak in the early morning and a nadir around midnight *(64)*. The normal range for morning plasma cortisol is broad; patients with Cushing's syndrome, pseudo-Cushing's states, and normals have an overlap of their morning plasma cortisol levels, making this test unsuitable to diagnose Cushing's syndrome *(65)*. The diurnal serum cortisol test, which measures a midnight-serum-cortisol level, takes advantage of the fact that normal patients and patients with pseudo-Cushing's states have much lower levels in the evening and at night, whereas patients with Cushing's syndrome have high cortisol levels at night. Newell-Price et al. *(66)* described the use of this test to distinguish between patients with Cushing's syndrome and normal volunteers in subjects who were hospitalized for at least 2 d prior to sampling. A sleeping midnight plasma cortisol of greater than 50 nmol/L (1.8 μg/dL) was found in all patients with confirmed Cushing's syndrome, but none of the normal volunteers. This test was superior to the low-dose dexamethasone-suppression test in which three patients with Cushing's syndrome suppressed to low-dose dexamethasone with a morning plasma cortisol value of greater than 50 nmol/L (1.8 μg/dL). Unfortunately, no patients with pseudo-Cushing's states were included in this study, nor were patients with mild Cushing's syndrome particularly studied. Additionally, hospitalization of patients for 3 d to perform this test is impractical.

Papanicolaou et al. *(67)* used the midnight serum cortisol to distinguish patients with Cushing's syndrome from those with pseudo-Cushing's states. A midnight cortisol value greater than 7.5 μg/dL (208 nmol/L) correctly identified 225/234 patients with Cushing's syndrome, whereas a value less than this cutoff was found in all 23 patients with pseudo-Cushing's states. Thus, the specificity was 100% and the sensitivity was 96%. The test failed in a few patients with mild Cushing's syndrome (UFC less than 200 μg/d) and those who were episodic secretors of cortisol. This study compared the two groups needing differentiation, those with pseudo-Cushing's states and those with mild Cushing's syndrome. The study did, however, only examine hospitalized patients. Because of the timing of the required blood draw, this test may require a hospital admission as it is often difficult to obtain blood at midnight in an outpatient setting.

Because of the difficulty in obtaining blood at midnight, salivary cortisol was used to distinguish between Cushing's syndrome and pseudo-Cushing's states *(68)*. This test is based on the finding that salivary cortisol is in equilibrium with plasma-free cortisol and is independent of saliva production. This study examined 11 PM salivary cortisol in 39 patients with proven Cushing's syndrome, 39 patients referred for possible Cushing's syndrome, but in whom the diagnosis was excluded or not firmly established (RO) and 73 normal volunteers. The average 11 PM salivary cortisol was 20 times higher in the patients with Cushing's syndrome than the other two groups. Using a cutoff of 3.6 nmol/L (0.13 μg/dL), 36/39 patients with Cushing's syndrome had an elevated value, whereas 37/39 of the RO group and 38/39 of the normal volunteers had values less than the cutoff. The sensitivity and specificity of this test was 92% and 96%, respectively. Using a different assay and studying a smaller number of patients, Papanicolaou et al.

(69) also found that salivary cortisol levels can distinguish between patients with Cushing's syndrome and those with pseudo-Cushing's states. The fact that the upper limit of normal for this assay was 0.5 µg/dL, whereas that of the Raff et al. *(68)* study was 0.13 µg/dL, demonstrates that the salivary cortisol results have to be standardized at each laboratory. Recently, Dr. Findling has made the salivary cortisol test readily available to patients by distributing a packet which includes the salivet for collecting the saliva and instructions for mailing the sample to Aurora Laboratories. Samples are stable and can be collected in the patients' home and mailed. This test looks promising, however, it has not been tested on enough patients with pseudo-Cushing's states.

Dexamethasone-CRH Test

Another recommended test to distinguish between mild Cushing's syndrome and pseudo-Cushing's states in those patients with a mildly elevated UFC is the dexamethasone-CRH test. This test combines two tests, the low-dose dexamethasone suppression test (LDDST), and the CRH test, which individually are good, but not great at distinguishing between pseudo-Cushing's states and Cushing's syndrome. As discussed later, the dexamethasone test takes advantage of the fact that in patients with Cushing's syndrome, dexamethasone ineffectively suppresses the production of pituitary ACTH. CRH stimulates the pituitary to secrete ACTH, which leads to an increase in cortisol levels. Patients with Cushing's syndrome have a larger increase in plasma ACTH and cortisol levels than in normal individuals or those patients with pseudo-Cushing's states. Although these tests individually are helpful to diagnose Cushing's syndrome, many patients with pseudo-Cushing's states also respond to them in a similar manner as those with Cushing's syndrome, making them not the ideal tests to use individually. Yanovski et al. *(9)* elected to combine the two tests and gave 39 patients with Cushing's syndrome and 19 patients with pseudo-Cushing's states dexamethasone (0.5 mg) four times a day for two d starting at 12 PM (last dose at 6 AM). At 8 AM on the day of the last dose, the patients received intravenous ovine CRH (1 µg/kg) and cortisol and ACTH were measured at various times. All patients with Cushing's syndrome had mild hypercortisolemia (UFC between 250 and 1000 nmol/d; 90–362 µg/d) so that UFCs between patients with Cushing's syndrome and pseudo-Cushing's states completely overlapped. A plasma cortisol greater than 1.4 µg/dL (38 nmol/L) measured 15 min after the CRH injection correctly identified all patients with Cushing's syndrome, whereas a value less than 1.4 µg/d identified all patients with pseudo-Cushing's states (100% sensitivity and specificity). In contrast, the low-dose dexamethasone test, had a 74% specificity and 69% sensitivity when 17-OHS was measured on the second day of dexamethasone administration and 100% sensitivity and 56% sensitivity when UFCs were measured. The CRH stimulation test without dexamethasone pretreatment had 100% specificity and 64% sensitivity. This study has the advantage of comparing the dexamethasone-CRH test to other popular tests (LDDST and CRH test) in the same group of patients with mild Cushing's syndrome and pseudo-Cushing's states, and clearly showed the superiority of the dexamethasone-CRH test in this group of patients. The main drawback to this test is that it requires a lot of steps and the drug (CRH), while no longer investigational, is expensive. A subsequent paper *(70),* found, as expected, that the dexamethasone-CRH test completely distinguished patients with Cushing's syndrome from normal volunteers.

There are other tests (listed in Table 2) that may help distinguish between Cushing's syndrome or pseudo-Cushing's states. Although unable to completely distinguish these two groups, as well as the aforementioned diurnal cortisol tests and dexamethasone-CRH tests, low-dose dexamethasone tests, the insulin tolerance test, the desmopressin test, and the loperamide test can provide useful information. The IL-6 test is investigational, but may be helpful in the future. Low-dose dexamethasone tests are still widely performed.

Low-dose Dexamethasone Tests

These tests are based on the fact that patients with Cushing's syndrome are resistant to suppression by low-dose dexamethasone. Dexamethasone suppression is frequently abnormal in patients with depression (49–51), the very group designed to exclude. In the overnight dexamethasone suppression test (71,72), 1 mg of dexamethasone is given orally at 11 PM, and a plasma cortisol is drawn the following morning at 8 AM. A plasma cortisol greater than 5 µg/dL (138 nmol/L) suggests hypercortisolism. In the LDDST (73), dexamethasone (0.5 mg) is given every 6 h for 8 doses. A UFC greater than 10 µg/d (28 µmol/d) or a 17-OHS greater than 2.5 mg/d (6.90 µmol/d) on the second day of dexamethasone is consistent with Cushing's syndrome. These tests have been found to misclassify as many as 6% of patients with Cushing's syndrome and 15% of patients with pseudo-Cushing's state. Patients with major depression (43%), other psychiatric disorders (8–41%), obesity (13%), and the chronically ill (23%) do not suppress to overnight dexamethasone (74,75). An additional problem is the variable metabolism of dexamethasone in patients receiving medicines (such as rifampin, phenobarbital, or phenytoin) or in patients with renal or hepatic failure (76,77). Most importantly, estrogens raises CBG and because the RIA for cortisol measures total cortisol, high false-positive rates are seen in women taking estrogen (78). To increase the specificity of the overnight dexamethasone test, the cutoff of postdexamethasone serum cortisol was proposed to be 1.8 µg/dL (138 nmol/L) (79). However, it was recently reported that 19% of patients with Cushing's syndrome had a suppressed serum cortisol of less than 5 µg/dL (138 nmol/L) and a much larger percentage had a serum cortisol less than 1.8 µg/dL (80,81). Thus, the low-dose dexamethasone tests can neither be considered sensitive nor specific to distinguish between Cushing's syndrome or pseudo-Cushing's states. For these reasons, collection of urine for measurement of 24-h urinary-free cortisol excretion is likely to be a better screening test for Cushing's syndrome (81,82). For those patients already suspected of having Cushing's syndrome, the dexamethasone-CRH test is likely to be a better test than the LDDST to confirm Cushing's syndrome (9).

Insulin Tolerance Test

The insulin tolerance test (ITT) measures the pituitary corticotroph's ability to secrete ACTH in response to the stress of insulin-induced hypoglycemia. After an overnight fast, intravenous regular insulin (0.15 U/kg) is given as a bolus. Blood samples for glucose, ACTH, and cortisol are obtained at 0, 30, 60, and 90 min. An adequate level of hypoglycemia (a blood glucose concentration of less than 40 mg/dL or a decrease of more than 50% of the baseline concentration) needs to be obtained and a physician should be present during the test. An increase of plasma cortisol or ACTH by more than twofold compared to baseline is considered a normal response. Patients with pituitary Cushing's disease usually fail to respond to the stress of hypoglycemia and do not have an increase in ACTH and cortisol. This is perhaps a result of depressed CRH neurons in these patients. The corticotrophs of most patients with pseudo-Cushing's states respond appropriately to stimuli and an appropriate increase in ACTH and cortisol will occur. The ITT has about an 75% predictive value in discriminating between Cushing's syndrome and pseudo-Cushing's states (8,75,83) and is likely inferior than the dexamethasone-CRH test or diurnal cortisol tests. It is now rarely performed.

Desmopressin Test

Desmopressin, a vasopressin analog that stimulates corticotrophs, was found to stimulate ACTH in 14 of 14 patients with Cushing's syndrome, but not in 20 normal patients and 11 patients with depression (84). All the depressed patients lacked stigmata of hypercortisolism and most of them had normal cortisol excretion. Additionally, other studies have found that some patients with Cushing's syndrome do respond to desmopressin (85,86). Again, the lack of a true group of hypercortisolemic patients with pseudo-Cushing's state, preclude this study from being recommended.

Loperamide Test

The loperamide test is based on the fact that opiates decrease plasma ACTH and cortisol levels possibly because the precursor for ACTH, POMC, also contains the endogenous opiate, β-endorphin. Thus, opiates would be expected to decrease POMC levels and decrease ACTH secretion. It was postulated that patients with pseudo-Cushing's state would have this feedback intact, whereas those with Cushing's syndrome would lack this feedback. The opiate agonist, loperamide (immodium), a drug used to treat diarrhea, is given at one dose of 16 mg at 8:30 AM and three samples (basal, 180 and 210 min after drug) are obtained (87). In 41 patients with confirmed Cushing's syndrome, loperamide did not suppress the cortisol levels below 138 nmol/L (5 µg/dL), whereas in 104 of 110 patients referred for evaluation of Cushing's syndrome, which was subsequently ruled out, the cortisol value suppressed to less than 138 nmol/L (5 µg/dL) at either 150 or 210 min (88). However, in the group in which Cushing's syndrome was ruled out, it was unclear if the patients were hypercortisolemic. In a small study comparing the overnight dexamethasone test and the loperamide, the dexamethasone test was found to have higher specificity when patients with depression were evaluated (89). The loperamide test needs to be studied in more patients with mild Cushing's syndrome and pseudo-Cushing's state before it can be endorsed.

Interleukin 6 (IL-6) Test

IL-6 is a cytokine that stimulates the hypothalamic-pituitary axis via the CRH neuron in animals and was found to stimulate plasma cortisol and ACTH in normal volunteers (90). As pseudo-Cushing's states are marked by CRH excess, in Cushing's syndrome, there is a deficiency of CRH, therefore it was postulated that injection of IL-6 could distinguish between the two groups. The authors expected that IL-6 would stimulate plasma cortisol and ACTH in patients with pseudo-Cushing's states, but not in those patients with Cushing's syndrome. Thirty-four patients with Cushing's syndrome and nine patients with pseudo-Cushing's states received a single injection of IL-6 (3 µg/kg) (91). ACTH (maximum response at 90 min) and cortisol (maximum response at 120 min) rose in the patients with pseudo-Cushing's states, but not in those with Cushing's syndrome. An ACTH at 90 min and cortisol at 120 min was able to completely separate the groups. This study has only been reported in abstract form and IL-6 is an investigational drug, making its use limited. We await further studies using this interesting agent.

Tests Not Recommended to Distinguish Between Cushing's Syndrome and Pseudo-Cushing's States

There are also tests (Table 2) that are not helpful in making the distinction between Cushing's syndrome or pseudo-Cushing's states and may actually be confusing if done before the diagnosis of Cushing's syndrome is made. Inferior petrosal sinus sampling (IPSS), an excellent test to differentiate the etiologies of confirmed Cushing's syndrome, measures ACTH in the petrosal sinuses draining the pituitary compared to simultaneously drawn levels from the periphery. The test is usually given with CRH. Yanovski et al. *(92)* proposed that IPSS would be able to separate patients with Cushing's syndrome from those with pseudo-Cushing's states and speculated three findings in patients with Cushing's syndrome compared to those with pseudo-Cushing's states: (1) that the ACTH concentrations in the petrosal sinus compared to the periphery would be higher; (2) that there would be more of a difference in the ACTH concentrations between the petrosal sinuses; and (3) that CRH administration would not stimulate ACTH concentrations in the suppressed petrosal sinus. They studied 7 normal volunteers, 9 patients with pseudo-Cushing's states, and 40 patients with Cushing's syndrome. Contrary to their expectations, all three groups had elevated petrosal to central ACTH concentrations, had lateralization of one petrosal sinus and responded similarly to CRH administration. Thus, IPSS can not be used to distinguish patients with Cushing's syndrome from those with pseudo-Cushing's states and may actually be misleading if performed before the diagnosis of Cushing's syndrome is made.

Pituitary MRI is also very good for localizing a pituitary tumor once the diagnosis of Cushing's syndrome is made, however, it is not recommended to distinguish between Cushing's syndrome and pseudo-Cushing's states. This is because up to 10% of normal individuals have what radiologists read as a pituitary tumor on MRI (incidentalomas) *(93)*. If a patient without Cushing's syndrome only has a pituitary MRI performed that shows an adenoma, she/he may be inappropriately diagnosed as having CD and undergo unnecessary surgery.

As aforementioned, a morning plasma cortisol is also not able to distinguish between mild Cushing's syndrome and pseudo-Cushing's state. Similarly, a plasma-free cortisol, although higher in patients with Cushing's syndrome than those with pseudo-Cushing's state, also exhibited too much overlap between the two groups to be used clinically to exclude pseudo-Cushing's state *(65)*.

TREATMENT OF PSEUDO-CUSHING'S STATES AND CONCLUSIONS

The distinction between Cushing's syndrome and pseudo-Cushing's states is often difficult, leading to frustration for both patient and physician. To prevent this frustration, working closely with a good endocrinologist who sees many patients with Cushing's syndrome is needed. Patience is also needed. With time, most patients will "declare themselves" and develop a clearer picture consistent with either Cushing's syndrome or a pseudo-Cushing's state. While waiting, treating the underlying psychiatric condition (if present) is often helpful. In some patients, a trial of low-dose ketoconazole (200 mg twice a day) may be helpful in that if the patient improves on this treatment, clinically relevant hypercortisolism is probably present, whereas if the patient does not improve, most likely the patient's symptoms are unrelated to hypercortisolism. This trial cannot reliably be used to distinguish between Cushing's syndrome and pseudo-Cushing's states as both groups may improve on ketoconazole. Liver function tests and signs of adrenal insufficiency need to be monitored on this drug. The tincture of time is the best cure!

REFERENCES

1. Yanovski JA, Cutler G, Jr. Glucocorticoid action and the clinical features of Cushing's syndrome. Endocrinol Metab Clin North Am 1994; 23:487–509.
2. Orth DN. Cushing's syndrome. N Engl J Med 1995; 332:791–803.
3. Ross EJ, Linch DC. Cushing's syndrome-killing disease: discriminatory value of signs and symptoms aiding early diagnosis. Lancet 1982; 2:646–649.
4. Missed Diagnosis. Family Circle February 2nd 1993; 68–73.
5. Rosmond R, Dallman MF, Bjorntorp P. Stress-related cortisol secretion in men: relationships with abdominal obesity and endocrine, metabolic and hemodynamic abnormalities [see comments]. J Clin Endocrinol Metab 1998; 83:1853–1859.
6. Rees LH, Besser GM, Jeffcoate WJ, Goldie DJ, Marks V. Alcohol-induced pseudo-Cushing's syndrome. Lancet 1977; 1:726–728.
7. Smalls AG, Kloppenborg PW, Njo KT, Knoben JM, Ruland CM. Alcohol-induced Cushing's syndrome. Br Med J 1976; 2:1298.
8. Besser GM, Edwards CRW. Cushing's syndrome. Clin Endocrinol Metab 1972; 1:451–490.
9. Yanovski JA, Cutler GB, Jr, Chrousos GP, Nieman LK. Corticotropin-releasing hormone stimulation following low-dose dexamethasone administration: a new test to distinguish Cushing's syndrome from pseudo-Cushing's states. J Am Med Assoc 1993; 269:2232–2238.
10. Tsigos C, Young RJ, White A. Diabetic neuropathy is associated with increased activity of the hypothalamic-pituitary-adrenal axis. J Clin Endocrinol Metab 1993; 76:554–558.
11. Roy MS, Roy A, Gallucci WT, Colliler B, Young K, Kamilaris TC, et al. The ovine corticotropin-releasing hormone-stimulation test in type I diabetic patients and controls: suggestion of mild chronic hypercortisolism. Metabolism 1993; 42:696–700.
12. Paton A. Alcohol-induced cushingoid syndrome. Br Med J 1976; 2:1504.
13. Lamberts SW, Klijn JG, de Jong FH, Birkenhager JC. Hormone secretion in alcohol-induced pseudo-Cushing's syndrome. Differential diagnosis with Cushing's disease. JAMA 1979; 242:1640–1643.
14. Jeffcoate W. Alcohol-induced pseudo-Cushing's syndrome. Lancet 1993; 341:676, 677.
15. Wand GS, Dobs AS. Alterations in the hypothalamic-pituitary-adrenal axis in actively drinking alcoholics. J Clin Endocrinol Metab 1991; 72:1290–1295.
16. Jain S, Sakhuja V, Bhansali A, Gupta KL, Dash RJ, Chugh KS. Corticotropin-dependent Cushing's syndrome in a patient with chronic renal failure—a rare association. Ren Fail 1993; 15:563–566.
17. Otokida K, Fujiwara T, Oriso S, Kato M. Cortisol and its metabolites in the plasma and urine in Cushing's syndrome with chronic renal failure (CRF), compared to Cushing's syndrome without CRF. Nippon Jinzo Gakkai Shi 1989; 31:651–656.
18. Sharp NA, Devlin JT, Rimmer JM. Renal failure obfuscates the diagnosis of Cushing's disease. JAMA 1986; 256:2564, 2565.
19. Arai K, Chrousos GP. Syndromes of glucocorticoid and mineralocorticoid resistance. Steroids 1995; 60:173–179.
20. de Lange P, Koper JW, Huizenga NA, Brinkmann AO, de Jong FH, Karl M, et al. Differential hormone-dependent transcriptional activation and—repression by naturally occurring human glucocorticoid receptor variants. Mol Endocrinol 1997; 11:1156–1164.
21. Lamberts SW. The glucocorticoid insensitivity syndrome. Horm Res 1996; 1:2–4.
22. Friedman TC, Papanicolaou DA. Comment on high urinary free cortisol excretion in a patient with psychogenic polydipsia. J Clin Endocrinol Metab 1998; 83:3378, 3379.
23. Cizza G, Nieman LK, Doppman JL, Passaro MD, Czerwiec FS, Chrousos GP, et al. Factitious Cushing syndrome. J Clin Endocrinol Metab 1996; 81:3573–3577.

24. Friedman TC, Mastorakos G, Newman TD, Mullen NM, Horton EG, Costello R, et al. Carbohydrate and lipid metabolism in endogenous hypercortisolism: shared features with metabolic syndrome X and NIDDM. Endocr J 1996; 43:645–655.

25. Reaven GM. Role of insulin resistance in human disease. Diabetes 1988; 37:1595–1607.

26. Peeke PM, Chrousos GP. Hypercortisolism and obesity. Ann NY Acad Sci 1995; 771:665–676.

27. Kreze A, Veleminsky J, Spirova E. Low-dose dexamethasone suppression of urinary-free cortisol in the differential diagnosis between Cushing's syndrome and obesity. Klin Wochenschr 1985; 63:188, 189.

28. Pasquali R, Cantobelli S, Casimirri F, Capelli M, Bortoluzzi L, Flamia R, et al. The hypothalamic-pituitary-adrenal axis in obese women with different patterns of body fat distribution. J Clin Endocrinol Metab 1993; 77:341–346.

29. Mårin P, Darin N, Amemiya T, Andersson B, Jern S, Björntorp P. Cortisol secretion in relation to body fat distribution in obese premenopausal women. Metabolism 1992; 41:882–886.

30. Gibney J, Wallace JD, Spinks T, Schnorr L, Ranicar A, Cuneo RC, et al. The effects of 10 years of recombinant human growth hormone (GH) in adult GH-deficient patients. J Clin Endocrinol Metab 1999; 84:2596–2602.

31. Ho TT, Chan KC, Wong KH, Lee SS. Abnormal fat distribution and use of protease inhibitors. Lancet 1998; 351:1736, 1737.

32. Massip P, Marchou B, Bonnet E, Cuzin L, Montastruc JL. Lipodystrophia with protease inhibitors in HIV patients. Therapie 1997; 52:615.

33. Carr A, Samaras K, Burton S, Law M, Freund J, Chisholm DJ, et al. A syndrome of peripheral lipodystrophy, hyperlipidaemia and insulin resistance in patients receiving HIV protease inhibitors. Aids 1998; 12:F51–58.

34. Viraben R, Aquilina C. Indinavir-associated lipodystrophy. Aids 1998; 12:F37–39.

35. Yanovski JA, Miller KD, Kino T, Friedman TC, Chrousos GP, Tsigos C, et al. Endocrine and metabolic evaluation of human immunodeficiency virus-infected patients with evidence of protease inhibitor-associated lipodystrophy. J Clin Endocrinol Metab 1999; 84:1925–1931.

36. Hadigan C, Miller K, Corcoran C, Anderson E, Basgoz N, Grinspoon S. Fasting hyperinsulinemia and changes in regional body composition in human immunodeficiency virus-infected women. J Clin Endocrinol Metab 1999; 84:1932–1937.

37. Fujii H, Iida S, Gomi M, Tsugawa M, Kitani T, Moriwaki K. Augmented induction by dexamethasone of metallothionein IIa messenger ribonucleic acid in fibroblasts from a patient with cortisol hyperreactive syndrome. J Clin Endocrinol Metab 1993; 76:445–449.

38. Iida S, Moriwaki K, Fujii H, Gomi M, Tsugawa M, Nakamura Y, et al. Quantitative comparison of aromatase induction by dexamethasone in fibroblasts from a patient with familial cortisol resistance and a patient with cortisol hyperreactive syndrome. J Clin Endocrinol Metab 1991; 73:192–196.

39. Iida S, Nakamura Y, Fujii H, Nishimura J, Tsugawa M, Gomi M, et al. A patient with hypocortisolism and Cushing's syndrome-like manifestations: cortisol hyperreactive syndrome. J Clin Endocrinol Metab 1990; 70:729–737.

40. Huizenga NA, Koper JW, De Lange P, Pols HA, Stolk RP, Burger H, et al. A polymorphism in the glucocorticoid receptor gene may be associated with and increased sensitivity to glucocorticoids in vivo. J Clin Endocrinol Metab 1998; 83:144–151.

41. Stewart PM. 11 beta-Hydroxysteroid dehydrogenase: implications for clinical medicine. Clin Endocrinol 1996; 44:493–499.

42. Bujalska IJ, Kumar S, Stewart PM. Does central obesity reflect "Cushing's disease of the omentum"? Lancet 1997; 349:1210–1213.

43. Bujalska IJ, Kumar S, Hewison M, Stewart PM. Differentiation of adipose stromal cells: the roles of glucocorticoids and 11beta-hydroxysteroid dehydrogenase. Endocrinology 1999; 140:3188–3196.

44. Stewart PM, Boulton A, Kumar S, Clark PM, Shackleton CH. Cortisol metabolism in human obesity: impaired cortisone→cortisol conversion in subjects with central adiposity. J Clin Endocrinol Metab 1999; 84:1022–1027.

45. Gold PW, Goodwin FK, Chrousos GP. Clinical and biochemical manifestations of depression. Relation to the neurobiology of stress (1). N Engl J Med 1988; 319:348–353.

46. Chrousos GP, Schuermeyer TH, Doppman J, Oldfield EH, Schulte HM, Gold PW, et al. NIH conference. Clinical applications of corticotropin-releasing factor. Ann Intern Med 1985; 102:344–358.

47. Gold PW, Loriaux DL, Roy A, Kling MA, Calabrese JR, Kellner CH, et al. Responses to corticotropin-releasing hormone in the hypercortisolism of depression and Cushing's disease. Pathophysiologic and diagnostic implications. N Engl J Med 1986; 314:1329–1335.

48. Gold PW, Goodwin FK, Chrousos GP. Clinical and biochemical manifestations of depression. Relation to the neurobiology of stress (2). N Engl J Med 1988; 319:413–420.

49. Arana GW, Mossman D. The dexamethasone suppression test and depression. Approaches to the use of a laboratory test in psychiatry. Endocrinol Metab Clin North Am 1988; 17:21–39.

50. Carroll BJ. The dexamethasone suppression test for melancholia. Br J Psych 1982; 140:292–304.

51. Carroll BJ, Feinberg M, Greden JF, Tarika J, Albala AA, Haskett RF, et al. A specific laboratory test for the diagnosis of melancholia. Standardization, validation, and clinical utility. Arch Gen Psych 1981; 38:15–22.

52. Rubin RT, Phillips JJ, McCracken JT, Sadow TF. Adrenal gland volume in major depression: relationship to basal and stimulated pituitary-adrenal cortical axis function. Biol Psych 1996; 40:89–97.

53. Rivier C, Imaki T, Vale W. Prolonged exposure to alcohol: effect on CRF mRNA levels, and CRF- and stress-induced ACTH secretion in the rat. Brain Res 1990; 520:1–5.

54. Redei E, Branch BJ, Gholami S, Lin EY, Taylor AN. Effects of ethanol on CRF release in vitro. Endocrinology 1988; 123:2736–2743.

55. Groote Veldman R, Meinders AE. On the mechanism of alcohol-induced pseudo-Cushing's syndrome. Endocr Rev 1996; 17:262–268.

56. Johnson DA, Lee NM, Cooke R. Adaptation to ethanol-induced fluidization of brain lipid bilayers. Drug Alcohol Depend 1979; 4:197–202.

57. Dave JR, Eiden LE, Karanian JW, Eskay RL. Ethanol exposure decreases pituitary corticotropin-releasing factor binding, adenylate cyclase activity, proopiomelanocortin biosynthesis, and plasma beta-endorphin levels in the rat. Endocrinology 1986; 118:280–286.

58. Dave JR, Krieg R, Jr, Witorsch RJ. Modulation of prolactin binding sites in vitro by membrane fluidizers. Effects on male prostatic and female hepatic membranes in alcohol-fed rats. Biochim Biophys Acta 1985; 816:313–320.

59. Hiramatsu R, Nisula BC. Effect of alcohol on the interaction of cortisol with plasma proteins, glucocorticoid receptors and erythrocytes. J Steroid Biochem 1989; 33:65–70.

60. Stewart PM, Burra P, Shackleton CH, Sheppard MC, Elias E. 11 beta-Hydroxysteroid dehydrogenase deficiency and glucocorticoid status in patients with alcoholic and non-alcoholic chronic liver disease. J Clin Endocrinol Metab 1993; 76:748–751.

61. Lex BW, Ellingboe JE, Teoh SK, Mendelson JH, Rhoades E. Prolactin and cortisol levels following acute alcohol challenges in women with and without a family history of alcoholism. Alcohol 1991; 8:383–387.

62. Schuckit MA, Risch SC, Gold EO. Alcohol consumption, ACTH level, and family history of alcoholism. Am J Psych 1988; 145:1391–1395.

63. Nieman LK, Cutler GB, Jr. The sensitivity of the urine free cortisol measurement as a screening test for Cushing's syndrome. Endocrine Soc (abstract) 1990; 72:822.

64. Krieger DT, Allen W, Rizzo F, Krieger HP. Characterization of the normal temporal pattern of plasma corticosteroid levels. J Clin Endocrinol Metab 1971; 32:266–284.

65. Friedman TC, Yanovski JA. Morning plasma-free cortisol: inability to distinguish patients with mild Cushing's syndrome from patients with pseudo-Cushing states. J Endocrinol Invest 1995; 18:696–701.

66. Newell-Price J, Trainer P, Perry L, Wass J, Grossman A, Besser M. A single sleeping midnight cortisol has 100% sensitivity for the diagnosis of Cushing's syndrome. Clin Endocrinol 1995; 43:545–550.

67. Papanicolaou DA, Yanovski JA, Cutler G, Jr, Chrousos GP, Nieman LK. A single midnight serum cortisol measurement distinguishes Cushing's syndrome from pseudo-Cushing states. J Clin Endocrinol Metab 1998; 83:1163–1167.

68. Raff H, Raff JL, Findling JW. Late-night salivary cortisol as a screening test for Cushing's syndrome. J Clin Endocrinol Metab 1998; 83:2681–2686.

69. Papanicolaou DA, Mullen N, Nieman LK. Diurnal salivary cortisol determination: an accurate and convenient test for the diagnosis of Cushing syndrome. Endocrine Soc (abstract) 1995; 77:OR10-4.

70. Yanovski JA, Cutler G, Jr, Chrousos GP, Nieman LK. The dexamethasone-suppressed corticotropin-releasing hormone stimulation test differentiates mild Cushing's disease from normal physiology. J Clin Endocrinol Metab 1998; 83:348–352.

71. Pavlatos FC, Smilo RP, Forsham PH. A rapid screening test for Cushing's syndrome. JAMA 1865; 193:720–723.

72. Nugent CA, Nichols T, Tyler FH. Diagnosis of Cushing' syndrome-single dose dexamethasone. Arch Intern Med 1965; 116:172–176.

73. Liddle GW. Tests of pituitary-adrenal suppressibility in the diagnosis of Cushing's syndrome. J Clin Endocrinol Metab 1960; 20:1539–1561.

74. Murphy BE. Steroids and depression. J Steroid Biochem Mol Biol 1991; 38:537–559.

75. Crapo LM. Cushing's syndrome: a review of diagnostic tests. Metabolism 1979; 28:955–977.

76. Terzolo M, Borretta G, Ali A, Cesario F, Magro G, Boccuzzi A, et al. Misdiagnosis of Cushing's syndrome in a patient receiving rifampicin therapy for tuberculosis. Horm Metab Res 1995; 27:148–150.

77. Meikle AW, Lagerquist LG, Tyler FH. Apparently normal pituitary-adrenal suppressibility in Cushing's syndrome: dexamethasone metabolism and plasma levels. J Lab Clin Med 1975; 86:472–478.

78. Tiller JW, Maguire KP, Schweitzer I, Biddle N, Campbell DG, Outch K, et al. The dexamethasone suppression test: a study in a normal population. Psychoneuroendocrinology 1988; 13:377–384.

79. Wood PJ, Barth JH, Freedman DB, Perry L, Sheridan B. Evidence for the low-dose dexamethasone suppression test to screen for Cushing's syndrome—recommendations for a protocol for biochemistry laboratories. Ann Clin Biochem 1997; 34:222–229.

80. Findling JW, Shaker JL, Brickner RC, Magill SB, Lalande BM, Raff H. Low-dose dexamethasone suppression testing cannot be used to exclude Cushing's syndrome. Endocrin Soc 1999; 81:OR21–23 (abstract).

81. Findling JW, Raff H. Newer diagnostic techniques and problems in Cushing's disease. Endocrinol Metab Clin North Am 1999; 28:191–210.

82. Tsigos C, Papanicolaou DA, Chrousos GP. Advances in the diagnosis and treatment of Cushing's syndrome. Baillieres Clin Endocrinol Metab 1995; 9:315–336.

83. James VH, Landon J, Wynn V, Greenwood FC. A fundamental defect of adrenocortical control in Cushing's disease. J Endocrinol 1968; 40:15–28.

84. Malerbi DA, Fragoso MC, Vieira Filho AH, Brenlha EM, Mendonca BB. Cortisol and adrenocorticotropin response to desmopressin in women with Cushing's disease compared with depressive illness. J Clin Endocrinol Metab 1996; 81:2233–2237.

85. Colombo P, Passini E, Re T, Faglia G, Ambrosi B. Effect of desmopressin on ACTH and cortisol secretion in states of ACTH excess. Clin Endocrinol 1997; 46:661–668.

86. Malerbi DA, Mendonca BB, Liberman B, Toledo SP, Corradini MC, Cunha-Neto MB, et al. The desmopressin stimulation test in the differential diagnosis of Cushing's syndrome. Clin Endocrinol 1993; 38:463–472.

87. Ambrosi B, Bochicchio D, Ferrario R, Colombo P, Faglia G. Effects of the opiate agonist loperamide on pituitary-adrenal function in patients wiht suspected hypercortisolism. J Endocrinol Invest 1989; 12:31–35.

88. Ambrosi B, Bochicchio D, Colombo P, Fadin C, Faglia G. Loperamide to diagnose Cushing's syndrome. J Am Med Assoc 1993; 270:2301, 2302.

89. Bernini GP, Argenio GF, Cerri F, Franchi F. Comparison between the suppressive effects of dexamethasone and loperamide on cortisol and ACTH secretion in some pathological conditions. J Endocrinol Invest 1994; 17:799–804.

90. Tsigos C, Papanicolaou DA, Defensor R, Mitsiadis CS, Kyrou I, Chrousos GP. Dose effects of recombinant human interleukin-6 on pituitary hormone secretion and energy expenditure. Neuroendocrinology 1997; 66:54–62.

91. Papanicolaou DA, Lotsikas AJ, Torpy DJ, Tsigos C, Chrousos GP. A single injection of interleukin-6 accurately distinguishes Cushing syndrome from pseudo-Cushing states. Endocrine Soc 1998; 80:OR12-3 (abstract).

92. Yanovski JA, Cutler GB, Jr, Doppman JL, Miller DL, Chrousos GP, Oldfield EH, et al. The limited ability of inferior petrosal sinus sampling with corticotropin-releasing hormone to distinguish Cushing's disease from pseudo-Cushing states or normal physiology. J Clin Endocrinol Metab 1993; 77:503–509.

93. Hall WA, Luciano MG, Doppman JL, Patronas NJ, Oldfield EH. Pituitary magnetic resonance imaging in normal human volunteers: occult adenomas in the general population. Ann Intern Med 1994; 120:817–820.

16 Adrenocortical Tumors and Oncogenes

Martin Reincke, MD

CONTENTS

INTRODUCTION

Adrenocortical carcinoma is a highly malignant tumor with an incidence of case per 1.7 million/yr *(1)*. At the time of diagnosis, 70% of the patients suffer from an advanced tumor stage with local invasion or distant metastasis and can rarely be cured *(2)*. In contrast, benign adrenal lesions are much more frequent. Most of these tumors are clinically silent and are incidentally detected by ultrasound or computed tomography *(3)*. The prevalence of asymptomatic adrenal mass is 1–2% of abdominal CT's *(4)*. The majority of these tumors are nonfunctional adrenal adenomas, their pathogenesis being largely unknown.

Unfortunately, progress in the understanding of adrenal tumorigenesis has been slow. Studies using the "candidate gene approach" suggest a low prevalence of mutations in tumor suppressor genes and oncogenes in adenomas. Mutations in G-protein coupled receptors and G-proteins identified in growth-hormone-secreting pituitary tumors and thyroid adenomas have not been found in adrenal cortex neoplasms. This supports the concept that the signal-transduction cascade controlling tumor growth in adrenocortical neoplasms is different from that of pituitary and thyroid tumors. This chapter will, therefore, focus on recent developments in the field of adrenal-specific mechanisms of tumorigenesis.

From: *Contemporary Endocrinology: Adrenal Disorders*
Edited by: A. N. Margioris and G. P. Chrousos © Humana Press, Totowa, NJ

HEREDITARY TUMOR SYNDROMES

Several hereditary tumor syndromes are associated with the formation of benign or malignant adrenocortical tumors.

Li–Fraumeni Syndrome

The Li–Fraumeni syndrome was first described in 1969 *(5)*. It is a rare familial tumor syndrome associated with a high incidence of breast cancer, leukemias, soft-tissue sarcomas, gliomas, and adrenocortical carcinomas. Affected patients generally develop the first tumor before age 30, and the second or third neoplasias are frequently observed in patients previously treated with chemotherapy or irradiation *(6)*. The molecular basis of this disease has been recently elucidated by identification of germ-line point mutations in the *p53* tumor suppressor gene *(7,8)*. The second *p53* allele is inactivated in tumor tissue by deletion of the short arm of chromosome 17 (17p) eliminating all wild-type *p53* activity *(9)*. Recently, *p53* germ-line mutations have been found in children with adrenocortical carcinomas without a classical family history of the Li-Fraumeni syndrome *(10,11)*. Because of the consequences of germ-line *p53* mutations for these individuals and their relatives, genetic testing has been recommended for risk assessment in childhood adrenocortical carcinoma.

Beckwith–Wiedemann Syndrome (BWS)

The BWS is a rare condition (1/13.700 live births) characterized by macroglossia, gigantism, earlobe pits or creases, abdominal wall defects, and an increased risk for the development of Wilms tumors of the kidney, rhabdomyosarcoma, hepatoblastoma, and adrenal carcinoma *(12,13)*. Although most BWS cases are sporadic, families have been reported in which the disease segregates as an autosomal dominant trait with incomplete penetrance. BWS maps to chromosome 11p15.5 *(14)*. Uniparental paternal isodisomie for this locus, which includes the *IGF* II gene, has been identified in affected individuals *(15)*. The complete loss of one *IGF* II allele and a duplication of the remaining allele in association with *IGF* II overexpression has been demonstrated in tumors of the BWS and in sporadic adrenocortical tumors *(15,16)*.

Multiple Endocrine Neoplasia Type 1

The genetic defect responsible for multiple endocrine neoplasia type 1 (MEN 1) has been mapped to chromosome 11q13 *(17)*. Tumorigenesis results from unmasking of a recessive mutation in an as yet unidentified tumor suppressor gene with development of parathyroid adenomas, pituitary adenomas, and tumors of the endocrine pancreas. Involvement of the adrenal gland has been reported in a considerable proportion of patients (36–41%) with MEN 1. This lesion is often characterized as bilateral hyperplasia or adenomas, and occasionally, even carcinomas *(18)*. Recently, in 12 patients with adrenocortical tumors out of a series of 33 patients with MEN 1, loss of constitutional heterozygosity for chromosome 11q13 was demonstrated only in a patient with adreno-cortical carcinoma, but not in 11 patients with benign adrenal lesions *(18)*. This suggests that adrenocortical tumorigenesis is probably not a primary lesion in the MEN 1 syndrome. In the same study, insulin- or proinsulin-secreting pancreatic endocrine tumors were significantly overrepresented in patients with MEN 1 and adrenal tumors suggesting that adrenocortical tumorigenesis may be stimulated by insulin and insulin-related peptides in these patients.

Familial Hyperaldosteronism Type II (FH-II)

Familial hyperaldosteronism type I is characterized by primary hyperaldosteronism with hypertension and hypokaliemic alkalosis, which responds to dexamethasone treatment *(19)*. The genetic basis recently elucidated is a hybrid gene that involves the fusion of the regulatory region of the *CYP11B1* gene encoding 11β-hydroxylase with the coding region of another gene (*Cyp11B2*) encoding aldosterone synthase *(20)*. Whereas tumor formation has not been described in FH-I, Stowasser et al. *(21)* reported recently five families with familial occurrence of primary hyperaldosteronism that was not glucocorticoid-suppressible, but was associated with aldosterone-producing adenomas or bilateral adrenal hyperplasia. The genetic basis of this so-called familial hyperaldosteronism type II has not been elucidated yet.

PROOPIOMELANOCORTIN (POMC) PEPTIDES AND OTHER GROWTH FACTORS

Long-standing excess of adrenocorticotropic hormone (ACTH) and related peptides is associated with the development of nodular adrenal hyperplasia. Macronodular adrenal disease has been observed in 17–40% of patients with ACTH-dependent Cushing's syndrome. These nodules generally remain ACTH-dependent and regress after successful treatment of the source of ACTH excess. Rarely, transition from pituitary dependent to ACTH independent Cushing's syndrome has been observed *(22,32)*.

Congenital adrenal hyperplasia (CAH) can cause adrenocortical nodular hyperplasia. Indeed, 80% of patients with classical 21-hydroxylase deficiency have uni- or bilateral nodular adrenal hyperplasia *(24,25)*. This has been explained by chronic stimulation of the adrenal cortex by elevated ACTH and related peptides. Macronodular adrenal disease in patients with CAH is generally clinically silent, but functional adrenal neoplasms, mainly androgen-secreting tumors, have been described in patients with CAH (Table 1). Surprisingly, 45% of heterozygote relatives of patients with 21-hydroxylase deficiency also have macronodular adrenal disease *(25)*. This indicates that ACTH and POMC peptides may not be the only player in this condition, because these peptides are generally within the normal range. In these patients, the mild impairment of steroid biosynthesis causing intraadrenal accumulation of steroid precursors may interfere with auto- and paracrine feedback mechanisms, inducing "compensatory" adrenal hyperplasia.

CYTOGENETIC ASPECTS OF ADRENOCORTICAL TUMORIGENESIS

The genetic aberrations involved in sporadic primary adenocortical tumors are not completely understood. Previous studies have focused on selected chromosome regions. Yano et al. studied the loss of heterozygosity in one primary and eight recurrent adrenocortical carcinomas and eight sporadic benign lesions *(37)*. The carcinomas showed loss of heterozygosity on 17p, 11p, and 13q. No genetic changes were found in any of the benign lesions. Karyotype analysis of two sporadic adrenocortical carcinomas have revealed alterations at 11p *(38,39)*. In 5 of 12 aldosterone-producing adenomas, abnormal karyotypes involving loss of chromosome Y (*n*=5), loss of chromosome 19 (*n*=1), and partial trisomy 7q were found *(40)*. Using fluorescence *in situ* hybridization, trisomy of chromosome 1, 8, 11, 12, and 15 was detected in an adrenocortical carcinoma

Table 1
Functional Adrenocortical Tumors in Patients with Congenital Adrenal Hyperplasia:
Review of the Literature

Author	Year of Publication	Age (years)	Sex	Steroid Block	Histology	Tumor Size (cm)
Hamwi (26)	1957	39	F	21-OHD	carcinoma	10
Daeschner (27)	1965	13	F	21-OHD	adenoma	9
Van Seters (28)	1981	61	F	21-OHD	adenoma	13
Pang (29)	1981	16	F	21-OHD	adenoma	3
Baumann (30)	1982	11	F	21-OHD	carcinoma	8
Shinohara (31)	1986	21	F	21-OHD	adenoma	?
Takayama (32)	1988	37	F	21-OHD	adenoma	7
Jaursch (33)	1989	41	M	21-OHD	carcinoma	10
Sunaga (34)	1989	34	M	21-OHD	adenoma	5
Touitou (35)	1989	61	F	11β-OHD	adenoma	4
Shimshi (36)	1992	51	F	21-OHD	adenoma	4

F=Female; M=male; 21-OHD=21-hydroxylase deficiency; 11β-OHD=11β-hydroxylase deficiency

(41). More recently, using comparative genomic hybridization (CGH), a high frequency of genetic abberations was detected in adrenocortical carcinomas (42). Losses most often involved the chromosomal regions 2, 11q, and 17p (four of eight tumors), whereas gains took place at chromosome 4 and 5 (four of eight tumors). These results differ from our own experience using CGH in 7 adenomas and 14 carcinomas (43). Chromosomal gains were much more prevalent than losses and affected chromosomes 5, 7, 9q, 12q, 14q, 16p, 20q (Fig. 1). Total gains and losses were less frequent in large adenomas (tumor diameter > 4.0 cm) and absent in small adenomas (< 4 cm). These studies show that adrenal carcinoma tumorigenesis involves amplifications of chromosomes, not commonly affected in other human tumors, indicating the presence of new and possibly adrenal-specific oncogenes. This may give new insights into the mechanisms of adrenocortical tumorigenesis.

ONCOGENES AND TUMOR SUPPRESSOR GENES

Clonal Analysis of Adrenocortical Tumors

The pathogenesis of cancer is generally considered to be a multistep process, during which an initiating event is followed by tumor promotion. The initiative event is widely regarded as a somatic mutation occurring in a single cell, which, because of a selective growth advantage, proliferates to produce a monoclonal tumor (44,45). Adrenocortical steroid secretion is a complex process that is regulated by several hormones and growth factors, which also control adaptative processes like hypertrophy and hyperplasia of the adrenal cortex. Determination of the clonal composition of neoplastic adrenal tissues is instrumental in establishing the cellular origin of adrenocortical tumors. A polyclonal tumor would favor the idea that it developed from a group of cells under the common stimulus of growth factors of extra- or intraadrenal origin. Conversely, a monoclonal tumor would suggest that it developed from a single genetically aberrant cell. Two recent publications investigated the clonal composition of adrenocortical tumors using

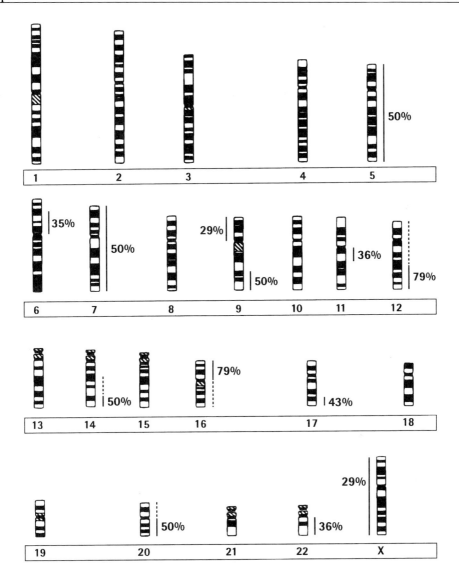

Fig. 1. Chromosomal losses (left) and gains (right) in 14 (= 100%) sporadic adrenocortical carcinomas.

X chromosome inactivation analysis. Gicquel et al *(46)* found a monoclonal pattern in all four carcinomas studied. Of 14 benign adenomas, 8 tumors were monoclonal, whereas 6 adenomas showed a polyclonal pattern. The study of Beuschlein et al. *(47)* revealed monoclonality in all carcinomas (*n*=3) and in 7 of 8 adenomas. One cortisol-producing adenoma in this study was polyclonal. These data demonstrate that adrenocortical carcinomas are generally monoclonal as the result of oncogenic mutations of single cells with transformation and expansion into a malignant clone. Most of the adenomas also arise from oncogenic mutations, whereas a minority of benign adenomas is genetically heterogeneous. These adenomas may have an oligo- or multicellular origin under the putative action of extraadrenal or local growth factors. However, monoclonal and polyclonal adenomas might represent different stages of a common multistep process *(48)*. In this notion, the growth of polyclonal tumor tissue arise either from the proliferation of cells with a constitutive intrinsic growth potential or by stimulation of mitogens, followed by a secondary mutational event conferring a growth advantage of a particular clone leading to monoclonality.

ACTH Receptor Mutations and Adrenal Tumors

Cyclic AMP is a key second messenger involved in both hormone hypersecretion and/or increased cell proliferation in a variety of endocrine tissues. Constitutive activation of key regulatory proteins of cAMP, such as G-protein-coupled receptors and GTP-binding proteins, have been implicated in the pathogenesis of such diseases as acromegaly and toxic thyroid adenomas *(49,50)*. Oncogenic transformation of the TSH receptor gene by point mutations was found in approx 30% of hyperfunctioning thyroid adenomas *(50)*. These mutations caused amino acid substitutions in the carboxy-terminal portion of the third cytoplasmic loop of this receptor in 3 of 11 hyperfunctioning thyroid adenomas. The mutant receptors conferred constitutive activation of adenylyl cyclase, when tested by transfection in COS cells. An alternative pathway increasing intracellular cAMP and associated with tumorigenesis are constitutive activating mutations in the α-chain of the stimulatory G-proteins (Gs) found in growth hormone-producing adenomas and thyroid adenomas *(49)*. The mutant G proteins in these tumors remain in the activated state, stimulating the adenylyl cyclase and, hence, cAMP production.

Adrenocortical tumorigenesis differs from pituitary and thyroid tumorigenesis because activation of the cAMP/protein kinase A pathway seems to be of little importance in the development of adrenocortical neoplasms. ACTH is the main hormone regulating steroid-hormone secretion, however, it fails to cause adrenocortical hypertrophy in the absence of innervation by the splanchnic nerve. ACTH in physiologic concentrations does not stimulate cell proliferation of adrenocortical cells in vitro, and even pharmacologic doses of ACTH induce only a moderate cell growth *(51)*. In keeping with this findings, activating mutations of neither the ACTH receptor nor the α-chain of the Gs have been identified in benign or malignant adrenocortical tumors *(49,52–54)*. On the contrary, activating mutations of the Gi2, one of the adenylyl cyclase inhibitory G proteins, were found in very few adrenocortical tumors, but not in a variety of other endocrine and nonendocrine tumors *(49,54,55)*.

These data suggest that in the adrenal cortex, the ACTH/Gs/protein kinase A signaling pathway is preferentially important for steroid hormone secretion and, hence, maintenance of a highly differentiated cellular phenotype, but is of relatively low importance for cellular proliferation. This is supported by the recent finding of deletions of the *ACTH* receptor gene in undifferentiated adrenocortical tumors. Of 16 patients with benign lesions, mutational loss of the *ACTH-R* gene by deletion was present in one oncocytic nonfunctional adenoma, but not in 15 hyperfunctioning adenomas. Of four informative patients with adrenocortical carcinomas, loss of heterozygosity (LOH) of the ACTH receptor gene was present in two cases. Both patients had advanced tumor stages and showed a more rapid course than carcinoma patients without LOH. Northern blot experiments showed reduced expression of *ACTH-R* mRNA in the tumors with LOH of the *ACTH-R* gene, suggesting functional significance of this finding at the transcriptional level *(56,57)*. These data demonstrate that the ACTH receptor may act

Table 2
Mutations in Oncogenes and Tumor-Suppressor Genes in Adrenocortical Tumors

Gene	Prevalence of Mutations	Author	Year
Signal Transduction			
constitutive activating	0/25 tumors	Latronico et al. *(52)*	1995
ACTH receptor mutations	0/16 tumors	Light et al. *(53)*	1995
ACTH receptor deletions	1/16 adenomas	Reincke et al. *(54,55)*	1996
	2/4 carcinomas		
constitutive activating	0/55 adenomas	Sachse et al. *(56)*	1997
angiotensin II	0/1 carcinomas		
type 1 receptor mutations			
G-Protein mutations (Gαs)	0/11 tumors	Lyons et al. *(49)*	1990
	0/18 tumors	Reincke et al. *(57)*	1993
G-Protein mutations (Gαi2)	3/11 tumors	Lyons et al. *(49)*	1990
	0/18 tumors	Reincke et al. *(54)*	1993
	0/18 tumors	Gicquel et al. *(58)*	1995
Calcium-dependent	Normal in 17/17 tumors	Latronico et al. *(59)*	1994
proteinkinase C activity			
Ras mutations	0/17 tumors	Moul et al. *(60)*	1993
	0/33 tumors	Ohgaki et al. *(61)*	1993
	3/24 carcinoma (N-*ras*)	Yashiro et al. *(62)*	1994
	4/32 adenomas (N-*ras*)		
Growth Factors			
IGF II overexpression	5/16 carcinomas	Giquel et al. *(12)*	1994
	2/17 adenomas		
	5/6 carcinomas	Ilvesmäki et al. *(63)*	1993
	0/15 adenomas		
Tumor Suppressor Genes			
p53 exon 4	11/15 adenomas	Lin et al. *(64)*	1994
	0/19 adenomas	Reincke et al. *(65)*	1996
p53 exon 5–8	3/15 carcinoma	Ohkagi et al. *(61)*	1993
	0/18 adenomas		
	5/13 carcinomas	Reincke et al. *(65)*	1994
	0/5 adenomas		

as a tumor suppressor gene. Allelic loss of the *ACTH* receptor gene in adrenocortical tumors can result in loss of differentiation, a characteristic feature of human tumorigenesis that is associated with clonal expansion of a malignant cell clone.

IGF II, p53, and Other Oncogenes

Using the candidate gene approach, several studies have investigated the prevalence of putative adrenal oncogenes and tumor suppressor genes (Table 2). Most of these studies showed a low prevalence of mutations. However, *IGF* II overexpression and mutations in the *p53* tumor suppressor gene have frequently be demonstrated in adrenocortical carcinomas.

IGF II

IGF II overexpression is frequent in adrenocortical tumors [see, for review, *(48)*], particularly in adrenocortical carcinomas (84%) compared to adenomas (6%) strongly suggesting a determinant role for this factor in tumor progression and/or acquisition of the malignant phenotype. *IGF* II overexpression has been demonstrated at the mRNA and at the protein level, and both receptors for *IGF* I and *IGF* II are present in adrenocortical tumors *(52,67)*. Thus, all components of the machinary required for auto- and paracrine action of IGFs are present in adrenocortical tumors. Structural abnormalities of the *IGF* II gene locus at chromosome 11p15 is frequently demonstrable in adrenal carcinomas *(12)*. The *IGF* II gene is maternally imprinted with the sole expression of the paternal allele. Nearly 80% of all carcinomas show loss of constitutive heterozygosity of the 11p15 region, probably by paternal isodisomy. However, the genetic events causing *IGF* II hypersecretion appear to be heterogeneous and complex, involving additional mechanisms like loss of maternal imprinting of the *IGF* II gene and changes in the putative *IGF* II repressor H19 *(48)*.

p53 Tumor Suppressor Gene

Mutations in the *p53* tumor suppressor gene are the most common genetic alterations in humans identified to date *(5,68)*. The *p53* gene functions as a tumor suppressor gene and more specific as a cell-cycle regulator. Inactivation of *p53* by point mutations and/ or deletions results in loss of tumor suppressor function. *p53* mutations are rarely observed in benign tumors, are generally a late event in tumorigenesis, and are associated with a malignant phenotype *(69–71)*. More than 90% of *p53* mutations found in human tumors are located within exon 5 to 8 *(71)*. These exons contain four highly conserved domains essential for a normal function of the protein. Mutations outside of these areas are scattered throughout the remaining exons, and their pathophysiological significance has been a matter of some debate *(71)*. Several lines of evidence suggest that mutant *p53* is involved in adrenal tumorigenesis. First, allelic loss of the chromosomal locus of the *p53* gene, 17p, has been demonstrated by Yano et al. in adrenal carcinomas, but not in adenomas *(37)*. Second, the aforementioned Li–Fraumeni syndrome, which is caused by germ-line *p53* mutations is associated with development of adrenocortical carcinomas *(3,4)*. Third, we and others recently identified *p53* mutations in approx 30% of sporadic adrenal carcinomas *(60,66)*.

Recently, Lin et al. in a study from Taiwan reported a new mutational hot spot within exon 4 in benign adrenal tumors, with 9 of 15 (60%) adenomas having evidence for *p53* mutations by SSCP *(64)*. Sequencing confirmed the presence of point mutations at codon 100, 102, or 104, within exon 4. We reexamined the prevalence of *p53* mutations in exon 4 and could not find any mutation in a series of 27 tumors from Europe and the United States *(65)*. This casts considerable doubt on the significance of the finding of Lin et al., which are, most likely, explained by geographic differences or technical factors.

In summary, recent progress in the understanding of adrenal tumorigenesis shows that the genetic events associated with adrenocortical carcinoma involve loss of heterozygosity at chromosome 11p, 13q, and 17p, and amplification of chromosomal areas 5, 7, 9, 12, 16, 22. *IGF*-II hypersecretion is often present in adrenal cancer, whereas *p53* mutations and ACTH receptor deletions seem to be a late event in cancer formation associated with a malignant phenotype (Fig. 2). The majority of adrenal adenomas is monoclonal in cell composition, however, the genetic events involved in clonal expansion and hormone excess remain to be elucidated.

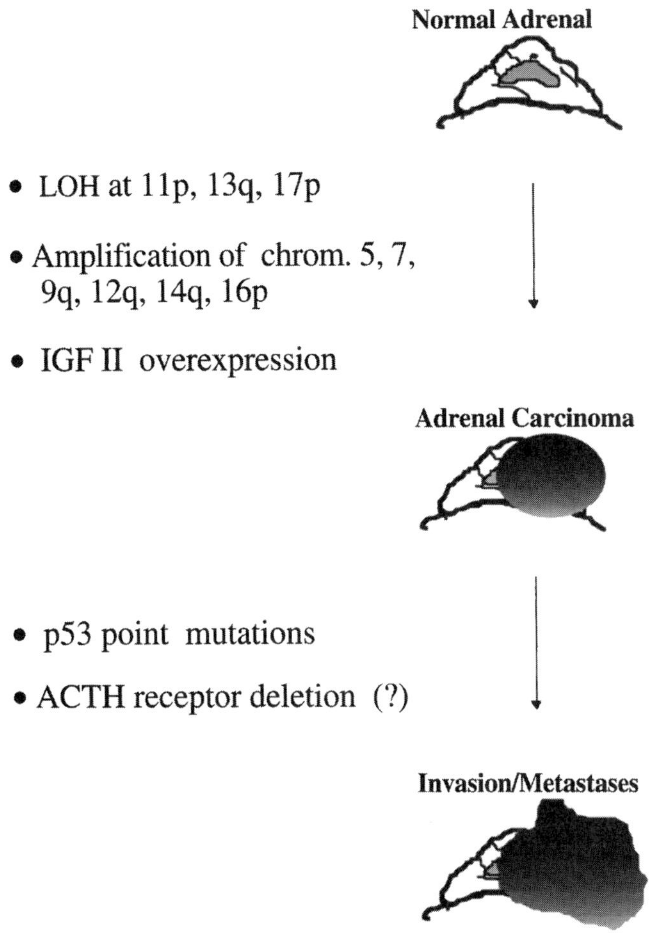

Normal Adrenal

- LOH at 11p, 13q, 17p

- Amplification of chrom. 5, 7, 9q, 12q, 14q, 16p

- IGF II overexpression

Adrenal Carcinoma

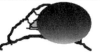

- p53 point mutations

- ACTH receptor deletion (?)

Invasion/Metastases

Fig. 2. A model of adrenal carcinogenesis. For details, see text.

REFERENCES

1. Lipset MB, Hertz R, Ross GT. Clilnical and pathophysiologic aspects of adrenocortical carcinoma. Am J Med 1963; 35:374.
2. Søreide JA, Braband K, Thoresen SØ. Adrenal cortical carcinoma in Norway, 1970–1984. World J Surg 1992; 16:663–668.
3. Reincke M, Allolio B. Das nebennierneninzidentalom: die kunst der beschänkung in diagnostik und therapie. Dtsch Ärzteblatt [A] 1995; 92:764–770.
4. Copeland PM. The incidentally discovered adrenal mass. Ann Int Med 1983; 98:940–945.
5. Li FP, Frauemeni JF. Soft-tissue sarcomas, breast cancer, and other neoplasms: a familial syndrome? Ann Int Med 1969; 71:747–752.
6. Malkin D, Jolly KW, Barbier N, Look AT, Friend SH, Gebhardt MC, et al. Germline mutations of the p53 tumor suppressor gene in children and young adults with second malignant neoplasms. N Engl J Med 1992; 326:1309–1315.
7. Srivastava S, Zou Z, Pirollo K, Blattner W, Chang EH. Germ-line transmission of a mutated p53 gene in a cancer-prone family with Li-Fraumeni syndrome. Nature 1990; 348:747–749.
8. Malkin D, Li FP, Strong LC, et al. Germ line p53 mutations in a familial syndrome of breast cancer, sarcomas, and other neoplasms. Science 1990; 250:1233–1238.

9. Hollstein M, Sidransky D, Vogelstein B, Harris CC. p53 mutations in human cancers. Science 1991; 253:49–54.

10. Grayson GH, Moore S, Schneider BG, Saldivar V, Hensel CH. Novel germline mutation of the p53 tumor suppressor gene in a child with incidentally discovered adrenal cortical carcinoma. Am J Pediatr Hematol Oncol 1994; 16:341–347.

11. Wagner J, Portwine C, Rabin K, Leclerc JM, Narod SA, Malkin D. High frequency of germline p53 mutations in childhood adrenocortical cancer. J Natl Cancer Inst 1994; 86:1707–1710.

12. Wiedemann HR. Complex malformatif familial avec hernie ombilicale et macroglossie-un syndrome nouveau? J Genet Hum 1964; 13:223–232.

13. Beckwith JB. Macroglossia, omphalocoele, adrenal cytomegaly, gigantism and hyperplastic viscerome-galie. Birth Defects 1969; 5:188–196.

14. Koufos A, Grundy P, Morgan K, Aleck KA, Hadreos T, Lampkin BC, et al. Familial Wiedemann-Beckwith syndrome and a second Wilms tumor locus both map to 11p15.5. Am J Genet 1989; 44:711–719.

15. Henry I, Bonaiti-Pellie C, Chehensse V, Beldjord C, Schwartz C, Utermann G, et al. Uniparental paternal disomy in a genetic cancer-predisposing syndrome. Nature 191; 351:667–670.

16. Gicquel C, Xavier B, Schneid H, Francillard-Leblond M, Luton J-P, Girard F, et al. Rearrangement at the 11p15 locus and overexpression of IGF-II gene in sporadic adrenocortical tumors. J Clin Endocrinol Metab 1994; 78:1444–1453.

17. Larson C, Scogseid B, Öberg K, Nakamura Y, Nordenskjöld M. MEN type 1 gene maps to chromosome 11 and is lost in insulinoma. Nature 1988; 332:85–87.

18. Skogseid B, Larsson C, Lindgren P-G, Kvanta E, Rastad J, Theodorsson E, et al. Clinical and genetic features of adrenocortical lesions in MEN type 1. J Clin Endocrinol Metab 1992; 75:76–81.

19. Sutherland DJ, Ruse LJ, Laidlaw JC. Hypertension, increased aldosterone secretion and low plasma renin activity relieved by dexamethasone. Canad Med Assoc J 1966; 95:1109–1119.

20. Lifton RP, Dluhy RG, Powers M, Rich GM, Cook S, Ulick S, et al. A chimeric 11β-hydroxylase/aldosterone synthase gene causes glucocorticoid-remidiable aldosteronism and human hypertension. Nature 1992; 355:262–265.

21. Stowasser M, Gordon RD, Tunny TJ, Klemm SA, Finn WL, Krek AL. Familial hyperaldosteronism type II: Five families with a new variety of primary aldosteronism. Clin Experim Pharmacol Physiol 1992; 19:319–322.

22. Schteingart DE, Tsao HS. Coexistence of pituitary ACTH-dependent Cushing's syndrome with a solitary adrenal adenoma. J Clin Endocrinol Metab 1980; 50:961–966.

23. Hermus AR, Pieters GF, Smals AG, Pesman GJ, Lamberts SW, Benraad TJ, et al. Transition from pituitary-dependent to adrenal-dependent Cushing's syndrome. N Engl J Med 1988; 318:966–970.

24. Jaresch S, Schlaghecke R, Jungblut R, Krüskemper HL, Kley HK. Stumme Nebennierentumoren bei Patienten mit adrenogenitalem Syndrom Klin Wochenschr 1987; 65:627–633.

25. Jaresch S, Kornley E, Kley HK, Schlaghecke R. Adrenal incidentaloma and patients with homozygous and heterozygous congenital adrenal hyperplasia. J Clin Endocrinol Metab 1992; 74:658–669.

26. Hamwi GJ, Serbin RA, Kruger FA. Does adrenocortical hyperplasia result in adrenocortical carcinoma? N Engl J Med 1957; 257:1153–1155.

27. Daeschner GL. Adrenocortical adenoma arising in a girl with congenital adrenocortical syndrome. Pediatrics 1965; 36:141–144.

28. Van Seters AP, van Aalderen W, Moolenaar AJ, Gorsiro MCB, van Roon F, Backer ET. Adrenocortical tumor in untreated congenital adrenocortical hyperplasia associated with inadequate ACTH suppress-ibility. Clin Endocrinol 1981; 14:325–329.

29. Pang S, Becker D, Crotelingam J, Foley TP, Drah AL. Adrenocortical tumor in a patient with congenital adrenal hyperplasia due to 21-hydroxylase deficiency. Pediatrics 1981; 68:242–244.

30. Baumann A, Baumann CG. Virilizing adrenocortical carcinoma: development in a patient with salt-loosing congenital adrenal hyperplasia. JAMA 1982; 248:3140–3142.

31. Shinohara N, Sakashita S, Terasawe K, Nakanishi S, Koyanagi T. Adrenocortical adenoma associated with congenital adrenal hyperplasia. Jap J Urol 1986; 77:1519–152.

32. Takayama K, Ohashi M, Haji M, Matsumoto T, Mihara Y, Kumazawa J, et al. Adrenocortical tumor in a patient with untreated congenital adrenal hyperplasia owing to 21-hydroxylase deficiency: characterization of the steroidogenic lesion. J Urol 1988; 140:803–805.

33. Jaursch-Hancke C, Allolio B, Metzler U, Bidlingmaier F, Winkelmann W. Adrenocortical carcinoma in a patient with untreated congenital adrenal hyperplasia. Acta Endocrinol 1988; 117 (Suppl): 146–147.

34. Sunaga Y, Nishikawa M, Inaba K, Hirozane N. 21-hydroxylase deficiency associated with adrenal tumor: Case report of 2 brothers. Nippon Naibunpi. Gakkai. Zasshi. 1989; 65:525–536.
35. Touitou Y, Lecomte P, Auzeby A, Bogdan A, Besnier Y. Evidence of 11β-hydroxylase deficiency in a patient with cortical adrenal adenoma. Horm Metab Res 1989; 21:272–274.
36. Shimshi M, Ross F, Goodman A, Gabrilove JL. Virilizing adrenocortical tumor superimposed on congenital adrenocortical hyperplasia. Am J Med 1992; 93:338–342.
37. Yano T, Linehan M, Anglard P, Lerman MI, Daniel LN, Stein CA, et al. Genetic changes in human adrenocortical carcinoma. J Natl Cancer Inst 1989; 81:518–523.
38. Limon J, Dal Cin P, Gaeat J, Sandberg A. Translocation t(4;11)(q35;13) in an adrenocortical carcinoma. Cancer Genet Cytogenet 1987; 28:343–348.
39. Herrmann M, Rydstedt L, Talpos G, Ratner S, Wollman S, Lalley P. Chromosomal aberrations in two adrenocortical tumors, one with rearrangement at 11p15. Cancer Genet Cytogenet 1994; 75:111–116.
40. Gordon RD, Stowasser M, Martin N, Epping A, Conic S, Klemm SA, et al. Karyotypic abnormalities in benign adrenocortical tumors producing aldosterone. Cancer Genet Cytogenet 1993; 68:78–81.
41. Rosenberg C, Della-Rosa VA, Latronico AC, Mendoca BB, Vianna-Morgante AM. Selection of adrenal tumor cells in culture demonstrated by interphase cytogenetics. Cancer Genet Cytogenet 1994; 79:36–40.
42. Kjellman M, Kallioniemi OP, Karhu R, Höög A, Farnebo LO, Auer G, et al. Genetic abberations in adrenocortical tumors detected using comparative genomic hybridization correlate with tumor size and malignancy. Cancer Res 1996; 56:4219–4223.
43. Dohna M, Reincke M, Mincheva A, Allolio B, Solinas-Toldo S, Lichter P. Adrenocortical carcinoma is characterized by a high frequency of chromosomal gains and high-level amplifications. Genes Chromosomes Cancer. 2000; 28:145–152.
44. Fialkow PJ. Clonal origin of human tumors. Biochim Biophys Acta 1976; 458:283–321.
45. Knudson AG. Mutation and human cancer. Adv Cancer Res 1993; 17:317–352.
46. Gicquel C, Leblond-Francillard M, Bertagna X, Louvel A, Chapuls Y, Luton J-P, et al. Clonal analysis of human adrenocortical carcinomas and secreting adenomas. Clin Endocrinol 1994; 40:465–477.
47. Beuschlein F, Reincke M, Karl M, Travis W, Jaursch-Hancke C, Abdelhamid S, et al. Clonal composition of human adrenocortical neoplasms. Cancer Res 1994; 54:4927–4932.
48. Gicquel C, Bertagna B, Le Bouc Y. Recent advances in the pathogenesis of adrenocortical tumors. Eur J Endocrinol 1995; 133:133–144.
49. Lyons J, Landis CA, Harsh G, Vallar L, Grünewald K, Feichtinger H, et al. Two G protein oncogenes in human endocrine tumors. Science 1990; 249:655–659.
50. Parma J, Duprez L, Van Sande J, Cochaux P, Gervy C, Mockel J, et al. Somatic mutations in the thyrotropin receptor gene cause hyperfunctioning thyroid adenomas. Nature 1993; 365:649–651.
51. Estivariz FE, Iturriza F, Mclean C, Hope J, Lowry PJ. Stimulation of adrenal mitogenesis by N-terminal proopiomelanocortin. Nature 1982; 297:419–422.
52. Latronico AC, Reincke M, Mendonca BB, et al. No evidence for oncogenic mutations in the adrenocorticotropin receptor gene in human adrenocortical neoplasms. J Clin Endocrinol Metab 1995; 80:875–877.
53. Light K, Jenkins PJ, Weber A, Perrett C, Grossman A, Pistorello M, et al. Are activating mutations of the ACTH receptor involved in adrenal cortical neoplasia? Life Sci 1995; 56:1523–1527.
54. Reincke M, Mora P, Beuschlein F, Arlt W, Lehmann R, Allolio B. Allelic loss of the ACTH receptor gene in undifferentiated adrenocortical tumors. Exp Clin Endocrinol 1996; 104 (Suppl 1): 40.
55. Reincke M, Mora P, Beuschlein F, Arlt W, Chrousos GP, Allolio B. Deletion of the ACTH receptor gene in adrenocortical tumors: Implication for tumorigenesis. J Clin Endocrinol Metab 1996; submitted.
56. Sachse R, Shao X-J, Rico A, Finckh U, Rolfs A, Reincke M, et al. Absence of angiotensin II type 1 receptor gene mutations in human adrenal tumors. Eur J Endocrinol 1997; submitted.
57. Reincke M, Karl M, Travis W, Chrousos GP. No evidence for oncogenic mutations in guanine nucleotide binding proteins of human adrenocortical neoplasms. J Clin Endocrinol Metab 1993; 77:1419–1422.
58. Gicquel C, Dib A, Bertagna X, Amselem S, Le Bouc Y. Oncogenic mutations of alpha-Gi2 are not determinant for human adrenocortical tumorigenesis. Eur J Endocrinol 1995; 133:166–172.
59. Latronico AC, Mendonca BB, Bianco AC, Villares SM, Lucon MA, Nicolau W, et al. Calcium-dependent protein kinase-C activity in human adrenocortical neoplasms, hyperplastic adrenals, and normal adrenal tissue. J Clin Endocrinol Metab 1994; 79:736–739.
60. Moul JW, Bishoff JT, Theune SM, Chang EH. Absent ras gene mutations in human adrenal cortical neoplasms and pheochromocytomas. J Urol 1993; 149:1389–1394.

61. Ohgaki H, Kleihues P, Heitz PU. p53 mutations in sporadic adenocortical tumors. Int J Cancer 1993; 54:408–410.
62. Yashiro T, Hara H, Obara T, Kaplan EL. Point mutation of ras in human adrenal cortical tumor: absence in adrenocortical hyperplasia. World J Surg 1994; 18:455–460.
63. Ilvesmäki V, Kahri AI, Miettinen PJ, Voutilainen R. Insulin-like growth factors and their receptors in adrenal tumors: High IGF II expression in functional adrenocortical carcinomas. J Clin Endocrinol Metab 1993; 77:852.
64. Lin SR, Lee YJ, Tsai HJ. Mutations of the p53 gene in human functional neoplasms. J Clin Endocrinol Metab 1994; 78:483–491.
65. Reincke M, Wachenfeld C, Mora P, Thumser A, Jaursch-Hancke C, Abdelhamid S, et al. p53 mutations in adrenal tumors: Caucasian patients do not show the exon 4 "hot spot" found in Taiwan. J Clin Endocrinol Metab 1996; 81:3636–3638.
66. Reincke M, Karl M, Travis WH, Mastorakos G, Allolio B, Linehan HM. p53 mutations in human adrenocortical neoplasms: Immunohistochemical and molecular studies. J Clin Endocrinol Metab 1994; 78:790–794.
67. Kamio T, Shigematsu K, Kawai K, Tsuchiyama H. Immunoreactivity and receptor expression of IGF-I and insulin in human adrenal tumors. Am J Pathol 1991; 138:83–91.
68. Levine AJ, Momand J, Finlay CA. The p53 tumour suppressor gene. Nature 1991; 351:453–456.
69. Esrig D, Elmajian D, Cote RJ. Accumulation of nuclear p53 and tumor progression in bladder cancer. N Engl J Med 1994; 331:1259–1264.
70. Baker SJ, Preisinger AC, Jessup JM, Paraskeva C, Markowitz S, Willson JVK, et al. p53 gene mutations occur in combination with 17p allelic deletions as late events in colorectal tumorigenesis. Cancer Res 1990; 50:7717–7722.
71. Caron de Fromentel C, Soussi T. tp53 tumor suppressor gene: A model for investigating human mutagenesis. Genes Chrom Cancer 1992; 4:1–15.
72. Hartmann A, Blaszyk H, Sommer SS. p53 gene mutations inside and outside of exons 5–8: The patterns differ in breast and other cancers. Oncogene 1995; 10:681–688.
73. Yoshimoto K, Iwahana H, Fukuda A, Sano T, Saito S, Itakura M. Role of p53 in endocrine tumorigenesis: Mutation detection by polymerase chain reaction-single strand conformation polymorphism. Cancer Res 1992; 52:5061–5064.

17 Management of Adrenal Cancer

David E. Schteingart, MD
and Dominic Homan, MD

CONTENTS

INTRODUCTION

Primary adrenal cortical carcinoma is a rare but highly malignant tumor with generally poor prognosis. Life expectancy of afflicted patients depends on early diagnosis and treatment. An early diagnosis of functioning adrenocortical carcinomas depends on the physician's ability to recognize the clinical manifestations of excessive steroid-hormone production by the tumor. A definition of the biochemical abnormality present can be obtained with specific measurements of cortisol, aldosterone, androgen, or estrogen levels. Computerized tomography (T) or magnetic resonance imaging (MRI) helps to localize the tumor and define the presence or absence of local or distant metastases. For nonfunctioning tumors, their detection is frequently incidental to the investigation of nonspecific abdominal complaints. Attempts have been made to determine if an adrenal tumor is benign or malignant. Adrenal scintigraphy with ^{131}I-6-β-iodomethyl-19-norcholesterol (NP-59) showing uptake in most benign tumors and lack of uptake in most malignant tumors can be helpful. However, it is important to recognize that a few cases with positive imaging may still be malignant. Surgical resection of the

From: *Contemporary Endocrinology: Adrenal Disorders*
Edited by: A. N. Margioris and G. P. Chrousos © Humana Press, Totowa, NJ

primary tumor and recurrences, as well as hepatic or pulmonary metastases, may help increase life expectancy. Other methods of treatment including radiation therapy and chemotherapy have been less effective. Mitotane appears effective in extending survival of patients with adrenal carcinoma, particularly when administered as early as adjuvant therapy or when combined with repeated debulking resection of recurrent tumor. The toxicity associated with mitotane administration limits the use of larger and probably more effective doses in these patients. The synthesis of analogs with more limited toxicity may ultimately provide more effective tools in the pharmacologic management of this tumor.

INCIDENCE AND AGE OF PRESENTATION

Adrenocortical carcinomas are rare, highly malignant tumors that account for only 0.2% of deaths caused by cancer. Their incidence has been estimated at two per million population per year. Occasionally, children have been found to have adrenocortical carcinomas, but most cases occur between age 30–50 (1). Whereas the etiology of adrenal cancer remains unknown, some cases have been described in families with a hereditary cancer syndrome in whom mutations in tumor suppressor genes is an important factor in adrenal tumorigenesis. One such syndrome is the Li–Fraumeni, characterized by sarcoma, breast cancer, brain tumor, lung cancer, laryngeal carcinoma, leukemia, and adenocortical carcinoma. In these cases, the deleterious genotype has been expressed through several generations and found both in children and adults (2,3).

Several theories have been put forth to explain tumorigenesis in adrenal cortical carcinoma. They include development of chromosomal alterations leading to disregulation of a gene product or chronic stimulation of the gland. There are data supporting the presence of changes in the *p53* tumor suppressor gene located on chromosome 17p and its 53-kD protein. A germline mutation of the *p53* gene was found in a patient with an incidentally found adrenal cortical carcinoma (4). This mutation resulted in a premature stop codone. However, mutations at the *p53* loci have also been found in adrenal adenomas and pheochromocytomas (5). Others have shown allelic loss at the *p53* gene locus on chromosome 17p (6,7). In a study of 11 adrenal cortical carcinomas, 5 showed positive immunohistochemical staining for the *p53* protein (8), but 3 of these only had a small percentage of cells staining positive. In 2 of the 11 carcinomas, point mutations were shown in the *p53* gene in exons 5–8. These mutations resulted in a single amino acid change, presumably resulting in a protein with an altered half-life. There was also a deletion rearrangement in one adrenal cortical carcinoma. Another study (9) reported positive immunostaining for the *p53* gene product in 22 of the 42 cases of adrenal cortical carcinoma. However, they were unable to show that the *p53* status had any effect on long-term survival.

Changes in the *RB* gene have also been reported, but the nature of the changes in this gene and its regulation has not been completely worked out. As with the *p53* gene, allelic loss at the *RB* gene locus on chromosome 13q has been described in adrenal-cortical carcinoma (6). Other genetic markers examined included the *H19*, the insulin-like growth factor 2 (IGF-2), and the *p57^{kip2}* genes. These genes have been mapped to chromosome 11p15.5 (10) and appear to be important for fetal growth and development. The levels of *H19* and IGF-2 gene expression are very high in human fetal adrenal glands (11), but they subsequently decrease by 50% in adults. The gene product for

$p57^{kip2}$ is a member of the p21CIP1 cyclin-dependent kinase family and appear to regulate self-proliferation, exit from the cell cycle, and maintenance of differentiated cells. This gene product is usually found to be high in most normal human tissues. H19 and $p57^{kip2}$ gene expression is adrenocorticotropic hormone (ACTH)-dependent and regulation of the $p57^{kip2}$ gene appears to be related to cyclic adenosine monophosphate (cAMP)-dependent protein kinase pathway *(10)*. *H19* gene expression is markedly reduced in adrenal-cortical carcinomas, both nonfunctioning and functioning, especially in tumors producing cortisol and aldosterone *(10)*. There is also a loss of activity of the $p57^{kip2}$ gene product in virilizing adenomas and adrenal-cortical carcinomas *(10)*, suggesting that this gene product plays a role in the normal maintenance of adrenal cortical differentiation and function. In contrast, IGF-2 gene expression has been shown to be high in adrenal-cortical carcinomas.

Finally, the c-*myc* gene has also been evaluated for possible tumorigenesis. C-*myc* gene expression is relatively high in neoplasms and is often linked to poor prognosis. However, in adrenal-cortical carcinomas, the expression of c-*myc* is approx 10% of that found in normal adrenal tissues *(12)*. The c-*myc* gene is generally expressed in normal adrenal glands and is usually localized to the *zona fasiculata* and *zona reticularis*. The significance of a low c-*myc* gene expression in adrenal cortical carcinomas needs to be elucidated.

CLINICAL AND BIOCHEMICAL EVALUATION

Approx 50% of adrenal-cortical carcinomas are functioning and produce hormonal and metabolic syndromes leading to their discovery. The other 50% are silent and are only discovered when they attain large size and produce localized abdominal symptoms or metastases.

Cushing's syndrome is the most common clinical presentation in adult patients. Characteristically, these patients describe rapid development (3–6 mo) of the clinical manifestations of cortisol excess, including weight gain, muscle weakness, easy bruising, irritability, and insomnia. In addition, there are commonly manifestations of androgen excess, including hirsutism, acne, and irregular menses or amenorrhea in women. The androgen excess may decrease the severity of the catabolic effect of hypercortisolemia such that skin and muscle atrophy may not be as readily apparent as in those with benign tumors. Patients with metastatic disease have anorexia and weight loss, rather than weight gain. Adrenocortical carcinomas causing Cushing's syndrome are large with an average weight of 800 gm, but the clinical manifestations of hormone excess lead to earlier diagnosis and the finding of smaller tumors.

In patients with clinical manifestations of Cushing's syndrome, studies should include: measurement of urinary-free cortisol, serum cortisol, and DHEA-S at baseline and during dexamethasone suppression. Patients with cortisol secreting adrenocortical carcinomas demonstrate elevated baseline cortisol and DHEA-S levels and failure to suppress with a high (8 mg) dose of dexamethasone. ACTH levels are usually suppressed.

In patients with Cushing's syndrome secondary to adrenocortical carcinomas, the tumor may produce a mixture of steroid hormones, including cortisol and androgens. Whereas virilization frequently accompanies Cushing's syndrome, the main clinical manifestations occasionally are those of androgen excess with only subtle evidence of hypercortisolism. The steroid profile in serum or urine can sometimes help distinguish between benign and malignant adrenocortical tumors because of the presence of interme-diary precursors in the steroid biosynthetic pathway of their metabolites in patients with malignant neoplasms.

Sex hormone-producing carcinomas lead to virilization in women and manifestations of feminization in men. Women with virilizing adrenocortical carcinomas present with marked androgen-type hirsutism, male-pattern baldness, deepening voice, breast atro-phy, clitoral hypertrophy, decreased libido, and oligo or amenorrhea. Manifestations of androgen excess are less noticeable in men. In prepubertal boys, androgen excess causes precocious puberty without concomitant testicular enlargement. Feminizing tumors in women cause breast tenderness and dysfunctional uterine bleeding. Estrogen-secreting tumors in men are associated with gynecomastia, breast tenderness, testicular atrophy, and decreased libido. In prepubertal girls, feminizing tumors cause early breast and uterine development and onset of menarche.

Patients with virilizing tumors demonstrate elevated serum levels of testosterone, androstenedione, and DHEA-S, whereas patients with feminizing tumors have high serum estradiol levels. The level of these hormones is usually very high with total testosterone levels in women greater than 2.0 ng/ml (normal 0.3–0.6 ng/mL).

Aldosterone-producing adrenocortical carcinomas are extremely rare. They present with clinical manifestations of primary aldosteronism with hypertension and hypoka-lemia. Compared to patients with benign aldosterone-secreting adenomas, those with carcinoma have larger tumors, higher aldosterone levels, and more severe hypokalemia (13,14). Evaluation should include measurement of serum electrolytes, aldosterone, and plasma renin levels. The usual findings are severe hypokalemia with potassium levels below 2.5 mEq/L, hypernatremia, and metabolic alkalosis. Serum aldosterone levels are high, although plasma renin levels are suppressed.

A hormonal profile should also be obtained in patients with apparently nonfunctioning adrenal tumors. Some of these tumors produce biosynthetic steroid pathway intermedi-ates, such as progesterone and 11-deoxycortisol (15). It is important to determine the level of these steroids in patients with adrenocortical cancer prior to surgery because these hormones can be used as biochemical markers in the postoperative follow-up.

Silent adrenal cortical carcinomas do not present recognizable symptoms of excessive hormone production and are detected because of local symptoms. Some of these tumors, however, may be detected incidentally in the course of investigation of unrelated abdominal complaints. Incidentally discovered adrenal masses are found in 1–3% of computerized tomographic scanning (CT) of the abdomen. However, most of these masses are benign and adrenal cortical adenomas are 60 times more common than primary carcinomas (16). When adrenal masses are malignant, they are usually meta-static from extra adrenal neoplasms. In evaluating an incidentally found adrenal mass, size is an important consideration in determining if the mass is benign or malignant. Masses less than 3 cm are considered to be benign (17), whereas the probability that the mass is malignant is greatly increased when they measure >6 cm. Controversy remains on the probability that a mass measuring 3–6 cm is benign or malignant. Adrenal cortical carcinomas larger than 6 cm would have been small early in their development, and given the fact that early resection of these tumors offer the best chance for cure or long survival, recognizing and surgically resecting them is very important. The following case illustrates a circumstance in which an incidentally discov-ered small adrenal mass turned out to be malignant: A 45 yr-old woman was seen by a gastroenterologist 3 yr earlier for evaluation of a $2 \times 2 \times 7$-cm hemangioma in the right hepatic lobe found on CT. A 3-cm left adrenal mass was also found, but because of the small size, attention focused on the hepatic finding and the adrenal mass was not investigated further. She developed hirsutism, irregular menses, and obesity 3 yr later, and her serum testosterone and DHEA-S and urinary-free cortisol levels were high. A new CT scan showed the 3-cm lesion had grown to 7 cm with imaging characteristics of an adrenal cortical carcinoma. This diagnosis was confirmed histologically. The patient developed wide-spread metastases and died 2 yr later.

RADIOGRAPHIC DETECTION OF ADRENAL MASSES—EVALUATION OF WHETHER THEY ARE BENIGN OR MALIGNANT

A variety of imaging procedures can be used to localize and determine the possible benign or malignant character of an adrenal cortical mass.

1. *Computerized Axial Tomography (CT):* Malignant adrenal masses are usually larger than 5 cm and have an inhomogeneous pattern because of areas of necrosis within the tumor. The CT procedure will help determine the presence of involved lymph nodes and hepatic or pulmonary metastases. A definition of metastatic involvement is important in determining the treatment goals for a given patient. The tumors are frequently invasive of the upper pole of the adjoining kidney and of the inferior vena cavae. Unenhanced and 1-hr-enhanced CT have also been used to distinguish benign from malignant adrenal masses *(18,19)*. The distinction is based on the lipid content of the mass. Lipid-rich masses are usually benign, whereas lipid-poor masses are frequently malignant. Enhancement is measured in Hounsfield units (HU). Low-attenuation lesions have low HU values. Using unenhanced CT, it was shown that adenomas have values of less than +10 HU, whereas nonadenomas have values greater than +18 HU. Using these criteria, this method gives a sensitivity for distinguishing adenomas from nonadenomas of 73%, and a specificity of 96%. CT images obtained 1 hr after the injection of contrast show an enhancement of 11 ± 13 HU (<30) for adenomas and values of 49 ± 8.3 HU (>30) for nonadenomas with a sensitivity for distinguishing adenomas from malignant masses of 95%, and a specificity of 100%.
2. *Ultrasonography:* Malignant lesions vary in echo texture and are heterogeneous in appearance with focal or scattered echopenic or echogenic zones representing areas of tumor necrosis, hemorrhage and/or, calcification *(18,20)*.
3. *Magnetic Resonance Imaging (MRI):* Tumors appear as hypointense masses compared to the liver on T-1 weighted images and hyperintense compared to liver on T-2 weighted images. The MRI also demonstrates displacement or invasion of adjacent organs, as well as liver metastases. Superior blood vessel identification and the multiplanar capabilities of MRI may make it the imaging modality of choice in evaluating the extent of disease and in planning surgical excision *(21)*. The distinction between benign and malignant masses based on the presence of lipid can also be determined by chemical shift MRI. Lipid-rich adenomas show a 34% change in relative signaling intensity between in-phase and out-of-phase imaging, whereas nonadenomas do not change. This technique gives a specificity of 100%, and a sensitivity of 81% in distinguishing between these two types of lesions *(22)*.
4. *[131]I-6β-iodomethylnorcholesterol Scintigraphy:* Most adrenocortical carcinomas fail to image with this radionuclide. Because cortisol production suppresses ACTH secretion and the function of the contralateral adrenal gland, patients with cortisol-producing adrenocortical carcinomas fail to show an image either at the site of the tumor or the

contralateral gland. On the other hand, aldosterone-, androgen-, or estrogen-secreting tumors usually appear as an area of decreased uptake on the side of the tumor mass. The decreased or absent tracer uptake by adrenocortical carcinomas are in contrast with the increased concentration of radionuclide by benign tumors *(14)*. This distinction is not absolute. Patients with adrenocortical carcinoma may occasionally give positive nuclear scans. Based on these imaging characteristics, CT and iodocholesterol scintigraphy can be used together in the diagnosis of small (less than 4 cm) euadrenal masses. A study of 119 patients *(23)* found that concordant images (CT image and increased uptake on the same side) were 100% benign, whereas discordant images (a CT tumor image on one side and increased uptake on the contralateral side) were malignant in 73% of the cases.

CLINICAL ASSESSMENT OF EXTENT OF DISEASE

Adrenocortical carcinoma can be staged based on the size of the primary and extent of regional or distant tumor involvement according to the MacFarlane classification *(24)* as modified by Sullivan (Table 1) *(25)*. The sites of tumor spread in stage IV are summarized in Table 2. The most frequent sites for metastases are lung, liver, lymphnodes, and bone. The stage at which an adrenal cortical carcinoma is defined determines prognosis *(26,27)*. Whereas 50% of patients in stages I, II, and III are alive 40 mo after diagnosis, only 10% of patients in stage IV are alive at that time.

MANAGEMENT OF ADRENAL CORTICAL CARCINOMA

Therapeutic interventions used to treat patients with adrenal cancer include surgery, radiation therapy, nonspecific systemic chemotherapy, and mitotane *(28)*.

Surgical resection, even if incomplete, should be considered the initial step in therapy. Because most adrenal carcinomas are large, the surgical approach should be either transabdominal or thoracoabdominal with an incision of sufficient length to allow adequate exploration and resection of contiguous organs if necessary to remove gross tumor. The surgical goal should be the resection of the entire tumor mass when possible. Even if this is not possible because of local extension into other structures, tumor debulking should be carried out to the maximum degree possible. It is frequently necessary to remove the adjoining kidney in block with the tumor because of invasion by the tumor of the upper pole. In cases of liver metastases, a partial lobectomy with resection of the involved portion of the liver has led to long-term remission *(29)*. These aggressive efforts to excise all gross tumor are justified because adjuvant chemotherapy with mitotane appears to be most effective with minimal tumor burden.

Another approach to treatment is radiation therapy and nonspecific chemotherapy. Adrenocortical carcinomas have been reported as being resistant to radiation therapy that only causes transient reduction of local disease *(30)*. However, these earlier reports were based on techniques and equipment much less powerful than currently available, and it is possible that better responses could be obtained with newer methodology.

Nonspecific chemotherapy has caused only temporary improvement. Chemotherapeutic agents used in the treatment of metastatic adrenal carcinoma include: adriamycin cisplatin, etoposide, taxol, 5FU, oncovin, cyclosclophosphamide, and suramin. Although the consensus from several series is that systemic chemotherapy is not very effective at this stage of the disease, there are great difficulties in interpreting the response to therapy for the following reasons: (1) Series reported usually involves small number

Table 1
MacFarlane Classification of Adrenal-Cortical Carcinoma
Based on Size and Extent of Disease

Stage	Size	Lymphadenopathy	Local Invasion	Metastases
I	<5 cm	—	—	—
II	>5 cm	—	—	—
III	Any Size	+	+	—
IV	Any Size	+	+	+

Table 2
Sites of Spread in Stage 4 Adrenocortical Tumors *(1)*

Organ	Percent (N-33)
Lung	45
Liver	42
Lymph nodes	24
Bone	15
Pancreas	12
Spleen	6
Diaphragm	12
Miscellaneous (Brain, peritoneum skin, palate)	12

of patients; (2) There is great variability of treatment between series and within series; (3) The extent of the disease at which people are treated has been variable and not always well-defined; (4) There is also variable degrees of malignancy and series that include patients with low-grade malignancy, as well as patients with high-grade malignancy; (5) There is lack of uniformed definition of response; (6) The duration of response is not always stated clearly; (7) Patients within a series frequently receive multiple treatments in variable sequence so that treatments are difficult to compare; and (8) Radiation therapy is sometimes combined with chemotherapy.

Mitotane has been used consistently in the treatment of patients with metastatic adrenal cortical carcinoma, but not all agree with its efficacy *(31,32)*. In addition, it is associated with considerable toxicity when given in therapeutically effective doses. Mitotane is an adrenalytic drug with selective action on the adrenal cortex. When given to patients with pituitary ACTH-dependent adrenal-cortical hyperfunction, mitotane induces suppression of cortisol secretion and selective chemical ablation of the fasciculata and reticularis zones of the adrenal cortex. In a series of reports over the past 30 yr *(33)*, it appears that mitotane was associated with partial or complete response in 33% of patients with adrenal cancer. The timing of initiation of chemotherapy may influence patient survival. We *(34)* and others *(35)* have suggested that adjuvant mitotane therapy is associated with prolonged survival if it is given shortly after the primary tumor has been surgically excised and before local extension or additional metastases develop. However, other prospective studies in which patients have been randomly assigned to adjuvant therapy with mitotane, or without therapy have not shown a beneficial effect of mitotane on extending life expectancy *(36)*.

Suramin, a drug known to have antiparasitic effects, has been previously shown to have adrenocorticolytic effects in primates. When given to patients with adrenal carcinoma, a partial-to-minor response was observed in some patients. Suramin may have some therapeutic efficacy as a single agent in patients with metastatic adrenocortical carcinoma *(37)*. It has also been employed in combination with mitotane with better response than either drug alone.

LONG-TERM TREATMENT OUTCOME

Medical therapy for adrenocortical carcinoma is of limited effectiveness. The results of eight of the largest reported series *(38–45)* are summarized in Table 3. However, there is a significant number of patients on whom therapy can extend life expectancy without unacceptable morbidity. However, recurrence occurs even after long periods of remission. Surgical treatment in combination with medical treatment appears to be more effective than medical treatment alone, especially for patients with localized or regional disease (stages I–III).

Several series of patients receiving combined surgical-medical treatment for adrenocortical carcinoma have been evaluated: In a comparison of 18 patients treated with mitotane alone and 15 patients treated with combined surgical resection and mitotane chemotherapy, those who underwent surgical treatment had a more favorable response, with 33% of patients living more than 5 yr from the time of first recurrence *(46)*. In a study of 49 patients with adrenal carcinoma, surgical excision offered the best opportunity for prolonged survival. Forty-three percent of patients with a completely resectable tumor were alive with no evidence of disease an average of 7.3 yr postoperatively *(47)*. Comparing various types of therapy in 110 patients with adrenocortical carcinoma, it was noted that 56% of patients responded to surgery for localized and regional disease with a disease-free survival time of at least 2 yr. In contrast, abdominal radiation therapy was effective in 15%, systemic chemotherapy in 9%, and mitotane in 29% *(48)*. In a review of 82 patients, it was noted that survival in patients with metastatic disease was poor and not improved by treatment with mitotane, cytotoxic chemotherapy, or radiation therapy *(49)*. Thus, survival of patients with adrenal carcinoma with recurrent or metastatic disease is much better in patients receiving surgical treatment vs medical treatment. With surgical treatment, 50% of patients survive an average of 70 mo, whereas with medical treatment alone, less than 10% of patients are alive for this length of time. The surgical treatment involves not only resection of the primary lesion, but repeated resection of metastases.

THE USE OF INHIBITORS OF ADRENAL FUNCTION IN PATIENTS WITH FUNCTIONING ADRENAL CORTICAL CARCINOMA

In patients with residual disease who do not respond to antitumor therapy, the metabolic changes associated with excessive hormonal production can cause significant morbidity and shortened life expectancy. A variety of inhibitors of adrenal function have been used to suppress steroid hormone production and improve the clinical manifestations of the disease. The most commonly used inhibitors include ketoconazole, metyrapone, and aminoglutethimide.

Ketoconazole is an imidazole derivative that inhibits the synthesis of cortisol by inhibiting mitochondrial cytochrome *P450*-dependent enzymes, such as cholesterol side-chain cleavage and 11-β-hydroxylase in rat and mouse adrenal preparations. It

Table 3
Summary of Results of Medical Treatment of Adrenal-Cortical Carcinoma in
Eight of the Largest Series Reported

Study	Regimen	# Txd	# Resp	% Resp
Venkatesh, et al. (38)	opDDD	72	9E/12M/43N	29.2
	XRT	19	0E/3M/13N	15.8
	*Chemotherapy	31	0E/3M/24N	9.7
	XRT + op DDD	10	0E/3M/6N	30
	Chemo + op DDD	23	0E/5M/16N	21.7
	adjuvant op DDD	7	6E/1U	—
Kasperlik-Zaluska, et al. (39)	Local/regional dz c			
	early p op/op DDD	13	10 surviving 2–10 yr	
	† late p op/op DDD	13	2 surviving	
	CP/ET	3	1–20 mo remission	
	5FU/op DDD	4	10–24 mo remission	
	XRT	2	5 & 12 mo remissions	
Magee, et al. (40)	XRT (4 lost to F/U)	10	0E/4M/2N	40
	OP DDD	3	0E/2M/1N	66.7
Teinturier, et al. (41)	op DDD	20	6	30
	5FU/AD/CP	3	1	33.3
	op DDD/5FU/AD/CP	1	1	100
	CP/ET	3	2	66.7
	CP/AD	1	1	100
	CY/ET	1	0	0
	CY/CP/VM-26	1	0	0
	CP/ET/AD	1	0	0
Didolkar, et al. (42)	**Chemotherapy	28	3	11
	XRT	10	4	40
Nader et al. (43)	op DDD	49	9 E & M	19.1
	XRT	10	2M	22.2
	**Chemotherapy	28	3M	11.5
Schlumberger (44)	5FU/AD/CP	14		23
	5FU/AD/CP/op DDD	3	2M	66.7
Bukowski, et al. (45)	op DDD/CP	37	1E/10M	30

*Chemotherapy consisted of AD/CY/VI/melphalan/peptochemio
**Chemotherapy was not indicated
†late p op = 15 mo postoperative
op′-DDD = Mitotane; XRT = radiation therapy; CP = *cis* Platin; ET = etoposide; 5FU = 5 fluorouracil;
AD = adriamycin; CY = cytoxan; VI = vincristine; E = effective response; M = moderate response; N = no response; U = unknown response

has been found to be an important inhibitor of gonadal and adrenal steroidogenesis in vivo when given in doses as low as 200–600 mg/d. Ketoconazole has been used to treat several cases of Cushing's syndrome and virilization caused by adrenal tumor *(50)*. Clinical improvement occurs frequently, but regression of metastatic disease is rare *(51)*. When patients are treated with ketoconazole, adrenal insufficiency is avoided by decreasing the dose sufficiently to maintain normal cortisol levels. The most frequent adverse reactions with ketoconazole are nausea and vomiting, abdominal pain, and pruritus in 1–3% of patients. Hepatotoxicity, primarily of the hepatocellular type, has been associated with its use *(50)*.

Metyrapone is a 11-β-hydroxylase inhibitor. In doses of 250 mg twice daily to 1 gm twice daily, patients experience biochemical and clinical improvement. Nausea, vomiting, and dizziness can occur in association with treatment. Because of the high cost and side effects, metyrapone should be used only as a temporary therapy in patients with severe cortisol-secreting adrenocortical carcinomas.

Aminoglutethimide inhibits cholesterol side-chain cleavage and the conversion of cholesterol to delta-5-pregnenolone in the adrenal cortex. As a consequence, the synthesis of cortisol, aldosterone, and androgens is suppressed. The drug has been used both in adults and children in doses of 0.5–2.0 gm/d. Cortisol levels fall gradually with regression of the clinical manifestations of Cushing's syndrome (52). Eventually, patients may need glucocorticoid replacement. The effect of aminoglutethimide is promptly reversed by interruption of therapy. Aminoglutethimide causes gastrointestinal (anorexia, nausea, vomiting) and neurologic (lethargy, sedation, blurred vision) side effects and can cause hypothyroidism in 5% of patients. Skin rash is frequently observed during the first 10 d of treatment; this usually subsides despite continuation of treatment. Headaches have also been observed with larger doses.

UNDERSTANDING THE ROLE OF MITOTANE IN THE TREATMENT OF ADRENAL CANCER

We have studied the mechanism of the adrenalytic action of mitotane in order to determine which patients might benefit the best from this type of treatment, and the possibility of developing better compounds for the treatment of adrenal cancer. Mitotane belongs to the class of drugs that require metabolic transformation into active metabolites for therapeutic action. The active metabolite either covalently combines to specific targets in the cells responsive to the drugs, and/or induce oxygen activation leading to toxicity. We have shown that mitotane is transformed to an acyl chloride by a mitochondrial $P450$-mediated hydroxylation and that the acyl chloride covalently combines to specific bionucleophiles within the adrenal cortical cell for the adrenalytic effect to take place (Fig. 1). The requirement for metabolic transformation for adrenalytic effect was shown by the testing of an analog of mitotane, in which methylation at the β-carbon blocks metabolic transformation (Fig. 2). When administered to dogs, an animal species very sensitive to mitotane, methylated mitotane is without effect (53). In preliminary studies, we have characterized the $P450$ enzyme involved in mitotane metabolism as being different to the well-known steroidogenic enzymes. It is likely that this $P450$ is a novel hydroxylating enzyme, perhaps involved in drug metabolism. We have also characterized the protein targets to which the mitotane metabolite binds, and shown it to be a 49.5 and an 11.5 molecular-weight protein whose role in the cell cycle still needs to be determined.

The requirement for metabolic transformation for activity has led us to develop a tritium-release assay (54). For this assay, tritiated mitotane is incubated with adrenal homogenates or cell suspensions. Unreacted substrate is removed on the amount of tritium released to the acrea medius determined. The tritium-released assay correlates with the ability of the tissue to transform to the acyl chloride. A comparison of the metabolic activity of various adrenal cortical tumors, using the tritium-release assay, shows significant variability in this activity (Table 4). The possibility that the response to mitotane depends on the metabolic activity of the neoplastic tissue was studied using

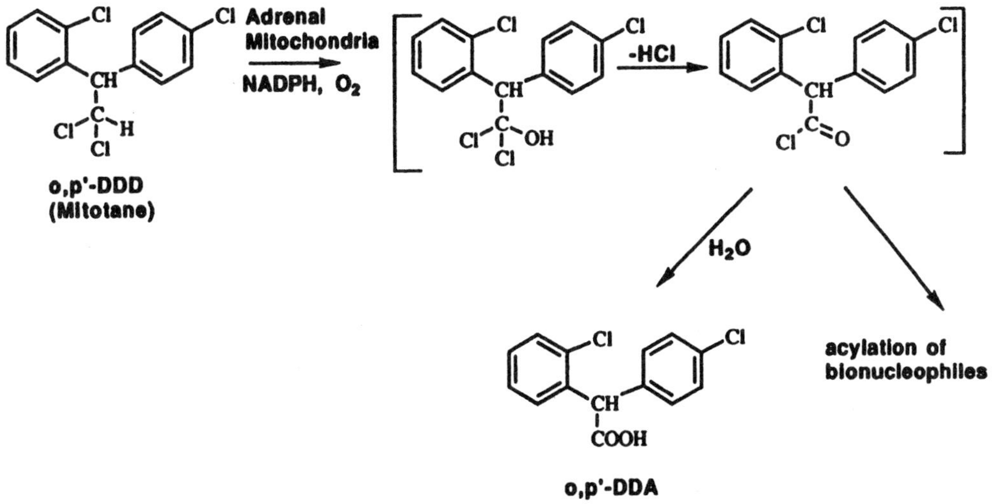

Fig. 1. Metabolic transformation of mitotane by adrenal mitochondria. Steps involved include: (1) Hydroxylation at the β carbon; (2) Dehydrochlorination; (3) Formation of an acyl chloride, a reactive intermediate; (4) Covalent binding to specific bionucleophiles; or (5) Conversion to o,p'-DDA, the acetic acid derivative.

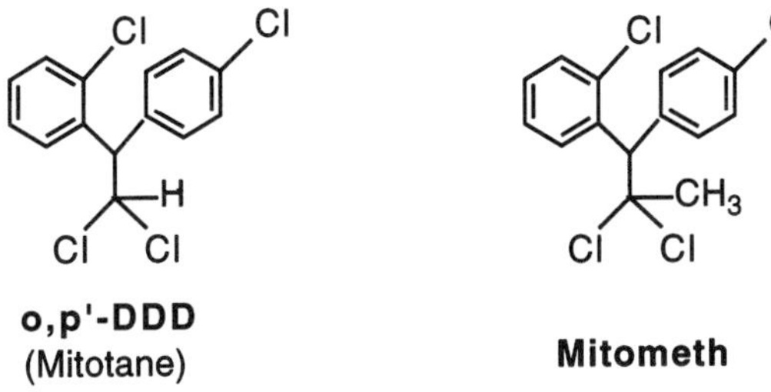

Fig. 2. Structure of mitometh, the inactive methylated analog of mitotane.

C14-labeled mitotane. The patient who had the greatest ability to metabolize mitotane by the tumor was also the one who had the longest survival (Table 5). In addition to metabolic transformation, another mechanism of action is oxidative damage through formation of free radicals, which induces cytotoxicity. Preliminary evidence for this mechanism has been developed in vitro in adrenal-cortical cancer cells to which mitotane was added with or without alpha tocopherol, an antioxidant. The addition of alpha tocopherol decreases the action of mitotane, suggesting oxidative damage as another mechanism (Fig. 3).

We have proposed that adrenal tumors vary in their ability to effect metabolic transformation or initiate free-radical production, and may therefore express variable sensitivity to mitotane. The ability of tumors to transform mitotane could predict the clinical response to the drug. Prospective studies of the relationship between the ability to transform mitotane using the tritium-release assay and the clinical response could help determine which patients with adrenal cancer should be treated with mitotane as an antitumor drug.

Table 4
Comparison of the Ability of Adrenocortical Tumors to
Metabolize Mitotane

Tissue	% H_3 Released
Normal Adrenal	0.510 ± 0.034
Adrenal Carcinoma	
MC	0.106 ± 0.002
RL	0.016 ± 0.006
MS	1.776 ± 0.046
JM	0.702 ± 0.156
Adrenal Adenoma	
FB	0.0173 ± 0.004

*Pineiro-Sanchez, et al.
#Unpublished Data
[3]H Mitotane was incubated with tumor homogenates and the percent ^{3}H released was measured after transformation.

Table 5
Correlation Between In Vitro Metabolic Activity of Neoplastic Tissue and the Patient's
Response to Mitotane Therapy

Patient	Total % Transformation[a]	Treatment Response
RF	0.2	—
GE	0.25, 0.34	—
LS	1.21, 1.32	+
Blank (boiled adrenal)	0.10, 0.35, 0.38	

[a]Metabolites separated by HPLC and counted by LSC. Expressed as % of total radioactivity added.

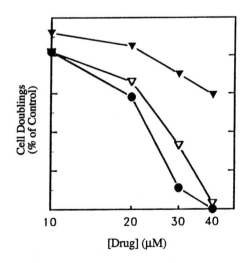

Fig. 3. Reversal by α-tocopherol acetate of the antitumor effect of mitotane on a chemokine-secreting human adrenocortical carcinoma cell line in vitro.

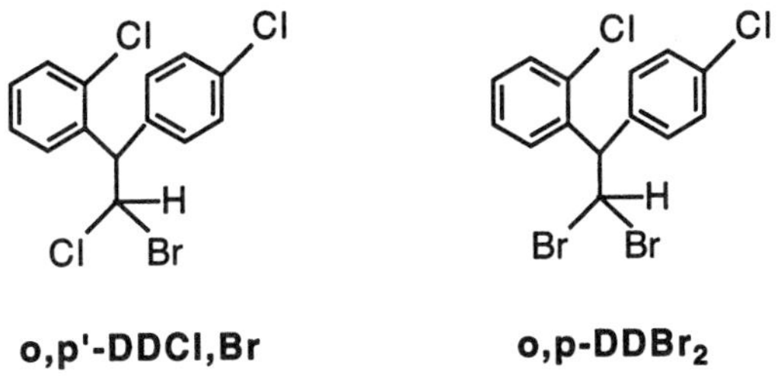

Fig. 4. Chemical structure of two mitotane analogs in which bromine was substituted for chlorine at the β carbon.

The limited efficacy of mitotane as an adrenalytic drug in the treatment of adrenal cancer has prompted investigation into the development of analogs with greater antitumor effects. We investigated the possibility that by enhancing the formation of the acyl chloride, the activity of mitotane on adrenal tumor cells could be increased. Various halides have different reactivity and potential ability to induce transformation into the active metabolite. For example, bromine may be more reactive than chlorine in inducing metabolism at the β-carbon. Thus, two compounds were synthesized in which one or both chlorides at the β-carbon were replaced by bromine. One is an o,p′-DDchlorobromo compound, the other, an o,p-DDdibromo analog (Fig. 4). The activity of these two analogs were compared to mitotane in vivo and in vitro. In vivo, dogs received mitotane or the chlorobromo and dibromo compounds. The adrenalytic activity was measured in terms of the histologic change in the glomerulosa/fasciculata + reticularis ratio. A higher ratio indicates greater atrophy of the fasciculata and reticularis, the main site of action of these compounds. The adrenalytic activity was also estimated in terms of inflammatory change in the adrenal glands of dogs receiving these compounds. The chlorobromo and dibromo analogs appear to have a greater effect. This was also tested in vitro by examining the antiproliferative effect of mitotane and the two brominated analogs in equimolar amounts on the growth and cortisol secretion of a steroid-secreting human adrenal cortical carcinoma cell line (NCI-H295). A greater effect was noted both on cell growth and cortisol production (Fig. 5). Further preclinical studies are needed before the clinical efficacy and toxicity of these analogs can be determined.

Another potentially important effect of mitotane is that of inhibiting the expression of the multidrug resistant gene and production of the MDR-1/P glycoprotein (55). This glycoprotein is highly expressed in normal adrenal and in adrenal cortical carcinomas, potentially leading to decreased responsiveness to chemotherapeutic agents. Treatment with mitotane has been reported to increase the accumulation of chemotherapeutic drugs in adrenal-cortical carcinoma cells. The possibility of combining mitotane with other therapeutic agents in the treatment of adrenal cortical carcinomas is currently being studied.

Mitotane causes significant toxicity in therapeutically effective doses. The adverse effects of mitotane are dose-dependent and usually intolerable at doses above 6 g daily, a dosage may be required to achieve blood levels greater than 14 µg/dL, which has been reported to be associated with therapeutic response (56). Treatment should begin with lower doses such as 1 g twice daily, and gradually increased to tolerance. The drug is best administered with fat-containing foods, because its absorption and transport

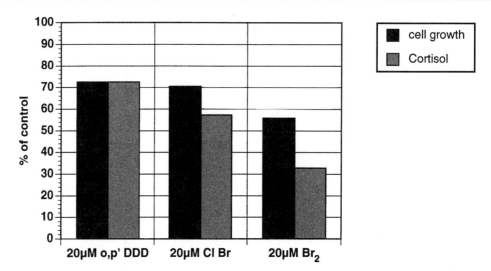

Fig. 5. Comparison of the effect of mitotane and two brominated analogs on NCI-H295 human adrenal cancer cell growth and cortisol production.

appears coupled to lack of proteins. The cortisol response to mitotane therapy should be followed by measuring the urinary-free cortisol. Mitotane increased binding of cortisol to cortical-steroid binding globulin, and the serum cortisol levels can be elevated even when circulating free cortisol is not *(57)*. The tumor response to mitotane should be followed by CT. Treatment with mitotane inhibits the function and causes destruction of the contralateral adrenal gland. Thus, patients should be covered with hydrocortisone 25–35 mg. daily. Synthetic glucocorticoids such as prednisone and dexamethasone are less desirable because their metabolism may be enhanced by mitotane, rendering determination of the optimum replacement dose less certain. In low doses (2–4 g daily), mitotane has less adrenalytic effects on the *zona glomerulosa,* and is less likely to suppress aldosterone production. With larger doses, replacement with fludrocortisol may be necessary.

Prominent early side effects of large doses of mitotane are anorexia and nausea. These side effects can be minimized by administering the largest dose at bedtime so that patients sleep through the most uncomfortable period. Side effects can be reversed by interrupting therapy for several days, and restarting the drug at a lower dose. A macular-papular exanthem and exfoliative dermatitis can occur, but both are rare. Hepatoxicity interruption in therapy is also unusual.

In summary, although new understanding of adrenal tumorigenesis and drug metabolism may help design more effective treatment for adrenal cancer, mitotane, either by itself or in combination with other chemotherapeutic agents, still remains an important component of medical treatment for patients with adrenal-cortical cancer.

REFERENCES

1. Brennan MF. Adrenocortical carcinoma. Ca—A Cancer J Clinicians 1987; 37:348–365.
2. Lynch HT, Katz DA, Bogard PJ, Lynch JF. The sarcoma, breast cancer, lung cancer and adrenocortical carcinoma syndrome revisited. Childhood cancer. Am J Dis Child 1985; 139:134–136.
3. Hartley AL, Birch JM, Marsden HB, Reid H, Harris M, Blair U. Adrenal cortical tumors: Epidemiological and familial aspects. Arch Dis Child 1987; 62:683–689.

4. Grayson GH, Moore S, Schneider BG, Saldivar V, Hensel CH. Novel germline mutation of the p53 tumor suppressor gene in a child with incidentally discovered adrenal cortical carcinoma. Am J Pediatr Hematol Oncol 1994; 16:341–347.

5. Lin SR, Lee YJ, Tsai HJ. Mutations of the p53 gene in human functional adrenocortical neoplasms. J Clin Endocrinol Metab 1994; 78:483–491.

6. Miyamoto H, Kubota Y, Shuin T, Shiozaki H. Bilateral adrenocortical carcinoma showing loss of heterozygosity at the p53 and RB gene loci. Cancer Genet Cytogenet 1966; 88:181–183.

7. Yano T, Linehan M, Anglard P, Lermaan MI, Daniel LN, Stein CA, et al. Genetic changes in human adrenocortical carcinomas. J Natl Cancer Inst 1989; 81:518–523.

8. Reincke M, Karl M, Travis WH, Mastorakos G, Allolio B, Linehan HM, et al. p53 mutations in human adrenocortical neoplasms: immunohistochemical and molecular studies. J Clin Endocrinol Metab 1994; 78:790–794.

9. McNicol AM, Nolan CE, Struthers AJ, Farquharson MA, Hermans J, Haak HR. Expression of p53 in adrenocortical tumours: Clinicopathological correlations. J Pathol 1997; 181:146–152.

10. Liu J, Kahri AI, Heikkilä P, Voutilainen R. Ribonucleic acid expression of the clustered imprinted genes p57[kip2] insulin-like growth factor-II and H19 in adrenal tumors and cultured adrenal cells. J Clin Endocrinol Metab 1997; 82:1766–1771.

11. Liu J, Kahri AI, Heikkilä P, Ilvesmäki V, Voutilainen R. H19 and insulin-like growth factor-II gene expression in adrenal tumors and cultured adrenal cells. J Clin Endocrinol Metab 1995; 80:492–496.

12. Liu J, Voutilainen R, Kahri AI, Heikkilä P. Expression patterns of the c-myc gene in adrenocortical tumors and pheochromocytomas. J Endocrinol 1997; 152:175–181.

13. Farge D, Chatellier G, Pagny YJ, Jeunemaitre X, Plouin PF, Corvol P. Isolated clinical syndrome of primary aldosteronism in four patients with adrenocortical carcinoma. Am J Med 1987; 83:635–640.

14. Arteaga E, Biglieri EG, Kater CE, Lopez JM, Schambelan M. Aldosterone-producing adrenocortical carcinoma. Preoperative recognition and course in three cases. Ann Intern Med 1984; 101:316–321.

15. Grondal S, Curstedt T. Steroid profile in serum: Increased levels of sulphated pregnenolone and pregn5-ene-3 beta, 20 alpha-diol in patients with adrenocortical carcinoma. Acta Endocrinol 1991; 124:381–385.

16. Copeland PM. The incidentally discovered adrenal masses. Ann Surg 1984; 199:116–122.

17. Bencsik Z, Szaboles I, Goth M, Voros A, Kaszas J, Kovacs L. Incidentally detected adrenal tumors (incidentalomas): Histological heterogeneity and differentiated therapeutic approach. J Intern Med 1995; 237:585–589.

18. Korobkin M, Francis IR, Kloos RT, Dunnick NR. The incidental adrenal mass. Radiol Clin N Am 1996; 34:1037–1054.

19. Korobkin M, Brodeur FJ, Francis IR, Quint LE, Dunnick NR, Goodsitt M. Delayed enhanced CT for differentiation of Benign from Malignant adrenal masses. Radiology 199; 200:737–742.

20. Hamper UM, Fishman EK, Hartman DS, Roberts JL, Sanders RC. Primary adrenocortical carcinoma: sonographic evaluation with clinical and pathologic correlation in 26 patients. Am J Roentgenol 1987; 148:915–919.

21. Smith SM, Patel SK, Turner DA, Matalon TA. Magnetic resonance imaging of adrenal cortical carcinoma. Urol Radiol 1989; 11:1–6.

22. Korobkin M, Lombardi TJ, Aisen AM, Francis IR, Quint LE, Dunnick NR, et al. Characterization of adrenal masses with chemical shift and Gadolinium enhanced imaging. Radiology 1995; 197:414–418.

23. Gross MD, Shapiro B, Bouffard JA, Glazer GM, Francis IR, Wilton GP, et al. Distinguishing benign and malignant euadrenal masses. Ann Intern Med 1988; 109:613–618.

24. MacFarlane DA. Cancer of the adrenal cortex: The natural history, prognosis and treatment in the study of fifty five cases. Ann R Coll Surg Engl 1958; 23:155–186.

25. Sullivan M. Adrenal cortical carcinoma. Urology 1978; 120:660.

26. Hogan T. A clinical and pathological study of adrenocortical carcinoma; therapeutic implications. Cancer 1980; 45:2880.

27. Bradley E. Primary and adjunctive therapy in carcinoma of the adrenal cortex. Surg Gynecol Obstet 1975; 141:507.

28. Schteingart DE. Treating adrenal cancer. The Endocrinologist 1992; 2:149–157.

29. Thompson NW. Adrenocortical carcinoma. (Thompson NW, Vinik AI, eds) 1983, pp. 119–128.

30. Percarpio B, Knowlton AH. Radiation therapy of adrenal cortical carcinoma. Acta Rad Ther 1976; 15:288–292.

31. Hogan TF, Citrin DL, Johnson BM, Nakamura S, Davis TE, Borden EC. o,p'-DDD (mitotane) therapy

of adrenal cortical carcinoma: Observations on drug dosage, toxicity and steroid replacement. Cancer 1978; 42:2177–2181.

32. Luton JP, Cerdas S, Billaud L, Thomas G, Guilhaume B, Bertagna X, et al. Clinical features of adrenocortical carcinoma, prognostic factors, and the effect of mitotane therapy. N Engl J Med 1990; 3322:1195–1201.

33. Wooten MD, King DK. Adrenal cortical carcinoma. Epidemiology and treatment with mitotane and a review of the literature. Cancer 1993; 72:3145–3155.

34. Schteingart DE, Motazedi A, Noonan RA, Thompson NW. The treatment of adrenal carcinoma. Arch Surg 1982; 117:1142.

35. Kasperlik-Zaluska A. Impact of adjuvant mitotane on the clinical course of patients with adrenocortical carcinoma. Cancer 1994; 73:1533–1534.

36. Vassilopoulou-Sellin R, Guinee VF, Klein MJ, Taylor SH, Hess KR, Schultz PN, et al. Impact of adjuvant mitotane on the clinical course of patients with adrenocortical cancer. Cancer 1993; 71:3119–3123.

37. LaRocca RV, Stein CA, Danesi R, Jamis-Dow CA, Weiss GH, Myers CE. Suramin in adrenal cancer: modulation of steroid hormone production, cytotoxicity in vitro, and clinical antitumor effect. J Clin Endocrinol Metab 1990; 71:497–504.

38. Venkatesh S, Hickey RC, Sellin RV, Fernanadez JF, Samaan NA. Adrenal cortical carcinoma. Cancer 1989; 64:765–769.

39. Kasperlik-Zaluska A, Migdalska BM, Zgliczynski S, Markowska AM. Adrenocortical carcinoma: a clinical study and treatment results of 52 patients. Cancer 1995; 75:2587–2591.

40. Magee BJ, Gattamaneni HR, Pearson D. Adrenal cortical carcinoma: Survival after radiotherapy. Clin Rad 1987; 38:587–588.

41. Teinturier C, Brugières L, Lemerle J, Chaussain JL, Bougnères PF. Corticoserrénalomes de l'enfant: Analyse rétrospective de 54 cas. Arch Pédiatr 1996; 3:235–240.

42. Didolkar MS, Bescher RA, Elias EG, Moore RH. Natural history of adrenal cortical carcinoma: a clinicopathologic study of 42 patients. Cancer 1981; 47:2153–2161.

43. Nader S, Hickey RC, Sellin RV, Samaan NA. Adrenal cortical carcinoma: a study of 77 cases. Cancer 1983; 52:707–711.

44. Schlumberger M, Brugieres L, Gicquel C, Travagli JP, Droz JP, Parmentier C. 5-Fluorouracil, doxorubicin and cisplatin as treatment for adrenal cortical carcinoma. Cancer 1991; 67:2997–3000.

45. Bukowski RM, Montie J, Crawford D, Wolf M. Cisplatin (CDDP) and mitotane in metastatic adrenal carcinoma: a southwest oncology group study. Proc Am Soc Clin Oncol 1990; 9:296.

46. Jensen JC, Pass HI, Sindelar WF, Norton JA. Recurrent or metastatic disease in select patients with adrenocortical carcinoma: aggressive resection vs. chemotherapy. Arch Surg 1991; 126:457–461.

47. King D, Lack E. Adrenal cortical carcinoma; a clinical and pathological study of 49 cases. Cancer 1979; 44:239.

48. Bodie B, Novick AC, Pontes JE, Straffon RA, Montie JE, Babiak T, et al. The Cleveland Clinic experience with adrenal cortical carcinoma. J Urol 1989; 141:257–260.

49. Bradley EL. Primary and adjunctive therapy in carcinoma of the adrenal cortex. Surg Gynecol Obstet 1975; 141:507–516.

50. Kruimel JW, Smals AG, Beex LU, Swinkels LM, Pieters GF, Kloppenborg PW. Favorable response of a virilizing adrenocortical carcinoma to preoperative treatment with ketoconazole and postoperative chemotherapy. Acta Endocrinol 1991; 124:492–496.

51. Contreras P, Rojas A, Biagini L, et al. Regression of metastatic adrenal carcinoma during palliative ketoconazole treatment. Lancet 1985; 2:151.

52. Schteingart DE, Cash R, Conn JW. Aminoglutethimide and metastatic adrenal cancer. Maintained reversal (six months) of Cushing's syndrome. JAMA 1966; 198:1007.

53. Schteingart DE, Sinsheimer JE, Counsell RE, Abrams GD, McClellan N, Djanegara T, et al. Comparison of the adrenalytic activity of mitotane and a methylated homolog on normal adrenal cortex and adrenal cortical carcinoma. Cancer Chemother Pharmacol 1993; 31:459–466.

54. Pineiro-Sanchez ML, Vaz ADN, Counsell RE, Ruyan M, Schteingart DE, Sinsheimer JE. Synthesis of β^3H-mitotane for use in a rapid assay for mitotane metabolism. J Labeled Compds XXXVI 1995; 2:121–127.

55. Bates SE, Shien CY, Mickley LA, Dichek NL, Gazdar A, Loriaux L, et al. Mitotane enhances cytotoxicity of chemotherapy in cell lines expressing a multidrug resistance gene (mdr-1/P-glycoprotein) which is also expressed by adrenocortical carcinomas. J Clin Endocrinol Metab 1991; 78:18–29.

56. Haak HR, Hermans J, VandeVelde CJH, Lentjes EGWM, Goslings BM, Fleuren GJ, et al. Optimal treatment of adrenal cortical carcinoma with mitotane: results in a consecutive series of 96 patients. Brit J Cancer 1994; 69:947–951.

57. VanSeters AP, Moolenaar AJ. Mitotane increases the blood levels of hormone-binding proteins. Acta Endocrinol 1991; 124:526–533.

18 Adrenal Incidentalomas

Bruno Allolio, MD

CONTENTS

INTRODUCTION

Several decades ago, the collection of adrenals for anatomical studies and large autopsy series have both demonstrated a high incidence of adrenal nodules *(1–5)*. Today, modern imaging techniques like ultrasound, computerized tomography (CT), and magnetic resonance imaging (MRI) enable the detection of adrenal tumors during their lifetime with increasing frequency. Adrenal tumors incidentally discovered by modern imaging techniques have been termed adrenal incidentalomas.

Definition

An adrenal incidentaloma is defined as an adrenal mass not suspected prior to the imaging procedure, which led to its discovery. Thus, by definition, patients undergoing an abdominal CT scan for staging of malignant disease never harbor an incidentaloma, as adrenal metastases are a robust possibility prior the investigation. Nevertheless, some adrenal adenomas may be discovered by tumor staging. In patients with adrenal hypertension, it is sometimes difficult to assess whether an adrenal mass detected by abdominal ultrasound has been found incidentally. However, investigation of endocrine hypertension usually requires biochemical evidence before imaging procedures are ordered.

Epidemiology

No population-based studies are available to precisely define the incidence and prevalence of adrenal nodules. However, postmortem investigations *(1–7)* and large

From: *Contemporary Endocrinology: Adrenal Disorders*
Edited by: A. N. Margioris and G. P. Chrousos © Humana Press, Totowa, NJ

Table 1
Prevalence of Adrenal Tumors in Autopsy Series and CT Studies

First Author	Year	Design	N	Adrenal Tumors%
Russi *(1)*	1944	retrospective autopsy study	9000	1.45
Commons *(2)*	1948	retrospective autopsy study	7437	2.86
Shamma *(3)*	1958	retrospective autopsy study	220	1.8
Kokko *(4)*	1967	retrospective autopsy study	1495	1.41
Hedeland *(5)*	1968	prospective autopsy study	739	8.7
Reinhard *(6)*	1994	prospective autopsy study	498	5.0
Total			19,389	$x = 2.38$
Glazer *(8)*	1982	retrospective CT-study	2200	0.6
Garz *(9)*	1985	retrospective CT-study	12,000	0.5
Kley *(10)*	1990	prospective CT-study	2568	4.4
Stark *(11)*	1994	prospective CT-study	13,818	0.8
Total			30,586	$x = 1.0$

studies using CT *(8–11)* give consistent results: Autopsy series reported adrenal tumors in 1.4–8.7% of cases *(1,5)*. Most of these tumors were small adenomas. The prevalence of tumors with a diameter >1.5 cm is still 1.8%, and tumors with a diameter >6 cm have been reported in 0.025% of patients *(1)*. Using CT, a prevalence between 0.6–4.4% has been found *(8–11)*. When pooling the data of several studies representing more than 30,000 patients, the mean prevalence is around 1% (Table 1). Thus, more than 2 million subjects in the United States harbor an adrenal tumor easily detected by CT. Most of these tumors are very small (diameter ≤ 1 cm) and 79% of these tumors have a diameter < 2 cm *(10)*.

Both sexes are equally affected *(1,2,5,12)*, although in some studies a slight female preponderance has been reported *(13)*. The prevalence of incidentalomas increases with age, peaking in the seventh decade *(1,2,12,14)*. Autopsies and CT indicate that both adrenals are affected with equal frequency. Some studies have reported a higher prevalence of incidentalomas in the right adrenal *(13)*. However, this observation can be explained by the fact that the right adrenal nodules are more easily detected by ultrasound.

CLINICAL FINDINGS

By definition, patients with an incidentaloma have no clinical signs or symptoms of adrenal disease present. However, more-detailed questioning and a careful second physical examination may reveal subtle evidence for hormone excess (such as recent weight gain, skin atrophy, episodic headaches). Moreover, arterial hypertension and obesity are significantly more prevalent in patients with incidentaloma *(14,15)*. The association of hypertension and adrenal nodules has already been observed in autopsy studies and thus cannot be explained by an increased likelihood of imaging procedures in patients with hypertension *(7,16)*. In addition, patients with incidentaloma more frequently suffer from diabetes mellitus type II *(1,5)*. Taking these findings together, there seems to be a clear association with features of the metabolic syndrome (obesity, primary arterial hypertension, diabetes mellitus type II b) *(17)*.

Table 2
Differential Diagnosis of Adrenal Incidentalomas and
Specific Diagnosis in 267 Cases *(14)*

	n
Adrenal adenoma	
inactive	206
cortisol producing	23
aldosteronoma	1
androgen producing	—
estrogen producing	—
Adrenocortical carcinoma	1
Nodular hyperplasia	3
Pheochromocytoma	7
Ganglioneuroma	3
Ganglioneuroblastoma	—
Angiomyolipoma	—
Lipoma	—
Liposarcoma	—
Myelolipoma	9
Lymphangioma	1
Hemangioma	1
Hematoma/hemorrhage	1
Abscess	—
Adrenal cyst	6
Metastasis	3
Renal cell carcinoma	1
Retroperitoneal sarcoma	—
Gastric leiomyoma	—
Neurilemmoma	1
Accessory spleen	—

DIFFERENTIAL DIAGNOSIS

While benign adrenal adenomas are, by far, the most frequent cause for adrenal incidentalomas, numerous other causes have to be considered (Table 2). As only a minority of patients require surgical removal of the tumor, the true prevalence of the different causes is not known. Large extraadrenal tumors are sometimes misclassified as tumors of adrenal origin. This concerns mostly primary retroperitoneal neoplasms.

PATHOGENESIS

The increase in adrenal nodularity with age has led to the assumption that adrenocortical nodular hyperplasia is a manifestation of the aging adrenal *(7)*. This view is supported by the observation that, in the majority of older subjects, both adrenals are affected and that the occurrence of nodules is associated with capsular arteriopathy. It was suggested that adrenal nodules represent focal hyperplasia in response to focal ischemic loss of cortical tissue *(7)*.

However, clonal analysis of adrenal tumors showed that the vast majority is of monoclonal origin, although consistently, some polyclonal nodules were also found *(18,19)*. Thus, at least the larger adrenal nodules are the result of clonal expansion following somatic oncogenic mutations. Nevertheless, to date, it cannot be excluded that some of these true neoplasias arise from polyclonal focal nodular hyperplasia.

Another line of evidence links congenital adrenal hyperplasia (CAH) caused by 21-hydroxylase deficiency to the occurrence of incidentalomas. Macronodular adrenals are a frequent finding in patients with classical CAH and may be found in more than 80% of the cases (20). Patients not receiving adequate steroid therapy are at an even increased risk of developing adrenocortical cancer (21,22). Interestingly, macronodular hyperplasia is not restricted to homozygotes of 21-hydroxylase deficiency. Using abdominal CT scans in families with CAH, Jaresch et al. (23) found adrenal nodules in 45% of heterozygous carriers. A causal relationship between adrenal enzyme defects and incidentalomas is suggested by the fact that the population frequency of CAH heterozygosity (2%) and the prevalence of incidentalomas (1–2%) are very similar. Moreover, it has been shown in several studies that 30–70% of patients with adrenal tumors exhibit an exaggerated response of 17α-hydroxyprogesterone after stimulation with adrenocorticotropic hormone (ACTH) as is seen in heterozygous carriers of CAH (24,26). However, using multisteroid analysis, we and others have found that patients with adrenal incidentaloma have increased secretion of multiple precursors of the mineralcorticoid and glucocorticoid pathway after an ACTH challenge indicating impaired 11β-hydroxylase and 17,20-lyase activity in the tumor itself, rather than heterozygosity for 21-hydroxylase deficiency (27,28). Most importantly, recent molecular analysis of a series of adrenal tumors revealed that mutations in the 21-hydroxylase gene are rare and not linked to the ACTH-induced 17α-hydroxyprogesterone increase (29). Thus, heterozygosity for CAH is of minor importance for the majority of adrenal incidentalomas and the cause for the exaggerated steroid response resides only in the tumor and, hence, disappears after surgery.

The high incidence of arterial hypertension, obesity, and even frank diabetes mellitus type II in patients with incidentaloma suggests a relationship to the metabolic syndrome (15). In a recent prospective series of patients with adrenal incidentalomas, we found that all 13 consecutive cases exhibited elevated insulin in the fasting state or after a glucose challenge (17). Moreover, a high prevalence (61%) of disturbed glucose tolerance was found more recently in a series of 64 consecutive patients with nonfunctioning adrenal adenomas (30). Insulin is a potent mitogen and acts specifically on the adrenal cortex by stimulation of steroidogenesis and cell proliferation through both insulin and insulin-like growth factor 1 (IGF 1) receptors (31–33). Thus, a significant proportion of adrenal nodules may be regarded as a manifestation of the metabolic syndrome.

DIAGNOSTIC APPROACH

Careful diagnostic evaluation holds the potential of early detection and prevention of disease. On the other hand, as most lesions are benign, hormonally silent, and do not require surgery, it is important to limit costs by avoiding all unnecessary diagnostic tests. Two questions must be answered: Is the lesion truly hormonally inactive? What is the probability of malignancy?

Endocrinological Investigation

The aim is the detection of subclinical adrenal hypersecretion by selecting the most informative tests (Table 3). Relevant endocrine activity is related to tumor size (Fig. 1).

Table 3
Stepwise Endocrinological Investigation in Adrenal Incidentalomas

Step I

a) 24-h urinary catecholamine excretion

plus

b) serum cortisol after dexamethasone suppression (3 mg dexamethasone at 23.00 h orally)

plus

c) serum potassium and repeated blood pressure measurements, only in case of spontaneous hypokalemia or arterial hypertension, also measurement of PRA and serum aldosterone at rest, 24-h urinary potassium excretion

plus

d) serum DHEAS

Step II (only if corresponding test results in Step I are abnormal)

a) 123 I-MIBG scintigraphy

or

b) CRH-test, analysis of diurnal cortisol secretion, and high-dose (8 mg) dexamethasone suppression

or

c) Orthostasis test with measurement of PRA and serum aldosterone, 24-h urinary aldosterone 18-glucoronide excretion.

in selected cases: bilateral adrenal vein catheterization with determination of aldosterone and cortisol

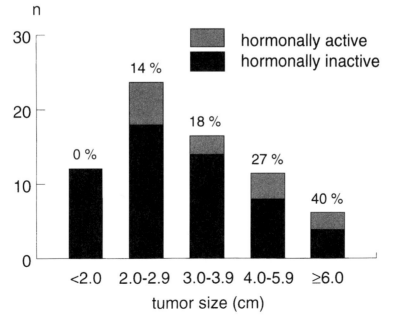

Fig. 1. Tumor size and endocrine activity in adrenal incidentalomas.

Incidentalomas with a diameter <1 cm require no work up, as significant hypersecretion is exceptionally rare. Such a cutoff allows to reduce diagnostic costs substantially. However, as small aldosteronomas may cause severe hypertension, this approach is restricted to normotensive and normokalemic patients.

Pheochromocytoma has been reported in a frequency ranging from 0–11% *(13,15,25,34–38)* among adrenal incidentalomas. Patients with pheochromocytoma may develop life-threatening hypertensive crisis and are at high risk during surgery without proper precautions *(39,40)*. Thus, it is mandatory to exclude or confirm pheochromocytoma in all incidentalomas by determination of 24-h urinary catecholamines or metanephrines. Measurement of plasma catecholamines is inferior and suppression tests (clonidine-test) are seldom required. In patients with elevated catecholamine excretion, we advocate 123-I metaiodobenzylguanidine (MIGB) szintigraphy for preoperative detection of metastatic disease *(40)*.

Autonomous cortisol secretion by adrenal incidentalomas is reported with increasing frequency *(13–15,25,34,35,41–44)*. Depending on the amount of glucocorticoids secreted by the tumor, the clinical significance ranges from a slightly attenuated diurnal cortisol rhythm to complete atrophy of the contralateral adrenal with lasting adrenal insufficiency after unilateral adrenalectomy *(44,45)*. Thus, subclinical Cushing's syndrome must be ruled out in every patient scheduled for surgery to avoid postoperative adrenal crisis *(45)*. The best means to uncover autonomous cortisol secretion is the short dexamethasone suppression test. As the adrenal origin of a pathological cortisol secretion is anticipated, we prefer a higher dexamethasone dose (3 mg instead of 1 mg) to reduce false positive results. A suppressed serum cortisol (<3 µg/dL) excludes significant cortisol secretion by the tumor. Serum cortisol >3 µg/dL requires further investigation including a corticotropin-releasing-hormone (CRH) test and analysis of the diurnal rhythm. Determination of urinary-free cortisol is less useful, as increased values are a late finding, usually associated with emerging clinical signs of Cushing's syndrome *(44)*. Patients with ACTH and cortisol not responding to CRH may develop adrenal insufficiency after surgery and require adequate substitution therapy (Fig. 2).

Conn adenoma is rare among adrenal incidentalomas *(15)*. In normotensive patients with a serum potassium above 3.9 mmol/L, no specific measurements are necessary. Otherwise, determination of plasma renin activity (PRA), together with plasma aldosterone, is required. Unfortunately, antihypertensive medication frequently interferes with mineralocorticoid regulation and hampers the interpretation of the measurements. Often, it is necessary to discontinue the medication for some time or switch to a less-interfering substance (e.g., prazosin) *(46)*. Patients with suppressed PRA require further evaluation in a specialized center, which may even include bilateral adrenal catheterization to prove that the incidentaloma is indeed the source of the mineralocorticoid excess.

Low serum dehydroepiandrosterone-sulfate (DHEAS) has been reported in a high percentage of patients with adrenal tumors and may be used as evidence of an adrenocortical origin of the tumor *(25,35,47)*. Moreover, as high DHEAS concentrations are found in a substantial proportion of adrenocortical carcinomas, measurement of DHEAS can contribute to the characterization of incidentalomas. The pathogenesis of low DHEAS levels in adrenal adenomas has not been elucidated. Suppression of ACTH by silent hypercortisolism has been suggested, but remains to be proven *(25)*. Unpublished results of our own group in three patients with a Conn adenoma indicate that low DHEA(S) secretion is not confined to the tumor-bearing side arguing against altered

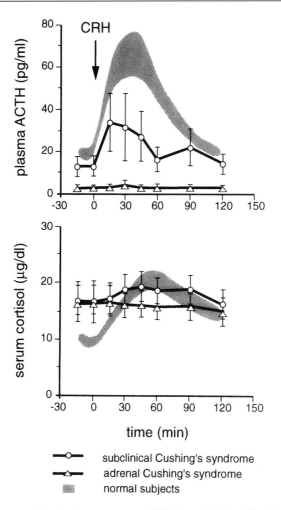

Fig. 2. Impaired ACTH and Cortisol response to CRH in subclinical Cushing's syndrome (*n*=6). Data from patients with adrenal Cushing's syndrome (*n*=6) are also given.

enzyme activity in the tumor or a paracrine action of the neoplastic tissue. Possibly low DHEAS merely indicates premature adrenal aging favoring the development of adrenal nodules *(7)*.

The value of DHEAS in the assessment of adrenal tumors should not be overestimated, as DHEAS shows a steep age-related decrease in normal subjects with wide intersubject variation *(48)*. Moreover, some adrenocortical cancers may also exhibit decreased serum DHEAS suggestive of a benign adenoma *(13)*.

Adrenal Imaging

Adrenal imaging is not only the first step in the discovery of the incidentaloma, but may also contribute to its characterization *(49)*. As incidentalomas are difficult to evaluate by ultrasound alone, additional imaging with CT is usually performed with the exception of the highly echogenic adrenal myelolipoma. Using CT, adrenal adenomas typically appear homogeneous and exhibit lower-than-water density (< 0–15 HU) and well-defined margins *(15)*. In contrast, adrenal carcinomas are generally larger, inhomogeneous, and show soft tissue density. Irregular margins and central necrosis or hemorrhage increase the probability of malignancy. However, benign pheochromocytoma may also present as large inhomogeneous tumor with hemorrhage *(49)*. In difficult cases, MRI may be helpful to further differentiate benign from malignant adrenal tumors, although, again, complete separation is not achieved *(50–52)*. Malignant lesions and pheochromocytomas typically demonstrate increased intensity on T_2-weighted MRI compared to liver. Gadolinium-enhanced dynamic studies have found strong enhancement and slow wash out in malignant neoplasms, whereas adenomas showed rapid wash out *(53,54)*. More recently, chemical-shift MRI has been used for characterization of adrenal tumors. Benign tumors like adrenal adenomas with high lipid content demonstrate a typical signal intensity loss on chemical shift imaging relative to the liver *(55,56)*. However, to better evaluate the potential of this new technique, more malignant neoplasms need to be investigated. Adrenocortical szintigraphy with NP-59 has been advocated for analysis of adrenal incidentalomas *(15)*. Benign adrenal adenomas typically exhibit a "concordant" pattern with uptake of the radiotracer on the side of the known adrenal mass, whereas in malignant neoplasms, the uptake is decreased or missing leading to a "discordant" pattern. However, some adrenal carcinomas may mimic benign lesions with a "concordant" uptake. In our opinion, adrenal scintigraphy should be restricted to larger (>3 cm) nonfunctioning lesions with HU-values in CT above those expected for adrenal adenomas *(15)*. Newer methods using positron emission tomography (PET) and 11C-metomidate may become useful tools for characterization of incidentalomas *(57)*.

Tumor Size

Most management strategies for incidentalomas have used tumor size as an important tool to discriminate benign from malignant lesions *(58)*. The rationale behind this approach is the observation that most adrenal carcinomas are very large at the time of diagnosis *(59,60)*. Several studies have shown that the probability of malignancy increases with tumor size *(13–15,25,37,58,61)*. However, as malignant lesions also start small, it is obvious that some smaller carcinomas will be misclassified using only tumor size for discrimination (Fig. 3). Thus, follow-up imaging is mandatory to analyze tumor growth. As a rule, follow-up imaging is performed by CT 3–6 mo after initial evaluation. The interval depends on the degree of suspicion of malignancy. If clear tumor growth is demonstrated, surgical removal of the tumor is suggested.

Interestingly, in the majority of cases, no tumor growth is detected *(14)* suggesting either a very slowly growing neoplasm or ceased tumor growth. Probably both mechanisms contribute to the high percentage of unchanged adrenal masses during follow-up.

Fine Needle Aspiration (FNA)

FNA is of limited value as histological differentiation between benign and malignant adrenal tumors is difficult *(62)*. Moreover, FNA is not free of side effects and may lead to pneumothorax or frank retroperitoneal bleeding *(63)*.

Thus, we restrict FNA to patients with known malignancy, in whom the adrenal mass is the only evidence of possible metastatic disease *(64)*. As aforementioned, adrenal masses in these patients do not qualify as incidentaloma sensu strictu. Malignant adrenal disease (metastases) is much more frequent in this patient group. In addition,

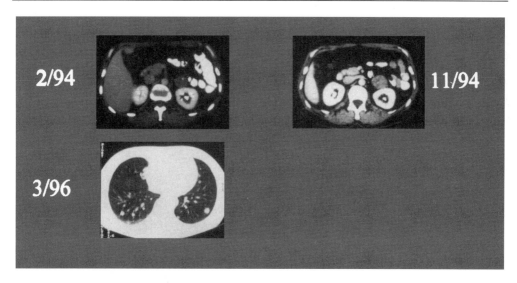

Fig. 3. Case of a patient with an incidentally discovered pheochromocytoma. The initial evaluation (2/94) showed normal urinary catecholamine excretion. Follow-up imaging (11/94) revealed tumor enlargement and adrenalectomy was performed. The histological diagnosis was phechromocytoma. Further follow-up demonstrated metastatic disease (3/96) and elevated urinary catecholamine excretion.

pheochromocytoma has to be excluded prior FNA as it may cause hypertensive crisis and even death *(65,66)*.

THERAPEUTIC CONSIDERATIONS

As a rule, hormonally active tumors are surgically removed to prevent serious morbidity. This strategy is undisputed for Conn adenomas and pheochromocytoma. However, it remains doubtful that all patients with subclinical Cushing's syndrome benefit from adrenal surgery, as progress from subclinical disease to overt Cushing's syndrome may occur only in a minority of cases *(44,67)*. No prospective studies have investigated the influence of adrenal surgery on body weight, hypertension, or bone mineral density (BMD) in these patients. However, despite subclinical disease, patients with autonomous cortisol secretion may have reduced BMD and altered bone turnover *(68)*.

As autonomous cortisol secretion by the tumor may range from a small percentage of the daily requirements to borderline hypersecretion with suppression of the contralateral adrenal, it is likely that the metabolic benefits of surgery will vary accordingly. Adrenal surgery has significant morbidity and mortality *(63)*, which have to be taken into account in decision-making. Thus, the newly developed endoscopic adrenalectomy *(64–66)* with its low morbidity may justify earlier intervention. However, more data on morbidity and mortality after adrenalectomy using modern techniques are urgently needed.

Because of the high risk of malignancy, tumors with a diameter ≥ 5 cm are surgically removed after adequate endocrinological investigation (Fig. 4). Smaller tumors (3–5 cm) may also be removed, if there is strong suspicion of malignancy after adrenal imaging *(15)* or because of clearly elevated serum DHEAS. All tumors demonstrating

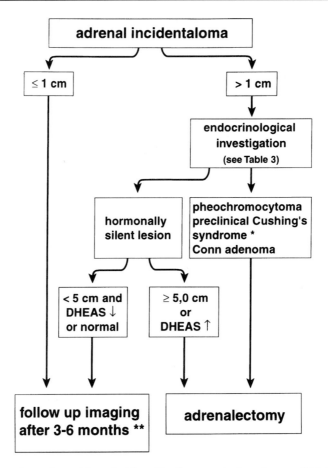

Fig. 4. Approach to the patient with an incidentally discovered adrenal mass. * Not all patients with subclinical Cushing's syndrome may need adrenalectomy (see text). ** Time to follow-up imaging should be inversely related to tumor size.

growth during follow-up should also be removed. As in all these cases, malignancy is a robust possibility, adrenal surgery should use the conventional approach.

SUMMARY

Adrenal incidentalomas are detected with increasing frequency by modern refined imaging techniques. Their prevalence rises with advancing age and is particularly high in patients with features of the metabolic syndrome (arterial hypertension, obesity, insulin resistance). Endocrinological investigation (24-h urinary catecholamines, dexa-methasone suppression test, serum DHEAS, and PRA) will reveal a significant percentage of hormonally active tumors with subclinical disease (e.g., pheochromocytoma, subclinical Cushing's syndrome). The risk of malignancy is low and increases with tumor diameter. In hormonally inactive tumors, tumor size remains the most useful parameter for clinical decision-making: All tumors with a maximum diameter ≥ 5 cm should be surgically removed. Smaller tumors require follow-up imaging and should be removed if tumor growth is detected. No endocrinological investigation is required for adrenal incidentalomas with a diameter < 1 cm.

REFERENCES

1. Russi S, Blumenthal HT. Small adenomas of the adrenal cortex in hypertension and diabetes. Arch Intern Med 1945; 76:284–291.
2. Commons RR, Callway CP. Adenomas of the adrenal cortex. Arch Intern Med 1948; 81:37–41.
3. Shamma AH, Goddard JW, Sommers SC. A study of the adrenal status in hypertension. J Chron Dis 1958; 8:587–595.
4. Kokko JP, Brown TC, Bermann MM. Adrenal adenoma and hypertension. Lancet 1967; 1:468–470.
5. Hedeland H, Östberg G, Hökfelt B. On the prevalence of adrenocortical adenomas in an autopsy material in relation to hypertension and diabetes. Acta Med Scand 1968; 184:211–214.
6. Reinhard C, Saeger W, Schubert B. Nodules and adenomas in the adrenal cortex: incidence in post-mortem series and correlation with clinical data. Exp Clin Endocrinol 1994; 102 (Suppl 1):192.
7. Dobbie JW. Adrenocortical nodular hyperplasia: the aging adrenal. J Pathol 1969; 99:1–18.
8. Glazer HS, Weymann PJ, Sagel SS, Levitt RG, McClennan BL. Nonfunctioning adrenal masses: incidental discovery on computed tomography. Am J Roentgenol 1982; 139:81–85.
9. Garz G, Luning M, Melzer B. Computertomographische Zufallsbefunde von hormoninaktiven Nebennierenadenomen. Radiol Diagn (Berlin) 1985; 26:761–766.
10. Kley HK, Wagner H, Jaresch S, Jungblut R, Schlaghecke R. Endokrin inaktive Nebennierentumoren. In: Allolio B, Schulte HM, eds. Moderne Diagnostik und therapeutische Strategien bei Nebennierenerkrankungen. Schattauer, New York, 1990; pp. 189–197.
11. Stark S, Pavel M, Sachse R, Cidlinski K, Riel R, Hahn EG, et al. Endocrine inactive adrenocortical adenomas (ACA) are a condition of the elderly. Exp Clin Endocrinol 1994; 102 (Suppl 1): 193.
12. Russell RP, Masi AT, Richter ED. Adrenal cortical adenomas and hypertension. A clinical pathologic analysis of 690 cases with matched controls and a review of the literature. Medicine (Baltimore) 1972; 51:211–225.
13. Kasperlik-Zaluska AA, Roslonowska E, Slowinska-Srzednicka, Migdalska B, Jeske W, Malowska A, et al. Incidentally discovered adrenal mass (incidentaloma): investigation and management of 208 patients. Clin Endocrinol 1997; 46:29–37.
14. Reincke M, Allolio B. Das Nebenniereninzidentalom: Die Kunst der Beschränkung in Diagnostik und Therapie. Dtsch Ärzteblatt 1995; 92:764–770.
15. Kloos RT, Gross MD, Francis IR, Korobkin M, Shapiro B. Incidentally discovered adrenal masses. Endocr Rev 1995; 16:460–484.
16. Neville AM. The nodular adrenal. Invest Cell Pathol 1978; 1:99–111.
17. Reincke M, Faßnacht M, Väth S, Mora P, Allolio B. Adrenal Incidentalomas: a manifestastion of the metabolic syndrome? Endocr Res 1996; 22(4):755–761.
18. Beuschlein F, Reincke M, Karl M, Travis W, Jaursch-Hancke C, Abdelhamid S, et al. Clonal composition of human adrenocortical neoplasms. Cancer Res 1994; 54:4927–4932.
19. Gicquel C, Leblond-Francillard M, Bertagna X, Louvel A, Chapuls Y, Luton JP, et al. Clonal analysis of human adrenocortical carcinomas and secreting adenomas. Clin Endocrinol 1994; 40:465–477.
20. Jaresch S, Schlaghecke R, Jungblut R, Krüskemper HL, Kley HK. Stumme Nebennierentumoren bei Patienten mit adrenogenitalem Syndrom. Klin Wochenschr 1987; 65:627–633.
21. Jaursch-Hancke C, Allolio B, Metzler U, Bidlingmaier F, Winkelmann W. Adrenocortical carcinoma in a patient with untreated congenital adrenal hyperplasia. Acta Endocrinol 1988; 177 (Suppl):146–147.
22. Hamwi GJ, Serbin RA, Kruger FA. Does adrenocortical hyperplasia result in adrenocortical carcinoma? N Engl J Med 1957; 257:1153–1155.
23. Jaresch S, Kornely E, Kley HK, Schlaghecke R. Adrenal incidentaloma and patients with homozygous or heterozygous congenital adrenal hyperplasia. J Clin Endocrinol Metab 1992; 74:685–689.
24. Seppel T, Schlaghecke R. Augmented 17-alpha-hydroxyprogesterone response to ACTH stimulation as evidence of decreased 21-hydroxylase activity in patients with incidentally discovered adrenal incidentalomas. Clin Endocrinol 1994; 41:445.
25. Terzolo M, Osella G, Ali A, Boretta M, Magro G, Piovesan A, et al. Different patterns of steroid secretion in patients with adrenal incidentalomas. J Clin Endocrinol Metab 1996; 81:740–744.
26. New MI, Lorenzen F, Lerner AJ, Kohn B, Oberfield SE, Pollack MS, et al. Genotyping steroid 21-hydroxylase deficiency: Hormonal reference data. J Clin Endocrinol Metab 1983; 57:320–326.
27. Reincke M, Peter M, Sippel WG, Allolio B. Impairment of 11β-hydroxylase, but not 21-hydroxylase, in adrenal "incidentalomas." Eur J Endocrinol 1997; 136:196–200.
28. Sadoul JL, Kezachian B, Altare S, Hadjali Y, Canivet B. Apparent activities of 21-hydroxylase,

17alpha-hydroxylase and 17,20-lyase are impaired in adrenal incidentalomas. Eur J Endocrinol 1999;141:238–245.

29. Beuschlein F, Schulze E, Mora P, Gensheimer HP, Maser-Gluth C, Allolio B, et al. Steroid 21-hydroxylase mutations and 21-hydroxylase messenger ribonucleic acid expression in human adrenocortical tumors. J Clin Endocrinol Metab 1998; 83:2585–2588.

30. Fernandez-Real JM, Engel WR, Simo R, Salinas I, Webb SM. Study of glucose tolerance in consecutive patients harboring incidental adrenal tumours. Study Group of Incidental Adrenal Adenomas. Clin Endocrinol 1998; 49:53–61.

31. Mesiano S, Mellon SH, Jaffe RB. Mitogenic action, regulation, and localization of insulin-like growth factors in the human fetal adrenal gland. J Clin Endocrinol Metab 1993; 76:968–976.

32. Penhoat A, Chatelain PG, Jaillard C, Saez JM. Characterization of insulin-like growth factor I and insulin receptors on cultured bovine adrenal fasciculata cells. Role of these peptides on adrenal cell function. Endocrinology 1988; 122:2518–2626.

33. Pillion DJ, Arnold P, Yang M, Stockard CR, Grizzle WE. Receptors for insulin and insulin-like growth factor—I in the human adrenal gland. Biochem Biophys Res Com 1989; 165:204–211.

34. Hensen J, Buhl M, Bahr V, Oelkers W. Endocrine activity of the "silent" adrenocortical adenoma is uncovered by response to corticotropin-releasing hormone. Klin Wochenschr 1990; 68:608–614.

35. Osella G, Terzolo M, Boretta G, Magro G, Ali A, Piovesan A, et al. Endocrine evaluation of incidentally discovered adrenal masses (incidentalomas). J Clin Endocrinol Metab 1994; 79:1532–1539.

36. Herrera MF, Grant CS, van Heerden PF, Ilstrup DM. Incidentally discovered adrenal tumors: an institutional perspective. Surgery 1991; 110:1014–1021.

37. Siren JE, Haapiainen RK, Huikuri KT, Sivula AH. Incidentalomas of the adrenal gland: 36 operated patients and review of literature. World J Surg 1993; 17:634–639.

38. Ross NS, Aron DC. Hormonal evaluation of the patient with an incidentally discovered adrenal mass (see comments). N Engl J Med 1990; 323:1401–1405.

39. Samaan NA, Hickey RC, Shutts PE. Diagnosis, localization and management of pheochromocytoma. Pitfalls and follow-up in 41 patients. Cancer 1988; 62:2451–2460.

40. Bravo EL. Evolving concepts in the pathophysiology, diagnosis, and treatment of pheochromocytoma. Endocr Rev 1994; 15:356–368.

41. Beyer HS, Doe RP. Cortisol secretion by an incidentally discovered nonfunctional adrenal adenoma. J Clin Endocrinol Metab 1986; 62:1317–1321.

42. Bogner U, Eggens U, Hensen J, Oelkers W. Incidentally discovered ACTH-dependent adrenal adenoma presenting as "pre-Cushing's syndrome". Acta Endocrinol (Copenh) 1986; 111:89–92.

43. Charbonnel B, Chatal JF, Ozanne P. Does the corticoadrenal adenoma with "pre-Cushing's syndrome" exist? J Nucl Med 1981; 22:1059–1061.

44. Reincke M, Nieke J, Krestin GP, Saeger W, Allolio B, Winkelmann W. Preclinical Cushing's syndrome in adrenal "incidentalomas": comparison with adrenal Cushing's syndrome. J Clin Endocrinol Metab 1992; 75:826–832.

45. Huiras CM, Pehling GB, Caplan RH. Adrenal insufficiency after operative removal of apparently nonfunctioning adrenal adenomas. JAMA 1989; 261:894–898.

46. Young Jr WF, Hogan MJ, Klee GG, Grant CS, van Heerden JA. Primary aldosteronism: diagnosis and treatment. Mayo Clin Proc 1990; 65:96–110.

47. Flecchia D, Mazza E, Carlini M, et al. Reduced serum levels of dehydroepiandrosterone sulphate in adrenal incidentalomas: a marker of adrenocortical tumor. Clin Endocrinol 1995; 42:129–134.

48. Orentreich N, Brind JL, Rizer RL, Vogelman JH. Age changes and sex differences in serum dehydroepiandrosterone sulfate concentrations throughout adulthood. J Clin Endocrinol Metab 1984; 59:551–555.

49. Rezneck RH, Armstrong P. Imaging in endocrinology. The adrenal gland. Clin Endocrinol 1994; 40:561–576.

50. Reinig JW, Stutley JE, Leonhardt CM, Spicer KM, Margolis M, Caldwell CB. Differentiation of adrenal masses with MR imaging: comparison of techniques. Radiology 1994; 192:41–46.

51. Doppman JL, Reinig JW, Dwyer AJ, Frank JP, Norton J, Loriaux DL, et al. Differentiation of adrenal masses by magnetic resonance imaging. Surgery 1987; 102:1018–1026.

52. Baker ME, Blinder R, Spritzer C, Leight CS, Herfkens RJ, Dunnick NR. MRI evaluation of adrenal masses at 1.5 T. AJR. Am J Roentgenol 1989; 153:307–312.

53. Semelka RC, Shoenut JP, Lawrence PH, Greenberg HM, Maycher B, Madden TP, et al. Evaluation of adrenal masses with gadolinium enhancement and fat-suppressed MR imaging. J Magn Reson Imaging 1993; 3:337–343.

54. Krestin GP, Friedmann G, Fischbach R, Neufang KF, Allolio B. Evaluation of adrenal masses in oncologic patients: dynamic contrast-enhancement MR vs. CT. Comput Assist Tomogr 1991; 15:104–110.

55. Tsushima Y, Ishizaka H, Matsumoto M. Adrenal masses: differentiation with chemical shift, fast low-angle shot MR imaging. Radiology 1993; 186:705–709.

56. Hood MN, Ho VB, Smirniotopoulos JG, Szumowski J. Chemical shift: the artifact and clinical tool revisited. Radiographics 1999; 19:357–371.

57. Juhlin C, Tornblom S, Rastad J, Bergstrom M, Bonasera T, Sundin A, et al. Differential diagnosis in adrenal gland tumors using PET and 11C-metomidate. Nord Med 1998; 113:306–307.

58. Copeland PM. The incidentally discovered adrenal mass. Ann Intern Med 1983; 98:940–945.

59. Nader S, Hickey RC, Sellin RV, Samaan NA. Adrenal cortical carcinoma. A study of 77 cases. Cancer 1983; 52:707–711.

60. Art W, Reincke M, Siekmann L, Winkelmann W, Allolio B. Suramin in adrenocortical cancer: limited efficacy and serious toxicity. Clin Endocrinol 1994; 41:299–307.

61. Prinz RA, Brooks MH, Churchill R, Graner JL, Lawrence AM, Paloyan E, et al. Incidental asymptomatic adrenal masses detected by computed tomography scanning. Is operation required? JAMA 1982; 248:701–704.

62. Lewinsky BS, Grigor KM, Symington T, Neville AM. The clinical and pathologic features of "non-hormonal" adrenocortical tumors. Report of twenty new cases and review of the literature. Cancer 1974; 33:778–790.

63. Yankaskas BC, Staab EV, Craven MB, Blatt PM, Sokhandan M, Carney CN. Delayed complications from fine-needle biopsies of solid masses of the abdomen. Invest Radiol 1986; 21:325–328.

64. Silvermann SG, Mueller PR, Pinkney LP, Koenker RM, Sletzer SE. Predictive value of image-guided adrenal biopsy: analysis of results of 101 biopsies. Radiology 1993; 187:715–718.

65. McCorkell SJ, Niles NL. Fine-needle aspiration of catecholamine-producing adrenal masses: a possibly fatal mistake. Am J Roentgenol 1985; 145:113–114.

66. Casola G, Nicolet V, van Sonnenberg E, Withers C, Bretagnolle M, Saba RM, et al. Unsuspected pheochromocytoma: risk of blood-pressure alterations during percutaneous adrenal biopsy. Radiology 1986; 159:733–735.

67. Terzolo M, Osella G, Ali A, Borretta G, Cesario F, Paccotti P, et al. Subclinical Cushing's syndrome in adrenal incidentaloma. Clin Endocrinol 1998; 48:89–97.

68. Torlontano M, Chiodini I, Pileri M, Guglielmi G, Cammisa M, Modoni S, et al. Altered bone mass and turnover in female patients with adrenal incidentaloma: the effect of subclinical hypercortisolism. J Clin Endocrinol Metab 1999; 84:23,812–2385.

69. Sellschopp C. Aktuelle Probleme der Nebennierenchirurgie. In: Allolio B, Schulte HM, eds. Moderne Diagnostik und therapeutische Strategien bei Nebennieren erkrankungen. Schattauer, New York, 1990, pp. 145–151.

70. Fletcher DR, Beiles CB, Hardy KY. Laparoscopic adrenalectomy. Aust N Z J Surg 1994; 64:427–430.

71. Dralle H, Scheumann GFW, Nashan B, Brabant G. Review: recent developments in adrenal surgery. Acta chir belg 1994; 94:137–140.

72. Gnazzoni G, Montorsi F, Bergamaschi F, Rigatti P, Cornaggia G, Lanzi R, et al. Effectiveness and safety of laparascopic adrenalectomy. J Urol 1994; 152:1375–1378.

73. Smith CD, Weber CJ, Amerson JR. Laparoscopic adrenalectomy: new gold standard. World J Surg 1999; 23:389–396.

19 Congenital Adrenal Hyperplasia

21-Hydroxylase Deficiency

Maria I. New, MD

CONTENTS

INTRODUCTION

Congenital adrenal hyperplasia (CAH) is a family of autosomal recessive disorders involving impaired enzymatic function at any of the various steps in the synthesis of cortisol from cholesterol by the adrenal cortex, with excessive secretion of adrenal androgens developing as a result of the defects. Blocks in cortisol synthesis impair the negative feedback control of adrenocorticotropin (ACTH) secretion, which leads to chronic stimulation of the adrenal cortex by ACTH. The enzyme deficiencies in CAH act as a dam behind which steroid precursors accumulate, which are then shunted through uninhibited pathways and result in excessive steroidogenesis. It is primarily the excess androgens and steroid precursors that determine the clinical presentation.

Over 90% of CAH cases are caused by 21-hydroxylase deficiency (less frequent causes are 11β-hydroxylase deficiency and 3β-hydroxysteroid dehydrogenase deficiency) *(1)*, which can occur in a classical (simple virilizing or salt wasting) or a nonclassical form. In classical CAH caused by 21-hydroxylase deficiency (21-OHD), prenatal exposure of female urogenital tissues to potent androgens such as testosterone and Δ^4-androstenedione at a critical stage of differentiation results in ambiguous external

From: *Contemporary Endocrinology: Adrenal Disorders*
Edited by: A. N. Margioris and G. P. Chrousos © Humana Press, Totowa, NJ

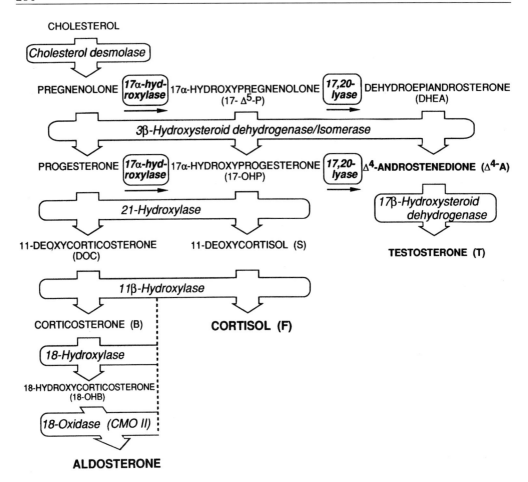

Fig. 1. Pathways of steroid biosynthesis.

genitalia in genetic females. Up to 75% of these patients will be salt wasters as well, lacking adequate aldosterone production *(2)*. In the nonclassical form of adrenal hyperplasia, patients are born with normal genitalia, and with a moderate enzyme deficiency, they present with signs of hyperandrogenism in childhood or later.

STEROIDOGENESIS

Aldosterone, cortisol, and testosterone are derived from cholesterol and utilize many of the same enzymes for their synthesis in the adrenal cortex (Fig. 1). Therefore, defects in any of the enzymes that are common to the synthesis pathway of these hormones can result in the loss of a combination of some or all of their production, or unchecked negative-feedback loops can lead to overproduction. In the case of 21-OHD, steroid precursors accumulate where the enzyme deficiency blocks their path, which then overflow into blocked biosynthetic pathways, resulting in the production of excess androgens.

The adrenal cortex produces cortisol and aldosterone by specific and largely separate regulatory systems. The cortex is divided into three distinct zones—the outer *zona*

NORMAL: ADRENOGENITAL:

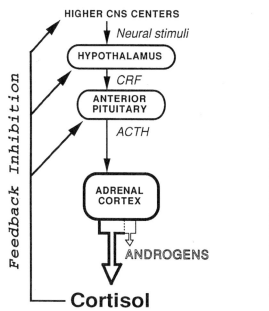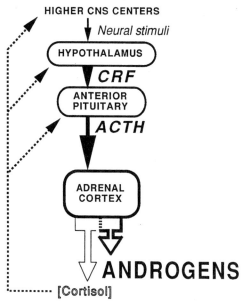

Fig. 2. Regulation of cortisol secretion in normal subjects and in patients with congenital adrenal hyperplasia. (From New MI, Levine LS. Congenital adrenal hyperplasia. In: Harris H, Hirschhorn K, eds. Advances in Human Genetics. Plenum, New York, 1973, p. 251.

glomerulosa (ZG), the middle *zona fasciculata* (ZF), and the inner *zona reticularis* (ZR)—defined by their different cellular arrangements and are functionally distinct. Mineralocorticoids are synthesized in the ZG, glococorticoids are produced by the ZF/ ZR, and androgenic steroids are synthesized in the ZR.

The production of cortisol in the ZF occurs in five steps: cleavage of the cholesterol side chain by the cholesterol desmolase enzyme, cytochrome *P450*scc, to yield pregnenolone; conversion of pregnenolone by 3β-dehydrogenation (with accompanying $\Delta^{5,4}$-isomerization) to progesterone by the short-chain dehydrogenase family enzyme 3β-hydroxysteroid dehydrogenase (3β-HSD); and successive hydroxylations at the 17α, 21, and 11β positions, each mediated by a distinct cytochrome *P450,* resulting in cortisol (Fig. 1) *(3).*

Cortisol synthesis is regulated by a negative-feedback loop in which high serum levels of cortisol inhibit the release of ACTH from the pituitary, whereas low serum levels of cortisol stimulate the release of ACTH. This defines the hypothalamo-pituitary-adrenal (HPA) axis (Fig. 2). The central nervous system (CNS) determines the hypothalamic setpoint for the plasma cortisol level, so that plasma cortisol levels lower than the hypothalamic-pituitary setpoint will increase the secretion (negative-feedback regulation). The adrenal 21-hydroxylase enzyme deficiency, causing impaired synthesis and decreased secretion of cortisol, thus leads to chronic elevations of ACTH with overstimulation and consequent hyperplasia of the adrenal cortex.

FETAL DEVELOPMENT

Without enzyme abnormalities, male genital differentiation in embryonic and fetal life is dependent on two functions of the testes *(4):* (1) the secretion from Leydig cells of sufficient quantities of testosterone (after it has undergone peripheral conversion to dihydrotestosterone [DHT]) to direct the formation of the internal male genital structures and external genitalia; and (2) the secretion from Sertoli cells of the nonsteroidal anti-Müllerian hormone (AMH) glycoprotein to suppress development of the mullerian ducts, so that normal males are born without a uterus and fallopian tubes.

Because there is no anomalous production of AMH in the gonadally normal female with CAH, and the 21-hydroxylase deficiency is only in the adrenals and not in the gonads, females presenting with even extreme virilization from DHT overexposure will have normal development of their internal reproductive structures. With proper treatment and reparative surgery of the external genitalia, childbearing is possible.

CLINICAL MANIFESTATIONS

The 21-hydroxylase deficiency syndrome presents in three forms: classical simple virilizing, classical salt-wasting, and nonclassical.

Classical Simple Virilizing

Excess adrenal androgen production coincides with the time of sexual development of the fetus and will result in varying degrees of genital ambiguity in newborn genetic females with CAH. In extreme cases, the urethra extends the full length of the phallus and cannot be distinguished from that of a normal male. In most cases, however, the excess androgens result in an enlarged clitoris with fusion of the labioscrotal folds, resulting in a urogenital sinus. For these females, the internal genitalia are normal with normal development of ovaries and müllerian structures.

Males affected with 21-OHD are born with normal genitalia. After birth, both females and males develop signs of androgen excess, such as precocious development of pubic and axillary hair, acne, phallic enlargement, rapid growth and musculoskeletal development, and advanced epiphyseal age. Though initial growth in the young child with CAH is rapid, potential height is reduced and short adult stature results because of premature epiphyseal fusion. Diagnosis is often times delayed in males, as the genital ambiguity that leads to diagnosis at birth in females is absent in males. However, even if diagnosis is not delayed and adrenal androgen excess is controlled, patients do not generally achieve their target height.

Classical Salt-Wasting

Depending on the severity of the loss of 21-hydroxylase function, adrenal aldosterone secretion may not be sufficient for sodium reabsorption by distal renal tubules. Patients with aldosterone deficiency suffer from salt-wasting 21-OHD. These patients are as virilized as those with simple virilizing 21-OHD and also have the potential of adrenal crisis (azotemia, vascular collapse, shock, and death) caused by renal salt-wasting. Adrenal crisis can occur as early as 1–4 weeks of life. Affected males are at high risk for salt-wasting adrenal crisis because their normal genitalia do not flag their condition; they are sometimes discharged from the hospital at birth without diagnosis and suffer a crisis at home.

Nonclassical

Nonclassical 21-OHD (NC21-OHD) may present at any time postnatally—in infancy, childhood, adolescence, or adulthood. Symptoms of NC21-OHD are those of androgen excess, including acne, premature development of pubic hair, advanced bone age, accelerated linear growth velocity, and, as in classical 21-OHD, reduced adult stature caused by premature epiphyseal fusion.

Females affected with NC21-OHD are born with normal genitalia, though postnatal symptoms may include hirsutism, temporal baldness, severe cystic acne, delayed menarche, menstrual irregularities, and infertility. A subset of female patients with NC21-OHD develop polycystic ovaries. Boys manifesting NC21-OHD may have early beard growth, acne, early growth spurt, premature pubic hair, an enlarged phallus, and advanced bone age resulting in short adult stature. Proportionately small testes as compared to that of the phallus is a reliable indication of adrenal androgen excess as opposed to testicular androgen excess. Adrenal androgen excess in men is not easily detectable and may only be manifested by short stature or oligozoospermia and diminished fertility.

No clinical signs are present in a limited number of males and females who are affected with NC21-OHD, as discovered during family studies. However, biochemically, they compare to affected patients.

EPIDEMIOLOGY

Analysis of CAH incidence data from almost 6.5 million newborns screened in the general population worldwide has demonstrated a consistent overall incidence of 1:15,000 live births for the severe classic form of CAH *(5–7)*. The incidence of CAH in either homogeneous or heterogeneous general populations has been as high as 1 in 7500 live births (Brazil).

The overall frequency of nonclassic 21-OHD is high. The study of Speiser et al. *(8)*, assessing the population genetics of the nonclassical disorder, found NC21-OHD to be the most common human autosomal recessive disease trait. The disease frequency in the general heterogeneous population of New York City was 1/100. The highest ethnic specific frequency was found among Ashkenazic Jews at 1/27. Other specific ethnic groups also exhibited high disease ferquency: 1/40 Hispanics, 1/50 Slavs, and 1/300 Italians. These results have also been confirmed by other reports *(9,10)*.

MOLECULAR GENETICS

The gene for adrenal 21-hydroxylase, *CYP21,* is located about 30 kb from an inactive cognate gene, *CYP21P* (P for pseudogene), on chromosome 6p in the area of *HLA* genes. The high degree of sequence similarity (96–98%) between *CYP21* and *CYP21P* permits two types of recombination events: (1) unequal crossing-over during meiosis, which results in complementary deletions/duplications of *CYP21* and the possible transmission of a null allele, and, (2) 9 noncorrespondences between the pseudogene and the coding gene *(11,12)* that, if transferred by "gene conversion," result in deleterious mutations. Deletions generally account for 20–25% of classic 21-OHD alleles, and small deletions and point mutations make up the rest.

Approx 40 mutations in the *CYP21* gene causing 21-OHD have been identified thus far *(13),* and of those, 8 mutations (9 including deletions) account for 90–95% of mutated alleles. Specific mutations may be correlated with a given degree of enzymatic compromise and the clinical form of 21-OHD *(14–20)*. The genotype for the classical form of CAH is predicted to be a severe mutation on both alleles at the 21-OH locus, with completely abolished enzymatic activity generally associated with salt wasting. The point mutation A (or C) to G near the end of Intron 2, which is the single most-frequent mutation in classic 21-OHD, causes premature splicing of the intron and a shift in the translational reading frame *(16,21)*. Most patients who are homozygous for this mutation have the salt-wasting form of the disorder *(22,23)*. One mutation in Exon 4 (I172N), specifically associated with simple virilizing 21-OHD *(24)*, has been shown using in in vitro-cell transfection assay to result in 1% of normal enzyme activity *(25)*. Adrenal production of aldosterone is normally in the range of 1/100–1/1000 that of cortisol. The very low residual activity of the I172N mutation apparently is still able to allow aldosterone synthesis and thus prevent significant salt wasting in most cases of the simple virilizing form of 21-hydroxylase deficiency.

Patients with NC21-OHD are predicted to have mild mutations on both alleles or one severe and one mild mutation of the 21-OH locus (compound heterozygote). Missense mutations in Exon 1 (P30L) and Exon 7 (V281L), which are predominantly associated with this form of the disease, reduce enzymatic activity in cultured cells to 20–50% of normal *(25)*. These patients do not have salt wasting.

In 1995, we published a study of genetic and clinical findings of over 200 patients with 21-OHD. We carefully assessed phenotypic characteristics by (1) genital status with respect to virilization in females; (2) ACTH stimulation tests to evaluate secretion of androgens and 17-hydroxyprogesterone; and (3) salt deprivation studies (whenever safe) to precisely describe the phenotype with respect to aldosterone deficiency and salt wasting. After dividing our patients into 26 mutation-identical groups, we found that in 11 groups, the genotype did not always predict the phenotype. One example of this nonconformity is the following: the V281L/Del genotype group consisted of 13 patients; while they had identical mutations, 11 were nonclassical, 1 was a simple virilizer, and 1 was a salt waster. Another example we found of nonconcordance of genotype to phenotype is illustrated in patients with Exon1 (P30L)/Intron2 (A or C to G) mutations, as some have the salt-wasting form, whereas the others have the nonclassical form. This unexplained phenotypic variability within each mutation group has important implications for prenatal diagnosis and treatment.

PRENATAL DIAGNOSIS AND TREATMENT

Prenatal diagnosis of 21-OHD has been performed for several decades *(26)*, 1995 #232). Diagnosis by 17-OHP levels and HLA serotyping were attempted, but found to be diagnostically limited and inaccurate. The method generally used at the present time is direct DNA analysis of the 21-OH gene *(CYP21)* with molecular genetic techniques.

An algorithm has been developed for prenatal diagnosis and treatment (Fig. 3). Dexamethasone (20 µg/kg/d) is administered to the pregnant mother as early as 4 wk gestation (ideally, by 8 wk gestation), blind to the affected status of the fetus, to suppress excess adrenal androgen secretion and prevent virilization should the fetus be an affected female. Diagnosis by DNA analysis requires chorionic villus sampling in the 9th to 11th wk gestation, or later, in the second trimester, by sampling of amniotic fluid cells obtained by amniocentesis (wk 15–18). The fetal DNA is then used for specific

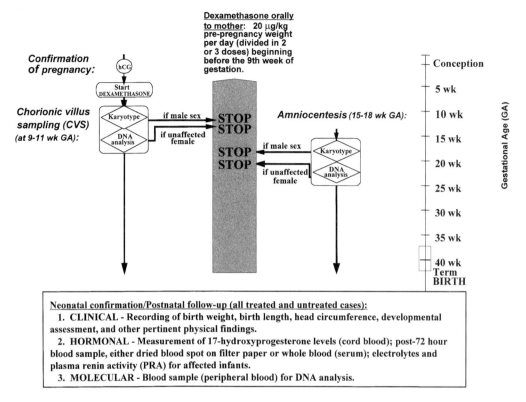

Fig. 3. Algorithm depicting prenatal management of pregnancy in families at risk for a fetus with 21-OHD.

amplification of the *CYP21* gene utilizing the polymerase chain reaction (PCR). The PCR products are dot blotted, followed by hybridization with radiolabeled allele-specific probes. We developed a method that only requires PCR with allele-specific primers, which reduces the time for prenatal diagnosis from about 2 wk to only a few days, thus allowing unnecessary prenatal treatment to be terminated promptly *(27)*.

If the fetus is determined to be a male upon karyotype or an unaffected female upon DNA analysis, treatment is discontinued. Otherwise, treatment is continued to term. When properly administered, dexamethasone is effective in preventing ambiguous genitalia in the affected female, and also is generally well-tolerated by both the mother (except for, by report, statistically greater weight gain in dexamethasone-treated mothers) and by the fetus *(28,29)*. The largest human studies have shown no congenital abnormalities and that the birth weight, birth length, and head circumference were not different in offspring of dexamethasone-treated pregnancies and those not treated *(28–31)*, provided patients and physicians adhered to the recommended therapeutic protocol. This is the first instance of an inborn metabolic error to be successfully treated prenatally.

FUTURE DIRECTIONS

As the sophistication of computers continues to grow, the ability to store large amounts of clinical data and to explore and statistically evaluate relationships between clinical and genetic variables, response to treatment, and so on, is greatly enhanced. Medical informatics encompasses all applications of computer science to medicine, and has the potential to expand the scope of clinical and molecular research, as well as to the quality of patient care. With thorough databases, we can obtain complex clinical queries that formerly were cumbersome and error-prone. Data integrity is maximized through feedback mechanisms and controled data entry. These new tools will amplify the study of genotype/phenotype correlations.

ACKNOWLEDGMENT

The author would like to express her appreciation to Laurie Vandermolen for editorial assistance.

REFERENCES

1. New MI, Dupont B, Grumbach K, Levine LS. Congenital adrenal hyperplasia and related conditions. In: Stanbury JB, Wyngaarden JB, Frederickson DS, Goldstein JL, Brown MD, eds. The Metabolic Basis of Inherited Disease. McGraw-Hill, New York, 1982, 973–1000.
2. New MI, Ghizzoni L, Speiser PW. Update on congenital adrenal hyperplasia. In: Lifshitz F, ed. Pediatric Endocrinology. Marcel Dekker, New York, 1985; 16: pp. 305–320.
3. New MI, White PC. Genetic disorders of steroid metabolism. In: R.V. Thakker, ed. Genetic and Molecular Biological Aspects of Endocrine Disease. Bailliere Tindall, London, 1995; pp. 525–554.
4. Jost A. Embryonic sexual differentiation. In: Hermaphroditism, Genital Anomalies and Related Endocrine Disorders. H.W. Jones, and W.W. Scott, eds. Wilkins & Wilkins, Baltimore, MD, 1971; p. 16.
5. Pang S, Clark A. Congenital adrenal hyperplasia due to 21-hydroxylase deficiency: Newborn screening and its relationship to the diagnosis and treatment of the disorder. Screening 1993; 2:105–139.
6. Pang S, Clark A. Newborn screening, prenatal diagnosis, and prenatal treatment of congenital adrenal hyperplasia due to 21-hydroxylase deficiency. Trends Endocrinol Metab 1990; 1:300–307.
7. Pang SY, Wallace MA, Hofman L, Thuline HC, Dorche C, Lyon IC, et al. Worldwide experience in newborn screening for classical congenital adrenal hyperplasia due to 21-hydroxylase deficiency. Pediatrics 1988; 81:866–874.
8. Speiser PW, Dupont B, Rubinstein P, Piazza A, Kastelan A, New IM. High frequency of nonclassical steroid 21-hydroxylase deficiency. Am J Hum Genet 1985; 37:650–667.
9. Sherman SL, Aston CE, Morton NE, Speiser P, New MI. A segregation and linkage study of classical and nonclassical 21-hydroxylase deficiency. Am J Hum Genet 1988; 42:830–838.
10. Zerah M, Ueshiba H, Wood E, Speiser PW, Crawford C, McDonald T, et al. Prevalence of nonclassical steroid 21-hydroxylase deficiency based on a morning salivary 17-hydroxyprogesterone screening test: a small sample study. J Clin Endocrinol Metab 1990; 70:1662–1667.
11. Higashi Y, Yoshioka H, Yamane M, Gotoh O, Fujii-Kuriyama Y. Complete nucleotide sequence of two steroid 21-hydroxylase genes tandemly arranged in human chromosome: a pseudogene and a genuine gene. Proc Natl Acad Sci USA 1986; 83:2841–2845.
12. White PC, New MI, Dupont B. Structure of the human steroid 21-hydroxylase genes. Proc Natl Acad Sci USA 1986; 83:5111–5115.
13. Krawczak M, Cooper DN. The human gene mutation database. Trends Genet 1997; 13:121–122.
14. Werkmeister JW, New MI, Dupont B, White PC. Frequent deletion and duplication of the steroid 21-hydroxylase genes. Am J Hum Genet 1986; 39:461–469.
15. Mornet E, Crete P, Kuttenn F, Raux-Demay MC, Boue J, White PC, et al. Distribution of deletions and seven point mutations on CYP21B genes in three clinical forms of steroid 21-hydroxylase deficiency. Am J Hum Genet 1991; 48:79–88.
16. Higashi Y, Hiromasa T, Tanae A, Miki T, Nakura J, Kondo T, et al. Effects of individual mutations in the P-450(C21) pseudogene on the P-450(C21) activity and their distribution in the patient genomes of congenital steroid 21-hydroxylase deficiency. J Biochem 1991; 109:638–644.
17. Speiser PW, Dupont J, Zhu D, Serrat J, Buegeleisen M, Tusie LM, et al. Disease expression and molecular genotype in congenital adrenal hyperplasia due to 21-hydroxylase deficiency. J Clin Invest 1992; 90:584–595.

18. Wedell A, Ritzen EM, Haglund SB, Luthman H. Steroid 21-hydroxylase deficiency: three additional mutated alleles and establishment of phenotype-genotype relationships of common mutations. Proc Natl Acad Sci USA 1992; 89:7232–7236.

19. White PC, Tusie-Luna MT, New MI, Speiser PW. Mutations in steroid 21-hydroxylase (CYP21). Hum Mutat 1994; 3:373–378.

20. New MI, Crawford C, Wilson RC. Genetic disorders of the adrenal steroidogenic enzymes. In: AEH Emery and D Rimoin, eds. Principles and Practice of Medical Genetics. Churchill Livingstone, New York, 1996; pp. 1441–1476.

21. Higashi Y, Tanae A, Inoue H, Hiromasa T, Fujii-Kuriyama Y. Aberrant splicing and missense mutations cause steroid 21-hydroxylase [P-450(C21)] deficiency in humans: possible gene conversion products. Proc Natl Acad Sci USA 1988; 85:7486–7490.

22. Speiser PW, New MI, Tannin GM, Pickering D, Yang SY, White PC. Genotype of Yupik Eskomos with congenital adrenal hyperplasia due to 21-hydroxylase deficiency. Hum Genet 1992; 88:647,648.

23. Wilson RC, Mercado AB, Cheng KC, New MI. Steroid 21-hydroxylase deficiency: genotype may not predict phenotype. J Clin Endocrinol Metab 1995; 80:2322–2329.

24. Amor M, Parker KL, Globerman H, New MI, White PC. Mutation in the CYP21B gene (Ile-172-Asn) causes steroid 21-hydroxylase deficiency. Proc Natl Acad Sci USA 1988; 85:1600–1607.

25. Tusie-Luna M, Traktman P, White PC. Determination of functional effects of mutations in the steroid 21-hydroxylase gene (CYP21) using recombinant vaccinia virus. J Biolog Chem 1990; 265:20,916–20,922.

26. Speiser PW, New MI. Prenatal diagnosis and treatment of congenital adrenal hyperplasia. J Pediatr Endocrinol 1994; 7:183–191.

27. Wilson RC, Wei JQ, Cheng KC, Mercado AB, New MI. Rapid DNA analysis by allele-specific PCR for detection of mutations in the steroid 21-hydroxylase gene. J Clin Endocrinol Metab 1995; 80:1635–1640.

28. Mercado AB, Wilson RC, Cheng KC, Wei JQ, New MI. Extensive personal experience: Prenatal treatment and diagnosis of congenital adrenal hyperplasia owing to steroid 21-hydroxylase deficiency. J Clin Endocrinol Metab 1995; 80:2014–2020.

29. Carlson AD, Obeid JS, Kanellopoulou N, Wilson RC, New MI. Congenital adrenal hyperplasia: update on prenatal diagnosis and treatment. In: F Labrie, ed. Xth International Congress on Hormonal Steroids. J Steroid Biochem Mol Biol, Quebec, Canada, June 17–20, 1998; 69:19–29.

30. Forest MG, Betuel H, David M. Prenatal treatment in congenital adrenal hyperplasia due to 21-hydroxylase deficiency: update 88 of the French multicentric study. Endocr Rers 1989; 15:277–301.

31. Forest MG, David M, Morel Y. Prenatal diagnosis and treatment of 21-hydroxylase deficiency. [Review]. J Steroid Biochem Molec Biol 1993; 45:75–82.

20 Steroid 11β-Hydroxylase Deficiency

Perrin C. White

CONTENTS

INTRODUCTION
STEROID 11β-HYDROXYLASE ISOZYMES
REGULATION OF CYP11B1
BIOCHEMICAL ABNORMALITIES IN 11β-HYDROXYLASE
    DEFICIENCY
CLINICAL PRESENTATION
THERAPY
GENETIC ANALYSIS
REFERENCES

INTRODUCTION

Inherited defects in cortisol biosynthesis are collectively termed congenital adrenal hyperplasia [reviewed in *(1)*]. Steroid 21-hydroxylase deficiency is, by far, the most common of these defects; it is reviewed elsewhere in this volume. This chapter reviews a related disease, steroid 11β-hydroxylase deficiency [reviewed in greater detail in *(2)*].

The steroidogenic defects that cause congenital adrenal hyperplasia are often considered to occur in "classic" forms that are apparent at birth and in milder "nonclassic" forms that either remain asymptomatic or present with signs of androgen excess during childhood or at puberty. Both forms of 11β-hydroxylase deficiency will be discussed.

Whereas more than 90% of patients with classic congenital adrenal hyperplasia have 21-hydroxylase deficiency (*see* Chapter 22), 11β-hydroxylase deficiency comprises approx 5–8% of cases in most populations *(3)* and thus occurs in approx 1 in 200,000 births. A large number of cases of 11β-hydroxylase deficiency has been reported in Israel among Jewish immigrants from Morocco, a relatively inbred population. The incidence in this group is currently estimated to be 1/5000–1/7000 births *(4)*.

STEROID 11β-HYDROXYLASE ISOZYMES

Cortisol is synthesized from cholesterol in the *zona fasciculata* of the adrenal cortex. This process requires five enzymatic conversions (*see* Chapter 5): cleavage of the cholesterol side chain to yield pregnenolone, 17GRα-hydroxylation and 3β-dehydrogenation to 17-hydroxyprogesterone, and successive hydroxylations at the 21 and 11β

From: *Contemporary Endocrinology: Adrenal Disorders*
Edited by: A. N. Margioris and G. P. Chrousos © Humana Press, Totowa, NJ

positions. A "17-deoxy" pathway is also active in the *zona fasciculata,* in which 17-hydroxylation does not occur and the final product is normally corticosterone.

The same 17-deoxy pathway is active in the adrenal *zona glomerulosa,* which contains no 17-hydroxylase activity. However, corticosterone is not the final product in the *zona glomerulosa;* instead, corticosterone is successively hydroxylated and oxidized at the 18 position to yield aldosterone.

Whereas the cholesterol side-chain cleavage, 3β-dehydrogenase, and 21-hydroxylase steps are each catalyzed by the same enzyme in the *zonae fasciculata* and *glomerulosa,* humans have two 11β-hydroxylase isozymes that are, respectively, responsible for cortisol and aldosterone biosynthesis, CYP11B1 (P450c11, 11β-hydroxylase) and CYP11B2 (P450c18, P450cmo, P450aldo, or aldosterone synthase). These isozymes are mitochondrial cytochromes *P450* located in the inner membrane on the matrix side. Each is synthesized with 503 amino acid residues, but a signal peptide is cleaved in mitochondria to yield the mature protein of 479 residues *(5).* The sequences of the proteins are 93% identical *(6).*

The CYP11B1 isozyme 11β-hydroxylates 11-deoxycorticosterone to corticosterone and 11-deoxycortisol to cortisol, as determined by expressing the corresponding cDNAs in cultured cells *(7–9)* and after actual purification from aldosterone secreting tumors *(10).* It 18-hydroxylates corticosterone poorly and has no 18-oxidase activity. In contrast, *CYP11B2* has strong 11β-hydroxylase activity, but also 18-hydroxylates and then 18-oxidizes corticosterone to aldosterone. Only two amino acid residues are responsible for the differences in activities of these isozymes; changing Ser-288 to Gly and Val-320 to Ala is sufficient to confer 18-oxidase activity on CYP11B1 *(11).*

In humans, CYP11B1 and CYP11B2 are encoded by two genes *(6)* on chromosome 8q21–q22 *(12,13)* (Fig. 1). Each contains nine exons spread over approx 7000 basepairs (7 kb) of DNA. The nucleotide sequences of these genes are 95% identical in coding sequences and about 90% identical in introns. The two genes are approx 40-kb apart *(14,15)* and *CYP11B2* is on the left if the genes are pictured as being transcribed left to right.

REGULATION OF *CYP11B1*

Cortisol synthesis is primarily controled by ACTH (corticotropin) *(16),* which acts through a specific G-protein-coupled receptor *(17)* to increase levels of cAMP (adenosine 3′,5′ monophosphate). Cyclic AMP has short-term (minutes to hours) effects on cholesterol side-chain cleavage activity, but longer-term (hours to days) effects on transcription of genes encoding the enzymes required to synthesize cortisol *(18).* The transcriptional effects occur at least in part through increased activity of protein kinase A *(19),* which phosphorylates transcriptional regulatory factors.

The human *CYP11B1* gene is expressed at high levels in normal adrenal glands *(6),* and transcription of this gene is appropriately regulated by cAMP *(20).* The 5′ flanking region of the gene includes *(6)* a TATA box variant, a palindromic cAMP response element, and several recognition sites for steroidogenic factor-1 (SF-1). SF-1 sites appear in the regulatory regions of all steroid hydroxylase genes expressed in the adrenal cortex and the gonads *(21,22).* Although the human transcriptional regulatory region has not yet been analyzed in detail, all of these sequences are required for

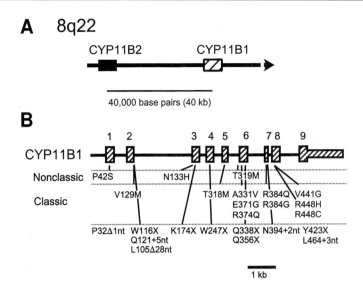

Fig. 1. Mutations involving the 11β-hydroxylase (CYP11B1) gene. **A,** the location of the CYP11B1 genes is diagramed, relative to the aldosterone synthase (CYP11B2) gene. **B,** mutations in CYP11B1 causing nonclassic or classic 11β-hydroxylase deficiency. These are arranged in the diagram so that those causing increasing enzymatic compromise are arrayed from top to bottom. Dotted lines divide mutants into groups with similar activities. As an example of mutation terminology, P42S is Proline-42 to Serine. Δ, deletion, +, insertion. Other single letter amino acid codes: A, alanine; C, cysteine; D, aspartic acid; E, glutamic acid; F, phenylalanine; G, glycine; H, histidine; I, isoleucine; K, lysine; L, leucine; M, methionine; N, asparagine; P, proline, Q, glutamine; R, arginine; S, serine; T, threonine; V, valine; W, tryptophan; Y, tyrosine.

normal transcription of murine and bovine *CYP11B* genes *(23–26)*. Factors binding TATA boxes *(27)* and cAMP response elements *(28)* have previously been identified. SF-1 (also called Ad4BP) is an orphan nuclear receptor that is required for steroidogenic gene expression in the adrenal cortex and the gonads *(29,30)*.

BIOCHEMICAL ABNORMALITIES IN 11β-HYDROXYLASE DEFICIENCY

In 11β-hydroxylase deficiency, 11-deoxycortisol (compound S) and deoxycorticosterone are not efficiently converted to cortisol and corticosterone, respectively. Decreased production of glucocorticoids results in poor feedback inhibition on the hypothalamus and anterior pituitary, causing increased secretion of ACTH. This stimulates the *zona fasciculata* of the adrenal cortex to overproduce steroid precursors proximal to the blocked 11β-hydroxylase step. A large proportion of these precursors is excreted in the urine as tetrahydro metabolites, but some are shunted (through the activity of 17-hydroxylase/17,20-lyase) into the pathway of androgen biosynthesis.

Therefore, the specific hormonal diagnosis of 11β-hydroxylase deficiency can be made by detecting high basal or ACTH-stimulated levels of deoxycorticosterone and/or 11-deoxycortisol in the serum, or increased excretion of the tetrahydro-metabolites of these compounds in a 24-h urine collection. Although most classic cases of 11β-hydroxylase deficiency will have greatly elevated levels of both of these hormones, some patients will have selective elevation of either one alone *(3)*. Urinary 17-ketosteroids are also elevated, reflecting increased shunting of precursors into the sex-steroid pathway. Possibly because deoxycorticosterone and certain metabolites are mineralocorticoid agonists, plasma renin activity is usually suppressed in older children and levels of aldosterone are consequently low even though the ability to synthesize aldosterone is actually unimpaired *(31)*. The diagnosis of 11β-hydroxylase deficiency may be missed in neonates, who often lack the diagnostic features of hypertension and suppressed renin. Another potential source of error is that mild to moderate elevations of 17-hydroxyprogesterone are often detected, and if deoxycorticosterone and 11-deoxycortisol are not specifically measured, an erroneous diagnosis of 21-hydroxylase deficiency is possible *(32)*.

Obligate heterozygous carriers of 11β-hydroxylase deficiency alleles (e.g., parents) have no consistent biochemical abnormalities detectable even after stimulation of the adrenal cortex with intravenous ACTH *(33)*. This is in contrast to carriers of 21-hydroxylase deficiency alleles, who usually have mildly elevated serum levels of the substrate, 17-hydroxyprogesterone, demonstrable in serum samples taken after administration of corticotropin *(34)*.

Appropriate biochemical criteria for diagnosis of nonclassic 11β-hydroxylase deficiency have not been established. It has been suggested that the diagnosis should be suspected in patients with ACTH-stimulated levels of 11-deoxycortisol that are >3 times the 95th percentile for age *(35,36)*. As discussed below, this criterion is probably not sufficiently stringent and leads to false positive diagnoses.

CLINICAL PRESENTATION

Androgen Excess

Females affected with classic 11β-hydroxylase deficiency are born with masculinization of their external genitalia similar to that seen in females affected with 21-hydroxylase deficiency. Clitoromegaly may occasionally be so severe as to be indistinguishable from a normal male penis *(4,37,38)*. The urethral and genital openings move anteriorly and may fuse into a urogenital sinus. Depending on the severity of masculinization, this sinus may open on the perineum, at the base of the phallus, or even at the tip of the glans. Additionally, the labioscrotal folds fuse partially or completely; if fusion is complete, the resulting structure is indistinguishable from the male scrotum although, of course, testes are not present. Because their external genitalia can be very difficult to distinguish from those of a cryptorchid male, affected females have occasionally been reared to adulthood as males.

In contrast to the external genitalia, the gonads and the internal genital structures (Fallopian tubes, uterus, and cervix) arising from Müellerian ducts are normal in affected females because the substance that normally causes involution of these structures in males, Müellerian inhibitory factor, is not produced by the fetal ovary *(39)*. Therefore, affected females have intact reproductive potential if their external genital abnormalities are corrected surgically and excessive adrenal androgen secretion is controlled with glucocorticoids. For this reason, affected females will usually be reared from infancy as girls even if the degree of masculinization of the external genitalia is severe.

Other signs of androgen excess that occur postnatally include rapid somatic growth in childhood and accelerated skeletal maturation leading to premature closure of the epiphyses and short adult stature. Additionally, patients may have premature development of sexual and body hair (premature adrenarche) and acne. Androgens may affect the hypothalamic-pituitary-gonadal (HPA) axis leading to amenorrhea or oligomenorrhea in females and true precocious puberty or, conversely, poor spermatogenesis in males *(40)*.

Patients with nonclassic 11β-hydroxylase deficiency are born with normal genitalia (some affected females may have mild clitoromegaly) and present with signs and symptoms of androgen excess as children. Previously asymptomatic adult women may present with hirsutism and oligomenorrhea *(41–44)*. This clinical presentation is similar to that of nonclassic 21-hydroxylase deficiency.

Mineralocorticoid Excess

Because the 11β-hydroxylation step required for aldosterone biosynthesis is mediated by a distinct isozyme, CYP11B2, signs of aldosterone deficiency are rarely seen. Instead, approximately two-thirds of patients with the severe, "classic" form of 11β-hydroxylase deficiency have high blood pressure *(4,45)*, often beginning in the first few years of life *(46)*. Although the hypertension is usually of mild to moderate severity, left ventricular hypertrophy and/or retinopathy have been observed in up to one-third of patients, and deaths from cerebrovascular accidents have been reported *(4,47)*. Other signs of mineralocorticoid excess such as hypokalemia and muscle weakness or cramping occur in a minority of patients and are not well correlated with blood pressure. Plasma renin activity is usually suppressed and levels of aldosterone are consequently low even though the ability to synthesize aldosterone is actually unimpaired.

The cause of hypertension in 11β-hydroxylase deficiency is not well understood. It might be assumed that it is caused by elevated serum levels of deoxycorticosterone, but blood pressure and deoxycorticosterone levels are poorly correlated in patients *(3,45)*. In addition, this steroid has only weak mineralocorticoid activity when administered to humans or other animals. Perhaps other metabolites of deoxycorticosterone are responsible for the development of hypertension. The 18-hydroxy and 19-nor metabolites of deoxycorticosterone are thought to be more potent mineralocorticoids *(48)*, but consistent elevation of these steroids in 11β-hydroxylase deficiency has not been documented. Moreover, synthesis of these steroids requires hydroxylations within the adrenal (19-nor-deoxycorticosterone is synthesized via 19-hydroxy and 19-oic intermediates) that are probably mediated primarily by CYP11B1 *(49)*. This is unlikely to take place efficiently in 11β-hydroxylase deficiency.

Patients with mild ("late onset" or "nonclassic") 11β-hydroxylase deficiency have normal or, at most, mildly elevated blood pressure *(3,50)*.

THERAPY

Glucocorticoid administration replaces cortisol and thus reduces ACTH secretion, suppressing excessive adrenal androgen production and preventing further virilization. It should be utilized in all patients with classic 11β-hydroxylase deficiency and in nonclassic patients with significant signs of androgen excess. Such therapy should also suppress ACTH-dependent production of mineralocorticoid agonists in patients with hypertension. Overdosing should be avoided because it may cause Cushing's syndrome. Oral hydrocortisone is most often used for maintenance therapy in children because it is identical to the endogenous glucocorticoid, cortisol. The usual mode of treatment is with 10–20 mg/m^2/d (average dose approx 15 mg/m^2/d) in divided doses. If epiphyseal maturation is complete, the regimen may be changed to a longer acting agent such as prednisone or dexamethasone.

Abnormal external genitalia in females with the classic form of the disease should be reconstructed with clitoral recession and vaginoplasty (51,52).

Although glucocorticoids should also suppress excessive production of mineralocorticoids, adjunctive antihypertensive drugs may be required if hypertension has been long-standing prior to treatment. Calcium channel blockers represent first-line therapy, as these drugs are effective in the treatment of hypertension in primary aldosteronism (53) and in low-renin essential hypertension (54). In contrast, angiotensin-converting enzyme (ACE) inhibitors (effective in high or normal renin hypertension) do not mitigate sodium retention or hypertension in the face of exogenously administered mineralocorticoids (55) and are, thus, less likely to be helpful.

GENETIC ANALYSIS

Deficiency of 11β-hydroxylase results from mutations in *CYP11B1*. Mutations in *CYP11B2* cause aldosterone deficiency, and recombinations between *CYP11B1* and *CYP11B2* lead to abnormal regulation of aldosterone biosynthesis, a condition termed glucocorticoid suppressible hyperaldosteronism. These conditions are reviewed elsewhere in this volume.

At this time, 20 mutations in *CYP11B1* have been identified in patients with classic 11β-hydroxylase deficiency (56–60). In Moroccan Jews, a group that has a high prevalence of 11β-hydroxylase deficiency, almost all affected alleles carry the same mutation, *Arg*-448 to *His* (R448H) (56). This probably represents a founder effect, but this mutation has occurred independently in other ethnic groups, and another mutation of the same residue (R448C) has also been reported (60). This apparent mutational "hotspot" contains a CpG dinucleotide. Such dinucleotides are prone to methylation of the cytosine followed by deamidation to TpG; several other mutations in *CYP11B1* (T318M, R374Q, R384Q) are of this type.

These and almost all other missense mutations identified thus far are in regions of known functional importance 6162 (63) and abolish enzymatic activity (58). For example, R448 is adjacent to *Cys-450,* which is a ligand of the heme iron atom of this cytochrome *P450* enzyme. T318M (*Thr-318* to *Met*) modifies an absolutely conserved residue that is thought to be critical for proton transfer to the bound-oxygen molecule (63). E371G (*Glu-371* to *Gly*) and R374Q (*Arg-374* to *Gln*) also mutate highly conserved residues and may affect binding of adrenodoxin. R384Q is in a region that may form part of the substrate binding pocket (63). Almost all *P450*s have a basic residue (H15 or Arg) at this or the immediately adjacent position (61). Finally, V441G (*Val-441* to *Gly*) is adjacent to the highly conserved heme binding region, and this mutation may change the secondary structure of the protein.

Other mutations found in patients with the classic form of the disease are nonsense or frameshift mutations that also abolish enzymatic activity. One, a nonsense mutation of *Trp-247* (W247X) has been identified in several unrelated kindreds in Austria and also probably represents a founder effect (60).

Although patients with the classic form of the disease apparently completely lack 11β-hydroxylase activity, they differ significantly in the severity of the various signs and symptoms of their disease. There is not a strong correlation between severity of hypertension and biochemical parameters such as plasma levels of the 11β-hydroxylase substrates, deoxycortisol and deoxycorticosterone, and urinary excretion of tetrahydrodeoxycortisol *(4,56)*. Moreover, there is no consistent correlation between the severity of hypertension and degree of virilization. These phenotypic variations must be governed by factors outside the *CYP11B1* locus.

Thus far, five patients with putative nonclassic 11β-hydroxylase deficiency have been genetically analyzed *(64)*. Three patients were diagnosed in childhood because of advanced bone age, accelerated growth, acne, and precocious adrenarche. Two of these were found to be compound heterozygotes for different mutations. One patient carried two missense mutations, *Asn-133* to *His* (N133H) and *Thr-319* to *Met* (T319M), whereas the other carried a nonsense mutation, *Tyr-423* to *Stop* (Y423X), and a missense mutation, *Pro-42* to *Ser* (P42S).

Recombinant enzymes carrying each of the three missense mutations were partially active when expressed in cultured cells; the nonsense mutation was presumed to destroy enzymatic activity. One male did not have any mutations detected, and the genetic basis for his disease is not known.

Thus, nonclassic 11β-hydroxylase deficiency is associated with missense mutations that decrease, but do not destroy enzymatic activity. Patients can carry either two such mutations or a mutation on one chromosome that encodes a partially active enzyme and a mutation on the other chromosome that encodes an inactive enzyme. Patients with two chromosomes encoding inactive enzymes have the classic form of the disease. The same correspondence between genotype and phenotype is seen in 21-hydroxylase deficiency.

No mutations were detected in two patients aged 32 and 25 yr who were participants in a study screening for CAH in hyperandrogenic women. Both patients had 11-deoxycortisol levels after ACTH stimulation that were >3 times the upper limit of normal, and thus this diagnostic criterion is insufficiently stringent. The patients with true nonclassic 11β-hydroxylase deficiency had 11-deoxycortisol levels >5 times the upper limit of normal, and this threshold should be used in diagnosing this disorder.

The frequency of nonclassic 11β-hydroxylase deficiency is not known. Few cases have been published, suggesting that it is rare, but many cases may not be ascertained because the signs of androgen excess are mild. Nevertheless, nonclassic 11β-hydroxylase deficiency is clearly not a significant cause of androgen excess in adult women. The two women with possible nonclassic 11β-hydroxylase deficiency in whom we found no mutations were the only such subjects identified in a study of 260 women with signs and symptoms of hyperandrogenism *(65)*.

Thus, genuine nonclassic 11β-hydroxylase deficiency must account for much less than 1% of cases of hyperandrogenism in women. In contrast, a large proportion (30–87%) of women with hyperandrogenism have mildly elevated (>95th percentile) levels of 11-deoxycortisol *(65–67)*. They also have elevated levels of cortisol and adrenal androgens, suggesting that they are in a state of adrenocortical hyperactivity. This apparently does not usually involve a discrete defect in steroid biosynthesis.

REFERENCES

1. White PC. Genetic diseases of steroid metabolism. Vitam Horm 1994; 49:131–195.
2. White PC, Curnow KM, Pascoe L. Disorders of steroid 11 beta hydroxylase isozymes. Endocr Rev 1994; 15:421–438.
3. Zachmann M, Tassinari D, Prader A. Clinical and biochemical variability of congenital adrenal hyperplasia due to 11 beta-hydroxylase deficiency. A study of 25 patients. J Clin Endocrinol Metab 1983; 56:222–229.
4. Rosler A, Leiberman E, Cohen T. High frequency of congenital adrenal hyperplasia (classic 11 beta-hydroxylase deficiency) among Jews from Morocco. Am J Med Genet 1992; 42:827–834.
5. Yanagibashi K, Haniu M, Shively JE, Shen WH, Hall P. The synthesis of aldosterone by the adrenal cortex. Two zones (fasciculata and glomerulosa) possess one enzyme for 11 beta-, 18-hydroxylation, and aldehyde synthesis. J Biol Chem 1986; 261:3556–3562.
6. Mornet E, Dupont J, Vitek A, White PC. Characterization of two genes encoding human steroid 11 beta-hydroxylase (P-450(11) beta). J Biol Chem 1989; 264:20,961–20,967.
7. Kawamoto T, Mitsuuchi Y, Toda K, Yokoyama Y, Miyahara K, Miura S, et al. Role of steroid 11 beta-hydroxylase and steroid 18-hydroxylase in the biosynthesis of glucocorticoids and mineralocorticoids in humans. Proc Natl Acad Sci USA 1992; 89:1458–1462.
8. Curnow KM, Tusie-Luna MT, Pascoe L, Natarajan R, Gu JL, Nadler JL, et al. The product of the CYP11B2 gene is required for aldosterone biosynthesis in the human adrenal cortex. Mol Endocrinol 1991; 5:1513–1522.
9. Kawamoto T, Mitsuuchi Y, Ohnishi T, Ichikawa Y, Yokoyama Y, Sumitomo H, et al. Cloning and expression of cDNA for human cytochrome P-450aldo as related to primary aldosteronism. Biochem Biophys Res Commun 1990; 173:309–316.
10. Ogishima T, Shibata H, Shimada H, Mitani F, Suzuki H, Saruta T, et al. Aldosterone synthase cytochrome P-450 expressed in the adrenals of patients with primary aldosteronism. J Biol Chem 1991; 266:10,731–10,734.
11. Curnow KM, Mulatero P, Emeric-Blanchouin N, Aupetit-Faisant B, Corvol P, Pascoe L. The amino acid substitutions Ser288Gly and Val320Ala convert the cortisol producing enzyme, CYP11B1, into an aldosterone producing enzyme [letter]. Nat Struct Biol 1997; 4:32–35.
12. Chua SC, Szabo P, Vitek A, Grzeschik KH, John M, White PC. Cloning of cDNA encoding steroid 11 beta-hydroxylase (P450c11). Proc Natl Acad Sci USA 1987; 84:7193–7197.
13. Wagner MJ, Ge Y, Siciliano M, Wells DE. A hybrid cell mapping panel for regional localization of probes to human chromosome 8. Genomics 1991; 10:114–125.
14. Pascoe L, Curnow KM, Slutsker L, Connell JM, Speiser PW, New MI, et al. Glucocorticoid-suppressible hyperaldosteronism results from hybrid genes created by unequal crossovers between CYP11B1 and CYP11B2. Proc Natl Acad Sci USA 1992; 89:8327–8331.
15. Lifton RP, Dluhy RG, Powers M, Rich GM, Gutkin M, Fallo F, et al. Hereditary hypertension caused by chimaeric gene duplications and ectopic expression of aldosterone synthase. Nat Genet 1992; 2:66–74.
16. Waterman MR, Simpson ER. Regulation of steroid hydroxylase gene expression is multifactorial in nature. Recent Prog Horm Res 1989; 45:533–563.
17. Mountjoy KG, Robbins LS, Mortrud MT, Cone RD. The cloning of a family of genes that encode the melanocortin receptors. Science 1992; 257:1248–1251.
18. John ME, John MC, Boggaram V, Simpson ER, Waterman MR. Transcriptional regulation of steroid hydroxylase genes by corticotropin. Proc Natl Acad Sci USA 1986; 83:4715–4719.
19. Wong M, Rice DA, Parker KL, Schimmer BP. The roles of cAMP and cAMP-dependent protein kinase in the expression of cholesterol side chain cleavage and steroid 11 beta-hydroxylase genes in mouse adrenocortical tumor cells. J Biol Chem 1989; 264:12867–12871.
20. Kawamoto T, Mitsuuchi Y, Toda K, Miyahara K, Yokoyama Y, Nakao K, et al. Cloning of cDNA and genomic DNA for human cytochrome P-45011 beta. FEBS Lett 1990; 269:345–349.
21. Morohashi K, Honda S, Inomata Y, Handa H, Omura T. A common transacting factor, Ad4-binding protein, to the promoters of steroidogenic P-450s. J Biol Chem 1992; 267:17913–17919.
22. Rice DA, Mouw AR, Bogerd AM, Parker KL. A shared promoter element regulates the expression of three steroidogenic enzymes. Mol Endocrinol 1991; 5:1552–1561.
23. Hashimoto T, Morohashi K, Takayama K, Honda S, Wada T, Handa H, et al. Cooperative transcription

activation between Adl, a CRE-like element, and other elements in the CYP11B gene promoter. J Biochem (Tokyo) 1992; 112:573–575.

24. Honda S, Morohashi K, Omura T. Novel cAMP regulatory elements in the promoter region of bovine P-450(11 beta) gene. J Biochem (Tokyo) 1990; 108:1042–1049.

25. Mouw AR, Rice DA, Meade JC, Chua SC, White PC, Schimmer BP, et al. Structural and functional analysis of the promoter region of the gene encoding mouse steroid 11 beta-hydroxylase. J Biol Chem 1989; 264:1305–1309.

26. Rice DA, Aitken LD, Vandenbark GR, Mouw AR, Franklin A, Schimmer BP, et al. A cAMP-responsive element regulates expression of the mouse steroid 11 beta-hydroxylase gene. J Biol Chem 1989; 264:14011–14015.

27. Kao CC, Lieberman PM, Schmidt MC, Zhou Q, Pei R, Berk AJ. Cloning of a transcriptionally active human TATA binding factor. Science 1990; 248:1646–1650.

28. Meyer TE, Habener JF. Cyclic adenosine 3′,5′-monophosphate response element binding protein (CREB) and related transcription-activating deoxyribonucleic acid-binding proteins. Endocr Rev 1993; 14:269–290.

29. Lala DS, Rice DA, Parker KL. Steroidogenic factor I, a key regulator of steroidogenic enzyme expression, is the mouse homolog of fushi tarazu-factor I. Mol Endocrinol 1992; 6:1249–1258.

30. Honda S, Morohashi K, Nomura M, Takeya H, Kitajima M, Omura T. Ad4BP regulating steroidogenic P-450 gene is a member of steroid hormone receptor superfamily. J Biol Chem 1993; 268:7494–7502.

31. Levine LS, Rauh W, Gottesdiener K, Chow D, Gunczler P, Rapaport R, et al. New studies of the 11 beta-hydroxylase and 18-hydroxylase enzymes in the hypertensive form of congenital adrenal hyperplasia. J Clin Endocrinol Metab 1980; 50:258–263.

32. Honour JW, Anderson JM, Shackleton CH. Difficulties in the diagnosis of congenital adrenal hyperplasia in early infancy: the 11 beta-hydroxylase defect. Acta Endocrinol (Copenh) 1983; 103:101–109.

33. Pang S, Levine LS, Lorenzen F, Chow D, Pollack M, Dupont B, et al. Hormonal studies in obligate heterozygotes and siblings of patients with 11 beta-hydroxylase deficiency congenital adrenal hyperplasia. J Clin Endocrinol Metab 1980; 50:586–589.

34. New MI, Lorenzen F, Lerner AJ, Kohn B, Oberfield SE, Pollack MS, et al. Genotyping steroid 21-hydroxylase deficiency: hormonal reference data. J Clin Endocrinol Metab 1983; 57:320–326.

35. Lashansky G, Saenger P, Dimartino-Nardi J, Gautier T, Mayes D, Berg G, et al. Normative data for the steroidogenic response of mineralocorticoids and their precursors to adrenocorticotropin in a healthy pediatric population. J Clin Endocrinol Metab 1992; 75:1491–1496.

36. Lashansky G, Saenger P, Fishman K, Gautier T, Mayes D, Berg G, et al. Normative data for adrenal steroidogenesis in a healthy pediatric population: age- and sex-related changes after adrenocorticotropin stimulation. J Clin Endocrinol Metab 1991; 73:674–686.

37. Harinarayan CV, Ammini AC, Karmarkar MG, Prakash V, Gupta R, Taneja N, et al. Congenital adrenal hyperplasia and complete masculinization masquarading as sexual precocity and cryptorchidism. Indian Pediatr 1992; 29:103–106.

38. Bistritzer T, Sack J, Eshkol A, Zur H, Katznelson D. Sex reassignment in a girl with 11 beta-hydroxylase deficiency. Isr J Med Sci 1984; 20:55–58.

39. Donahoe PK. Mullerian inhibiting substance in reproduction and cancer. Mol Reprod Dev 1992; 32:168–172.

40. Hochberg Z, Schechter J, Benderly A, Leiberman E, Rosler A. Growth and pubertal development in patients with congenital adrenal hyperplasia due to 11-beta-hydroxylase deficiency. Am J Dis Child 1985; 139:771–776.

41. Birnbaum MD, Rose LI. Late onset adrenocortical hydroxylase deficiencies associated with menstrual dysfunction. Obstet Gynecol 1984; 63:445–451.

42. Lucky AW, Rosenfield RL, McGuire J, Rudy S, Helke J. Adrenal androgen hyperresponsiveness to adrenocorticotropin in women with acne and/or hirsutism: adrenal enzyme defects and exaggerated adrenarche. J Clin Endocrinol Metab 1986; 62:840–848.

43. Cathelineau G, Brerault JL, Fiet J, Julien R, Dreux C, Canivet J. Adrenocortical 11 beta-hydroxylation defect in adult women with postmenarchial onset of symptoms. J Clin Endocrinol Metab 1980; 51:287–291.

44. Brodie BL, Wentz AC. Late onset congenital adrenal hyperplasia: a gynecologist's perspective. Fertil Steril 1987; 48:175–188.

45. Rosler A, Leiberman E, Sack J, Landau H, Benderly A, Moses SW, et al. Clinical variability of congenital adrenal hyperplasia due to 11 beta-hydroxylase deficiency. Hormone Res 1982; 16:133–141.

46. Mimouni M, Kaufman H, Roitman A, Morag C, Sadan N. Hypertension in a neonate with 11 beta-hydroxylase deficiency. Eur J Pediatr 1985; 143:231–233.

47. Hague WM, Honour JW. Malignant hypertension in congenital adrenal hyperplasia due to 11 beta-hydroxylase deficiency. Clin Endocrinol (Oxf) 1983; 18:505–510.

48. Griffing GT, Dale SL, Holbrook MM, Melby JC. 19-nor-deoxycorticosterone excretion in primary aldosteronism and low renin hypertension. J Clin Endocrinol Metab 1983; 56:218–221.

49. Ohta M, Fujii S, Ohnishi T, Okamoto M. Production of 19-oic-11-deoxycorticosterone from 19-oxo-11-deoxycorticosterone by cytochrome P-450(11)beta and nonenzymatic production of 19-nor-11-deoxycorticosterone from 19-oic-11-deoxycorticosterone. J Steroid Biochem 1988; 29:699–707.

50. de Simone G, Tommaselli AP, Rossi R, Valentino R, Lauria R, Scopacasa F, et al. Partial deficiency of adrenal 11-hydroxylase. A possible cause of primary hypertension. Hypertension. 1985; 7:204–210.

51. Donahoe PK, Powell DM, Lee MM. Clinical management of intersex abnormalities. Curr Probl Surg 1991; 28:513–579.

52. Mulaikal RM, Migeon CJ, Rock JA. Fertility rates in female patients with congenital adrenal hyperplasia due to 21-hydroxylase deficiency. N Engl J Med 1987; 316:178–182.

53. Nadler JL, Hsueh W, Horton R. Therapeutic effect of calcium channel blockade in primary aldosteronism. J Clin Endocrinol Metab 1985; 60:896–899.

54. Resnick LM, Nicholson JP, Laragh JH. Calcium, the renin-aldosterone system, and the hypotensive response to nifedipine. Hypertension 1987; 10:254–258.

55. Biollaz J, Durr J, Brunner HR, Porchet M, Gavras H. Escape from mineralocorticoid excess: the role of angiotensin II. J Clin Endocrinol Metab 1982; 54:1187–1193.

56. White PC, Dupont J, New MI, Leiberman E, Hochberg Z, Rosler A. A mutation in CYP11B1 (Arg-448—His) associated with steroid 11 beta-hydroxylase deficiency in Jews of Moroccan origin. J Clin Invest 1991; 87:1664–1667.

57. Helmberg A, Ausserer B, Kofler R. Frame shift by insertion of 2 basepairs in codon 394 of CYP11B1 causes congenital adrenal hyperplasia due to steroid 11 beta-hydroxylase deficiency. J Clin Endocrinol Metab 1992; 75:1278–1281.

58. Curnow KM, Slutsker L, Vitek J, Cole T, Speiser PW, New MI, et al. Mutations in the CYP11B1 gene causing congenital adrenal hyperplasia and hypertension cluster in exons 6, 7, and 8. Proc Natl Acad Sci USA 1993; 90:4552–4556.

59. Naiki Y, Kawamoto T, Mitsuuchi Y, Miyahara K, Toda K, Orii T, et al. A nonsense mutation (TGG [Trp116]—TAG [Stop] in CYP11B1 causes steroid 11beta-hydroxylase deficiency. J Clin Endocrinol Metab 1993; 77:1677–1682.

60. Geley S, Kapelari K, Johrer K, Peter M, Glatzl J, Vierhapper H, et al. CYP11B1 mutations causing congenital adrenal hyperplasia due to 11β-hydroxylase deficiency. J Clin Endocrinol Metab 1996; 81:2896–2901.

61. Nelson DR, Strobel HW. On the membrane topology of vertebrate cytochrome P-450 proteins. J Biol Chem 1988; 263:6038–6050.

62. Poulos TL. Modeling of mammalian P450s on basis of P450cam X-ray structure. Meth Enzymol 1991; 206:11–30.

63. Ravichandran KG, Boddupalli SS, Hasemann CA, Peterson JA, Deisenhofer J. Crystal structure of hemoprotein domain of P450BM-3, a prototype for microsomal P450's. Science 1993; 261:731–736.

64. Johrer K, Geley S, Strasser-Wozak EM, Azziz R, Wollmann HA, Schmitt K, et al. CYP11B1 mutations causing nonclassic adrenal hyperplasia due to 11b-hydroxylase deficiency. Hum Mol Genet 1997; 6:1829–1834.

65. Azziz R, Boots LR, Parker CR Jr, Bradley E Jr, Zacur HA. 11 beta-hydroxylase deficiency in hyperandrogenism. Fertil Steril 1991; 55:733–741.

66. Gibson M, Lackritz R, Schiff I, Tulchinsky D. Abnormal adrenal responses to adrenocorticotropic hormone in hyperandrogenic women. Fertil Steril 1980; 33:43–48.

67. Guthie GP, Wilson EM, Quillen DL, Jawad MJ. Adrenal androgen excess and defective 11β-hydroxylation in women with idiopathic hirsutism. Arch Intern Med 1982; 412:729–735.

21 Micronodular Adrenal Disease and the Syndrome of Myxomas, Spotty Skin Pigmentation, and Endocrine Overactivity

Constantine A. Stratakis, MD, DMSc

INTRODUCTION

In recent years, two primary adrenal disorders affecting the adrenal cortex have been implicated in the pathogenesis of corticotropin (ACTH)-independent Cushing's syndrome (CS) *(1)*. Primary pigmented adrenocortical disease (PPNAD), also known as "micronodular adrenal disease," is a congenital disorder, which, in the majority of the reported cases, is associated with Carney complex. The complex is a multiple endocrine neoplasia (MEN) syndrome that affects the adrenal cortex and other endocrine glands, and is associated with abnormal pigmentation of the skin and mucosae, myxomas, and other neoplasms *(2)*. Massive macronodular adrenocortical disease is another form of bilateral adrenal hyperplasia, which leads to CS, but is not associated with any other clinical findings. Macronodular disease should be contrasted with PPNAD: It is not congenital, almost always occurs in older patients, and its etiology is unclear. Other forms of bilateral adrenocortical hyperplasia distinct from PPNAD and not always associated with hypercortisolism include the lesions of the adrenal glands described in patients with the McCune-Albright and MEN type-1 syndromes *(3,4)*. In this chapter, we will focus on PPNAD and Carney complex.

From: *Contemporary Endocrinology: Adrenal Disorders*
Edited by: A. N. Margioris and G. P. Chrousos © Humana Press, Totowa, NJ

FEATURES OF PPNAD

In case reports dating back as early as 1949, children and young adults were described with pituitary-independent CS and a unique type of adrenal pathology in common: a bilateral form of adrenal hyperplasia, characterized by multiple, small, pigmented, adrenocortical nodules that were surrounded by internodular cortical atrophy (5,6). Various names were given to this peculiar lesion, the most common of which was "micronodular adrenal disease" (6); this was later replaced by "primary pigmented nodular adrenal disease" (PPNAD), a term that was first coined by Dr. J. Aidan Carney in 1984 (7).

PPNAD may occur independently or, more commonly, as part of the complex of "spotty skin pigmentation, myxomas, and endocrine overactivity" or Carney complex, which was described in 1985 (8–10). This syndrome also encompasses several familial cases of cutaneous and cardiac myxomas associated with lentigines and blue nevi of the skin and mucosae, which have been described under the acronyms NAME (for nevi, atrial myxoma, myxoid neurofibromata, and ephelides) and LAMB (for lentigines, atrial myxoma, mucocutaneous myxoma, blue nevi) syndromes (11,12).

In PPNAD, the glands are most commonly normal-sized or small and peppered with black or brown nodules set in a cortex that is usually atrophic (10). This atrophy is pathognomonic and reflects the autonomous function of these nodules and the suppressed levels of pituitary ACTH. Despite their small size (less than 6 mm), the nodules are visible with computed tomography (CT-scan) or magnetic resonance imaging (MRI) of the adrenal glands, most likely because of the surrounding atrophy (13). The combination of atrophy and nodularity gives the glands an irregular contour, which is distinctly abnormal and diagnostic, especially in younger patients with CS. Occasionally, one or both of the glands may be larger and harbor adenomas with a calcified center, while macronodules larger than 10 mm may be present in older patients (14).

Patients with PPNAD often present with a variant CS called "atypical" (ACS) (15), which is characterized by an asthenic, rather than obese, body habitus. This phenotype is caused by severe osteoporosis, short stature, and severe muscle and skin wasting. ACS was recognized as early as 1956 and has since been described in several cases of patients with CS (15–18). Only recently, however, was this condition associated with PPNAD (14,19). A recent review of the literature indicated that almost all the reported cases of ACS could be attributed to PPNAD, including that of a patient who presented 27 years after unilateral adrenalectomy (14). Patients with ACS tend to have normal or near-normal 24-h urinary-free cortisol (UFC) production, but this is characterized by the absence of the normal circadian rhythmicity of cortisol (14–18). Occasionally, normal cortisol production is interrupted by days or weeks of hypercortisolism, which gives rise to yet another variant called "periodic CS" (PCS). PCS is frequently found in children and adolescents with PPNAD (19). In both ACS and PCS, as well as in classic CS, caused by PPNAD, paradoxical increase of UFC and/or 17-hydroxy-corticosteroids (17-OHS) is seen during the second phase (high-dose dexamethasone administration) of the Liddle's test (20). This feature may be useful diagnostically for PPNAD (20); it reflects, perhaps, a tendency that these nodules have for increased responsiveness to other steroids (21).

PPNAD only rarely is present isolated. At the National Institutes of Health (NIH), where vigorous screening for Carney complex signs has been instituted under a research

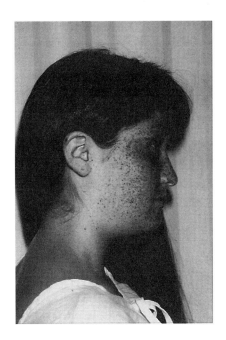
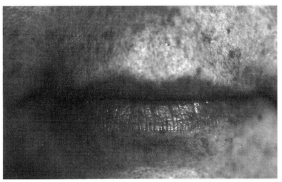
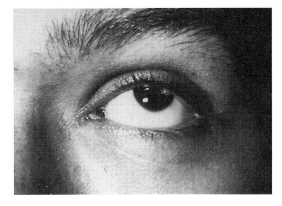

Fig. 1. Pigmented lesions and an eyelid myxoma in patients with Carney complex. These findings can be absent in patients with PPNAD because the syndrome has an extremely variable phenotype.

protocol, more than 20 patients have been treated for PPNAD since 1968. All of these patients met the diagnostic criteria for Carney complex that was developed by Stratakis et al. *(22),* with the exception of a 32-yr-old patient, who had PPNAD in her mid-twenties, underwent adrenalectomy, and has had no other tumors or skin pigmentation characteristic of the complex. Thus, we believe fewer than 10% of the PPNAD cases represent isolated forms of the disease; most of these patients have Carney complex, a syndrome that has a well-defined, but extremely variable, phenotype.

CARNEY COMPLEX

Among the individual components of Carney complex, the cardiac myxoma is the one most responsible for the significant morbidity and mortality associated with the syndrome. This tumor occurs often at multiple sites (affecting any or all cardiac chambers), at a relatively young age, and is equally distributed between the sexes *(23).* The cutaneous myxomas have a predilection for the eyelids and external ear canals, although they may affect any part of the skin *(24,25).* Mammary myxoid tumors may also occur at multiple sites and be bilateral; even the clinically "normal" breast of patients with the complex commonly shows microscopic foci of myxomatous masses, which can be identified by MRI *(26,27).*

The centrofacial spotty pigmentation of Carney complex involves the vermilion border of the lips and the conjunctiva (Fig. 1). The pigmented spots may be tanned, irregularly shaped, and poorly outlined, or small, sharply delineated, and dark brown to black. The conjunctival pigmentation typically affects the lacrimal caruncle and the conjunctival semilunar fold, and may involve the sclera. Five to 10% of patients with Carney complex have one or more intraoral pigmented spots, and the female external genitalia are commonly heavily pigmented. Blue nevi (the usual type, as well as the exceptionally rare epithelioid type) and combined and common junctional, dermal, and compound nevi, as well as café-au-lait spots also occur in the syndrome (28,29).

About 10% of patients with Carney complex have a growth hormone (GH)-secreting pituitary adenoma that results in acromegaly (22). Although most of the known patients with this condition had macroadenomas, a number of recently investigated cases show that abnormal 24-h GH secretion can precede the development of a pituitary tumor in the complex. The disorder, therefore, provides the unusual opportunity for prospective screening of affected patients without clinical acromegaly. In one such case, serial measurements of GH or somatomedin C, or both, became progressively abnormal over several years; recently, a pituitary mass was identified on computed tomography, and partial hypophysectomy revealed minute foci of a GH-producing adenoma.

Endocrine involvement in Carney complex also includes three types of testicular tumors: large-cell calcifying Sertoli cell tumor (among the rarest testicular neoplasms), adrenocortical rests, and Leydig cell tumor (30). About one-third of affected male patients have these masses. The large-cell calcifying Sertoli cell tumor, a bilateral, multicentric, and benign neoplasm, may secrete estrogens and cause precocious puberty, gynecomastia, or both (30). Finally, three new components of the syndrome have been identified: psammomatous melanotic schwannoma, epithelioid blue nevus, and ductal adenoma of the breast (22,31–33). Because thyroid follicular neoplasms, both benign and malignant, have been found in a number of patients, it is possible that thyroid involvement will prove to be a component of the syndrome (34).

GENETICS OF CARNEY COMPLEX AND PPNAD

Like the other MEN syndromes, Carney complex is inherited in an autosomal dominant manner. Sporadic cases constitute approximately half of the known patients (10,22). Interestingly, parent-of-origin effects in the inheritance of the disease have been observed (35). A genetic locus was determined for Carney complex by linkage analysis of polymorphic markers from likely areas of the genome (22). Positive lod scores were obtained for nine markers on the short arm of chromosome 2, identifying an approx 4 centiMorgan (cM)-long area in the cytogenetic band 2p16 (CNC locus), which is likely to contain the gene(s) responsible for the complex (36). This region includes the D2S123 locus, where another genetic syndrome, hereditary nonpolyposis colorectal cancer (HNPCC), was recently mapped (37). The gene for HNPCC (hMSH2) codes for a protein that plays a direct role in DNA mismatch repair, increasing microsatellite stability and enhancing mutation avoidance in human cells (38). Linkage analysis excluded this gene from being a candidate for the complex (22).

The mapping of the Carney complex gene at a locus where genes responsible for regulating DNA stability reside is of particular interest, since several lines of evidence indicate that chromosomal instability may be a feature of the tumor cell lines established from patients with the lentiginosis syndromes. Indeed, the formation of telomeric associations and dicentric chromosomes is a frequent feature of fibroblasts derived from the myxoid tumors excised from patients with Carney complex *(39–41)*. Also, a recent study found similar features in cultured in vitro adrenocortical cells derived from PPNAD nodules *(42);* microsatellite analysis of the tumors excised from patients with Carney complex confirmed the significant genomic instability that accompanies tumorigenesis in this syndrome *(42)*. Numerous areas of loss or gain of heterozygosity, and/or deletions, involving all 22 autosomal chromosomes were found. These changes did not include the *CNC* locus on chromosome 2p16, a finding that suggests that alterations of the heterozygosity of the responsible gene(s) may not be necessary for oncogenesis in this condition. Although mutations of the *gsp* protooncogene were not present in Carney complex tumors *(43)*, and the locations of several genes that code for components of the guanine nucleotide-binding proteins (G-proteins) were excluded by linkage analysis *(22,44)*, it seems likely that the gene or genes responsible for this condition may participate in G-protein-controled or -related signaling systems. Recently, a family with Carney complex that does not map to chromosome 2p16 was reported *(45)*. This finding has been confirmed by our laboratory in another large kindred that had a number of recombinant genotypes with the first locus *(46)*. Thus, it appears likely that genetic heterogeneity exists in the syndrome; the second locus is on chromosome 17 (17a22–24) *(47)*.

TREATMENT OF PPNAD

At this time, the suggested therapy for PPNAD is bilateral adrenalectomy. This is performed, not only for the treatment of CS, but also to prevent the development of an adrenocortical neoplasm (although there are no reports in the literature of such a transformation occurring). Because bilateral adrenalectomy is generally considered to be an operation with many long-term potential consequences, some physicians have opted to treat patients with PPNAD with unilateral adrenalectomy, reserving a second operation until the time when CS recurs. Although this position is defensible, it is important to recall that even if frank CS is clinically absent, patients with PPNAD do not regain normal cortisol dynamics after unilateral adrenalectomy, and as such, they are at risk for other secondary complications *(14)*.

SUMMARY

This is currently an exciting time for clinicians and basic scientists interested in primary diseases of the adrenal glands. As the molecular basis of these conditions becomes better understood, basic researchers will be provided with a detailed insight into adrenocortical function and early differentiation, and clinicians will offer better therapies to patients affected by these disorders.

REFERENCES

1. Stratakis CA, Chrousos GP. Cushing's syndrome and disease. In: Finberg L, ed. Saunder's Manual of Pediatric Practice. Saunders, Philadelphia, 1998, p. 807–809.
2. Stratakis CA. Genetics of Carney complex and related familial lentiginoses, and other multiple tumor syndromes. Front Biosci. 2000; 5:D353–D366.
3. Boston BA, Mandel S, LaFranchi S, Bliziotes M. Activating mutation in the stimulatory guanine nucleotide-binding protein in an infant with Cushing's syndrome and nodular adrenal hyperplasia. J Clin Endocrinol Metab 1994; 79:890–893.
4. Skogseid B, Larsson C, Lindgren P-G, Kvanta E, Rastad J, Theodorsson E. Clinical and genetic

features of adrenocortical lesions in multiple endocrine neoplasia type-1. J Clin Endocrinol Metab 1992; 75:76–81.

5. Schweizer-Cagianut M, Salomon F, Hedinger CE. Primary adrenocortical nodular dysplasia with Cushing's syndrome and cardiac myxomas. A peculiar familial disease. Virchows Arch A Pathol Anat Histol 1982; 397:183–192.

6. Schweizer-Cagianut M, Froesch ER, Hedinger CE. Familial Cushing's syndrome with primary adrenocortical microadenomatosis (primary adrenocortical nodular dysplasia). Acta Endocrinol (Copenh) 1980; 94:529–535.

7. Shenoy BV, Carpenter PC, Carney JA. Bilateral primary pigmented nodular adrenocortical disease. Rare cause of the Cushing's syndrome. Am J Surg Pathol 1984; 8:335–344.

8. Carney JA, Gordon H, Carpenter PC, Shenoy BV, Go VLW. The complex of myxomas, spotty pigmentation, and endocrine overactivity. Medicine (Baltimore) 1985; 64:270–283.

9. Carney JA, Hruska LS, Beauchamp GD, Gordon H. Dominant inheritance of the complex of myxomas, spotty pigmentation and endocrine overactivity. Mayo Clin Proc 1986; 61:165–172.

10. Carney JA, Young WF. Primary pigmented nodular adrenocortical disease and its associated conditions. Endocrinologist 1992; 2:6–21.

11. Atherton DJ, Pitcher DW, Wells RS, Macdonald DM. A syndrome of various cutaneous pigmented lesions, myxoid neurofibromata and atrial myxoma: the NAME syndrome. Br J Dermatol 1980; 103:421–429.

12. Rhodes AR, Silverman RA, Harrist TJ, Perez-Atayde AR. Mucocutaneous lentigines, cardiomucocutaneous myxomas, and multiple blue nevi: the "LAMB" syndrome. J Am Acad Dermatol 1984; 10:72–82.

13. Doppman JL, Travis WD, Nieman L, Miller DL, Chrousos GP, Gomez TM. Cushing's syndrome due to primary pigmented nodular adrenocortical disease: findings at CT and MRI imaging. Radiology 1989; 172:415–420.

14. Sarlis NJ, Chrousos GP, Doppman JL, Carney JA, Stratakis CA. Primary pigmented nodular adrenocortical disease (PPNAD): re-evaluation of a patient with Carney complex 27 years after unilateral adrenalectomy. J Clin Endocrinol Metab 1997; 82:2037–2043.

15. Mellinger RC, Smith RW. Studies of the adrenal hyperfunction in 2 patients with atypical Cushing's syndrome. J Clin Endocrinol Metab 1955; 16:350–366.

16. Kracht J, Tamm J. Bilaterale kleinknotige Adenomatose der Nebennierenrinde bei Cushing-Syndrom. Virchows Arch path Anat 1960; 333:1–9.

17. Levin ME. The development of bilateral adenomatous adrenal hyperplasia in a case of Cushing's syndrome of eighteen years' duration. Am J Med 1966; 40:318–324.

18. De Moor P, Roels H, Delaere K, Crabbe J. Unusual case of adrenocortical hyperfunction. J Clin Endocrinol Metab 1965; 25:612–620.

19. Gomez-Muguruza MT, Chrousos GP. Periodic Cushing's syndrome in a short boy: usefulness of the ovine corticotropin releasing hormone test. J Pediatr 1989; 115:270–273.

20. Sarlis NJ, Papanicolaou DA, Chrousos GP, Stratakis CA. Paradoxical increase of urinary-free cortisol and 17-hydroxy-steroids to dexamethaosone during Liddle's test: a diagnostic test for primary pigmented adrenocortical disease. [Abstract P2-76]. In: Proc 79th Ann Meet Endocrine Soc, Minneapolis, MN, Endocrine Society Press, Bethesda, 1997, p. 303.

21. Caticha O, Odell WD, Wilson DE, Dowdell LA, Noth RH, Swislocki ALM. Estradiol stimulates cortisol production by adrenal cells in estrogen-dependent primary adrenocortical nodular dysplasia. J Clin Endocrinol Metab 1993; 77:494–497.

22. Stratakis CA, Carney JA, Lin J-P, Papanicolaou DA, Karl M, Kastner DL, et al. Carney complex, a familial multiple neoplasia and lentiginosis syndrome: analysis of 11 kindreds and linkage to the short arm of chromosome 2. J Clin Invest 1996; 97:699–705.

23. Carney JA. Differences between nonfamilial and familial cardiac myxoma. Am J Surg Pathol 1985; 9:53–55.

24. Kennedy RH, Flanagan JC, Eagle RC Jr, Carney JA. The Carney complex with ocular signs suggestive of cardiac myxoma. Am J Ophthalmol 1991; 111:699–702.

25. Ferreiro JA, Carney JA. Myxomas of the external ear and their significance. Am J Surg Pathol 1994; 18:274–280.

26. Carney JA, Toorkey BC. Myxoid fibroadenoma and allied conditions (myxomatosis) of the breast. A heritable disorder with special associations including cardiac and cutaneous myxomas. Am J Surg Pathol 1991; 15:713–721.

27. Courcoutsakis NA, Chow CK, Shawker T, Carney JA, Stratakis CA. Breast imaging findings in the

complex of myxomas, spotty pigmentation, endocrine veracity, and schwannomas (Carney complex). Radiology 1997; 205:221–227.

28. Carney JA, Ferreiro JA. The epithelioid blue nevus. A multicentric familial tumor with important associations, including cardiac myxoma and psammomatous melanotic schwannoma. Am J Surg Pathol 1996; 20:259–272.

29. Carney JA. Carney complex: the complex of myxomas, spotty pigmentation, endocrine veractivity, and schwannomas. Semin Dermatol 1995; 14:90–98.

30. Premkumar A, Stratakis CA, Shawker TH, Papanicolaou DA, Chrousos GP. Testicular ultrasound in Carney complex. J Clin Ultrasound 1997; 25:211–214.

31. Carney JA. Psammomatous melanotic schwannoma. A distinctive, heritable tumor with special associations, including cardiac myxoma and the Cushing's syndrome. Am J Surg Pathol 1990; 14:206–222.

32. Carney JA, Toorkey BC. Ductal adenoma of the breast with tubular futures. A probable component of the complex of myxomas, spotty pigmentation, endocrine overactivity, and schwannomas. Am J Surg Pathol 1991; 15:722–731.

33. Carney JA, Stratakis CA. Ductal adenoma of the breast [letter]. Am J Surg Pathol 1996; 20:1154–1155.

34. Stratakis CA, Courcoutsakis N, Abati A, Filie A, Doppman JL, Carney JA, et al. Thyroid gland abnormalities in patients with the "syndrome of spotty skin pigmentation, myxomas, and endocrine overactivity" (Carney complex). J Clin Endocrinol Metab 1997; 82:2037–2043.

35. Stratakis CA, Pras E, Tsigos C, Karl M, Papanicolaou DA, Kastner DL, et al. Genetics of Carney complex: parent of origin effects and putative non-Mendelian features in an autosomal dominant disorder; absence of common defects of the ACTH receptor and RET genes. Pediatr Res 1995; 37:99A.

36. Stratakis CA, Pras E, Lin J-P, Kastner DL, Carney JA, Chrousos GP. Carney complex, a multiple endocrine neoplasia and familial lentiginosis syndrome: clinical analysis and linkage to the D2S123 locus (chromosome 2p16). Am J Hum Genet 1995; 57:A54.

37. Leach FS, Nicolaides NC, Papadopoulos N, Liu B, Jen J, Parsons R, et al. Mutations of a *mut*S homolog in hereditary nonpolyposis colorecteal cancer. Cell 1993; 75:1215–1225.

38. Fishel R, Ewel A, Lee S, Lescoe MK, Griffith J. Binding of mismatched microsatellite DNA sequences by the human MSH2 protein. Science 1994; 266:1403–1405.

39. Dewald GW, Dahl RJ, Spurbeck JL, Carney JA, Gordon H. Chromosomally abnormal clones and nonrandom telomeric translocations in cardiac myxomas. Mayo Clin Proc 1987; 62:558–567.

40. Dijkhuizen T, van der Derg E, Molenaar WM, Meuzelaar JJ, de Jong B. Cytogenetics of a case of cardiac myxoma. Cancer Genet Cytogenet 1992; 63:73–75.

41. Richkind KE, Wason D, Vidaillet HJ. Cardiac myxoma characterized by clonal telomeric association. Genes Chrom Cancer 1994; 9:68–71.

42. Stratakis CA, Jenkins RB, Pras E, Mitsiades CS, Raff SB, Stalboerger P, et al. Cytogenetic and microsatellite alterations in tumors from patients with the syndrome of myxomas, spotty skin pigmentation, and endocrine overactivity (Carney complex). J Clin Endocrinol Metab 1996; 81:3607–3614.

43. DeMarco L, Stratakis CA, Boson WL, Yakbovitz O, Carson E, Adrade LM, et al. Sporadic cardiac myxomas and tumors from patients with Carney complex are not associated with activating mutations of the Gsα gene. Hum Genet 1996; 98:185–188.

44. Stratakis CA, Pras E, Papanicolaou DA, Karl M, Kastner DL, Carney JA, et al. Carney complex and primary pigmented nodular adrenocortical disease: segregation, simulation and linkage analysis using the candidate gene approach. [Abstract] Presented at the 77th Endocrine Soc Meet 1995; (P3)28.

45. Basson CT, MacRae CA, Korf B, Merliss A. Genetic heterogeneity of familial atrial myxoma syndromes (Carney complex). Am J Cardiol 1997; 79:994–995.

46. Taymans S, Macrae CA, Casey M, Merliss A, Lin J-P, Rocchi M, et al. A refined genetic, radiation hybrid, and physical map of the Carney complex (CNC) locus on chromosome 2p16; evidence for genetic heterogeneity in the syndrome. Am J Hum Genet (Suppl) 1997; 61:A:84.

47. Casey M, Mah C, Merliss AD, Kirschner LS, Taymans SE, Denio AE, Korf B, et al. Identification of a novel genetic locus for familial cardiac myxomas and carney complex. Circulation. 1998; 98: 2560–2566.

22 Congenital Lipoid Adrenal Hyperplasia

Walter L. Miller

CONTENTS

INTRODUCTION

Congenital lipoid adrenal hyperplasia (lipoid CAH) is a rare disorder, especially in non-Japanese populations, and, hence, some may regard it as a mere medical curiosity. This chapter shows how the curiosity of investigators from Europe, Japan, and the United States led to the solution of this unusual disease, and, in turn, how the solution of this disease provided novel fundamental insights into the regulation of steroid hormone biosynthesis and into developmental endocrinology.

HISTORY

Lipoid CAH was first described in detail as an inherited endocrine disorder by Prader et al. *(1–3)*, although several autopsy cases appeared earlier in the pathology literature *(4–7)*. Prader et al. described male pseudohermaphroditism, an apparent lack of adrenal steroids and accumulation of lipid deposits in the adrenal, inherited in an autosomal recessive fashion. Camacho et al. then showed that affected tissues accumulated cholesterol esters, and suggested that the disorder was in one of the enzymes involved in the conversion of cholesterol to pregnenolone *(8)*. However, the nature of the defect was unclear, in part because the enzymology of the conversion of cholesterol to pregnenolone was unclear. At that time, it was thought that a series of enzymes constituted a "20,22 desmolase complex," and that lipoid CAH was caused by a defect in one of these enzymes that sequentially catalyzed the hydroxylation of cholesterol on carbons 20 and 22, followed by scission of the C20-22 bond. When Degenhart et al. incubated mitochondria from affected tissue with cholesterol, they obtained no pregnenolone. However, pregnenolone was produced *(9)* when they incubated the mitochondria with 20α-hydroxycholesterol. They logically concluded that the defect was in a specific 20α-hydroxylase. This conclusion was incorrect, but the experimental design was

291

prescient: 23 years later, a similar experiment helped to prove that lipoid CAH was caused by a mutation in a nonenzymatic protein *(10)*. Koizumi et al. confirmed Degenhart's finding that affected mitochondria failed to convert cholesterol to pregnenolone *(11)*. However, by this time it was known that the conversion of cholesterol to pregnenolone was catalyzed by a mitochondrial cytochrome *P450* enzyme, termed *P450scc*, (where *scc* denotes *s*ide-*c*hain *c*leavage), which was the terminal oxidase in a mitochondrial electron-transfer chain where NADPH donated electrons to a flavoprotein (adrenodoxin reductase), which then transferred them to an iron-sulfur protein (adrenodoxin), which in turn donated them to *P450scc (12,13)* [for review, see *(14)*]. Thus, Koizumi examined *P450scc* in the affected adrenal mitochondria in the only fashion then available, by carbon monoxide-induced difference spectra, and concluded that affected mitochondria had roughly half of the normal amount of total cytochrome *P450*. At that time, it was known that steroid 11β/18-hydroxylase activities were also catalyzed by a mitochondrial *P450*, and as 11β/18-hydroxylase activity was normal in the affected mitochondria, but failed to convert cholesterol to pregnenolone, Koizumi et al. logically concluded that the defect was an absence of cytochrome *P450scc*. This belief persisted for another 14 yr, and was supported by our own reports *(15,16)*. The cloning of the human *P450scc* cDNA *(17)* and gene *(18)* permitted testing of this hypothesis. Although our preliminary examinations of the *P450scc* gene in affected patients revealed no gross abnormalities *(16)*, it was not until we found normal sequences for the *P450scc* gene and cDNA from affected patients that it became clear that lipoid CAH was not caused by mutations in *P450scc* or a component of the hypothetical "20,22 desmolase complex" *(19)*.

Upon finding normal *P450scc* gene and cDNA sequences in lipoid CAH, examination of RNA from affected tissue also suggested that the transcripts for adrenodoxin reductase and adrenodoxin were of normal size and abundance *(19)*. Although we did not sequence these, it seemed clear that subtle mutations in these proteins could not cause lipoid CAH, as these proteins also transferred electrons to the mitochondrial *P450s* involved in vitamin D and in bile acid biosynthesis, and these functions were normal in lipoid CAH patients, thus we began to consider that lipoid CAH might be caused by disruption of a factor involved in the transport of cholesterol into mitochondria *(19)*. Unfortunately then, as now, it was not know exactly how cholesterol traveled from lipid droplets to mitochondria.

SEARCH FOR THE ACUTE REGULATOR OF STEROIDOGENESIS

From 1980 to 1995, substantial effort was expended in many laboratories searching for the "acute regulator" of steroidogenesis [for review, see *(20)*]. It was clear that ACTH could induce adrenal steroidogenesis in a very rapid, cycloheximide-inhibitable fashion: the "acute response" *(21–24)*. Work in the later 1980s showed that ACTH through cAMP induced the transcription of the genes for *P450scc* and other steroidogenic enzymes *(25,26)*. It was proposed that a short-lived cyclohexamide-sensitive steroid hormone-inducing protein (SHIP) was involved in this process as a transcription factor *(25)*, but it soon became clear that the action of cycloheximide did not affect transcription of the steroidogenic enzyme genes or the accumulation of their cognate mRNAs *(27–30)*.

Several candidates for the "acute regulator" were proposed, including sterol carrier protein 2 *(31,32)*, so-called steroidogenesis-activator peptide and its resumed precursor, GRP-78 *(33–35)*, and the peripheral benzodiazepine receptor (PBR) *(36,37)* and its presumed endogenous ligand termed endozepine or diazepam-binding inhibitor (DBI) *(38, 39)*. However, the size and abundance of the mRNAs for all of these proteins were normal in lipoid CAH tissues *(19)*. Although it still appears likely that PBR plays a major role in cholesterol movement into mitochondria *(40)* the *PBR* gene sequence was wholly normal in lipoid CAH *(41)*. Thus, none of these factors were involved in lipoid CAH, and, on closer examination, none of them possessed the three required features of the "acute regulator": (1) rapid inducibility by cAMP; (2) short half-life evidenced by cycloheximide sensitivity; (3) capacity to induce steroidogenesis. However, another family of peptides, initially termed pp30, pp32, and pp37 *(42–44)* appeared to possess the needed characteristics. Stocco's purification of one of these proteins led to its cloning from mouse Leydig MA-10 cells; when its cDNA expression vector was transfected back into MA-10 cells it enhanced their steroidogenesis, engendering the name "steroidogenic acute regulatory protein," or StAR *(45)*. Yet these studies were done in a cell system that contained endogenous StAR, so that some major questions remained.

At this point, the study of lipoid CAH and the study of StAR came together, illuminating both fields. Our clinical studies showed that not all steroidogenic tissues were affected in lipoid CAH, as had been previously thought, but that the placenta's ability to synthesize progesterone from cholesterol was not disrupted in this disease *(46)*. Thus, a further characteristic of the protein disrupted in lipoid CAH had to be that it was expressed in the adrenals and gonads, but not in the placenta (or possibly the brain also) *(46)*. After its initial cloning from mouse MA-10 cells *(45)* work on StAR progressed rapidly (for review, *see* Chapter 7 in this volume). When Sugawara et al. showed that StAR was expressed in the adrenals and gonads, but not in the placenta or brain *(47)*, StAR immediately became the foremost candidate for the cause of lipoid CAH. At this time, (fall 1994) our laboratory still had some of the cDNA that we had prepared from the gonadal tissue of a lipoid CAH patient, which we had used to show that *P450scc* was unaffected *(19)*. Based on the then-unpublished sequence of human StAR cDNA obtained by our collaborator Dr. Jerome F. Strauss III, we synthesized human StAR oligonucleotides and PCR-amplified the StAR cDNA from our index patient. We quickly found that the StAR cDNA was mutated in this patient, and then found mutations in the genomic DNA of three more patients, thus establishing that StAR mutations caused lipoid CAH *(10,48)*. By this time, it was known that soluble hydroxysterols were freely accessible to mitochondrial *P450scc (49)*. Thus, we showed that cells transfected with the *P450scc* system *(50)* had their steroidogenic capacity increased eight-fold by cotransfection with StAR, and that this action of StAR could be bypassed by providing the transfected cells with the soluble hydroxysterol 22OH-cholesterol *(10,48)*. This showed that StAR acted to facilitate the movement of cholesterol into mitochondria, but that StAR's action was not required by hydroxysterols. This experiment essentially recapitulated Degenhart's experiment published in 1972; both the 22OH-cholesterol we used *(10,48)* and the 20-OH cholesterol used by Degenhart et al. in 1972 *(9)* bypassed the absent action of StAR. However, Degenhart et al. could not interpret their results accurately as it was not then known that cholesterol required a cycloheximide-sensitive factor to enter mitochondria, or that the action of this factor could be circumvented by use of soluble hydroxysterol analogs of cholesterol.

CLINICAL FINDINGS IN LIPOID CAH

The initial clinical reports of lipoid CAH appeared sporadically. Hauffa et al. published the first comprehensive review of this disease in 1985, 30 yr after Prader's first report, and found only 32 proven cases in search of the worldwide literature (only six of which were in English-language publications), thus suggesting that lipoid CAH was very rare *(15)*. The true incidence of lipoid CAH is unknown, but it is clearly very high in people of Japanese, Korean, and Palestinian ancestry *(51)*. Hauffa's review found that all patients had normal phenotypically female external genitalia irrespective of chromosomal sex (indicating a severe defect in fetal testicular synthesis of testosterone), hyponatremia, hyperkalemia, low urinary 17-hydroxycorticosteroids and 17-ketosteroids (indicating a profound lesion in adrenal steroid biosynthesis), hyperpigmentation (caused by overproduction of ACTH), and an excellent response to glucocorticoid and mineralocorticoid replacement *(15)*. Fourteen of 28 patients had male gonads (as indicated by karyotype, buccal smear, gonadal appearance, or gonadal histology), consistent with autosomal recessive inheritance. Although only 11 of these first patients survived, both Kirkland et al. *(52)* and Hauffa et al. *(15)* showed that patients with lipoid CAH could survive to adulthood if diagnosed early in infancy and provided with appropriate glucocorticoid and mineralocorticoid replacement therapy. Hauffa et al. also pointed out the genetic clustering of lipoid CAH, with a remarkable 56% of the initial 32 patients being of Japanese heritage.

Hauffa et al. noted certain oddities in the clinical presentations and hormonal findings in their review. Only 15 of 28 patients manifested clinical signs of adrenal insufficiency by 2 wk of age, the time at which the salt-wasting crisis of conventional 21-hydroxylase deficiency is usually apparent, and some affected patients did not become clinically ill until more than 3 mo of age. Nevertheless, until quite recently, the conventional view of lipoid CAH was that it was caused by a severe disorder in the cholesterol side-chain cleavage system, leading to the common alternative name "20–22 desmolase deficiency." This disorder was thought to ablate all adrenal and gonadal steroidogenesis, consistent with the wholly female external genitalia of affected 46,XY individuals. The low, but measurable, adrenal steroids found in many affected newborns were unexplained, and dismissed as transplacental maternal steroids, crossreacting materials, or the result of "partial blocks" in the enzymatic step. The generally later age of onset of the salt-wasting crisis in lipoid CAH compared to 21-hydroxylase deficiency was dismissed as caused by the unproven putative salt-wasting effects of the high concentrations of 17OH-progesterone in 21-hydroxylase deficiency.

The clinical view of lipoid CAH has changed dramatically in the past few years. The demonstration that *P450scc* was not disordered in this disease *(19)* was the first step in revising views of lipoid CAH. In 1994, Matsuo et al. presented astonishing findings, published only in abstract form, reporting that only 16 of 63 Japanese patients with lipoid CAH were 46,XX genetic females, and that all five who were over 13 yr of age had spontaneous breast development and vaginal bleeding associated with serum estradiol levels ranging from 22 to 85 pg/mL *(53)*. This preliminary report was largely overlooked until the demonstration that StAR mutations caused lipoid CAH *(10)* triggered intensive study of the disease. We recently summarized the clinical findings in our index cases *(10,46,48)* and described the clinical and molecular genetic findings in 15 additional, previously undescribed, cases of lipoid CAH *(51)*. These and additional hormonal data are summarized in Table 1. The 20 affected infants were all of term gestation and of appropriate size for gestational age. Five infants had hypoglycemia and six infants had some form of neonatal respiratory difficulties, but true respiratory distress syndrome or hyaline membrane disease caused by diminished production of pulmonary surfactant was not documented. The age of onset of symptoms of hyponatremia and hyperkalemia varied dramatically, from 1 d to 2 mo of age, and most infants who were tested had measurable levels of cortisol and, (in 46,XY males) testosterone, which failed to rise following tropic stimulation. Even more remarkable, many infants survived for an extended time without hormonal replacement therapy: treatment did not begin until after age 2 mo in seven infants, and one survived for 6 mo without glucocorticoid or mineralocorticoid replacement. Thus, although the adrenal lesion in lipoid CAH eventually becomes the most severe of any of the forms of CAH, some steroidogenic activity persists and the onset of clinical symptoms may be delayed for quite some time. By contrast, 46,XY patients with lipoid CAH reported to date have had wholly normal female external genitalia, even though the age of onset of glucocorticoid and mineralocorticoid deficiencies varies substantially. Thus, the testicular lesion appears to be more severe and manifests at a much earlier stage of development than the adrenal lesion.

Because we could show that virtually all of these infants had genetic lesions that were genetically and biochemically equivalent (i.e., had nonfunctional StAR proteins) (51), we hypothesized that the variation in onset of symptoms had to reflect some other phenomenon that was secondary to the genetic lesion. The clues came from our in vitro studies of the biology of P450scc and StAR, and from Matsuo's preliminary report of ovarian function in lipoid CAH patients. We, and others, had previously shown that nonsteroidogenic cells (e.g., African green monkey kidney COS-1 cells) only needed to be transfected with vectors expressing P450scc to acquire the ability to convert cholesterol to pregnenolone (50,54) [for review see (55)]. As all cells and tissues express the mRNAs for adrenodoxin (28) and adrenodoxin reductase (56), it was initially not surprising that COS-1 cells exhibited cholesterol side-chain cleavage activity when transfected with a P450scc cDNA expression vector. It was also clear that incubating cells with soluble hydroxysterols resulted in far more pregnenolone production than arose from endogenous cellular cholesterol (47,54). Soluble hydroxysterols provide maximal substrate availability to the P450scc system, and, in fact result in two- to three-fold greater production of pregnenolone than can be achieved in cells transfected with a StAR expression vector and stimulated with cAMP (10,47,51,57). However, the key point was that some steroidogenesis persisted in these transfected cells in the absence of StAR. Thus, we reasoned that the steroidogenic tissues of patients with StAR mutations should retain a modest degree of steroidogenic capacity. This led us to introduce the concept that there were distinct StAR-dependent and StAR-independent modes of steroidogenesis. In addition to transfected cells in vitro, the placenta (46) and brain (58) represent examples of StAR-independent steroidogenesis in vivo. This conceptualization permitted us to theorize why some infants with lipoid CAH do not manifest clinical evidence of mineralocorticoid deficiency for several months, and why 46,XX genetic females with lipoid CAH undergo spontaneous feminization at the age of puberty (53,59).

We envision the pathophysiology of lipoid CAH as resulting from two different cellular events (51). First, mutant StAR prevents the acute steroidogenic response in

Table 1
Lipoid CAH Patients

Pt. No.	Gest. Age (wk)	Birth Wt (gm)	Age at Onset of Sx[+]	Age at Onset of Rx[+]	Na (mEq/L)	K (mEq/L)	ACTH (pg/mL)	PRA (ng/mL/h)	ACTH Test Cortisol (μg/dL) Pre	ACTH Test Cortisol (μg/dL) Post	hCG Test Testosterone (ng/dL) Pre	hCG Test Testosterone (ng/dL) Post	Pigment	Glucose (mg/dL)	Pulmonary Problems
1	—	2550	19 d	19 d	—	—	—	—	"low"	"low"	10.5	20.3	Yes	—	—
2	40	2580	1 mo	2 mo	137	5.8	4600	11.6	9.5	9.4	4.4	4.0	Yes	92	—
3	41	2900	4 d	3 mo	130	6.7	—	—	<1.0	<1.0	27.2	27.0	Yes	—	—
4	41	2765	1 d	1 d	124	7.8	—	>60	1.7	<1.0	nil	—	Yes	56	Resp Distress
5	37	2240	1 d	5 mo	117	7.1	—	136*	1.1	1.1	—	—	No	"low"	Resp Distress
6	40	3200	5 d	5 d	133	6.6	>570	22*	14.5	19.6	—	—	No	—	Resp Distress
7	42	5000	7 d	12 d	120	8.0	—	—	nil	—	8.0	nil	Yes	13	—
8	40	3500	10 d	22 d	123	8.1	—	—	—	—	—	—	No	70	Asphyxia
9	40	4400	2 wk	3 wk	126	6.8	—	—	—	—	—	—	No	36	Asphyxia
10	41	3380	8 d	6 wk	126	5.6	—	12.3	0.9	1.0	2.7	—	Yes	11	—
11	38	2700	10 d	35 d	132	7.2	1400	>50	11.3	—	—	—	No	—	—
12	42	4250	—	6 mo	118	5.9	384	>60	9.1	9.2	3.2	—	No	88	—
13	36	2270	2 mo	4 mo	123	6.9	—	—	0	<1.4	<3	<3	Yes	63	—
14	39	2800	2–4 wk	2 mo	107	7.3	—	"high"	0	0	—	—	No	—	—
15	40	3460	1 wk	16 d	124	8.9	—	—	3.5	3.6	—	—	Yes	—	Retained fluid
16	40	3320	10 d	—	113	9.0	585	>12.6	2.2	<1.0	—	<3.0	Yes	"normal"	—
17	—	—	4 wk	—	—	—	—	—	1.3	2.4	—	—	—	—	—
18	—	—	abortus	—	—	—	—	—	—	—	—	—	—	—	—
19	—	—	4 wk	4 wk	128	6.9	—	—	—	—	—	—	Yes	—	—
20	36	2750	1 d	9 d	128	7.1	—	—	—	—	—	—	Yes	13	Apnea
21	42	3290	4 wk	10 wk	118	8.9	2450	120	<1	—	<3	—	Yes	92	—

+Sx–clinical symptoms; Rx–hormonal treatment
*Plasma renin concentrations in mIU/mL

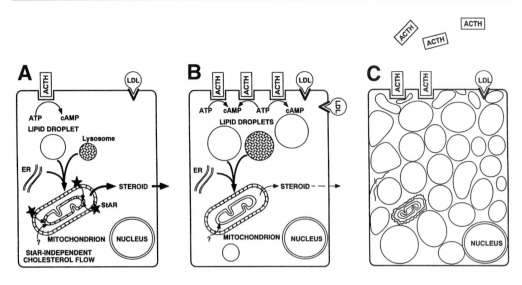

Fig. 1. Model of lipoid CAH in an adrenal cell. **(A)** In the normal cell, cholesterol is derived from endogenous synthesis from acetyl CoA in the endoplasmic reticulum (ER), from cholesterol esters stored in lipid droplets, and from low-density lipoprotein (LDL) cholesterol which, after receptor-mediated endocytosis, is processed in lysosomes before it is used or stored in lipid droplets. Cholesterol is transported to the outer mitochondrial membrane by ill-defined processes involving the cytoskeleton [for review, see *(68)*]. The rate-limiting step in steroidogenesis is the movement of cholesterol from the outer to the inner mitochondrial membrane; this can be promoted by StAR, but may also be mediated by StAR-independent mechanisms. Thus, the net synthesis of steroid is caused by both StAR-dependent and StAR-independent means. **(B)** In the absence of StAR, as in early lipoid CAH or in a placental cell, StAR-independent mechanisms can still move some cholesterol into the mitochondria, resulting in a low level of steroidogenesis. In an affected adrenal cell this results in increased corticotropin secretion, stimulating further production of cholesterol and its accumulation as cholesterol esters in lipid droplets. **(C)** As lipid droplets accumulate, they engorge the cell, damaging its cytoarchitecture both through physical displacement and by the chemical action of cholesterol autooxidation products. Steroidogenic capacity is destroyed and consequently tropic stimulation continues. In the ovary, follicular cells remain unstimulated and, hence, undamaged until they are recruited at the beginning of each cycle. Small amounts of estradiol are produced, analogously to panel **B**, effecting phenotypic feminization and withdrawal bleeding, but the cycles are anovulatory, resulting in infertility and progressive hypergonadotropic hypogonadism.

the fetal testis and adrenal. This ablates StAR-dependent steroidal responsiveness to tropic stimulation, but permits a modest level of StAR-independent basal steroidogenesis, as seen in the placenta or in cells transfected with vectors expressing the *P450scc* system without StAR. Second, the accumulation of unused cholesterol esters in affected steroidogenic cells may damage the cell, either through physical engorgement with lipid droplets or as a consequence of toxic effects of sterol autooxidation products, and eventually disrupt the basal, StAR-independent steroidogenesis (Fig. 1). Thus, the fetal testis, which undergoes profound tropic stimulation by human chorionic gonadotropin in early gestation, is severely affected early in gestation, so that there is no evidence of any virilization, even in a patient with partial StAR activity [e.g., as patient 13 in ref. *(51)*]. Similarly, the fetal zone of the adrenal, which normally makes huge amounts of dehydroepiandrosterone for conversion to estriol by the placenta, is also profoundly affected, leading to the minimal estriol concentrations in the plasma of women carrying a lipoid CAH fetus *(46)*. By contrast, the definitive zone of the fetal adrenal makes relatively small amounts of steroids *in utero*, but probably develops into the adrenal *zonas glomerulosa* and *fasciculata* (which, respectively, produce mineralocorticoids and glucocorticoids) following birth *(60)*. These zones are variably affected by the accumulation of cholesterol esters, leading to the modest, but detectable, levels of steroid hormones typically seen in affected infants, and permitting survival for up to several months, until the accumulation of cholesterol esters finally ablates all residual StAR-independent adrenal steroidogenesis. In contrast to the testis and adrenal, the fetal ovary lacks steroidogenic enzymes and steroidogenic capacity *(61)*. As it remains unstimulated until puberty, the affected ovary does not accumulate cholesterol esters. The onset of puberty, which is an event in the CNS, independent of sex steroids *(62)* produces the gonadotropins that stimulate the maturation of individual ovarian follicles, leading to low levels of ovarian estrogen synthesis in affected 46,XX females. The accumulation of ovarian cholesterol esters eventually destroys the StAR-independent steroidogenic capacity of the affected follicles, but previously unstimulated follicles are recruited in subsequent cycles, permitting a low level of estrogen synthesis to continue. This will result in clinical feminization, with breast development and minimal amounts of pubic and axillary hair that result from low levels of ovarian androgens in the absence of adrenal androgens. This estrogen synthesis will cycle normally, so that estrogen withdrawal bleeding of the uterus will occur monthly in the pattern of normal menses. However, the amount of estrogen produced is low with consequently hyper-gonadotropic hypergonadism. This hypergonadotropic state may induce the formation of large ovarian cysts, which can undergo torsion leading to a fatal outcome. Thus, we recommend that 46,XX genetic female patients with lipoid CAH receive treatment with oral contraceptives and/or medroxyprogesterone to suppress the gonadotropins and cyst development *(59)*.

UNANSWERED QUESTIONS

The identification of StAR as the factor responsible for lipoid CAH ends the 40-year quest for the cause of the disease and will permit rapid accurate diagnosis in the newborn and ascertainment of the heterozygous, carrier state in those populations in which lipoid CAH is common (i.e., Japanese, Koreans, and Palestinians) *(51)*. However, some questions remain. In our survey of 15 previously unstudied lipoid CAH patients, we found one who had no StAR mutation *(51)*. Although it remains possible that we missed a StAR mutation in the unsequenced introns or regulatory regions of this patient's *StAR* gene, this also raises the possibility that there may be other factors which, when mutated, create a syndrome that is clinically indistinguishable from lipoid CAH. We now have identified a second as-yet unreported patient without an identifiable StAR mutation, further suggesting this possibility. As more patients are diagnosed, it remains crucial to perform imaging studies of the adrenals, as the diagnosis of lipoid CAH cannot be made in the absence of massive adrenal enlargement *(15)*. If such imaging studies are not performed, other disorders may be misdiagnosed as lipoid CAH. The most likely would be congenital adrenal hypoplasia *(63,64)*, but hypothetical lesions in the transcription factor SF-1, which is required for adrenal and gonadal development in the rodent *(65)*, might also be expected to produce a similar phenotype. Thus, whereas finding StAR mutations in all but one patient examined certainly establishes StAR as the predominant cause of the lipoid CAH phenotype, it remains possible that mutations in other genes may produce a similar phenotype, identifying genes would be of substantial interest.

Second, the mechanism of StAR's action remains wholly unknown. The early suggestion that it facilitated cholesterol movement from the outer to inner mitochondrial membrane by forming contact sites between the two *(20)* has been disproven. Although StAR has a mitochondrial leader peptide and is imported into mitochondria, it remains wholly active when this peptide is removed, prohibiting StAR's entry into the mitochondria *(66)*. It seems likely that cytoplasmic StAR interacts with proteins on the outer mitochondrial membrane, possibly in a fashion analogous to a ligand and its receptor. What might that receptor be, and what would be the clinical consequences of mutations in such a receptor? The abundant evidence that the mitochondrial benzodiazepine receptor complex participates in steroidogenesis [for review, see *(37, 40)*] indicates that a careful examination of potential interactions between StAR and this receptor complex is needed.

Third, the sex ratio of lipoid CAH remains confusing. The StAR gene is on chromosome 8p11.2 *(47)*, hence, lipoid CAH should exhibit autosomal recessive inheritance, affecting an equal number of genetic males and females. Although Hauffa et al. *(15)* found a perfect 14:14 radio of 46,XX genetic males and 46,XX genetic females affected with lipoid CAH, Matsuo et al. *(53)* reported an XY/XX ratio of 47:16, we found a ratio of 18:3 *(51)* and Fujieda et al. *(67)* reported a ratio of 15:8. Thus, several large surveys have found a preponderance of affected 46,XY individuals. There is no apparent reason for this: as affected individuals of both genetic sexes will have the same phenotypic appearance and hormonal findings in infancy, we would not expect there to be bias in ascertainment. An effect of StAR on 23,X sperm cannot be excluded, and could lead to further understanding of fertilization. Thus, the syndrome of congenital lipoid adrenal hyperplasia has yet to reveal all of its secrets.

REFERENCES

1. Prader A, Gurtner HP. Das syndrom des pseudohermaphroditismus masculinus bei kongenitaler nebennierenrindenhyperplasie ohne androgenuberproduktion (adrenaler Pseudohermaphroditismus masculinus). Helv Paed Acta 1955; 10:397–412.
2. Prader A, Siebenmann RE. Nebenniereninsuffizienz bie kongenitaler lipoidhyperplasie der nebennieren. Helv Paed Acta 1957; 12:569–595.
3. Prader A, Anders CJPA. Zur genetik der kongenitalen lipoidhyperplasie der nebennieren. Helv Paed Acta 1962; 17:285–289.
4. Tilp A. Hochgradige Verfettung der nebenniere eines sauglings. Verhandlungen der deutschensch gesellschaft fur pathologie 1913; 16:305–307.
5. Brutschy P. Hochgradige lipoidhyperplasie beider nebennieren mit herdformigen kalkablagerunger bei einem fall von hypospadiasis penisscrotalis und doppelseitigem kryptorchismus mit unechter akzessorisher nebenniere am rechten hoden (pseudohermaphroditismus masculinus externus). Frankfurter Zeitschriff für Pathologie 1920; 24:203–240
6. Sandison AT. A form of lipoidosis of the adrenal cortex in an infant. Arch Dis Childh 1955; 30:538–541.
7. Zahn J. Ueber intersexualitat und nebennierenhyperplasie. Schweizerische Medizinische Wochenschrift 1948; 78:480–486.
8. Camacho AM, Kowarski A, Migeon CJ, Brough A. Congenital adrenal hyperplasia due to a deficiency of one of the enzymes involved in the biosynthesis of pregnenolone. J Clin Endocrinol Metab 1968; 28:153–161.

9. Degenhart HJ, Visser KHA, Boon H, O'Doherty NJD. Evidence for deficiency of 20α cholesterol hydroxylase activity in adrenal tissue of a patient with lipoid adrenal hyperplasia. Acta Endocrinol 1972; 71:512–518.

10. Lin D, Sugawara T, Strauss JF III, Clark BJ, Stocco DM, Saenger P, et al. Role of steroidogenic acute regulatory protein in adrenal and gonadal steroidogenesis. Science 1995; 267:1828–1831.

11. Koizumi S, Kyoya S, Miyawaki T, Kidani H, Funabashi T, Nakashima H, et al. Cholesterol side-chain cleavage enzyme activity and cytochrome P450 content in adrenal mitochondria of a patient with congenital lipoid adrenal hyperplasia (Prader disease). Clin Chem Acta 1977; 77:301–306.

12. Omura T, Sato R, Cooper DY, Rosenthal O, Estabrook RW. Function of cytochrome P450 of microsomes. Fed Proc 1965; 24:1181–1189.

13. Shikita M, Hall PF. Cytochrome P-450 from bovine adrenocortical mitochondria: an enzyme for the side chain cleavage of cholesterol. I. Purification and properties. J Biol Chem 1973; 248:5596–5604.

14. Miller WL. Molecular biology of steroid hormone synthesis. Endocr Rev 1988; 9:295–318.

15. Hauffa BP, Miller WL, Grumbach MM, Conte FA, Kaplan SL. Congenital adrenal hyperplasia due to deficient cholesterol side-chain cleavage activity (20,22 desmolase) in a patient treated for 18 years. Clin Endocrinol 1985; 23:481–493.

16. Matteson KJ, Chung B, Urdea MS, Miller WL. Study of cholesterol side chain cleavage (20,22 desmolase) deficiency causing congenital lipoid adrenal hyperplasia using bovine-sequence P450scc oligodeoxyribonucleotide probes. Endocrinology 1986; 118:1296–1305.

17. Chung B, Matteson KJ, Voutilainen R, Mohandas TK, Miller WL. Human cholesterol side-chain cleavage enzyme, P450scc: cDNA cloning, assignment of the gene to chromosome 15, and expression in the placenta. Proc Natl Acad Sci USA 1986; 83:8962–8966.

18. Morohashi K, Sogawa K, Omura T, Fujii-Kuriyama Y. Gene structure of human cytochrome P-450(scc), cholesterol desmolase. J Biochem 1987; 101:879–887.

19. Lin D, Gitelman SE, Saenger P, Miller WL. Normal genes for the cholesterol side chain cleavage enzyme, P450scc, in congenital lipoid adrenal hyperplasia. J Clin Invest 1991; 88:1955–1962.

20. Stocco DM, Clark BJ. Regulation of the acute production of steroids in steroidogenic cells. Endocr Rev 1996; 17:221–244.

21. Stone D, Hechter O. Studies on ACTH action in perfused bovine adrenals: aspects of progesterone as an intermediary in cortico-steroidogenesis. Arch Biochem Biophys 1955; 54:121–128.

22. Ferguson JJ. Protein synthesis and adrenocorticotropin responsiveness. J Biol Chem 1963; 238:2754–2759.

23. Garren LD, Ney RL, Davis WW. Studies on the role of protein synthesis in the regulation of corticosterone production by adrenocorticotropic hormone in vivo. Proc Natl Acad Sci USA 1965; 53:1443–1450.

24. Garren LD, Davis WW, Crocco RM. Puromycin analogs: action of adrenocorticotropic hormone and the role of glycogen. Science 1966; 152:1386–1388.

25. Waterman MR, Simpson ER. Regulation of steroid hydroxylase gene expression is multifactorial in nature. Recent Prog Horm Res 1989; 45:533–566.

26. Moore CCD, Miller WL. The role of transcriptional regulation in steroid hormone biosynthesis. J Steroid Biochem Mol Biol 1991; 40:517–525.

27. Golos TJ, Miller WL, Strauss JF III. Human chorionic gonadotropin and 8-bromo-cyclic adenosine mono phosphate promote an acute increase in cytochrome P450scc and adrenodoxin messenger RNAs in cultured human granulosa cells by a cycloheximide-insensitive mechanism. J Clin Invest 1987; 80:896–899.

28. Picado-Leonard J, Voutilainen R, Kao L, Chung B, Strauss JF III, Miller WL. Human adrenodoxin: Cloning of three cDNAs and cycloheximide enhancement in JEG-3 cells. J Biol Chem 1988; 263:3240–3244, corrected 11,016.

29. Ringler GE, Kao L-C, Miller WL, Strauss JF III. Effects of 8-bromo-cAMP on expression of endocrine functions by cultured human trophoblast cells. Regulation of specific mRNAs. Mol Cell Endocrinol 1989; 62:13–21.

30. Mellon SH, Vaisse C. cAMP regulates P450scc gene expression by a cycloheximide-insensitive mechanism in cultured mouse leydig MA-10 cells. Proc Natl Acad Sci USA 1989; 86:7775–7779.

31. Chandebhan R, Noland BJ, Scallen TJ, Vahouny GV. Sterol carrier protein 2: Delivery of cholesterol from adrenal lipid droplets to mitochondria for pregnenolone synthesis. J Biol Chem 1982; 257:8928–8934.

32. Vahouny GV, Chanderbhan R, Noland BJ, Irwin D, Dennis P, Labmeth JD, et al. Sterol carrier protein

2: identification of adrenal sterol carrier protein 2 and site of action for mitochondrial cholesterol utilization. J Biol Chem 1983; 258:11,731–11,737.

33. Pedersen RC, Brownie AC. Cholesterol side-chain cleavage in the rat adrenal cortex: Isolation of a cycloheximide-sensitive activator peptide. Proc Natl Acad Sci USA 1983; 80:1882–1886.

34. Pedersen RC, Brownie AC. Steroidogenesis activator polypeptide isolated from a rat Leydig cell tumor. Science 1987; 236:188–190.

35. Li X, Warren DW, Gregorie J, Pedersen RC, Lee AS. The rat 78000 dalton glucose regulated protein (GRP-78) as a precursor for the rat steroidogenesis activator polypeptide (SAP): the SAP coding sequence is homologous with the terminal end of GRP-78. Mol Endocrinol 1989; 3:1944–1952.

36. Iida S, Papadopoulos V, Hall PF. The influence of exogenous free cholesterol on steroid synthesis in cultured adrenal cells. Endocrinology 1989; 124:2619–2624.

37. Papadopoulos V. Peripheral-type benzodiazepine/diazepam binding inhibitor receptor. Biological role in steroidogenic cell function. Endocr Rev 1993; 14:222–240.

38. Yanagibashi K, Ohno Y, Kawamura M, Hall PF. The regulation of intracellular transport of cholesterol in bovine adrenal cells: purification of a novel protein. Endocrinology 1988; 123:2075–2082.

39. Besman MJ, Yanagibashi K, Lee TD, Kawamura M, Hall PF, Shively JE. Identification of des-(Gly-Ile)-endozepine as an effector of corticotropin-dependent adrenal steroidogenesis: stimulation of cholesterol delivery is mediated by the peripheral benzodiazepine receptor. Proc Natl Acad Sci USA 1989; 86:4897–4901.

40. Papadopoulos V, Amri H, Boujrad N, Cascio C, Culty M, Garnier M, et al. Peripheral benzodiazepine receptor in cholesterol transport and steroidogenesis. Steroids 1997; 62:21–28.

41. Lin D, Chang YJ, Strauss JF III, Miller WL. The human peripheral benzodiazepine receptor gene. Cloning and characterization of alternative splicing in normal tissues and in a patient with congenital lipoid adrenal hyperplasia. Genomics 1993; 18:643–650.

42. Pon LA, Orme-Johnson NR. Acute stimulation of steroidogenesis in corpus luteum and adrenal cortex by peptide hormones. J Biol Chem 1986; 261:6594–6599.

43. Stocco DM, Sodeman TC. The 30 kDa mitochondrial protein induced by hormone stimulation in MA-10 mouse Leydig tumor cells are processed from larger precursors. J Biol Chem 1991; 266:19,731–19,738.

44. Epstein LF, Orme-Johnson NR. Regulation of steroid hormone biosynthesis. Identification of precursors of a phosphoprotein targeted to the mitochondrion in stimulated rat adrenal cortex cells. J Biol Chem 1991; 266:19,739–19,745.

45. Clark BJ, Wells J, King SR, Stocco DM. The purification, cloning and expression of a novel luteinizing hormone-induced mitochondrial protein in MA-10 cells mouse Leydig tumor cells. Characterization of the steroidogenic acute regulatory protein (StAR). J Biol Chem 1994; 269:28,314–28,322.

46. Saenger P, Klonari Z, Black SM, Compagnone N, Mellon SH, Fleischer A, et al. Prenatal diagnosis of congenital lipoid adrenal hyperplasia. J Clin Endocrinol Metab 1995; 80:200–205.

47. Sugawara T, Holt JA, Driscoll D, Strauss JF III, Lin D, Miller WL, et al. Human steroidogenic acute regulatory protein (StAR): Functional activity in COS-1 cells, tissue-specific expression, and mapping of the structural gene to 8p11.2 and an expressed pseudogene to chromosome 13. Proc Natl Acad Sci USA 1995; 92:4778–4782.

48. Tee MK, Lin D, Sugawara T, Holt JA, Guiguen Y, Buckingham B, et al. T → A transversion 11 bp from a splice acceptor site in the gene for steroidogenic acute regulatory protein causes congenital lipoid adrenal hyperplasia. Hum Mol Genet 1995; 4:2299–2305.

49. Toaff ME, Schleyer H, Strauss JF III. Metabolism of 25-hydroxycholesterol by rat luteal mitochondria and dispersed cells. Endocrinology 1982; 111:1785–1790.

50. Harikrishna JA, Black SM, Szklarz GD, Miller WL. Construction and function of fusion enzymes of the human cytochrome P450scc system. DNA Cell Biol 1993; 12:371–379.

51. Bose HS, Sugawara T, Strauss JF III, Miller WL. The pathophysiology and genetics of congenital lipoid adrenal hyperplasia. N Engl J Med 1996; 335:1870–1878.

52. Kirkland RT, Kirkland JL, Johnson CM, Horning MG, Librik L, Clayton GW. Congenital lipoid adrenal hyperplasia in an eight-year-old phenotypic female. J Clin Endocrinol Metab 1973; 36:488–496.

53. Matsuo N, Tsuzaki S, Anzo M, Ogata T, Sato S. The phenotypic definition of congenital lipoid adrenal hyperplasia: analysis of the 67 Japanese patients (abstract). Horm Res 41 1994; (suppl): 106 (abstract)

54. Zuber MX, Mason JI, Simpson ER, Waterman MR. Simultaneous transfection of COS-1 cells with mitochondrial and microsomal steroid hydroxylases: incorporation of a steroidogenic pathway into non-steroidogenic cells. Proc Natl Acad Sci USA 1988; 85:699–703.

55. Miller WL. Mitochondrial specificity of the early steps in steroidogenesis. J Steroid Biochem Mol Biol 1995; 55:607–616.
56. Brentano ST, Black SM, Lin D, Miller WL. cAMP post-transcriptionally diminishes the abundance of adrenodoxin reductase mRNA. Proc Natl Acad Sci USA 1992; 89:4099–4103.
57. Sugawara T, Lin D, Holt JA, Martin KO, Javitt NB, Miller WL, et al. The structure of the human steroidogenic acute regulatory (StAR) protein gene: StAR stimulates mitochondrial cholesterol 27-hydroxylase activity. Biochemistry 1995b; 34:12,506–12,512.
58. Mellon SH. Neurosteroids: biochemistry, modes of action, and clinical relevance. J Clin Endocrinol Metab 1994; 78:1003–1008.
59. Bose HS, Pescovitz OH, Miller WL. Spontaneous feminization in a 46,XX female patient with congenital lipoid adrenal hyperplasia due to a homozygous frameshift mutation in the steroidogenic acute regulatory protein. J Clin Endocrinol Metab 1997.
60. Mesiano S, Coulter CL, Jaffe RB. Localization of cytochrome P450 cholesterol side-chain cleavage, cytochrome P450 17α-hydroxylase/17,20 lyase, and 3β-hydroxysteroid dehydrogenase-isomerase steroidogenic enzymes in human and rhesus monkey fetal adrenal glands: reappraisal of functional zonation. J Clin Endocrinol Metab 1993; 77:1184–1189.
61. Voutilainen R, Miller WL. Developmental expression of genes for the steroidogenic enzymes P450scc (20,22 desmolase), P450c17 (17α-hydroxylase/17,20 lyase) and P450c21 (21-hydroxylase) in the human fetus. J Clin Endocrinol Metab 1986; 63:1145–1150.
62. Grumbach MM, Styne DM. Puberty: ontogeny, neuroendocrinology, physiology, and disorders. In: Wilson JD and Foster DW, eds. Williams Textbook of Endocrinology, 8th Ed, WB Saunders, Philadelphia, PA, 1992, pp. 1139–1221.
63. Zanaria E, Muscatelli F, Bardoni B, Strom TM, Guioli S, Guo W, et al. An unusual member of the nuclear hormone receptor superfamily responsible for X-linked adrenal hypoplasia congenita. Nature 1994; 372:635–641.
64. Guo W, Burris TP, McCabe ERB. Expression of DAX-1, the gene responsible for X-linked adrenal hypoplasia congenita and hypogonadotropic hypogonadism, in the hypothalamic-pituitary-adrenal/gonadal axis. Biochem Mol Med 1994; 56:8–13.
65. Luo X, Ikeda Y, Parker KL. A cell-specific nuclear receptor is essential for adrenal and gonadal development and sexual differentiation. Cell 1994; 77:481–490.
66. Arakane F, Sugawara T, Nishino H, Liu Z, Holt JA, Pain D, et al. Steroidogenic acute regulatory protein (StAR) retains activity in the absence of its mitochondrial targeting sequence: implications for the mechanism of StAR action. Proc Natl Acad Sci USA 1996; 93:13,731–13,736.
67. Fujieda K, Tajima T, Nakae J, Sugawara T, Strauss JF III. Molecular analysis of the steroidogenic acute regulatory protein (StAR) gene from 23 Japanese patients with congenital lipoid adrenal hyperplasia. 10th Int Cong Endocrinol, Program and Abstr Vol 1 San Francisco, CA, (Abs #P2-728), 1996, p 586.
68. Hall PF. The roles of calmodulin, actin and vimentin in steroid synthesis by adrenal cells. Steroids 1997; 62:185–189.

23   Congenital Adrenal Hypoplasia

Michael Peter and Wolfgang G. Sippell

CONTENTS

INTRODUCTION

The enormous size of the newborn adrenal relative to the kidney was described by Morgagni in the beginning of the 18th century and later by Soemmering and Meckel who observed the absence of the adrenal cortex in anencephaly *(1)*. Fifty years after the first description of the primary or so-called cytomegalic form of congenital adrenal hypoplasia by Šikl *(2)*, the clinical features, hormonal findings, and diagnostic criteria, as well as the etiology and pathogenesis of this rare X-linked inherited disorder appear much more precisely defined.

EMBRYOLOGY AND DEVELOPMENT OF THE ADRENAL CORTEX

The adrenal cortex and the gonads rise from a particular cell population in the coelomic mesothelium termed adrenogenital primordium *(3)*. In the process of differentiation from the adrenogenital primordium to the mature adrenal cortex, upstream regulatory mechanisms and downstream target genes are involved. In their extensive study of the development of zonal patterns in the human adrenal gland, Sucheston and Cannon *(4)* described five landmark phases: (1) condensation of the coelomic epithelium (3–4 wk of gestation); (2) proliferation and migration of coelomic epithelial cells (4–6 wk of gestation); (3) morphological differentiation of fetal adrenal cortical cells into two distinct zones, termed the fetal zone and the definitive zone (8–10 wk of gestation); (4) decline and disappearance of the fetal zone (first three postnatal months); and (5) establishment and stabilization of the adult zonal pattern (10–20 yr of age). The fetal zone accounts for the bulk of the adrenal cortex (80–90%) and is the primary site of growth and steroidogenesis during fetal life. The definitive zone occupies the remainder of the cortex and comprises a narrow band of tightly packed cells surrounding the fetal zone. Soon after birth, the human adrenal cortex dramatically remodels. The fetal zone atrophies and the *zonas glomerulosa* and *fasciculata* develop. This remodeling is an apoptotic process *(5)*.

PATHOLOGY OF CONGENITAL ADRENAL HYPOPLASIA

Congenital hypoplasia of the adrenal glands is a rare cause of congenital adrenal insufficiency. Congenital adrenal hypoplasia has been described in association with other congenital abnormalities and may be primary, or secondary to anencephaly, microcephaly with occipital cephalomeningocele, or hydrocephalus with occipital defects. Congenital absence or hypoplasia of the pituitary, or neurohypophysial aplasia in the absence of other defects of the central nervous system, have also been reported. As in anencephaly, these secondary conditions are characterized by the small size of the fetal zone. The secondary form of congenital adrenal hypoplasia is also known as the miniature form. The definitive zone of the adrenal cortex is unremarkable. The miniature type occurs in sporadic and autosomal recessive forms. At birth, the weight of the adrenals in anencephaly is approx 10% of that in normal newborns *(6,7)*. Similar adrenal findings occur in infants of mothers who have been treated with high doses of corticosteroids during pregnancy.

The primary form of congenital adrenal hypoplasia is characterized by a fetal zone of large vacuolated cells. The definitive zone of the adrenal cortex is lacking. This condition has been first described by the Czech pathologist Šikl in 1948 *(2)*. The primary or cytomegalic form of congenital adrenal hypoplasia follows an X-linked mode of inheritance in most cases reported in the literature. However, some rare cases of affected female and male infants within the same family have been reported. Thus, a second form of cytomegalic congenital adrenal hypoplasia with autosomal recessive inheritance must be present *(8,9)*.

CLINICAL PRESENTATION

Clinical signs and symptoms in infants with congenital adrenal hypoplasia include poor feeding, failure to thrive, frequent vomiting, dehydration, and hyperpigmentation. Hyponatremia, hyperkalemia, metabolic acidosis, and hypoglycemia are common biochemical findings characteristic of combined glucocorticoid and mineralocorticoid deficiency *(10–14)*. Most of the reported cases are clinical case reports *(11–13,15–32)*. A large Greenlandic family comprising of 171 descendants in five generations with male patients suffering from X-linked congenital adrenal hypoplasia has been published by Petersen et al. *(33)*. The diagnosis of cytomegalic congenital adrenal hypoplasia is a histopathological diagnosis and can be made with certainty by postmorten examination only.

During the past 20 years, a total of 18 boys from 16 families were diagnosed by our laboratory as suffering from congenital adrenal insufficiency caused by congenital hypoplasia of the permanent adrenal cortex. All patients were of Caucasian origin. Clinical data of the 18 boys from our present series are summarized in Table 1. Fifteen boys presented with salt-wasting and failure to thrive in the first weeks of life (range 1 wk to 2 mo of age). One boy presented at age 5 mo with a hypoglycemic convulsion, while also showing laboratory and clinical signs of salt-wasting. His younger brother was prenatally diagnosed and treatment was initiated immediately after a diagnostic

Table 1
Clinical Characteristics of 18 AHC Boys

Case No.	Age at Onset of Symptoms	First Symptoms	Cryptorchidism/ Hypogonadotropic Hypogonadism	Phenotype	Family History	Remarks
1	1 mo	Salt-wasting	no/prepubertal	AHC	unknown	died at age 1 yr in Addisonian crisis
2	2 wk	Salt-wasting	yes/-	AHC, GKD, DMD	unknown	
3	2 mo	Salt-wasting	?/prepubertal	AHC	unknown	
4	3 wk	Salt-wasting	yes/prepubertal	AHC, GKD, DMD	yes	severe brain damage after convulsions, initial diagnosis CAH (21-hydroxylase def)
5	1 mo	Salt-wasting	yes/prepubertal	AHC	yes	died at age 6 yr in Addisonian crisis, initial diagnosis CAH (11-hydroxylase def)
6	3 wk	Salt-wasting	no/-	AHC	yes	died at age 4 mo
7	1 mo	Salt-wasting	?/-	AHC, GKD, DMD		
8	3 yr	Salt-wasting	no/prepubertal	AHC, GKD	yes	diagnosed after younger brother (case 9)
9	1 mo	Salt-wasting	no/prepubertal	AHC, GKD	yes	younger brother of case 8
10	2 wk	Salt-wasting	yes/prepubertal	AHC	unknown	low maternal estriol levels during pregnancy, initial diagnosis CAH (11-hydroxylase def)
11	1 mo	Salt-wasting	?/HH	AHC	unknown	initial diagnosis CAH (21-hydroxylase def)
12	2 wk	Salt-wasting	yes/HH	AHC	no	
13	2 wk	Salt-wasting	?/HH	AHC	unknown	initial CAH (21-hydroxylase def)
14	2 wk	Salt-wasting	?/prepubertal	AHC, GKD, DMD	no	
15	5 mo	Hypoglycemic convulsion	yes/prepubertal	AHC	yes	low maternal estriol levels during pregnancy, older brother of case no. 16
16	treatment started in the first wk	any	no/prepubertal	AHC	yes	low maternal estriol levels during pregnancy, younger brother of case no. 15
17	1 wk	Salt-wasting	yes/HH	AHC	yes	
18	2 wk	Salt-wasting	no/prepubertal	AHC	no	

AHC = congenital adrenal hypoplasia, GKD = glycerol kinase deficiency, DMA = Duchenne's muscular dystrophy adrenocorticotropic hormone (ACTH) test at 3 d of age *(34)*. One boy expressed no signs or symptoms of adrenal insufficiency until age 3 yr, when his younger brother was diagnosed as having congenital adrenal hypoplasia. Patients presenting with salt-wasting showed typical laboratory signs such as hyponatremia, hyperkalemia, metabolic acidosis, and elevated plasma renin activity. In these boys, blood glucose levels were normal at presentation. Seven boys had unilateral or bilateral cryptorchidism. Those patients who had already reached a postpubertal age, all suffered from delayed puberty caused by hypogonadotropic hypogonadism. From the total of 18 boys, 12 suffered exclusively from adrenal insufficiency, 6 had a contiguous gene syndrome (2 had congenital adrenal hypoplasia and glycerol kinase deficiency, and 4 had congenital adrenal hypoplasia, glycerol kinase deficiency, and Duchenne muscular dystrophy). In eight families, we found a history of unexplained deaths of male infants in the first months of life or of typical signs or symptoms of primary adrenal insufficiency such as hyperpigmentation. A primary diagnosis of congenital adrenal hyperplasia due to 21-hydroxylase or 11β-hydroxylase deficiency was assumed in four boys.

Postmorten examinations were performed on three boys who died at age 4 mo, 1 yr, and 6 yr, respectively. The findings in one case (death at age 4 mo), confirming the diagnosis of the cytomegalic type of adrenal hypoplasia, have been published by Kohlschütter *(30)*. The lack of the definitive zone of the adrenal cortex was confirmed in our two other cases during the postmortem examination. However, the characteristic large vacuolated cells resembling fetal adrenocortical cells were not visible in these two cases. This is not surprising because both patients died at an age when the involution of the fetocortex is completed.

Delayed onset of symptoms of congenital adrenal hypoplasia *(13,23,25,26,35,36)* as well as intrafamilial variability *(13,23,25,35–38)* has been described by several authors. Abnormalities in adrenal development seem to be variable, and less severe forms of this disorder could result in subclinical or late onset adrenal insufficiency.

The aforementioned signs and symptoms are indistinguishable from those observed in the salt-losing form of congenital adrenal hyperplasia because of 21-hydroxylase deficiency. A relatively common symptom occurring in boys with congenital adrenal hypoplasia that we observed in 7 out of 18 patients, is unilateral or bilateral cryptorchidism *(10)*. In general, a high rate of undescended testes is observed in patients with hypogonadotropic hypogonadism, which is a common feature of congenital adrenal hypoplasia patients *(23,36,39,40)*. It is now believed that all boys with congenital adrenal hypoplasia who reach a postpubertal age will have delayed puberty caused by hypogonadotropic hypogonadism. There is a clear phenotypic heterogeneity of hypogonadotropic hypogonadism in congenital adrenal hypoplasia patients reported in the literature with regard to the localization of the defects in the hypothalamus or in the pituitary. A primary pituitary defect was suggested by several studies *(13,41–43)* in which patients showed little or no response to prolonged treatment with pulsatile gonadotropin releasing hormone (GnRH). However, studies in two of our own patients who did respond to pulsatile GnRH suggested a primary defect in the hypothalamus *(44,45)*. More recent data from the literature suggest that *DAX-1* mutations impair gonadotropin production by acting at both the hypothalamic and the pituitary level *(38,46)*.

The interesting observation of an active hypothalamic-pituitary-gonadal axis in a congenital adrenal hypoplasia infant within the first 4 mo of life has been made by

Table 2
Hormonal Data of 18 AHC Boys Indicating an Active Hypothalamic-Pituitary-Gonadal
Axis within the First Months of Life

Hormone	Case 2	Case 4	Case 9	Case 10		Normal Ranges
	age 3 mo	age 3 mo	age 3 mo	age 1 mo	age 3 mo	1–3 mo
DHA-Sulfate (nmol/L)	<25	<25	<25	<25	<25	28–3000
Androstenedione (nmol/L)	0.66	3.7	0.94	10.0	0.31	0.77–5.7
Testosterone (nmol/L)	11.5	5.0	14.9	16.6	5.6	2.4–11.8
LH (mIU/mL)	—	2.1	0.5	7.3	—	1.5–7.1
FSH (mIU/mL)	—	3.6	3.8	2.0	—	1.5–3.9

Takahashi and coworkers *(47)*. Our data of four affected boys (Table 2) support this observation. All four boys had testosterone plasma levels within the midpubertal range. We did not perform GnRH testing in these boys, however, basal luteinizing hormone (LH) and follicle-stimulating hormone (FSH) were in the normal range for boys below age 3 mo (higher than prepubertal) indicating an active hypothalamic-pituitary-gonadal axis at this age. We propose the hypothesis that there might be a difference in the central regulation of hypothalamic-pituitary-gonadal activity between infant boys and pubertal boys.

Progressive high-frequency hearing loss starting during puberty has been observed in three patients by Zachmann et al. *(48)*. We did not observe this phenomenon in any of our adult patients.

Height development depends on the quality of substitution therapy with glucocorticoids. In our oldest patients, we observed slow growth during infancy and prepuberty. This was probably caused by relatively high glucocorticoid doses. The magnitude of the pubertal growth spurt depends on the induction of puberty by androgen administration. Final height is usually within genetic target height range.

One-third of our patients suffering from congenital adrenal hypoplasia had a contiguous gene syndrome. The phenotype, which includes congenital adrenal hypoplasia, glycerol kinase deficiency, and Duchenne muscular dystrophy, is relatively frequent. Glycerol kinase deficiency is an X-linked inborn error of metabolism characterized by hyperglycerolemia and glyceroluria. Duchenne muscular dystrophy is a severe muscle-wasting disorder, resulting in early confinement to a wheelchair and often death by age 20 caused by respiratory insufficiency. All patients with phenotypic involvement of the congenital adrenal hypoplasia, glycerol kinase deficiency, and Duchenne muscular dystrophy loci have some degree of developmental delay *(49)*. In patients with isolated congenital adrenal hypoplasia mental development is unimpaired if hypoglycemic brain damage has been avoided by proper substitution therapy.

FREQUENCY OF X-LINKED CONGENITAL ADRENAL HYPOPLASIA

The overall incidence of idiopathic adrenal hypoplasia has been estimated at 1/12,500 births or approx 0.2–0.26% in a large series of consecutive perinatal autopsies

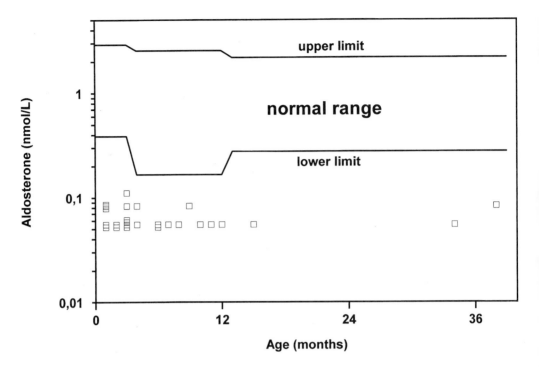

Fig. 1. Basal aldosterone plasma levels in congenital adrenal hypoplasia boys determined by multiste-roid analysis. Plasma aldosterone (open squares) was at or below the lower limit of detection of the assay (0.055 nmol/L) in all patients at first presentation.

(10,50). When comparing the frequency of congenital adrenal hyperplasia caused by 21-hydroxylase deficiency with that of congenital adrenal hypoplasia on the basis of the number of steroid analyses performed in our laboratory over the past decade, it can be stated that the diagnosis of congenital adrenal hypoplasia is much more rare. The frequency of congenital adrenal hyperplasia caused by 21-hydroxylase deficiency in the German population is approx 1/13,000 births *(51).* Thus, the frequency of congenital adrenal hypoplasia must be significantly less than 1/12,500 births.

HORMONAL FINDINGS AND DIAGNOSTIC RECOMMENDATIONS

The diagnosis of adrenal insufficiency in young infants depends on specific methods for the determination of steroids in plasma and/or urine. Our own data have been collected with the method of multisteroid analysis *(52),* using extraction and automated high-performance liquid gel chromatography (HPLC) prior to radioimmunoassay to avoid crossreactions with other abundant fetocortical steroids. In our present series *(14),* aldosterone deficiency preceded cortisol deficiency in all neonatal cases examined. When we determined plasma aldosterone in the salt-wasting infants between the first week of life and age 2 mo, plasma aldosterone was very low with no or little increase after ACTH stimulation (Fig. 1). At the same time, plasma cortisol was elevated or in the normal range in most of the patients, reflecting the still-active steroid production in the fetocortex. However, adrenal function subsequently declined, and at age 6 mo, all of the infants who presented with salt-wasting as neonates were cortisol deficient,

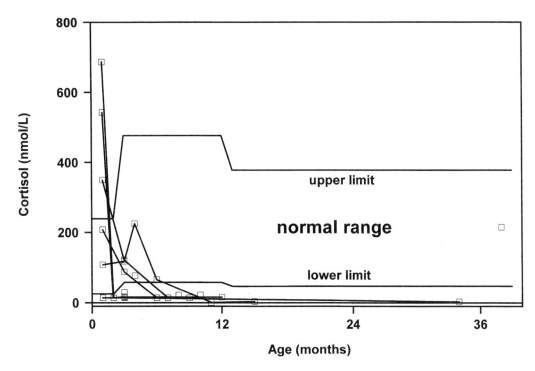

Fig. 2. Basal cortisol plasma levels in congenital adrenal hypoplasia boys determined by multisteroid analysis. Plasma cortisol (open squares) determined by our highly specific method was above the upper normal limit in some patients at first presentation. At age 6 mo, plasma cortisol was below normal except in one patient.

also (Fig. 2). However, some children showed a prolonged phase of glucocorticoid sufficiency *(14, 26)*. Thus, in the first weeks of life, an ACTH test is often necessary to prove cortisol deficiency. The diagnosis of adrenal insufficiency can also be made with a 24-h urine sample which is, however, difficult to collect in this very young age group.

Some of the boys with congenital adrenal hypoplasia were misdiagnosed as having congenital adrenal hyperplasia caused by 21-hydroxylase deficiency. The correct diagnosis depends on specific methods for the determination of steroids. We did not observe elevated 17-hydroxyprogesterone plasma levels in any of our patients. However, we detected elevated plasma levels of 11-deoxycortisol and 11-deoxycorticosterone in the first weeks of life, suggesting 11β-hydroxylase deficiency. This phenomenon was observed in 7 of our 18 patients and, in 1 patient, it disappeared even after age 6 mo (Table 3). We hypothesize that this might be caused by disturbed steroid production in the still-active fetocortex.

Prenatal diagnosis of congenital adrenal hypoplasia is not essential, but may be helpful in the management of the affected newborn because treatment can be started directly after birth. Congenital adrenal hypoplasia is one possible cause of low maternal plasma and/or urine estriol levels during pregnancy *(24)*. Thus, serial determinations of low plasma maternal estriol during pregnancy indicate congenital adrenal hypoplasia provided that other factors causing low estriol are excluded *(34)*.

Table 3
Serial Determinations of Plasma Steroids in the Same AHC Patient
Between 1 and 15 Mo of Age

Steroid (nmol/L)	Age 1 Mo	Age 3 Mo	Age 4 Mo	Age 6 Mo	Age 11 Mo	Age 15 Mo	Normal Children Age 3 Mo–1 Yr (Range)
Aldosterone	0.06	0.06	0.06	0.06	0.06	0.06	0.17–2.55
Corticosterone	2.63	5.80	8.14	3.52	1.01	0.14	0.14–15.9
11-Deoxycorti-costerone	0.48	0.88	4.48	0.09	0.09	0.09	0.09–1.0
Progesterone	0.35	0.35	0.35	0.10	0.10	0.10	0.10–4.01
17-OH-Progesterone	0.79	0.73	3.06	0.12	0.09	0.00	0.09–4.69
11-Deoxycortisol	13.68	15.68	33.78	4.50	0.75	0.09	0.61–4.16
Cortisol	107	118	225	66	<5	<5	58.5–477
Cortisone	47	34	74	8.90	4.2	3.10	19.4–127

Glycerol kinase deficiency and Duchenne muscular dystrophy should be excluded in every congenital adrenal hypoplasia boy by measuring plasma concentrations of glycerol and creatinine kinase. Glycerol kinase deficiency is routinely confirmed by documentation of the enzyme deficiency in leukocytes, fibroblasts, or liver.

We suggest the following diagnostic recommendations for congenital adrenal hypoplasia. Specific measurement of plasma cortisol and aldosterone (and precursor steroids) should be performed before and after ACTH stimulation. Direct radioimmunoassay (RIA) procedures without prior purification often give falsely elevated results for aldosterone, cortisol, and their precursors in young infants. During infancy, serial measurements of plasma steroids before and after ACTH may also be necessary for a correct diagnosis. Urinary steroid secretion pattern (gas chromatography) is an alternative tool for establishing the diagnosis of adrenal insufficiency. In addition, plasma-ACTH and plasma-renin activity should be determined. Glycerol kinase deficiency and Duchenne muscular dystrophy should be excluded in every congenital adrenal hypoplasia boy. At the time of normal onset of puberty, secretion of gonadotropins and sex steroids should be examined (e.g., GnRH test and spontaneous nocturnal LH and FSH).

Imaging techniques are not very important in the diagnosis of adrenal hypoplasia, however, they may be helpful to distinguish between adrenal hypoplasia and bilateral adrenal hemorrhage causing adrenal insufficiency.

MOLECULAR GENETICS

The *DAX*-1 gene encodes a protein that is very similar to members of the orphan nuclear receptor superfamily *(53)*. The *DAX*-1 gene is composed of two exons split by one 3.4-kb intron, and codes for a 470-amino acid protein. Putative DNA-binding and ligand-binding domains have been identified *(54)*. Little is known about the function of the *DAX*-1 gene product and its ligand. It has been suggested that *DAX*-1, together with the transcription factor SF-1, is part of a signal cascade required for the normal development of steroidogenic tissues *(55)*. The remarkable phenotype of the SF-1 knockout mouse, which is similar to that observed in patients with *DAX*-1 gene mutations, demonstrates that SF-1 is a key mediator in the development of the adrenal glands, gonads, and the ventromedial hypothalamic nucleus *(56)*. Recently, the mouse *DAX*-1 gene has been isolated *(57,58)*. The murine *DAX*-1 gene encodes for a 472-amino acid protein, with 75% overall nucleotide sequence homology to the human *DAX*-1 gene. The mouse model system of altered *DAX*-1 gene expression will give more insight into the role of the *DAX*-1 protein in tissue- and development-specific gene regulation.

In several studies, it has been proven that *DAX*-1 gene deletions or mutations are responsible for congenital adrenal hypoplasia *(14,35,37,38,47,53,54,59–62)*. It is now commonly agreed that *DAX*-1 gene mutations are also responsible for the frequent occurrence of hypogonadotropic hypogonadism in congenital adrenal hypoplasia patients.

Most of the reported point mutations are frameshift or stop mutations, which produce a truncated nonfunctioning protein. There are four exceptions, three amino acid substitutions, R267P *(37)*, A300V *(47)*, and N440I *(61)*, and one deletion of a single amino acid V269 *(37)*. All of these mutations are located in the putative ligand-binding domain of the *DAX*-1 gene product.

DAX-1 binds to DNA hairpin structures. Binding of *DAX*-1 to the promoter of the gene encoding steroidogenic acute regulatory protein (StAR) results in the transcriptional repression of StAR expression and in the block of steroidogenesis *(63)*. Transcriptional repression by *DAX*-1 is exerted by a bipartite silencing domain present in the putative ligand binding domain of *DAX*-1. It has been shown that the point mutations R267P and ΔV269 impair silencing *(64)*.

In our series of 18 boys with congenital adrenal hypoplasia (Table 4), we found large deletions in the congenital adrenal hypoplasia—glycerol kinase—Duchenne muscular dystrophy gene locus in patients with a contiguous gene syndrome, whereas most of the patients with isolated congenital adrenal hypoplasia (with hypogonadotropic hypogonadism) had point mutations in the *DAX*-1 gene. Two patients with congenital adrenal hypoplasia and hypogonadotropic hypogonadism were found to have a complete deletion of the *DAX*-1 gene. The point mutations identified were all frameshift or stop mutations, which produce a truncated non-functioning protein. The stop codons were distributed over the entire gene *(14)*. In agreement with Nakae et al. *(60)*, we found that mutations even in the C-terminus of the *DAX*-1 protein cause congenital adrenal hypoplasia. The terminal 11 amino acids are particularly important for normal adrenal cortical embryogenesis.

Some male patients presenting with primary adrenal insufficiency in the first months of life have no *DAX*-1 gene deletion/mutation *(14,37)*. The diagnosis of primary adrenal insufficiency caused by the cytomegalic type of congenital adrenal hypoplasia is also made in girls *(8,9)*. It must be assumed that the human genome contains other unknown genes that are necessary for normal adrenal cortex development.

Because more and more monogenetic disorders are explained on a molecular level, an important question raised is the correlation of genotype to phenotype. As shown in our own *(14)* and other studies *(13)*, a wide phenotypic variability has been observed among congenital adrenal hypoplasia patients *(23,25,26,35–38)*. The structural differences in the presumptive *DAX*-1 gene product, as expected from the different point mutations within the gene, do not seem to explain different phenotypes regarding age at onset of symptoms, severity of symptoms, or occurrence of hypogonadotropic hypogonadism. For example, case No. 8 with complete deletion of the *DAX*-1 gene

Table 4
Deletions and Mutations in the AHC-GKD-DMD Gene Locus
Detected in 18 AHC Patients

Case No.	Phenotype	Result of Mutational Analysis
1	AHC	frameshift 546insACCC, first stop codon at codon 185
2	AHC, GKD, DMD	not done, dead, probably deletion of the AHC-GKD-DMD locus
3	AHC	Y130X
4	AHC, GKD, DMD	deletion of approx 1 Mb including the DAX-1-GKD-DMD locus
5	AHC	frameshift 1326delT, first stop codon at codon 461
6	AHC	not done, died at age 6 yr in Addisonian crisis
7	AHC, GKD, DMD	not done, dead, probably deletion of the AHC-GKD-DMD locus
8 (sib)	AHC, GKD	deletion of approx 650 kb including the DAX-1-GKD locus
9 (sib)	AHC, GKD	deletion of approx 650 kb including the DAX-1-GKD locus
10	AHC	Q420X
11	AHC	frameshift 585delTinsCC, first stop codon at codon 204
12	AHC	frameshift 544delG, first stop codon at codon 263
13	AHC	frameshift 477delT, first stop codon at codon 263
14	AHC, GKD, DMD	deletion of approx 1 Mb including the DAX-1-GKD-DMD locus
15 (sib)	AHC	no mutation in the DAX-1 gene
16 (sib)	AHC	no mutation in the DAX-1 gene
17	AHC	deletion of approx 350 kb including DAX-1 gene
18	AHC	deletion of approx 60 kb including DAX-1 gene

had a low normal cortisol plasma level with a blunted response to ACTH at age 3 yr, whereas another case, expressing a presumptive DAX-1 gene product only 10 basepairs shorter than normal, presented with a decreased cortisol plasma level at age 3 mo. These facts suggest that other epigenetic or nongenetic factors may influence the clinical course of congenital adrenal hypoplasia.

The pathophysiology of congenital adrenal hypoplasia is not well-understood. Studying the interplay between SF-1, DAX-1, and their downstream genes (for example, StAR) will provide us with a more-detailed understanding of the regulatory mechanisms functioning in the process of adrenal cortex differentiation.

TREATMENT

Careful clinical management of the affected children is important, because rapid and life-threatening deterioration of adrenal function frequently follows an asymptomatic period during infancy (13). Thus, early diagnosis ensures early start of mineralocorticoid and glucocorticoid treatment and prevents sudden death. Substitution therapy with glucocorticoids and mineralocorticoids should be started in every case with suspected adrenal insufficiency right after diagnostic blood samples have been taken. The doses for chronic substitution therapy during childhood are 10–15 mg/m² t.i.d. for hydrocortisone and 100–250 µg/m² b.i.d. or t.i.d. for fludrocortisone. In acute stress situations (e.g., intercurrent infections, surgery, accident, exams) elevated stress doses (three-to-five-fold) of both the glucocorticoid and the mineralocorticoid must be given without delay. Control of treatment should be made by clinical and laboratory parameters. Clinical parameters of adequate treatment are normal stress tolerance, normal height, and weight development, and normal bone maturation. Useful biochemical and hormonal parameters for adequacy of treatment are normal blood glucose, normal plasma and urine electrolytes, normal free-urinary cortisol, or salivary cortisol profile.

Induction of puberty may be achieved by androgens, hCG, pulsatile GnRH treatment. Induction of spermatogenesis is difficult to achieve and fertility has not yet been demonstrated in patients with X-linked congenital adrenal hypoplasia.

If these important therapeutic and management principles are not constantly met by physicians, parents, and later, the patients themselves, boys with isolated congenital adrenal hypoplasia, as well as those with a contiguous gene syndrome may have a poor prognosis, because we observed one death in Addisonian crisis and one case of severe brain damage after prolonged convulsions in our series of patients.

REFERENCES

1. Medvei VC. The history of clinical endocrinology. 2nd ed. Parthenon, Carnforth, 1993, p. 489.
2. Šikl H. Addison's disease due to congenital adrenal hypoplasia of the adrenals in an infant aged 33 days. J Pathol Bacteriol 1948; 60:323–326.
3. Morohashi K. The ontogenesis of the steroidogenic tissues. Genes Cells 1997; 2:95–106.
4. Sucheston ME, Cannon MS. Development of zonular patterns in the human adrenal gland. J Morphol 1968; 126:477–491.
5. Mesiano S, Jaffe RB. Developmental and functional biology of the primate fetal adrenal cortex. Endocr Rev 1997; 18:378–403.
6. Burke BA. The pituitary, pineal, adrenal thyroid, and parathyroid glands. In: Stocker JT, Dechner LP, eds. Pediatric Pathology. Lippincott, Philadelphia, 1992, pp. 941–1001.
7. Branchaud CL, Pearson Murphy BE. Physiopathology of the fetal adrenal. In: Pasqualini JR, Scholler R, eds. Hormones and Fetal Pathophysiology. Marcel Dekker, New York, 1992, pp. 53–85.
8. Burke BA, Wick MR, King R, et al. Congenital adrenal hypoplasia and selective absence of pituitary luteinizing hormone: a new autosomal recessive syndrome. Am J Med Genet 1988; 31:75–97.
9. Krüger G, Mix M, Pelz L, Dunker H. Cytomegalic type of congenital adrenal hypoplasia due to autosomal recessive inheritance. Am J Med Genet 1993; 46:475.
10. Kelch RP, Virdis R, Rappaport R, Greig F, Levine LS, New MI. Congenital adrenal hypoplasia. In: New MI, Levine LS, eds. Adrenal Diseases in Childhood. Pediatric and Adolescent Endocrinology. Karger, Basel, 1984; 13, pp. 156–161.
11. Brook CGD, Bambach M, Zachmann M, Prader A. Familial congenital adrenal hypoplasia. Helv Paediatr Acta 1973; 28:277–282.
12. Sperling MA, Wolfsen AR, Fisher DA. Congenital adrenal hypoplasia: an isolated defect of organogenesis. J Pediatr 1973; 82:444–449.
13. Kletter GB, Gorski JL, Kelch RP. Congenital adrenal hypoplasia and isolated gonadotropin deficiency. Trends Endocrinol Metab 1991; 2:123–128.
14. Peter M, Viemann M, Partsch CJ, Sippell WG. Congenital adrenal hypoplasia: Clinical spectrum, experience with hormonal diagnosis and report on new point mutations of the DAX-1 gene. J Clin Endocrinol Metab 1998; 83:2666–2674.
15. Williams A, Robinson MJ. Addison's disease in infancy. Arch Dis Child 1956; 31:265–269.
16. Mitchell RG, Rhaney K. Congenital adrenal hypoplasia in siblings. Lancet 1959; 1:488–492.
17. Boyd JF, MacDonald AM. Adrenal cortical hypoplasia in siblings. Arch Dis Child 1960; 35:561–568.
18. Uttley WS. Familial congenital adrenal hypoplasia. Arch Dis Child 1968; 43:724–730.

19. Zondek LH, Zondek T. Congenital adrenal hypoplasia in two infants. Acta Paediatr Scand 1968; 57:250–254.

20. Weiss L, Mellinger RC. Congenital adrenal hypoplasia—an X-linked disease. J Med Genet 1970; 7:27–32.

21. Favara BE, Franciosi RA, Miles V. Idiopathic adrenal hypoplasia in children. Am J Clin Pathol 1972; 57:287–296.

22. Pakravan P, Kenny FM, Depp R, Allen AC. Familial congenital absence of adrenal glands; evaluation of glucocorticoid, and estrogen metabolism in the perinatal period. J Pediatr 1974; 84:74–78.

23. Golden MP, Lippe BM, Kaplan SA. Congenital adrenal hypoplasia and hypogonadotropic hypogonadism. Am J Dis Child 1977; 131:1117–1118.

24. Hensleigh PA, Moore WV, Wilson K, Tulchinsky D. Congenital X-linked adrenal hypoplasia. Obstet Gynecol 1978; 52:228–232.

25. Hay ID, Smail PJ, Forsyth CC. Familial cytomegalic adrenocortical hypoplasia: an X-linked syndrome of pubertal failure. Arch Dis Child 1983; 56:715–721.

26. Sills IN, Voorhess ML, MacGillivray MH, Peterson RE. Prolonged survival without therapy in congenital adrenal hypoplasia. Am J Dis Child 1983; 137:1186–1188.

27. Virdis R, Levine LS, Levy D, Pang S, Rapaport R, New MI. Congenital adrenal hypoplasia: two new cases. J Endocrinol Invest 1983; 6:51–54.

28. Ferrandez A, Fuertes J, Martinez MP, Atares M, Zubillaga P. Congenital adrenal hypoplasia in a male with gonadotropin deficiency. Helv Paediatr Acta 1984; 39:379–384.

29. Rasmussen NH, Christoffersen J, Damkjaer Nielsen M. Congenital adrenal hypoplasia. Acta Paediatr Scand 1986; 75:870–871.

30. Kohlschütter A, Willig HP, Schlamp D, et al. Infantile glycerol kinase deficiency—a condition requiring prompt identification. Clinical, biochemical, and morphological findings in two cases. Eur J Pediatr 1987; 146:575–581.

31. Pillers DA, Weleber RG, Powell BR, Hanna CE, Magenis RE, Buist NR. Aland Island eye disease. (Forsius-Eriksson ocular albinism) and an Xp21 deletion in a patient with Duchenne muscular dystrophy, glycerol kinase deficiency, and congenital adrenal hypoplasia. Am J Med Genet 1990; 36:23–28.

32. Matfin G, Sheaves R, Muscatelli F, et al. Gene deletion causing adrenal hypoplasia congenital and hypogonadotropic hypogonadism. Clin Endocrinol 1994; 40:807–808.

33. Petersen KE, Bille T, Jacobsen BB, Iversen T. X-linked congenital adrenal hypoplasia. A study of five generations of a Greenlandic Family. Acta Paediatr Scand 1982; 71:947–951.

34. Peter M, Partsch CJ, Dörr HG, Sippell WG. Prenatal diagnosis of congenital adrenal hypoplasia. Horm Res 1996; 46:41–45.

35. Yanase T, Takayanagi R, Oba K, Nishi Y, Ohe K, Nawata H. New mutations of DAX-1 genes in two Japanese patients with X-linked congenital adrenal hypoplasia and hypogonadotropic hypogonadism. J Clin Endocrinol Metab 1996; 81:530–535.

36. Kelly WF, Joplin GF, Pearson GW. Gonadotropin deficiency and adrenocortical insufficiency in children: a new syndrome. Br Med J 1977; 9:98.

37. Muscatelli F, Strom TM, Walker AP, et al. Mutations in the DAX-1 gene give rise to both X-linked adrenal hypoplasia congenital and hypogonadotropic hypogonadism. Nature. 1994; 372:672–676.

38. Habiby RL, Boepple P, Nachtigall L, Sluss PM, Crowley-WF J, Jameson JL. Adrenal hypoplasia congenita with hypogonadotropic hypogonadism: evidence that DAX-1 mutations lead to combined hypothalamic and pituitary defects in gonadotropin production. J Clin Invest 1996; 98:1055–1062.

39. Prader A, Zachmann M, Illig R. Luteinizing hormone deficiency in hereditary congenital adrenal hypoplasia. J Pediatr 1975; 86:421–422.

40. Zachmann M, Illig R, Prader A. Gonadotropin deficiency and cryptorchidism in three prepubertal brothers with congenital adrenal hypoplasia. J Pediatr 1980; 97:255–257.

41. Gordon D, Cohen HN, Beastall GH, Hay ID, Thomson JA. Contrasting effects of subcutaneous pulsatile GnRH therapy in congenital adrenal hypoplasia and Kallmann's syndrome. Clin Endocrinol Oxf 1984; 21:597–603.

42. Kiluchi K, Kaji M, Momoi T, Mikawa H, Shigematsu Y, Sudo M. Failure to induce puberty in a man with X-linked congenital adrenal hypoplasia and hypogonadotropic hypogonadism by pulsatile administration of low-dose gonadotropin-releasing hormone. Acta Endocrinol Copenh 1987; 114:153–160.

43. Bovet P, Reymond MJ, Rey F, Gomez F. Lack of gonadotropic response to pulsatile gonadotropin-

releasing hormone in isolated hypogonadotropic hypogonadism associated to congenital adrenal hypoplasia. J Endocrinol Invest 1988; 11:201–204.

44. Kruse K, Sippell WG, von Schnakenburg K. Hypogonadism in congenital adrenal hypoplasia: evidence for a hypothalamic origin. J Clin Endocrinol Metab 1984; 58:12–17.

45. Partsch CJ, Sippell WG. Hypothalamic hypogonadism in congenital adrenal hypoplasia. Horm Metab Res 1989; 21:623–625.

46. Guo W, Burris TP, McCabe ERB. Expression of DAX-1, the gene responsible for X-linked adrenal hypoplasia congenita and hypogonadotropic hypogonadism, in the hypothalamic-pituitary-adrenal/gonadal axis. Biochem Mol Med 1995; 56:8–13.

47. Takahashi T, Shoji Y, Haraguchi N, Takahashi I, Takada G. Active hypothalamic-pituitary-gonadal axis in an infant with X-linked adrenal hypoplasia congenita. J Pediatr 1997; 130:485–488.

48. Zachmann M, Fuchs E, Prader A. Progressive high frequency hearing loss: an additional feature in the syndrome of congenital adrenal hypoplasia and gonadotrophin deficiency. Eur J Pediatr 1992; 151:167–169.

49. McCabe ERB. Disorders of glycerol metabolism. In: Scriver CB, Beaudet AL, Sly WS, Valle D, eds. The Metabolic and Molecular Bases of Inherited Disease. McGraw-Hill, New York, 1995; pp. 1631–1652.

50. Laverty CRA, Fortune DW, Beischer NA. Congenital idiopathic adrenal hypoplasia. Obstet Gynecol 1973; 41:655–663.

51. Mauthe I, Laspe H, Knorr D. Zur Häufigkeit des kongenitalen adrenogenitalen Syndroms (AGS): München 1963–72. Klin Pädiat 1976; 189:172–176.

52. Sippell WG, Bidlingmaier F, Becker H, et al. Simultaneous radioimmunoassay of plasma aldosterone, corticosterone, 11-deoxycorticosterone, progesterone, 17-hydroxyprogesterone, 11-deoxycortisol, cortisol, and cortisone. J Steroid Biochem 1978; 9:63–67.

53. Zanaria E, Muscatelli F, Bardoni B, et al. An unusual member of the nuclear hormone receptor superfamily responsible for X-linked adrenal hypoplasia congenita. Nature 1994; 372:635–641.

54. Guo W, Burris TP, Zhang YH, et al. Genomic sequence of the DAX1 gene: an orphan nuclear receptor responsible for X-linked adrenal hypoplasia congenita and hypogonadotropic hypogonadism. J Clin Endocrinol Metab 1996; 81:2481–2486.

55. Burris TP, Guo W, Le T, McCabe ERB. Identification of a putative steroidogenic factor-1 response element in the DAX-1 promoter. Biochem Biophys Res Commun 1995; 214:576–581.

56. Caron KM, Clark BJ, Ikeda Y, Parker KL. Steroidogenic factor 1 acts at all levels of the reproductive axis. Steroids 1997; 62:53–56.

57. Swain A, Zanaria E, Hacker A, Lovell BR, Camerino G. Mouse Dax1 expression is consistent with a role in sex determination as well as in adrenal and hypothalamus function. Nat Genet 1996; 12:404–409.

58. Bae DS, Schaefer ML, Partan BW, Muglia L. Characterization of the mouse DAX-1 gene reveals evolutionary conservation of a unique amino-terminal motif and widespread expression in mouse tissue. Endocrinology 1996; 137:3921–3927.

59. Guo W, Mason JS, Stone CG, et al. Diagnosis of X-linked adrenal hypoplasia congenita by mutation analysis of the DAX1 gene. JAMA 1995; 274:324–330.

60. Nakae J, Tajima T, Kusuda S, et al. Truncation at the C-terminus of the DAX-1 protein impairs its biological actions in patients with X-linked adrenal hypoplasia congenita. J Clin Endocrinol Metab 1996; 81:3680–3685.

61. Schwartz M, Blichfeldt S, Müller J. X-linked adrenal hypoplasia in a large Greenlandic family. Detection of a missense mutation (N4401) in the DAX-1 gene; implication for genetic counseling and carrier diagnosis. Hum Genet 1997; 99:83–87.

62. Kinoshita E, Yoshimoto M, Motomura K, et al. DAX-1 gene mutations and deletions in Japanese patients with adrenal hypoplasia congenita and hypogonadotrophic hypogonadism. Horm Res 1997; 48:29–34.

63. Zazopoulos E, Lalli E, Stocco DM, Sassone-Corsi P. DNA binding and transcriptional repression by DAX-1 blocks steroidogenesis. Nature 1997; 390:311–315.

64. Lalli E, Bardoni B, Zazopoulos E, et al. A transcriptional silencing domain an DAX-1 whose mutation causes adrenal hypoplasia congenita. Mol Endocrinol 1997;13:1950–1960.

24 The HPA Axis and HIV Infection

Daniel S. Donovan, Jr., MD and Robert G. Dluhy, MD

CONTENTS

INTRODUCTION

Various changes in endocrine function have been described in association with human immunodeficiency virus (HIV) infection. Alterations in hypothalamic-pituitary-adrenal (HPA) axis function have been the most thoroughly investigated. Manifestations of HPA axis dysfunction usually correlate with the degree of immune compromise or stage of HIV illness. Studies investigating endocrine function during the course of HIV illness have used either the revised CDC or Walter Reed criteria *(1)*. Newer markers of HIV disease status or progression, such as viral load, have not been used. On the other hand, CD4+ cell counts do reliably predict the risk of various opportunistic infections *(2)*. The spectrum of endocrine dysfunction observed during the course of HIV infection is also likely to be altered by new-generation antiretroviral agents and medications to treat opportunistic illness that will prolong life.

OVERVIEW OF PATHOGENETIC MECHANISMS

Beyond the normal adaptive reactions to stress, there are unique HPA axis responses to HIV infection. For example, cytokines may interact at a number of loci in the HPA axis (e.g., direct action on the adrenal cortex) although levels of these mediators are not usually systemically elevated. An exception is interferon alpha (INF-α) for which levels correlate both with disease progression and hypertriglyceridemia *(3)*.

Direct destruction of adrenal or pituitary tissue by opportunistic infection (fungal,

From: *Contemporary Endocrinology: Adrenal Disorders*
Edited by: A. N. Margioris and G. P. Chrousos © Humana Press, Totowa, NJ

viral, parasitic) as well as neoplastic infiltration have also been described *(4)*. Additional mechanisms of tissue damage include autoimmune destruction and hematologic abnormalities, such as thrombocytopenia, which may increase the risk for adrenal hemorrhage.

HIV infections *per se* may also cause direct injury to HPA axis cells. Although CD4+ T cells are the primary targets of the HIV virus, infection of non-CD4+ cells of various types has been reported *(5)*. HIV has direct cytopathic effects on CD4+ T cells and is one of the mechanisms leading to a dramatic decline in their number. The virus appears also to infect monocytes and macrophages, which then serve as a reservoir of infection. There is no direct evidence of HIV infection of endocrine tissues in vivo. However, alteration of endocrine cellular metabolism and/or function, such as adrenocortical resistance to adrenocorticotropic hormone (ACTH), without cytopathic destruction are possibilities.

HIV-infected patients are commonly treated with medications that can directly alter adrenocortical function, HPA responsiveness, or mimic signs and symptoms of adrenal insufficiency *(6)*. These include the azole antifungal agent, ketoconazole; the appetite stimulant megestrol acetate; antibiotics such as rifampin and trimethoprim; as well as opiates and anticonvulants. These will be discussed in more detail.

ANATOMIC FINDINGS

Adrenal Gland

Autopsy studies in patients dying of AIDS early in the epidemic commonly demonstrated involvement of the adrenal gland by opportunistic infection and less commonly by neoplasms. It was rare, however, to find total or near complete destruction of the gland. Although the adrenal gland often appeared grossly normal, histologic examination routinely revealed involvement by a variety of infectious pathogens, as well as other processes (Table 1).

The most frequently noted infectious agent is cytomegalovirus (CMV), which was found in 38–88% pathologic specimens. Such studies reveal the adrenal to be the most common extrapulmonary site of infection with CMV, so-called CMV "adrenalitis" *(6–13)*. The adrenal medulla appears to be more severely involved by CMV infection than the cortex with variable destruction reported in almost 100% of involved specimens. Histological findings include the presence of viral inclusions in both cortical and/or medullary cells with areas of focal inflammation, necrosis, necrotizing inflammation (so-called necrotizing adrenalitis), and fibrosis. In the few studies that have quantitated the degree of cortical destruction, less than 50% involvement was typical with up to a maximum of 60–70% noted. This is below the commonly accepted 80–90% cortical destruction criteria required to precipitate clinical adrenocortical insufficiency *(14)*. However, well-documented reports of adrenal insufficiency resulting from CMV adrenalitis as a result of extensive necrosis with viral inclusions have been reported *(15,16)*.

Other infectious agents including acid fast bacilli (AFB), primarily mycobacterium avium intracellular (MAI), and other pathogens including disseminated candida, cryptococcus, histoplasma, pneumocytis, and toxoplasmosis have been found *(17)*. In addition, malignant infiltration with Kaposis sarcoma, but unexplainably, not lymphoma, have been found with varying frequency. These conditions do not cause the degree of adrenal destruction seen with CMV; however, several processes may coexist. Hemorrhage or hemorrhagic infarction has been noted in 4–20% of cases raising the possibility of a

Table 1
Adrenal Pathologic Findings in Patients Dying of AIDS

Cytomegalovirus (CMV)
Lipid Depletion
Fibrosis
Hemorrhagic Infarction
Acid Fast Bacilli
Kaposi's Sarcoma
Cryptococcus
Massive Necrosis
Toxoplasma

Waterhouse-Friderichsen-like syndrome (18). Cortical lipid depletion, a lesion of unknown significance, has been noted in 30–100% of autopsy cases and has led to the hypothesis that substrate depletion may lead to decreased adrenal reserve.

Hypothalamus-Pituitary Gland

There have been relatively few pathological studies of the hypothalamus and pituitary gland. As in the adrenal, CMV has been the pathogen most commonly found but at a much lower frequency, about 3–5% of specimens examined (19,20). The incidence of pituitary microadenomas does not appear increased in HIV-infected patients compared to control specimens (20). Infarction and necrosis of the pituitary of varying degrees was found in 5–10% of specimens. Mosca noted an increase in cells with ACTH-immunohistochemical staining, with extension into the lateral wings, of the pituitary gland in a large number of specimens, 79%. Toxoplasma (21), pneumocysis, cryptococcus, and aspergillus have also been found in hypothalmic-pituitary specimens. Direct malignant infiltration of the hypothalmic-pituitary area has not been noted, but regional involvement has been seen.

CLINICAL FINDINGS

Adrenal Cortical Function

Several patterns of steroid hormone abnormalities have emerged during the study of adrenal function in patients with various stages of HIV infection. Alterations of adrenocortical function have included glucocorticoid, mineralocorticoid, and androgenic hormones (Table 2).

Glucocorticoids

The earliest studies of adrenal function attempted to correlate the frequent pathologic abnormalities found at autopsy with alterations in cortical function. In fact, the nonspecific symptoms seen in many patients with AIDS are similar to those in patients with frank adrenal insufficiency (e.g., anorexia, weight loss, profound lassitude and so on). In two studies, CMV adrenalitis was seen in approx 50% of the autopsied cases where functional information was available. Although nonspecific symptoms, potentially consistent with adrenal insufficiency were commonly noted, documented frank adrenocortical insufficiency was extremely uncommon. Elevated basal cortisol levels and/or blunted cortisol responses to ACTH stimulation were the rule. In the study by Pulakhandam,

Table 2
Patterns of Adrenal Cortical Abnormalities in HIV Infection

STAGE	Basal	ACTH Test (Rapid)*	ACTH Test (Long)*	CRH Test
ACTH				
CDC II, III	N, ↑, ↓	—	—	N, ↓, ↑
CDC IV	N, ↑, ↓	—	—	N, ↓, ↑
Cortisol				
CDC II, III	↑, N	N	N	N, ↓
CDC IV	↑	N, ↓	N, ↓	N, ↓
DHEA/DHEAS				
CDC II, III	↓	—	—	—
CDC IV	↓↓	—	—	—
Aldosterone				
CDC II, III	N, ↓	N, ↓	—	—
CDC II, III	N, ↓	N, ↓	—	—

Note: N, Normal; ↓, Decreased; ↑, Increased; — No data available
*Rapid—60 min cortisol level following 250 µg cosyntropin bolus
*Long—6–8 hours cosyntropin infusion.

all three patients with subnormal ACTH stimulation testing had severe adrenocortical fibrosis (13). In an early case report, adrenal insufficiency was documented 4 mo before the diagnosis of AIDS was established. Autopsy examination revealed complete cortical destruction (22). Overall, ACTH stimulation data were not available in the majority of autopsy cases.

Beyond autopsy-functional correlates, other studies have assessed adrenocortical function in patients infected with HIV at different stages of the disease. Testing included measurement of basal cortisol levels; the cortisol response over 30–60 min following the administration of ACTH[1-24] (the short cosyntropin stimulation test); and more recently, corticotropin-releasing hormone (CRH) testing. However, studies have been inconsistent in defining the criteria for adequate adrenal reserve.

One of the earliest studies, evaluating 20 AIDS patients with ACTH testing, found 4 with inadequate cortisol reserve of whom two had elevated ACTH levels (23). Subsequently, the most common finding in many series in patients with less-severe illness (CDC groups II and III) was either normal (24,25) or elevated basal and mean cortisol levels. The latter pattern was also seen frequently in symptomatic AIDS patients and/or later stages of HIV infection (26). Because concomitant elevations of ACTH levels were not common, these elevations in basal cortisol levels have been hypothesized to be secondary to increased cytokine production. For example, local production in the adrenal of cytokines or other mediators produced by activated monocytes have been postulated to directly increase cortisol secretion (Fig. 1). Accordingly, in vitro stimulation of cortisol secretion by interleukin 1 (IL-1) has been reported and this action in cultured, isolated adrenal cortical cells is blocked by prostaglandin inhibitors. It has also been postulated that there is local production of ACTH-like peptides from virally stimulated lymphocytes, which could lead to pituitary-independent release of cortisol (27,28).

Clinical adrenocortical insufficiency with hyperpigmentation and elevated ACTH

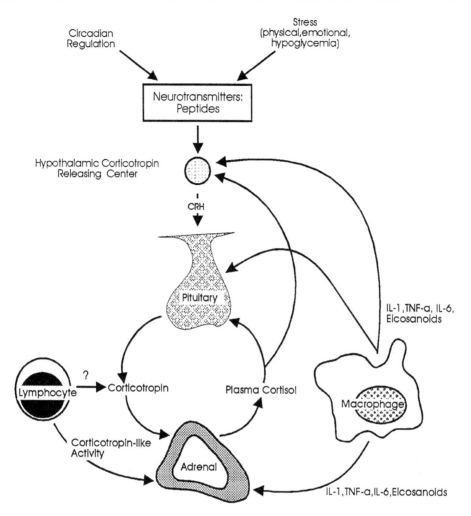

Fig. 1. Please supply figure caption. Please supply figure caption. Please supply figure caption. Please supply figure caption. Please supply figure caption. Please supply figure caption. Please supply figure caption.

levels is extremely uncommon in patients with frank AIDS. The majority of studies demonstrate subnormal cortisol responsiveness following ACTH stimulation in approx 5–10% of such subjects *(29)*. ACTH levels are usually normal, "inappropriately" low, or rarely, elevated. In a study of the circadian variation of cortisol, ACTH, and adrenal androgens, mean plasma ACTH levels were reduced, whereas the cortisol levels were elevated supporting a role for cytokine stimulated-adrenocortical secretion *(30)*. More recently, 32% of CDC stage IV patients had abnormal ACTH circadian rhythmicity *(31)*.

The response to corticotropic-releasing hormone (CRH) infusion was studied by Azar et al. in patients without AIDS, but with advanced HIV infection (less than 500 CD4+ T cells). Three patterns are well noted: 50% had normal ACTH-cortisol responses, 25% had normal ACTH, but reduced cortisol responses, and 25% had both reduced cortisol and ACTH responses. These findings point to loss of either pituitary or adrenal reserve in a substantial number of such subjects *(32)*. Freda et al., however, identified an additional patient group characterized by an exaggerated ACTH with a normal cortisol response to CRH *(33)*. The study of Lortholary et al. found 50% of CDC stage IVC patients, to have blunted responses of both ACTH and cortisol to CRH *(31)*, whereas Biglino et al. found almost absent ACTH and cortisol responses to CRH in six out of eight patients who were narcotic users; the remaining two exhibited blunted responses *(34)*. These results in opiate users must be interpreted carefully because opiates may impair ACTH release *(35)*.

Alterations in adrenal steroid biosynthesis may also occur in the setting of HIV infection. Membreno et al. reported deficiencies in the adrenal *zona fasiculata* synthesis of 17-deoxysteroids basally and after ACTH stimulation in almost all AIDS-related complex (ARC) and AIDS patients *(36)*. These abnormalities were more severe in the AIDS patients. In contrast, the 17-hydroxy pathway leading to cortisol synthesis remained intact or was elevated. It remains unclear whether these observed alterations in adrenal steroid metabolism represent an adaptive response, or whether this almost universal finding of selective, abnormal steroidogenesis in such patients with AIDS and ARC represents the harbinger of subsequent full-blown adrenocortical failure.

An acquired form of glucocorticoid resistance has been described in HIV-infected patients *(37,38)*. The first subject had classic signs and symptoms of adrenal insufficiency including weight loss, general weakness, anorexia, diarrhea, and mucocutaneous melanosis; however, the plasma and urine levels of cortisol were elevated in the setting of an elevated level of ACTH. A comparison of the glucocorticoid receptors of such HIV patients with glucocorticoid resistance to those from individuals with the classical hereditary form of glucocorticoid resistance reveal a difference in receptor binding characteristics suggesting a difference mechanism is responsible. HIV-glucocorticoid resistance is also accompanied by marked, persistent elevations in circulating INF-α levels. This may have either beneficial or adverse consequences on immune function and may also be partially responsible for the increased pigmentation such patients. In the original series, 17% of subjects exhibited glucocorticoid resistance with no symptoms or signs of adrenal androgen or mineralocorticoid deficiencies *(37,38)*.

Mineralocorticoids

Although hyponatremia and hyperkalemia are common findings in patients with advanced HIV disease, there are limited studies of the renin-angiotensin-aldosterone system. One patient who presented with hyperkalemia, had elevated plasma renin activity, but an abnormally low aldosterone level. Although the cortisol response to ACTH was submaximal, the mineralocorticoid deficiency was profound *(39)*. Two subsequent series found no significant differences in either the basal or stimulated aldosterone levels in patients with HIV disease. However, in one study of early HIV infection (corresponding to CDC groups II and III), basal aldosterone levels were significantly lower than control although the plasma renin activity (PRA) levels were elevated only in 18% of subjects *(40)*. In a longitudinal study of 53 patients, basal aldosterone and PRA remained unchanged over 2 yr; however, the aldosterone response to ACTH was abnormal in up to 26% of CDC stage II–III patients and up to 53% in CDC stage IV patients *(25)*. Although hyporeninenic hypoaldosteronism has been described in gravely ill patients with a variety of illnesses, this is an implausible explanation for the observed results because the study patients were not severely ill.

Hyporeninemic hypoaldosteronism has been reported in AIDS patients who presented with hyperkalemia. These subjects had normal cortisol and aldosterone responses to cosyntropin, but had low basal and stimulated PRA and aldosterone levels. Treatment with fludrocortisone in three of four subjects normalized their potassium levels *(41)*. However, all of the subjects were receiving sulfamethoxazole-trimethoprim. Trimethoprim is a known inhibitor of the distal sodium-epithelial channel, analogous to the action of the potassium-sparing diuretic amiloride *(42)*. Sulfa drugs may also cause interstitial nephritis *(43)* and subsequent hyporeninemic hypoaldosteronism. However, reports of isolated idiopathic hyporeninemic hypoaldosteronism in AIDS patients are extremely uncommon and the etiology of the hyporeninemic state remains obscure. Whether this relates to AIDS nephritis *per se* or is a complication of drug therapy, or both, is unknown. Thus, other causes should be sought before a diagnosis of idiopathic hyporeninemic hypoaldosteronism is made.

Androgens

Basal and stimulated adrenal androgen levels have been noted to be subnormal in HIV infection. Villette et al. in their study of circadian adrenocortical secretion in AIDS patients, found a marked decrease in the 24-h adjusted mean plasma levels of the adrenal androgens dehydroepiandrosterone (DHEA) and the sulfated compound (DHEA-S). The DHEA and DHEAS levels were 30% and 50% lower, respectively, in the CDC II patients than controls; levels were even lower, 46% and 65%, respectively, than controls in the CDC IV patients *(30)*. Other investigations have demonstrated a relationship between a fall in serum and urine androgen levels and a progressive decline of immune system function *(44,45)*. The physiologic significance of these changes is unclear, but an inverse relationship between DHEA-S levels and life expectancy and immune function has been suggested. DHEA has been demonstrated to have an antiproliferative effect on HIV in vitro *(46);* however, the clinical significance of this laboratory finding remains unclear. Increases in cortisol levels and decreases in DHEA and DHEA-S levels have been observed in a number of severe illnesses (such as burns and sepsis), leading to the hypothesis that this is an adaptive response of the adrenal cortex to severe stress *(47)*. The mechanism remains speculative. One possibility involves alteration of a non-ACTH adrenal regulatory factor or factors, whereas an alternative hypothesis is a shift in steroidogenic patterns toward cortisol during chronic ACTH stimulation.

Medulla

There have been no investigations of the prevalence of hypofunction of the adrenal medulla in AIDS. As previously noted, some autopsy studies have noted that the medulla is more commonly severely affected than the cortex. An abnormal norepinephrine response to the cold pressor test has been reported in HIV patients *(48)*. Whether abnormalities in adrenal medullary or sympathetic function contribute to morbidity or mortality by alterating homeostatic mechanisms under sympathoadrenal control is unknown.

MEDICATIONS

Concurrent medications are important confounding factors in the interpretation of adrenal function testing in patients with HIV infection *(49)* (Table 3). These patients often receive medications for related illnesses that are known to impair adrenal function.

Table 3
Medications and Possible Effects on Adrenal Function in HIV Infection

Medication	Mechanism	Effect
Rifampin	Accelerate cortisol metabolism	Reduce cortisol
Anticonvulsants (dilantin, phenobarbital)	Accelerate cortisol metabolism	Reduce cortisol
Ketoconazole	Impair adrenal steroidogenesis	Reduce cortisol
Opiates	Impair ACTH secretion Accelerate cortisol metabolism	Reduce cortisol
Megesterol acetate	Glucocorticoid agonist	Reduce cortisol
Trimethoprim	Renal sodium-epithelial channel receptor antagonist	Elevate potassium
Sulfonamides	Interstitial nephritis (decrease renin secretion)	Elevate potassium
Pentamidine	Renal toxicity	Elevate potassium

Moreover, the use of such agents in the setting of compromised adrenal reserve could conceivably precipitate overt adrenal insufficiency. For example, rifampin, used as antituberculous therapy in AIDS patients, is known to accelerate cortisol metabolism. Anticonvulsant therapy (such as dilantin and phenobarbital) not uncommonly prescribed in patients with central nervous system pathology, also accelerates the metabolism of cortisol, thus placing a patient with impaired adrenal reserve at risk for clinical adrenal insufficiency. Ketoconazole, an imidazole antifungal agent, which inhibits cortisol synthesis and blunts the cortisol response to ACTH in normal subjects, has been reported to cause adrenal insufficiency even in patients without previously known adrenal disease. Opiates have also been implicated as adrenal suppressive agents either by central (hypothalamic-pituitary) or direct adrenocortical mechanisms. Because many patients with HIV infection are either active or former drug users and many are on methadone maintenance, this potential interaction should be kept in mind. Pentamidine, used to treat pneumocystis infections, has been associated with hyperkalemia in the setting of renal disease. The appetite stimulant megesterol acetate has been associated with lowered cortisol levels and blunted HPA responsiveness, probably on the basis of the intrinsic glucocorticoid agonist properties of this steroid (50).

DIAGNOSIS AND MANAGEMENT

Our current state of knowledge regarding HIV infection and its impact on the adrenocortical function is incomplete. However, it is possible to make some recommendations for diagnosis and management of these patients based upon what is known. The incidence of overt adrenal insufficiency in patients with AIDS is low and is probably less than 5%. More frequent, occurring in approx 5–10% of patients with full-blown AIDS, are subclinical abnormalities in adrenocortical function usually demonstrated by submaximal cortisol responsiveness following cosyntropin stimulation. In addition, the degree of adrenal dysfunction in patients infected with HIV appears to be correlated with the stage of illness. As a correlate, more advanced HIV infection is usually associated pathologically with a greater degree of adrenal involvement.

Longitudinal data on HIV infection and its impact on adrenal function are limited.

Certainly, opportunistic infection and necrosis of the adrenal gland, especially by CMV, would likely be progressive. Thus, as newer therapies, such as combination regimens including protease inhibitors become more widespread and patients live longer, overt adrenal insufficiency would be expected to become more common.

Based upon the low prevalence of overt adrenal insufficiency in early HIV infection, routine screening of these patients is not warranted. Patients with more advanced HIV infection often have signs and symptoms suggestive of adrenal insufficiency. Despite the frequency of nonspecific complaints in these patients with advanced HIV infection, we recommend the performance of a rapid cosyntropin stimulation test in any patient with symptoms consistent with adrenal insufficiency, as well as in patients with known CMV infection. Any patient with a submaximal cosyntropin stimulation test should be considered at risk for overt adrenal crisis and treated with appropriate "stress dose" glucocorticoid therapy during episodes of severe illness, such as surgery or acute sepsis. Caution should be used, however, to prevent the indiscriminate use of potentially immunosuppressive doses of glucocorticoids. Whereas an early morning cortisol level would be expected to be elevated in patients with advanced HIV infection, a low level would mandate further evaluation. However, normal or only slightly elevated cortisol levels do not accurately predict adrenal reserve. Serial ACTH stimulation studies may be warranted in advanced HIV infection and in those with equivocal cortisol responses. The role of CRH testing is not yet clear and needs further study. Measurement of a plasma aldosterone/renin ratio and an ACTH-stimulated aldosterone level would be appropriate to screen for selective mineralocorticoid deficiency in the setting of hyperkalemia and hyponatremia.

Patients with symptomatic HIV infection about to be started on a medication known to impair adrenal function should also be tested prior to beginning the drug and again after dose stabilization (Table 3). Medications known to impair adrenal function should avoided if possible.

FUTURE DIRECTIONS

It is important to investigate the role of cytokines on HPA axis function in the setting of HIV illness and to define which alterations are adaptive or maladaptive. The possibility of a direct effect of HIV infection in adrenal tissue should be clarified. It will be important to attempt to predict which patients are at risk for adrenal insufficiency and to understand the longitudinal course of HIV infection on adrenal function. The prevalence and clinical importance of acquired glucocorticoid resistance also needs further study.

REFERENCES

1. Baltimore D and Feinberg MB. HIV revealed: toward a natural history of the infection. N Engl J Med 1989; 321:1673–1675.
2. Broder S, Merigan TC, Bolognesi D, eds. Textbook of AIDS Medicine, Williams & Wilkins, Baltimore, MD, 1994.
3. Grinspoon SK, Donovan Jr DS, Bilezikian JP. Aetiology and pathogenesis of hormonal and metabolic disorders in HIV infection. Baillière's Clin Endocrinol. Metab 1994; 8:735–755.
4. Ferreiro J, Vinters HV. Pathology of the pituitary gland in patients with the acquired immune deficiency syndrome (AIDS). Pathology 1988; 20:211–215.
5. Barboza A, Castro BA, Whalen M. Infection of cultured human adrenal cells by a different strains of HIV. AIDS 1992; 6:1437–1443.

6. Donovan Jr DS, Dluhy RG. AIDS and the adrenal gland. Endocrinologist 1991; 1:277–232.
7. Sellmeyer DE, Grunfeld C. Endocrine and metabolic disturbances in human immune deficiency virus infection and the acquired immune deficiency syndrome. Endocr Rev 1996; 17:518–532.
8. Reichert CM, O'Leary TJ, Levens DL, Simrell CR, Macher AM. Autopsy pathology in the acquired immune deficiency syndrome. Am J Pathol 1983; 112:357–382.
9. Weiss CD. The human immunodeficiency virus and the adrenal medulla. Ann Intern Med 1986; 105:300.
10. Glasgow BJ, Steinsapir KD, Anders K, Anders K, Layfield LJ. Adrenal pathology in the acquired immune deficiency syndrome. Am J Clin Pathol 1985; 84:594–597.
11. Welch K, Finkbeiner W, Aplers CE, Blumenfeld W, Davis RL. Autopsy findings in the acquired immune deficiency syndrome. JAMA 1984; 252:1152–1159.
12. Bricaire F, March C, Zoubi D, Matherson S, Rouveix E, Vittecoq D. Lesions surrenaliennes au cours du SIDA: etude anatomopathologique. Ann Med Intern 1987; 138:607–609.
13. Pulakhandam U, Dincsoy HP. Cytomegaloviral adrenalitis and adrenal insufficiency in AIDS. Am J Clin Pathol 1990; 93:651–656.
14. Barker NW. The pathologic anatomy in twenty-eight cases of Addison's disease. Arch Pathol 1929; 8:432–550.
15. Bleiweiss IJ, Pervez NK, Hammer GS, Dikman SH. Cytomegalovirus-induced adrenal insufficiency and associated renal cell carcinoma in AIDS. Mt Sinai J Med 1986; 53:676–679.
16. Angulo JC, Lopez JI, Flores N. Lethal cytomegalovirus adrenalitis in a case of AIDS. Scand J Urol Nephrol 1994; 28:105,106.
17. Tapper ML, Rotterdam HZ, Lerner CW. Adrenal necrosis in the acquired immunodeficiency syndrome. Ann Int Med 1984; 100:239–241.
18. Guarda LA, Luna MA, Smith Jr JL. Acquired immune deficiency syndrome: postmortem findings. Am J Clin Pathol 1984; 81:549–557.
19. Sano T, Kovacs K, Scheithauer BW, Rosenblum MK, Petito CK, Greco CM. Pituitary pathology in the acquired immunodeficiency syndrome. Arch Pathol Lab Med 1989; 113:1006–1070.
20. Mosca L, Costanzi G, Antonacci C, Boldorini R, Carboni N, Cristina S, et al. Hypophyseal pathology in AIDS. Histol Histopathol 1992; 7:291–300.
21. Croxson TS, Chapman WE, Miller LK. Toxoplasmosis presenting as panhypopituitarism in a patient with the acquired immune deficiency syndrome. Am J Med 1984; 77:760–764.
22. Guenthner EE, Rabinowe SI, Van Niel A, Naftilan A, Dluhy RG. Primary Addison's disease in a patient with the acquired immunodeficiency syndrome. Ann Intern Med 1984; 100:847–848.
23. Greene LW, Cole W, Greene JB, Levy B. Adrenal insufficiency as a complication of the acquired immunodeficiency syndrome. Ann Intern Med 1984; 101:497–498.
24. Raffi F, Brisseau JM, Planchon B, Remi JP, Barrier JH, Grolleau JY. Endocrine function in 98 HIV infected patients: a prospective study. AIDS 1991; 5:729–733.
25. Findling JW, Buggy BP, Gilson IH, Brummitt CF, Bernstein BM, Raff H. Longitudinal evaluation of adrenocortical function in patients infected with the human immunodeficiency virus. J Clin Endocrinol Metab 1994; 79:1091–1096.
26. Verges B, Chavanet P, Desgres J, Vaillant G, Waldner A, Brun JM, et al. Adrenal function in HIV infected patients. 1989; 121:633–637.
27. Darling G, Goldstein DS, Stull RL, Gorschboth CM, Norton JA. Tumor necrosis factor: immune endocrine interaction. Surgery 1989; 106:1155–1160.
28. Grinspoon SK, Bilezikian JP. HIV disease and the endocrine system. N Engl J Med 1992; 327:1360–1365.
29. Dobs A, Dempsey MA, Ladenson PW, Polk BF. Endocrine disorders in men infected with human immunodeficiency virus. Am J Med 1988; 84:611–616.
30. Villette JM, Bourin P, Doinel C, Mansour I, Fiet J, Boudou P, et al. Circadian variations in plasma levels of hypophyseal, adenocortical and testicular hormones in men infected with human immunodeficiency virus. J Clin Endocrinol Metab 1990; 70:572–577.
31. Lortholary O, Christeff N, Casassus P, Thobie N, Veyssier P, Trogoff B, et al. Hypothalamo-pituitary-adrenal function in human immunodeficiency virus-infected men. J Clin Endocrinol Metab 1996; 81:791–796.
32. Azar ST, Melby JC. Hypothalamic-pituitary-adrenal function in non-AIDS patients with advanced HIV infection. AM J Med Sci 1993; 305:321–325.
33. Freda PU, Wardlaw SL, Brudney K, Goland RS. Primary adrenal insufficiency in patients with the

acquired immunodeficiency syndrome: a report of five cases. J Clin Endocrinol Metab 1994; 79:1540–1545.

34. Biglino A, Limone P, Forno B, Pollono A, Cariti G, Molinatti GM, et al. Altered adrenocorticotropin and cortisol response to corticotropin-releasing hormone in HIV-1 infection. Eur J Endocrinol 1995; 133:173–179.

35. Dackis CA, Gurpegui M, Pottash ALC, Gold MS. Methadone induced hypoadrenalism. Lancet 1982; 1:1167.

36. Membreno L, Irony I, Dere W, Klein R, Biglieri EG, Cobb E. Adrenocortical function in acquired immunodeficiency syndrome. J Clin Endocrinol Metab 1987; 65:482–487.

37. Norbiato G, Bevilaxqua M, Bago T, Moroni M. Cortisol resistance in acquired immunodeficiency syndrome. J Clin Endocrinol Metab 1992; 74:608–613.

38. Norbiato G, Massimo G, Velella R, Mauro M. The syndrome of acquired glucocorticoid resistance in HIV infection. Baillière's Clin Endocrinol Metab 1994; 8:777–785.

39. Guy RJ, Turbert Y, Davidson RN. Mineralocorticoid deficiency in HIV infection. Br Med J 1989; 298:496–496.

40. Merenich JA, McDermott MT, Asp AA, Harrison SM, Kidd GS. Evidence of Endocrine involvement early in the course of human immunodeficiency virus infection. J Clin Endocrinol Metab 1990; 70:566–571.

41. Kalin MF, Poretsky L, Seres DS, Zumof. Hyporeninemic hypoaldosteronism associated with acquired immune deficiency syndrome. Am J Med 1987; 82:1035–1038.

42. Hsu I, Wordell CJ. Hyperkalemia and high-dose trimethoprim/sulfamethoxazole. Ann Pharmacother 1995; 29:427–429.

43. Appel GB, Neu HC. The nephrotoxicity of antimicrobial agents (third of three parts). N Engl J Med 1997; 296:784–787.

44. Jacobson MA, Fusaro RE, Galmarini M, Lang W. Deceased serum dehydroepiandrosterone is associated with an increased progression of human immunodeficiency virus infection in men with CD4 cell counts of 200–499. J Infect Dis 1991; 17:864–868.

45. Honor J, Schneider MA, Miller RF. Low adrenal androgens in men with HIV infection and the acquired immunodeficiency syndrome. Horm Res 1995; 44:35–39.

46. Henderson E, Yang JY, Schwartz A. Dehydroepiandrosterone (DHEA) and synthetic DHEA analogs are modest inhibitors of HIV-1B replication. 8:625–631.

47. Parker LN, Levin ER, Lifrak ET. Evidence for adrenocortical adaptation to severe illness. J Clin Endocrinol Metab 1985; 60:947–952.

48. Kumar M, Morgan R, Szapocznik J, Eisdorder C. Norepinephrine response in early HIV infection. J Acquir Immune Defic Syndr 1991; 6:61–65.

49. Opocher G, Manter F. Adrenal complications of HIV infection. Ballière's Clin Endocrinol Metab 1994; 8:769–776.

50. Loprinzi CI, Jensen MD, Jian N, Schaid DJ. Effect of megesterol acetate on the human pituitary-adrenal axis. Mayo Clin Proc 1992; 67:1160–1162.

25   Hypothalamic-Pituitary-Adrenal Axis and Obesity

Per Björntorp and Roland Rosmond

CONTENTS

INTRODUCTION
HUMAN STUDIES
METHODOLOGICAL DEVELOPMENTS
RESULTS
CONSEQUENCES OF THE ENDOCRINE PERTURBATIONS
SURROGATE MEASUREMENTS AND PROSPECTIVE STUDIES
HYPERTENSION
OBESITY
THE PATHOGENESIS OF THE DISTURBED HPA AXIS
GENETIC ASPECTS
CONCLUDING REMARKS
REFERENCES

INTRODUCTION

The origin of the concept of stress in biology and medicine is unknown. Investigations of stress rise from the recognition by Claude Bernard in 1878 that all living processes exist in a "milieu intériuer." Walter Cannon elucidated the mechanisms of maintaining physiological factors within certain limits and coined the term "homeostasis." As the homeostasis is constantly threatened by internal or external adverse factors, stressors, stress is usually defined as a state of threatened homeostasis. There are physical stressors such as cold, trauma, fever, and infection; psychological stressors such as social subordination, anxiety, and depression. The individual reaction to such stressors is highly dependent on the stressful stimulus, as well as the capability to habituate or adapt to the situation, so-called coping *(1)*.

The idea that frequent or persistent challenges of the hypothalamic-pituitary-adrenal (HPA) axis may constitute a base for pathophysiological consequences in the periphery of the body stems from the central role played by the HPA axis in the homeostatic processes. Although biologically plausible, this complex hypothesis has been difficult to study in humans *(2)*, presumably as a result of several inherent problems. First, because the impact of stress is dependent on the individual coping ability, the reported

From: *Contemporary Endocrinology: Adrenal Disorders*
Edited by: A. N. Margioris and G. P. Chrousos © Humana Press, Totowa, NJ

reaction is essentially subjective. Furthermore, although the extensive neural connections of the HPA axis have been greatly elicited throughout studies in animals, these pathways are far more complex in humans. Finally, the mechanisms of disease-generating processes in the periphery are still unclear. Consequently, studies in humans of the impact of stress on the HPA axis have provided inconsistent findings.

Animal Studies

In the 1950s, the idea emerged, under Selye's influence, that all noxious stimuli resulted in a series of metabolic changes, especially stimulation of the adrenals *(3)*. In 1955, Christian showed how the "social stress" of crowded conditions enlarges the adrenals, and, in 1964, Bronson and Eleftheriou demonstrated that exposure to aggressive behavior increases the adrenal weights *(4)*. In more recent decades, the central neurohormonal response pattern to stress has been greatly elicited throughout studies in both animals and humans *(5–7)*. There are two types of response patterns to stress of particular relevance for human health and disease *(6)*—namely, the defense (or fight–flight) reaction and the defeat reaction *(5–7)*. The defense or fight–flight reaction appears when the stressors can be controlled, an initial striving period results in full control of the situation. This reaction evokes primarily the locus coeruleus-sympathetic system, followed by increased levels of epinephrine-norepinephrine and testosterone, resulting in elevated blood pressure and heart rate during the striving phase. The defeat reaction, on the other hand, appears when the challenge is oppressive and unrestrained. This reaction is manifested in humans as deep sorrow and despair and a "no-way-out" or helplessness behavior. This type of reaction evokes primarily the HPA axis with resulting increase in adrenocorticotropic hormone (ACTH) and cortisol secretion. As the reproductive and growth axis is functionally influenced at many levels by the HPA axis, prolonged activation of the HPA axis leads to inhibition of sex steroids, as well as suppression of growth hormone (GH) secretion *(8,9)*. These endocrine perturbations, in turn, will be followed by consequences in the regulation of metabolism, growth, and the menstrual cycle.

The cortisol exerts a negative-endocrine feedback regulation on the pituitary and the hippocampus. The feedback is initiated by binding of steroid to regulatory gene elements *(10)*, and the feedback suppression is mediated by glucocorticoid receptors (GR) in the hippocampus *(11)*. Once cortisol is bound to these receptors, the HPA axis activity is controled. Studies in vivo and in vitro in cells from chronically stressed rats have shown that the sensitivity of the HPA axis to inhibition by cortisol is impaired *(12,13)*. When the HPA axis is subjected to prolonged elevated cortisol levels as in chronic stress, the GRs gradually lose their function, ending up in a presumably irreversible neurodegenerative condition *(11,14)*. Such hippocampal damage has been observed in individuals with Cushing's syndrome *(15)*, a condition also characterized by hypercortisolism.

HUMAN STUDIES

The neuroendocrine response patterns identified under experimental conditions in animals have also been observed in humans in standardized controlled laboratory stress tests. These results are, however, much more complex as compared to those in animals, probably because of the powerful control exerted by the central nervous system. For instance, the different characteristic reaction patterns seen in animals is considerably less clear, or even nonexisting in humans *(16)*. Furthermore, the individual variability is substantial, and there seems to be gender-specific types of endocrine responses to some extent *(5)*.

Although the pathophysiology of essential hypertension is still unclear, it has been demonstrated that activation of the central sympathetic nervous system by physical (exercise) or mental stressors can increase the blood pressure and heart rate, as well as cardiac output *(5–7)*. Such reactions may, when protracted, result in the characteristics of later stages of hypertension, including elevated peripheral circulatory resistance *(5–7)*.

It has been suggested that a corresponding frequent or persistent activation of one of the principal axes of neuroendocrine response in the human body—namely, the HPA axis, might result in similar pathophysiological consequences. However, this has not been established with certainty in humans, presumably as a result of methodological problems.

METHODOLOGICAL DEVELOPMENTS

A normal diurnal cortisol variation is a pattern in which cortisol levels are high and varying in the morning, and from 4 PM to midnight, less than 75% of the morning values. This secretory pattern is brought about by the central nervous system throughout complex neural connections. Cortisol is also secreted in short pulses, and increases proportionally when the HPA axis is provoked by physiological challenge (e.g., food intake) or perceived stress. To obtain a biochemical assessment of the HPA axis activity and regulation as complete as possible, these details need to be considered. The measurements of cortisol levels at various times of the day to determine the presence or absence of a circadian rhythm is important. The response to external stimuli is informative, and the physiological effect of food intake can be measured, provided that the stimulus is standardized. Various centrally occurring challenges of the HPA axis, in terms of psychological stress, are of fundamental importance, and as mental stressors are perceived differently, the individual coping ability has to be taken into account. In addition to these measurements of basal and stimulated HPA axis activity, the response to exogenous glucocorticoids is required to detect abnormal feedback regulation of cortisol secretion. Furthermore, the regulation of the cortisol secretion is highly affected by environmental disturbances. For instance, the artificial milieu of a laboratory or a hospital may distort the normal activity, and even minor trauma, such as venipuncture *per se* can significantly increase cortisol concentration in serum. Urinary cortisol measurements offers a tool to circumvent these difficulties. However, urinary measurements do not reveal the secretory pattern of cortisol, and the technique is usually restricted for practical reasons to inhospital patients.

The assessment of cortisol in saliva provides several advantages over blood cortisol measurements as the collection procedure is noninvasive and stress-free, making it ideal for use in psychoneuroendocrinological research *(17–20)*. Because salivary cortisol sampling is laboratory-independent, it can be applied under a variety of field settings. Cortisol is lipid-soluble, which enables the molecule to rapidly diffuse to the acinar cells of the salivary glands by the blood stream, and then easily pass through these cells into saliva. Neither maximal stimulation of saliva flow *(19)* nor minimal secretion of saliva following medication with anticholinergic side effects influences the concentration of cortisol in saliva *(17)*. Moreover, cortisol in saliva represents the unbound ("free") hormone fraction, and reflects accurately the free fraction of cortisol in plasma, despite the conversion of cortisol to cortisone in saliva by 11β-hydroxysteroid dehydrogenase *(20)*.

The different characteristics of the HPA axis activity and regulation during ordinary life conditions were measured by a series of saliva sampling over the day (n=7), in which cortisol levels were measured. The circadian rhythm of cortisol secretion was estimated as the variance of cortisol secretion. By addition of all measured values, a measurement of total cortisol secretion was obtained. Stress-related cortisol secretion was calculated as the response of cortisol to simultaneously reported perceived stress. The cortisol response to a physiological stimuli was estimated by a standardized lunch. In addition, a low-dose (0.5 mg × L) dexamethasone suppression test (DST) was performed. The feasibility of these measurements was tested and found adequate *(21,22)*.

The methods were then applied in samples of middle-aged men (51 yr, n=284) and women (42 yr, n=267), and set in relation to a number of anthropometric, endocrine, metabolic, and hemodynamic measurements. Furthermore, standardized questionnaires were utilized to obtain information on a number of issues.

RESULTS

Throughout these newly developed methods, we singled out subgroups of the functional status of the HPA axis. The first group was characterized by a high morning-cortisol peak, a normal circadian rhythm (variability), and feedback regulation (dexamethasone) along with a brisk cortisol response to lunch. Such individuals are, in general, lean, measured as body mass index (BMI, kg/m^2) and waist/hip circumference ratio (WHR), with higher values of insulin-like growth factor 1 (IGF-1) than average, and low total and low-density lipoprotein (LDL) cholesterol, as well as blood pressure.

The other group identified was characterized by the absence of a morning cortisol peak and circadian rhythm, a blunted suppression of cortisol by overnight low-dose dexamethasone and a poor lunch-induced cortisol response. Such individuals suffer from obesity with a predominance of centrally located body fat, low testosterone (in men) and IGF-1 concentrations, high insulin, glucose, triglycerides, total and LDL cholesterol, blood pressures, and heart rate, whereas high-density lipoprotein cholesterol is low. These relationships are all highly statistically significant (P<0.001), and consistent with the current opinion about the health consequences of an abnormal-functioning HPA axis *(2)*. Such individuals have abdominal obesity and insulin resistance, including hyperlipidemia and hypertension. This is in contrast to those with a normal HPA axis function, and further strengthens the importance of the HPA axis for human health *(21,22)*.

CONSEQUENCES OF THE ENDOCRINE PERTURBATIONS

The dysregulation of the HPA axis with additional inhibition of sex steroid and GH secretions *(9)*, are probably responsible for the multiple metabolic perturbations. Centralization of body fat is most likely an effect of cortisol, as clearly seen in Cushing's syndrome, exhibited as severe truncal obesity. Cortisol effects are counterbalanced by sex steroids and GH in several systems. Although cortisol promotes accumulation of visceral fat and insulin resistance in muscle tissue, the sex steroids and GH, often in concert, constitute the opposite. It should be noted that this may also occur with normal or low total-cortisol secretion, provided that the sex steroid and GHs are low. The cortisol and androgen effects are more pronounced in visceral fat depots because the density of specific hormonal receptors are higher in this adipose tissue region (23).

After adequate hormonal replacement therapy (HRT) in subjects with deficiency of sex steroids or GH, the anthropometric, metabolic, and circulatory abnormalities are successfully restored. In light of this clinical and experimental evidence, strengthened by interventional studies, it is thus obvious that the endocrine abnormalities plays a major role in the multitude of pathological processes in these systems (23–25).

SURROGATE MEASUREMENTS AND PROSPECTIVE STUDIES

Are there useful indicators of adaptations of the HPA axis activity for large-scale population and epidemiological studies when HPA axis activity measurements in a clinical setting are not feasible? Measurements of inhibited sex steroid and GH secretions are not sufficiently discriminative as they may cause essentially the same peripheral consequences as the primary HPA axis perturbations, and primary deficiencies of sex steroid and GH, not secondary to the HPA axis activity, might be involved. In previous studies, an elevated WHR was presumed to reflect an abnormal cortisol secretion (24). In support of this assumption, the results now available reveal strong correlations ($P<0.001$) between the WHR and abdominal sagittal diameter, an estimation of intraabdominal fat mass, and salivary cortisol measurements, particularly after stimulations of the HPA axis (food intake or perceived stress) (21,22). In conclusion, the WHR may thus be substituted theoretically by HPA axis abnormalities when interpreting studies where the WHR displays a powerful independent risk factor for cardiovascular disease, Type II diabetes, stroke, and premature mortality (24). This is not surprising, considering the vital function of the HPA axis for the overriding regulation of endocrine systems, which are responsible for the maintenance of normal energy storage and transport.

HYPERTENSION

The association of blood pressure to the syndrome requires a separate comment. It has been postulated that insulin resistance is linked to the hypertension (26) by a pathophysiological process that involves the sympathetic nervous system (27). Analyses in the cohort of men presented here suggest another possibility—namely, that visceral obesity and HPA axis perturbations are independently related to blood pressure, as well as heart rate, and that insulin and insulin resistance may account for only a part of this association (28). This suggests a simultaneous activation of the sympathetic nervous system and the HPA axis, mediated via a common arousal of hypothalamic centers. Results of other studies support this contention (29, Ljung et al., unpublished observations). Such a hypothalamic arousal syndrome may provide an excitatory influence on both the sympathetic nervous system, resulting in hypertension, and the HPA axis, resulting in abdominal obesity and its associated metabolic abnormalities. This would explain the statistical relationship between hypertension and insulin resistance, as well as the kinds of metabolic abnormalities that result.

OBESITY

Human obesity is characterized by a wide variation in the distribution of excess body fat, and the distribution of fat affects the risks associated with obesity, as well as the kinds of comorbidities that result. Central obesity is more strongly associated with comorbidities in various systems than peripheral obesity. This is abundantly evident, particularly when intraabdominal, visceral fat depots are enlarged *(24)*.

Elevated BMI and abdominal fat distribution (abdominal obesity) are closely related. The results of our recent studies suggest a possibility of interaction between the regulatory system of obesity and that of abdominal fat distribution. The BMI showed several significant relationships to the functional status of the HPA axis. This indicates an association between general obesity, measured as BMI, and the HPA axis. This is further supported by means of structural equation modeling (path analysis) where a direct link between the HPA axis function and BMI were found *(30)*. Given this information, together with previous studies *(31)*, suggesting leptin resistance in obesity, we performed analyses of leptin with similar results—namely, an increase in leptin concentration is associated with elevated BMI *(45)*. In addition, recent studies imply that cortisol may give rise to such a leptin resistance *(32)*. There is thus a prospect that the leptin sensitivity is influenced by the HPA axis. This would explain the well-known clinical observation that hypercortisolism, as in Cushing's syndrome or as an effect of corticosteroid therapy, is followed by obesity, whereas deficient secretion of cortisol, as in Addison's disease, is followed by anorexia. Moreover, in experimental models, obesity is frequently associated with an elevated adrenal secretion of cortisol, and upon adrenalectomy, weight loss is successfully achieved *(33)*.

THE PATHOGENESIS OF THE DISTURBED HPA AXIS

This overview has explored the pathophysiological consequences of an evoked, excessive perturbation of the HPA axis. In summary, there is considerable evidence of causal relationship between the HPA axis perturbations and endocrine, anthropometric, metabolic, and hemodynamic derangements. This then provides the missing link between the HPA axis and peripheral mechanisms influencing health and disease. In the following section, the environmental factors that influence the HPA axis will be reviewed.

Traits of anxiety and depression show associations with visceral obesity in both men and women *(34–36)*. We have recently identified a number of psychosocial and socioeconomic handicaps in subjects with the syndrome studied *(37,38)*. The most prominent factors, particularly in men, are divorce, solitude, poor economy, low education, unemployment, and problems at work when employed. These findings are consistent and give a picture of psychosocial and socioeconomic pressure, which would be expected to lead to a stress reaction of the depressive, uncontrollable type aforementioned. Moreover, we have identified a subgroup of abdominal obesity, where a blunted dexamethasone response is found, associated with traits of anxiety and depression *(36)*. We have, therefore, tentatively concluded that psychosocial and socioeconomic handicaps and pressures lead to a defeat reaction with HPA axis perturbations and endocrine, anthropometric, metabolic, and hemodynamic abnormalities as consequences, leading to highly prevalent and serious diseases.

In primates other than humans, exposure to standardized moderate psychosocial stress is followed by a diminished feedback regulation of the cortisol secretion, suppression of the reproductive axis, and depressive behavior *(39,40)*. Furthermore, such social stress is associated with visceral obesity, insulin resistance, dyslipidemia, hypertension, and coronary artery atherosclerosis *(39,40)*. Thus, these results bear a striking resemblance with that of humans subjected to psychosocial stress and socioeconomic subordination, followed by abdominal obesity and metabolic disturbances. These studies then provide a considerable support for a cause–effect relationship in susceptible individuals.

GENETIC ASPECTS

It is obvious that there is an individual variation in the sensitivity to environmental factors as those described in the preceding sections. Only susceptible individuals contract disease when subjected to environmental pressure. This probably depends on genetic background factors.

Of particular interest here is the regulatory mechanisms of the HPA axis. The circadian rhythm of cortisol secretion is strongly genetically controlled, and monozygotic twins show almost identical secretory pattern of cortisol *(41)*.

A dose-response study of the inhibition by dexamethasone administration has shown that the feedback regulation in subjects with visceral obesity is diminished *(42)*, parallel with a blunted function of peripheral GR in adipose tissue *(42a)*. The latter study indicates the possibilities of both a decreased responsiveness and sensitivity of the GRs. Consequently, the *GR* gene, located in chromosome 5 and consisting of 10 exons with a minimum size of 80 kb, has been partially sequenced. However, no abnormalities in the DNA-binding (exon 2) or steroid-binding (exon 9) domains of the *GR* gene have been revealed (unpublished data). Nevertheless, we have recently, in collaboration with Dr. Bouchard at Laval University in Canada, identified variants of the *GR* gene locus (GRL) in the form of restriction fragment length polymorphisms. With the restriction enzyme *Bcl*/I two alleles with fragment lengths of 4.5 and 2.3 kb were discoverable. The 4.5-kb allele is known to be associated with visceral obesity and insulin resistance *(43,44)*. In addition, the 4.5-kb allele was also directly associated with perturbations of the HPA axis, as well as visceral obesity *(45)*. Furthermore, this GRL polymorphism was found to be associated with higher leptin values (4.5/4.5 kb vs 2.3/2.3-kb genotype). The prevalence of 4.5/4.5-kb genotype of the male, Swedish population was 13.7%. The heterozygotes (2.3/4.5 kb) showed less of a relationship to abdominal obesity, insulin resistance, or HPA axis activity *(45)*.

The GRL polymorphism presented is localized at the known *Bcl*/I site in intron 1 and putative site in intron 2 near the upstream part of the coding exons of the *GR (46)*. As this GRL polymorphism is not located in a coding, regulatory, or splicing region of the *GR* gene, the functional role, if any, is uncertain, and is therefore currently under investigation.

CONCLUDING REMARKS

This chapter has addressed the complex and multifactorial association between the "negative" stress reaction and the periphery of the body. As a result, a clearer biological view of the impact of environmental stressors on human health may be defined. We suggest that stress that elicits a defeat reaction, activates hypothalamic centers in a

Hypothalamic Arousal Syndrome, which stimulates neuroendocrine-endocrine signals, and if prolonged, leads to the development of endocrine, anthropometric, metabolic, and hemodynamic risk factors for serious diseases. This has been possible to disclose by the development of new methods for the assessment of the HPA axis activity under ordinary, everyday life conditions. The peripheral consequences of this neuroendocrine arousal have been studied in detail with consistent results in a number of research designs, including intervention trials. Psychosocial and socioeconomic impairments with associated psychiatric symptoms are most likely important triggers for the perturbations of the HPA axis observed. This is supported by the striking resemblance of consequences in nonhuman primates subjected to psychosocial stress. This then would explain the long-sought connections between social handicaps and disease.

Environmental stressors may have a particularly strong impact on individuals with a predisposed genetical susceptibility. A locus for such susceptibility might be the GR control of the HPA axis, as indicated by the results presented in this chapter. The close relationship of general obesity with the syndrome can now also be visualized hypothetically. The *GR* gene polymorphism has a high prevalence in Swedish men (not yet examined in women). This opens up the possibility that among subjects exposed to social handicaps, only those with susceptibility of developing regulatory faults of the HPA axis become exposed to the pathogenic cascade of events. It seems, however, likely that a genetic predisposition to coping with social handicaps is also at hand in selected individuals at other than the GR level.

REFERENCES

1. Lazarus RS. Coping theory and research: past, present, and future. Psychosom Med 1993; 55:234–247.
2. Chrousos GP, Gold PW. A healthy body in a healthy mind—and vice versa—the damaging power of "uncontrollable" stress. J Clin Endocrinol Metab 1998; 83:1842–1845.
3. Selye H. The Stress of Life. McGraw-Hill, New York, 1956.
4. Krech D, Crutchfield RS, Livson N. Elements of Psychology. 2nd ed. Alfred A. Knopf, New York, 1969.
5. Henry JP, Stephens PM. Stress, Health, and the Social Environment. A Sociobiological Approach to Medicine. Springfield, New York, 1977.
6. Folkow B. Physiological organization of neurohormonal responses to psychosocial stimuli: implications for health and disease. Ann Behav Med 1993; 15:236–244.
7. Folkow B. Physiological aspects of the "defence" and "defeat" reactions. Acta Physiol Scand 161 1997; (Suppl. 640):34–37.
8. Laatikainen TJ. Corticotropin-releasing hormone and opioid peptides in reproduction and stress. Ann Med 1991; 23:489–496.
9. Chrousos GP, Gold PW. The concepts of stress and stress system disorders. Overview of physical and behavioral homeostasis. JAMA 1992; 267:1244–1252.
10. Dayanithi G, Antoni FA. Rapid as well as delayed inhibitory effects of glucocorticoid hormones on pituitary adrenocorticotropic hormone release are mediated by type II glucocorticoid receptors and require newly synthesized messenger ribonucleic acid as well as protein. Endocrinology 1989; 125:308–313.
11. McEwen BS, Cameron H, Chao HM, Gould E, Magarinos AM, Watanabe Y, et al. Adrenal steroids and plasticity of hippocampal neurons: toward an understanding of underlying cellular and molecular mechanisms. Cell Mol Neurobiol 1993; 13:457–482.
12. Young EA, Akil H. Paradoxical effect of corticosteroids on pituitary ACTH/β-endorphin release in stressed animals. Psychoneuroendocrinology 1988; 13:317–323.
13. Dallman MF, Akana SF, Scribner KA, Bradbury MJ, Walker C-D, Strack AM, et al. Stress, feedback and facilitation in the hypothalamo-pituitary-adrenal axis. J Neuroendocrinol 1992; 4:517–526.

14. Uno H, Tarara R, Else JG, Suleman MA, Sapolsky RM. Hippocampal damage associated with prolonged and fatal stress in primates. J Neurosci 1989; 9:1705–1711.
15. Starkman MN, Gebarski SS, Berent S, Schteingart DE. Hippocampal volume, memory dysfunction, and cortisol levels in patients with Cushing's syndrome. Biol Psychiatr 1992; 32:756–765.
16. Frankenhaeuser M. The sympathetic-adrenal and pituitary-adrenal response to challenge: comparison between the sexes. In: Dembroski TM, Schmidt TH, Blümchen G, eds., Biobehavioral Bases of Coronary Heart Disease, Human Psychophysiology. Karger, Basel, 1983, pp. 91–105.
17. Cook N, Harris B, Walker R, Hailwood R, Jones E, Johns S, et al. Clinical utility of the dexamethasone suppression test assessed by plasma and salivary cortisol determinations. Psychiatry Res 1986; 18:143–150.
18. Laudat MH, Cerdas S, Fournier C, Guiban D, Guilhaume B, Luton JP. Salivary cortisol measurement: a practical approach to assess pituitary-adrenal function. J Clin Endocrinol Metab 1988; 66:343–348.
19. Kahn JP, Rubinow DR, Davis C, Kling M, Post RM. Salivary cortisol: a practical method for evaluation of adrenal function. Biol Psychiatry 1988; 33:335–349.
20. Kirschbaum C, Hellhammer DH. Salivary cortisol in psychobiological research: an overview. Neuropsychobiology 1989; 22:150–169.
21. Rosmond R, Dallman MF, Björntorp P. Stress-related cortisol secretion in men: relationships with abdominal obesity and endocrine, metabolic and hemodynamic abnormalities. J Clin Endocrinol Metab 1998; 83:1853–1859.
22. Rosmond R, Holm G, Björntorp P. Food-induced cortisol secretion in men: relationships with abdominal obesity, hormones, metabolism, and circulation. Int J Obes Relat Metab Disord 2000; 24:4.
23. Björntorp P. The regulation of adipose tissue distribution in humans. Int J Obes Relat Metab Disord 1996; 20:291–302.
24. Björntorp P. Visceral obesity: a "civilization syndrome". Obes Res 1993; 1:206–222.
25. Björntorp P. Metabolic implications of body fat distribution. Diab Care 1991; 14:1132–1143.
26. Reisin E, Messerli FG, Ventura HO, Frohlich ED. Renal haemodynamic studies in obesity hypertension. J Hypertens 1987; 5:397–400.
27. Reaven GM, Lithell H, Landsberg L. Hypertension and associated metabolic abnormalities—the role of insulin resistance and the sympathoadrenal system. N Engl J Med 1996; 334:374–381.
28. Rosmond R, Björntorp P. Blood pressure in relation to obesity, insulin and the hypothalamic-pituitary-adrenal axis in Swedish men. J Hypertens 1998; 16:1721–1726.
29. Jern S, Bergbrant A, Björntorp P, Hansson L. Relation to central hemodynamics to obesity and body fat distribution. Hypertension 1992; 19:520–527.
30. Rosmond R, Björntorp P. The interactions between hypothalamic-pituitary-adrenal axis activity, testosterone, insulin-like growth factor I and abdominal obesity with metabolism and blood pressure in men. Int J Obes Relat Disord 1998; 22:1184–1196.
31. Considine RV, Sinha MK, Heiman ML, Kriauciunas A, Stephens TW, Nyce MR, et al. Serum immunoreactive-leptin concentrations in normal-weight and obese humans. N Engl J Med 1996; 334:292–295.
32. Zahrzewska KE, Cusin J, Sainbury A, Rohner-Jeanrenaud F, Jeanrenaud B. Glucocorticoids are counterregulatory hormones of leptin. Towards an understanding of leptin resistance. Diabetes 1997; 46:717–719.
33. York DA. Genetic models of animal obesity. In: Björntorp P, Brodoff BN, eds. Obesity. Lippincott, Philadelphia, PA, 1992, pp. 233–240.
34. Rosmond R, Lapidus L, Mårin P, Björntorp P. Mental distress, obesity and body fat distribution in middle-aged men. Obes Res 1996; 4:245–252.
35. Rosmond R, Björntorp P. Psychiatric ill-health of women and its relationship to obesity and body fat distribution. Obes Res 1998; 6:338–345.
36. Rosmond R, Björntorp P. Endocrine and metabolic aberrations in men with abdominal obesity in relation to anxio-depressive infirmity. Metabolism 1998; 47:1187–1193.
37. Rosmond R, Lapidus L, Björntorp P. The influence of occupational and social factors on obesity and body fat distribution in middle-aged men. Int J Obes Relat Metab Disord 1996; 20:599–607.
38. Rosmond R, Björntorp P. Psychosocial and socio-economic factors in women and their relationship to obesity and regional body fat distribution. Int J Obes Relat Metab Disord; 23:2.
39. Jayo JM, Shively CA, Kaplan JR, Manuck SB. Effects of exercise and stress on body fat distribution in male cynomolgus monkeys. Int J Obes Relat Metab Disord 1993; 17:597–604.

40. Shively CA, Laber-Laird K, Anton RF. Behavior and physiology of social stress and depression in female cynomolgus monkeys. Biol Psychiatry 1997; 41:871–882.
41. Linkowski P, Van Onderbergen A, Kerkhofs M, Bosson D, Mendlewicz J, Van Cauter E. Twin study of the 24-h cortisol profile: evidence for genetic control of the human circadian clock. Am J Physiol 1993; 264:173–181.
42. Ljung T, Andersson B, Bengtsson B-Å, Björntorp P, Mårin P. Inhibition of cortisol secretion by dexamethasone in relation to body fat distribution: a dose-response study. Obes Res 1996; 4:277–282.
42a. Lönn L, Stenlöf K, Ottosson M, et al. Body weight and body composition changes after treatment of hyperthyroidism. 1998; 83:4269–4273.
43. Weaver JU, Hitman GA, Kopelman PG. An association between a Bc11 restriction fragment length polymorphism of the glucocorticoid receptor locus and hyperinsulinemia in obese women. J Mol Endocrinol 1992; 9:295–300.
44. Buemann B, Vohl M-C, Chagnon M, Chagnon YC, Gagnon J, Pérusse L, et al. Abdominal visceral fat is associated with a *Bcl*I restriction fragment length polymorphism at the glucocorticoid receptor gene locus. Obes Res 1997; 5:186–192.
45. Rosmond R, Björntorp P. The interactions between hypothalamic-pituitary-adrenal axis activity, testosterone, insulin-like growth factor I and abdominal obesity with metabolism and blood pressure in men. 1998; 22:12.
46. Palmer LA, Hukku B, Harmon JM. Human glucocorticoid receptor gene deletion following exposure to cancer chemotherapeutic drugs and chemical mutagens. Cancer Res 1992; 52:6612–6618.

26   Aldosterone Synthase Deficiency

Michael Peter and Wolfgang G. Sippell

CONTENTS

INTRODUCTION

Children with congenital hypoaldosteronism present with a salt-wasting syndrome in the first weeks of life. Endocrine causes of salt-wasting can be easily differentiated by determination of aldosterone, cortisol, 17-hydroxyprogesterone, adrenocorticotropic hormone (ACTH), and plasma–renin activity or active renin (Table 1). For the interpretation of these parameters, valid reference data for infants are a prerequisite.

From: *Contemporary Endocrinology: Adrenal Disorders*
Edited by: A. N. Margioris and G. P. Chrousos © Humana Press, Totowa, NJ

Table 1
Differentiation of Endocrine Causes of Salt-Wasting by Determination of Aldosterone,
Cortisol, 17-OH-Progesterone, ACTH, and Plasma–Renin Activity

Diagnosis	Aldosterone	PRA	17-OH-Progesterone	Cortisol	ACTH
Aldosterone Synthase Deficiency	⇓	⇑	⇔	⇔	⇔
Pseudohypoaldosteronism	⇑	⇑	⇔	⇔	⇔
21-Hydroxylase Deficiency	⇓	⇑	⇑	⇓	⇑
Congenital Adrenal Hypoplasia	⇓	⇑	⇓	⇓	⇑

⇓ decreased
⇑ increased
⇔ normal

REGULATION OF ALDOSTERONE SECRETION

The major circulating mineralocorticoid is aldosterone, which is synthesized exclusively in the *zona glomerulosa*. Aldosterone secretion is governed by multiple factors that have complex regulatory interactions. The most important regulators of aldosterone secretion are the renin–angiotensin system and potassium. Corticotropin, sodium, and other agents such as vasopressin are minor regulators *(1)*.

METABOLIC PATHWAY OF ALDOSTERONE BIOSYNTHESIS

Aldosterone is synthesized in the *zona glomerulosa* of the adrenal cortex by the action of the transport protein steroidogenic acute regulatory (StAR) protein, which is responsible for the rapid transport of cholesterol into the mitochondrion, and by the subsequent action of four enzymes (Fig. 1). Cholesterol desmolase (or side-chain cleavage enzyme; *P450scc*), 21-hydroxylase (*P450c21*), and aldosterone synthase (*P450c11*Aldo) are cytochrome *P450* (CYP) enzymes, which are membrane-bound heme-containing proteins. The fourth enzyme, 3β-hydroxysteroid dehydrogenase (3β-HSD II), is a member of the short-chain dehydrogenase family *(2,3)*.

The first three steps of aldosterone biosynthesis (from cholesterol to progesterone) are identical to those required for biosynthesis of cortisol in the *zona fasciculata* and are mediated by the same enzymes in both zones (Fig. 1). However, the synthesis of cortisol requires 17α-hydroxylation of pregnenolone by 17α-hydroxylase (*P450c17*), which is expressed only in the *zona fasciculata (4)*. In contrast, aldosterone synthase is normally expressed only in the *zona glomerulosa (5–8)*. Thus, the specific patterns of expression of these two enzymes ensure that aldosterone and cortisol are synthesized appropriately.

STEROID 11β-HYDROXYLASE ISOENZYMES

The two 11β-hydroxylase isoenzymes that are responsible for cortisol (*P450c11*) and aldosterone (*P450c11*Aldo) biosynthesis in humans are mitochondrial cytochromes *P450,* located in the inner-mitochondrial membrane on the matrix side. Both have 503 amino acid residues, but a signal peptide is cleaved to yield the mature protein of

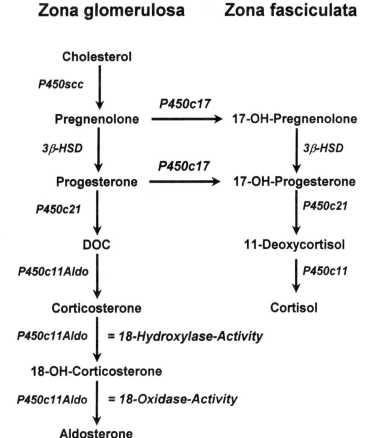

Fig. 1. Biosynthesis of aldosterone in the *zona glomerulosa* and of cortisol in the *zona fasciculata*. The two different biosynthetic defects in terminal aldosterone biosynthesis are shown (aldosterone synthase deficiency type I with low aldosterone and 18-hydroxycorticosterone; aldosterone synthase deficiency type II with low aldosterone and increased 18-hydroxycorticosterone).

479 residues *(9)*. The sequences of both proteins are 93% identical. *P450c11* and *P450c11*Aldo differ in 35 amino acids *(10)*.

CYP11B GENES

In humans, the two 11β-hydroxylase isoenzymes are encoded by two genes that are located on the long arm of chromosome 8 *(11,12)*. *CYP11B1* is the gene encoding *P450c11* and *CYP11B2* is that encoding *P450c11*Aldo.

Both genes are located approx 40 kb apart. Each gene contains 9 exons spread over 7 kb. The nucleotide sequences of both genes are 93% identical in coding sequences and about 90% identical in introns. Together with *CYP11A*, the gene encoding *P450scc, CYP11B1*, and *CYP11B2* are grouped into a single family within the cytochrome *P450* gene superfamily *(13)*.

CYP11B2 is regulated mainly by angiotensin II and potassium. The promoter region of *CYP11B1* and *CYP11B2* is strikingly different, underlining the fact that both genes are differentially regulated on the transcriptional level.

ACTION OF ALDOSTERONE

Mineralocorticoids regulate electrolyte transport across epithelial surfaces. The principal physiological mineralocorticoid is aldosterone. Its target tissues, which include kidney, colon, and salivary glands, have mineralocorticoid receptors that bind aldosterone with high affinity. Aldosterone regulates electrolyte excretion and intravascular volume mainly through its effect on the distal tubules and cortical collecting ducts of the kidneys, in which it increases sodium resorption from and potassium into the urine. Aldosterone increases the number of opened sodium-permeable channels. Aldosterone also increases potassium conductance through specific channels.

Aldosterone exerts most of its biological action on cells by occupying an intracellular receptor, the mineralocorticoid receptor, which then binds to DNA and thereby influences the transcription of various genes *(14)*.

HISTORICAL BACKGROUND OF ALDOSTERONE SYNTHASE DEFICIENCY

The most frequent cause of deficient aldosterone biosynthesis is congenital adrenal hyperplasia caused by 21-hydroxylase deficiency. Signs of androgen excess appear in these patients. However, a small group of patients do have aldosterone deficiency without any disturbances in cortisol and androgen biosynthesis. In the early 1960s, the diagnosis of a selective mineralocorticoid deficiency was established by urinary steroid metabolite determinations utilizing improved laboratory methods such as gas chromatography. In 1964, Visser and Cost *(15)* were the first to suggest a biosynthetic defect with autosomal recessive inheritance causing selective hypoaldosteronism caused by deficient 18-hydroxylation of corticosterone *(16)*. Subsequently, two patients with presumably deficient 18-oxidase were described by Ulick et al. *(17)* and Rappaport et al. *(18)*. A decade later, Ulick suggested the two biochemically different forms of selective aldosterone deficiency be termed corticosterone methyl oxidase (CMO) deficiency type I and type II *(19)*. In 1996, the nomenclature was changed to aldosterone synthase deficiency type I and type II *(20)*, because it was clear that one single *P450* enzyme, termed aldosterone synthase, catalyses all three steps of the terminal aldosterone biosynthesis. In both aldosterone synthase deficiency types, aldosterone biosynthesis is impaired, whereas corticosterone of *zona glomerulosa* origin, under the primary control of the renin–angiotensin system, is excessively produced. The two defects differ biochemically in that 18-hydroxycorticosterone is deficient in aldosterone synthase deficiency type I, but overproduced in aldosterone synthase deficiency type II.

PATHOPHYSIOLOGY OF ALDOSTERONE SYNTHASE DEFICIENCY

Aldosterone synthase deficiency is an autosomal recessively inherited disorder caused by mutations in the *CYP11B2* gene. Because of deficient adrenal *zona glomerulosa* aldosterone synthase activity, 11-deoxycorticosterone is not efficiently converted to aldosterone. Insufficient aldosterone secretion leads to decreased sodium resorption from and potassium secretion into the urine.

CLINICAL PRESENTATION OF
ALDOSTERONE SYNTHASE DEFICIENCY

All affected children present with frequent vomiting, failure to thrive, and severe, life-threatening salt loss in the first weeks of life (Table 2). In most of the published clinical case reports, no differences in the severity of clinical signs between young infants with aldosterone synthase deficiency types I and II have been observed. Rösler (21) has shown that in each affected individual the clinical severity of the disease decreases with age. Adolescents and adults may show only the abnormal steroid pattern which persists throughout life. The same natural course of the disease is observed in many patients with pseudohypoaldosteronism (21).

FREQUENCY OF ALDOSTERONE SYNTHASE DEFICIENCY

Precise data regarding the frequency of selective hypoaldosteronism and its two biochemical types in the general population are not available. It is generally assumed that aldosterone synthase deficiency type II is more frequent than aldosterone synthase deficiency type I. This is mainly because of the observation of Rösler who published data of 21 patients of Iranian Jewish origin with selective aldosterone deficiency caused by aldosterone synthase deficiency type II (21). This preponderance of aldosterone synthase deficiency type II is also reflected in the overall published case reports. In contrast to this, our material, which is the largest series of unrelated patients (Table 2) diagnosed by strictly the same methodology, indicates a comparable frequency of both aldosterone synthase deficiency types (22,23).

HORMONAL FINDINGS IN ALDOSTERONE SYNTHASE DEFICIENCY

The typical steroid profile in patients with aldosterone synthase deficiency consists of inadequate low (according to the sodium depletion) to undetectable aldosterone plasma levels and elevated mineralocorticoid precursor levels prior to the block (e.g., corticosterone and 11-deoxycorticosterone). Decreased aldosterone production leads to increased renin secretion via poor feedback control. Glucocorticoid biosynthesis is undisturbed, but because of stress, cortisol might be elevated in untreated patients in salt-losing state.

The biochemical criteria for the differentiation of the two aldosterone synthase deficiency-type variants are based on specific steroid determinations in urine and/or plasma. The criteria for differentiation of aldosterone synthase deficiency types I and II have been proposed by Ulick (19). The same author published revised and more precise biochemical criteria for the diagnosis of the two aldosterone synthase deficiency variants, based on urinary steroid measurements using gas chromatography/mass fragmentography (24). We have diagnosed 30 sporadic cases of congenital isolated hypoaldosteronism (21,22) using our method of multisteroid analysis by radioimmunoassay (RIA) after extraction and automated Sephadex LH-20 multicolumn chromatography (25).

Results of the plasma-steroid determinations in two of the patients originally described

Table 2
Clinical Data and Laboratory Findings in 16 Children with Aldosterone Synthase Deficiency

No.	Sex	Age at diagnosis (wks)	Birth weight (g)	Weight at diagnosis (g)	Na^+ (mmol/L)	K^+ (mmol/L)	PRA (ng/ml/h)	Population	Consanguinity	Type
1	f	4	3500	3550	125	7,5	55	Pakistan	+	I
2	f	11	2900	3180	131	6,7	68	Turkey	–	I
3	f	4	3050	2700	122	9,2	45	Turkey	–	I
4	m	8	3850	3380	123	6,0	67	Germany	–	I
5	m	3	3240	2950	128	7,2	176	Germany	–	I
6	m	8	3440	3500	128	6,2	>300	Turkey	–	I
7	m	screening	normal	—	132	5,2	7	Turkey	–	I
8	f	8	3500	3420	125	5,8	300	France	–	II
9	f	4	4020	3840	127	6,5	120	Lebanon*	+	II
10	f	20	4180	4680	129	6,5	265	Lebanon*	+	II
11	f	10	3440	3490	114	5,7	87	Germany	–	II
12	f	4	3200	2580	126	8,2	>300	Netherlands	–	II
13	m	4	3010	2760	127	5,9	46	Germany	–	II
14	m	24	3280	3520	107	6,4	72	Turkey	–	II
15	f	4	3700	3200	138	7,7	53	Italy	–	n.cl.**
16	m	8	3990	3860	126	6,4	27	Netherlands	–	n.cl.**

*siblings, **not classified

344

Table 3
Basal Plasma Steroids in Two Adult Patients with Aldosterone Synthase Deficiency
Type I Determined by Multisteroid Analysis

Steroid (nmol/L)	Patient 1	Patient 3	Normal (mean ± 1 SD)
Aldosterone	0.555	0.055	0.1 ± 0.02
18-OH-Corticosterone	0.17	0.055	0.9 ± 0.03
Corticosterone	32.9	23.6	11.4 ± 6.1
11-Deoxycorticosterone	2.3	1.8	0.14 ± 0.05
Progesterone	1.14	1.4	0.52 ± 0.22
17-OH-Progesterone	3.17	3.1	3.6 ± 1.1
11-Deoxycortisol	0.38	1.4	1.35 ± 0.61
Cortisol	154	196	287 ± 94
Cortisone	19.4	27.7	57.1 ± 7.5
Corticosterone/18-OHB*	194	429	—
18-OHB/Aldosterone	3.1	1	—

*18-OHB = 18-OH-Corticosterone

Table 4
Basal Plasma Steroids in an Untreated Patient with Aldosterone Synthase
Deficiency Type II at Age 4 mo and Normal Ranges Measured by our
Method of Multisteroid Analysis

Steroid (nmol/L)	Patient	Normal Range (<3 mo—1 yr)
Aldosterone (Aldo)	<0.055	0.17–2.55
18-OH-Corticosterone (18-OHB)	65.1	0.55–1.46
Corticosterone (B)	97.3	0.14–15.9
18-OH-11-Deoxycorticosterone	9.06	0.12–0.72
11-Deoxycorticosterone	2.23	0.09–0.99
Progesterone	0.29	0.09–4.01
17-OH-Progesterone	0.13	0.09–4.96
11-Deoxycortisol	6.03	0.43–5.66
Cortisol	221	58.5–477
B/18-OHB	1.5	—
18-OHB-Aldo	1184	—

by Visser and Cost (15) are given in Table 3. The two adult patients studied in an untreated state showed the typical steroid pattern of a defect in 18-hydroxylation of corticosterone. Aldosterone and 18-hydroxycorticosterone were decreased, whereas corticosterone and 11-deoxycorticosterone were increased. The corticosterone/18-OH-corticosterone ratio was elevated and the 18-hydroxycorticosterone/aldosterone ratio was decreased. According to the nomenclature proposed by Ulick, this defect is termed aldosterone synthase deficiency type I.

Results of plasma steroid determinations in a girl presenting with failure to thrive, feeding problems and mild dehydration at age 6 wk are shown in Table 4. Serum sodium was decreased (132 mEq/L) and potassium (6.4 mEq/L) and renin activity (52 ng/mL/h) were elevated. Plasma 17-hydroxyprogesterone and cortisol were normal with normal response to ACTH. The diagnosis of aldosterone synthase deficiency type II was made on the basis of specific plasma-steroid measurements (Table 4) with a markedly elevated ratio of 18-hydroxycorticosterone/aldosterone of 1180 (normal range 1–10) using our method of multisteroid analysis as described elsewhere (25).

Results of the determination of aldosterone, 18-hydroxycorticosterone and corticosterone by our method of multisteroid analysis in a large series of young infants with congenital hypoaldosteronism are shown in Fig. 2.

Using specific steroid determinations, the plasma level of 18-hydroxycorticosterone distinguishes between aldosterone synthase deficiency type I (where it is decreased or low-normal) and aldosterone synthase deficiency type II (where it is markedly elevated). The clearest distinguishing parameter between the two aldosterone synthase deficiency types reflecting impaired 18-hydroxylation is the ratio of plasma corticosterone/18-hydroxycorticosterone, which is elevated in aldosterone synthase deficiency type I and decreased in aldosterone synthase deficiency II. Moreover, the ratio of plasma 18-hydroxycorticosterone/aldosterone can also discriminate between the two aldosterone synthase deficiency variants (Table 5). The disadvantage of this ratio is that plasma aldosterone levels in these patients are often at or even below the lower limit of detection (22).

DIAGNOSTIC RECOMMENDATIONS FOR ALDOSTERONE SYNTHASE DEFICIENCY

For practical reasons, we recommend the following procedure for the diagnosis of aldosterone synthase deficiency in young infants. All salt-wasting neonates should be examined carefully. In female newborns with ambiguous genitalia and in all male neonates, first of all, 21-hydroxylase deficiency should be excluded by measuring basal 17-hydroxyprogesterone (RIA after extraction). Second, basal cortisol, aldosterone, and PRA should be determined. Highly specific methods (RIA after extraction and chromatography) for the determination of plasma steroids (particularly for aldosterone) are necessary in the early life period. In our own experience, many direct RIA methods yield far too-high results in newborns and young infants because vast amounts of interfering steroids from the fetoplacental unit and/or the still active fetal adrenal cortex. In children with low or undetectably low plasma aldosterone and elevated PRA, corticosterone should be determined next. A high ratio of corticosterone over aldosterone leads to the diagnosis of aldosterone synthase deficiency. The ratios of 18-hydroxycorticosterone/aldosterone and corticosterone/18-hydroxycorticosterone are necessary for further differentiation of aldosterone synthase deficiency types I and II. An ACTH test is not necessary for the diagnosis. The diagnosis can also be made by gas chromatography of a 24-h urine sample, which is, however, difficult to collect in this age group.

MOLECULAR GENETICS OF ALDOSTERONE SYNTHASE DEFICIENCY

Based on the biochemical findings, the existence of two different enzymes catalyzing the terminal aldosterone biosynthesis (corticosterone methyl oxidase type I = 18-hydroxylase and corticosterone methyl oxidase type II = 18-oxidase) has been postulated (19). However, the existence of these two different enzymes has been excluded. Investigations on cultured cells and in aldosterone-secreting tumors have shown that a single enzyme with 11β-hydroxylase, as well as 18-hydroxylase and 18-oxidase activity is expressed

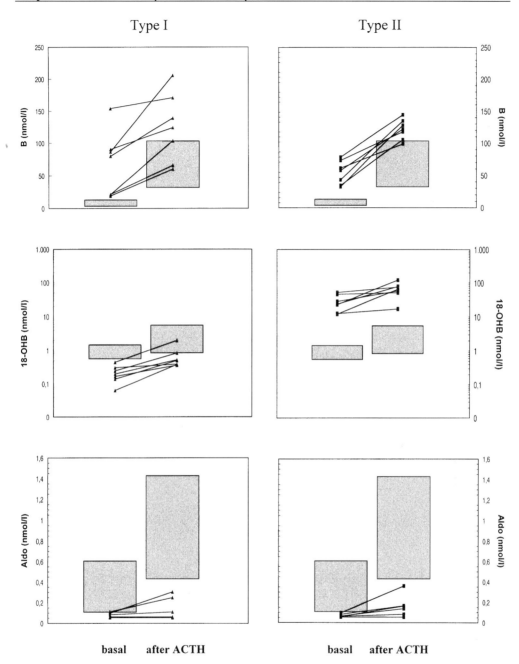

Fig. 2. Basal and ACTH-stimulated plasma levels of aldosterone (lower panel), 18-OH-corticosterone (middle panel), and corticosterone (upper panel) in normal infants and in untreated infants with congenital hypoaldosteronism (aldosterone synthase deficiency type I and type II); normal range (45–95. centile) shaded boxes.

Table 5
Ratios of 18-OHB/Aldo and B/18-OHB in 14 Children with
Aldosterone Synthase Deficiency

Aldosterone Synthase Deficiency	Patient No.	18-OHB/Aldo	B/18-OHB
Type I	1	5.5	67
	2	1.7	1068
	3	2.0	422
	4	1.1	1360
	5	2.2	314
	6	6.9	42
	7	2.7	124
Type II	8	310	2.4
	9	900	5.8
	10	191	1.1
	11	286	1.1
	12	836	2.5
	13	597	1.9
	14	346	1.4

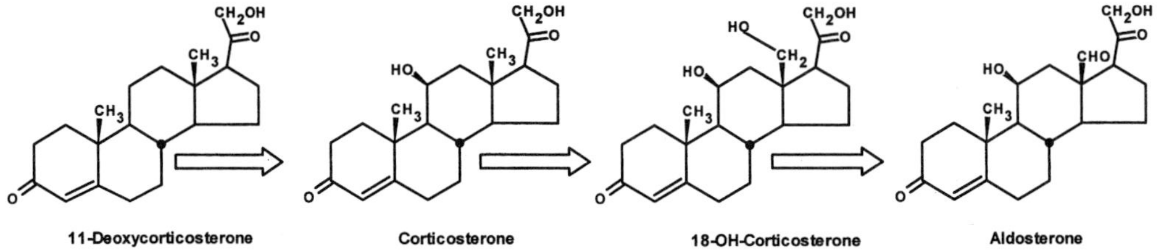

11-Deoxycorticosterone   Corticosterone   18-OH-Corticosterone   Aldosterone

Fig. 3. The terminal aldosterone biosynthesis in the *zona glomerulosa* of the human adrenal is catalyzed by one single *P450* enzyme termed aldosterone synthase. This enzyme exhibits three catalytic activities (11β-hydroxylase, 18-hydroxylase, and 18-oxidase).

in the adrenal zona glomerulosa (Fig. 3) *(5,7)*. This enzyme, termed aldosterone synthase (*P450c11*Aldo), is identical to corticosterone methyl oxidase I and II activity, and appears to catalyze exclusively the terminal aldosterone biosynthesis in humans *(5,9)*. It shows considerable homology with the enzyme 11β-hydroxylase *(P450c11)*, which catalyses the conversion of 11-deoxycortisol to cortisol in the *zona fasciculata* of the adrenal cortex *(10)*. *P450c11* can also convert 11-deoxycorticosterone to 18-OH-11-deoxycorticosterone, but it 18-hydroxylates corticosterone poorly. It cannot convert corticosterone into aldosterone *(9)*. Both enzymes are encoded by different genes in man, i.e., *CYP11B1* for *P450c11* and *CYP11B2* for *P450c11*aldo *(10)*. Both genes are located on chromosome 8q *(11,12)*.

So far, the molecular basis of aldosterone deficiency has been elucidated in patients with different genetic backgrounds (Fig. 4, Table 6).

In aldosterone synthase deficiency type I, five mutations of the *CYP11B2* gene have been described, all except one completely abolishing the activity of aldosterone synthase: Three patients of a consanguineous Amish kindred have a deletion of 5 nucleotides in exon 1 of *CYP11B2,* resulting in a frameshift to form a stop codon in the same exon

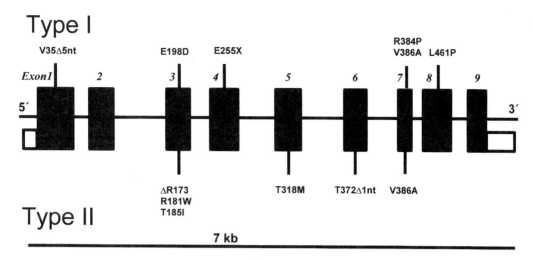

Fig. 4. Schematic representation of the genomic structure of the human *CYP11B2* gene and positions of mutations reported to date. Exons are represented by boxes; black boxes demarcate the coding regions, and open boxes represent the noncoding regions. The homozygous mutations *V35Δ5nt*, *E255X*, *R384P*, and *L461P* and the double-homozygous mutations *E198D* and *V386A* have been identified in patients with aldosterone synthase deficiency type I. The mutations *R181W* and *V386A* (double homozygous) and *T185I* (homozygous), the homozygous deletion *R173*, and the compound heterozygous mutations *T318M* and *T372Δ1nt* have been described in patients with aldosterone synthase deficiency type II.

(26). In a boy of a nonconsanguineous German family, we identified an R384P amino acid substitution in *CYP11B2 (27).* Another single-point mutation CTG (leucine) to CCG (proline) has been identified in a Turkish patient *(28).* In two of the three patients with congenital hypoaldosteronism originally published by Visser and Cost in 1964, we recently identified a homozygous single-base exchange (G to T) in codon 255 (GAG) causing a premature stop codon E255X *(TAG) (29).* Interestingly, we found the same mutation in a Turkish family with two affected brothers *(30).* One study in an individual carrying two homozygous mutations, E198D in exon 3 and V386A in exon 7, reported results for the hormonal phenotype suggesting aldosterone synthase deficiency type I (18-hydroxylase deficiency), which were inconsistent with the in vitro transfection data that indicated aldosterone synthase deficiency type II (18-oxidase deficiency) *(31).* We made the same observation in a patient from Spain carrying the same two homozygous mutations on his *CYP11B2* alleles.

Aldosterone synthase deficiency type II is frequently observed among Jews of Iranian origin. All affected individuals are homozygous for two missense mutations in *CYP11B2*, *R181W*, and *V386A*. Individuals homozygous for either mutation alone have no clinical symptoms *(32,33).* Zhang et al. *(34)* reported a patient with a typical clinical and hormonal picture of aldosterone synthase deficiency type II. Direct sequencing of PCR products showed that the mother's allele contributed *R181W* and the deletion/frameshift mutation *T372Δ1nt*, whereas the father's allele contributed *T318M* and *V386A*. Two further *CYP11B2* have been published, a single amino acid deletion of codon 173 in exon 3 and one single amino acid substitution *T185I* in exon 3 *(35,36).* Fardella et al. *(37)* described a gene-conversion event (between *CYP11B2* and *CYP11B1*) in three of

Table 6
CYP11B2 Gene Mutations in Aldosterone Synthase Deficiency Type I and Type II

Exon	Mutation	Sequence	Enzyme activity % of normal	Type	Ethnic group	Reference
Aldosterone synthase deficiency type I						
1	V35Δ5nt	—	0	I	Amish	Mitsuuchi, 1993
3	E198D	GAA → GAC	0*	I	Caucasian	Portrat-Doyen, 1998
7	V386A	GTG → GCG				
4	E255X	GAG → TAG	0	I	Caucasian	Peter, 1997
7	R384P	CGA → CCA	0	I	Caucasian	Geley, 1995
8	L461P	CTG → CCG	0	I	Caucasian	Nomoto, 1997
Aldosterone synthase deficiency type II						
3	R181W**	CGG → TGG	0–100***	II	Iranian Jews	Pascoe, 1992
7	V386A**	GTG → GCG				Mitsuuchi, 1992
5	T318M	ACG → ATG	0.1	II	not reported	Zhang, 1995
6	delC386X	delC372	0			
3	T185I	ACC → ATC	not determined	II	Caucasian	Peter, 1998
3	del R173	—	not determined	II	Caucasian	Peter, 1998

*Large decrease of 18-hydroxylase activity, no 18-oxidase activity in vitro.

**Individuals homozygous for both mutations are symptomatic.

***R181W has normal 11β-hydroxylase activity, decreased 18-hydroxylase activity, and undetectable 18-dehydrogenase activity in vitro. V386A has slightly decreased 18-hydroxylase activity in vitro.

four unrelated *P450c11*Aldo alleles from two unrelated patients with aldosterone synthase deficiency type II by which exon 3 and 4 of the *CYP11B2* gene encoding
*P450c11*Aldo were changed to the sequence of the nearby *CYP11B1* gene, which
encodes the related enzyme *P450c11*. This conversion resulted in a mutant *P450c11*Aldo
protein carrying three changes: *Asp*-141 → *Glu, Lys*-151 → *Asn, Ile*-248 → Thr.
Expression systems containing these mutants all retained normal 18-oxidase activity
of *P450c11*Aldo, indicating that the detected gene-conversion event is associated with,
but does not cause aldosterone synthase deficiency *(37)*. In the group of patients we
have collected over the past decade, we identified a wide spectrum of missense and
nonsense mutations in aldosterone synthase type I, as well as aldosterone synthase type
II-deficient patients *(35,36)*. Transfection experiments are currently under way in order
to determine the enzymatic activity of the mutant enzymes. However, we found three
patients with aldosterone synthase deficiency type II who did not carry any disease-
causing mutation in their *CYP11B2* gene *(30)*.

In vitro studies have shown a total loss of 18-hydroxylase activity of *P450c11*Aldo
in almost all aldosterone synthase type I-deficient alleles *(26–29)*. However, one study
reported inconsistent results between the hormonal phenotype and the in vitro transfection data *(31)*. In aldosterone synthase deficiency type II, the *R181W* mutation in
CYP11B2 does not impair 11β-hydroxylase activity, although it markedly decreases
18-hydroxylase activity, and abolishes 18-oxidase activity. The V386A mutation in
CYP11B2 causes a small, but consistent, reduction in 18-hydroxylase activity *(33)*. The
two *CYP11B2* mutations (*T372Δ1nt* and *T318M*) identified in a patient with aldosterone
synthase deficiency type II by Zhang et al. showed no measurable enzyme activity in
transfection experiments *(34)*.

The two variants of aldosterone synthase deficiency are caused by different mutations
within the same gene. In their review, White et al. *(9)* discussed the molecular genetic
differences between aldosterone synthase deficiency types I and II. They stated that
aldosterone synthase deficiency type I might be caused by a more severe reduction of
enzyme activity of aldosterone synthase. The high levels of corticosterone in both
aldosterone synthase deficiency types can be explained by upregulation of *P450c11* in
the *zona glomerulosa* under the control of elevated PRA *(7)*. It is, however, difficult
to explain the different 18-hydroxycorticosterone levels in both aldosterone synthase
deficiency types. In vitro, 11β-hydroxylase has 18-hydroxylase activity at a level of
about one-tenth of that of aldosterone synthase. If 11β-hydroxylase activity in the
zona glomerulosa is increased in both aldosterone synthase deficiency types, then 18-
hydroxycorticosterone should likewise be elevated in both. Another explanation for
increased 18-hydroxycorticosterone levels might be an overexpression of *CYP11B2* in
aldosterone synthase deficiency type II. However, the *R181W/V386A* mutant aldosterone
synthase from Iranian patients with aldosterone synthase deficiency type II has normal
11β-hydroxylase activity in vitro, but low 18-hydroxylase activity *(33)*. To clarify these
discrepancies, further molecular studies on a larger number of aldosterone-deficient
patients are necessary to elucidate the structure/function relationship of the enzyme
*P450c11*Aldo. Other factors besides *P450c11*Aldo might be involved in the genesis
of the distinctive phenotypes of aldosterone synthase deficiency types I and II.

The homologous *P450* enzymes aldosterone synthase and 11β-hydroxylase differ in 35
amino acids. Amino acid residues have been identified in a recent study using transfection
experiments with cDNAs, which encode hybrids between the highly homologous cyto-

Table 7
Amino Acid Differences Between *CYP11B1* (11β-Hydroxylase) and *CYP11B2*
(Aldosterone Synthase) (according to Curnow et al., Nature Structural Biology, 1997)

CYP11B1	Codon	CYP11B2	Exon
Met	11	Val	1
Val	13	Ala	1
Gln	22	Arg	1
Val	31	Ala	1
Arg	43	Gln	1
Arg	44	His	1
Asp	63	His	1
Val	68	Met	1
Asp	82	Asn	2
Ala	86	Pro	2
Gly	87	Arg	2
His	109	Cys	2
Ser	112	Ile	2
Glu	147	Asp	3
Asn	152	Lys	3
Lys	173	Arg	3
Thr	248	Ile	4
Ser	281	Asn	5
Gln	285	His	5
Ser*	**288**	**Gly**	**5**
Asn	296	Lys	5
Pro	301	Leu	5
Asp	302	Glu	5
Val*	**320**	**Ala**	**6**
Asn	335	Asp	6
Ala	339	Ile	6
Ala	386	Val	7
Arg	404	Gln	8
Pro	414	Ala	8
Tyr	439	His	8
Leu	471	Phe	9
Gln	472	Leu	9
Ser	492	Gly	9
Met	493	Thr	9
Phe	494	Ser	9

*Substitution of serine-288 by glycine and of valine-320 by alanine converts 11β-hydroxylase in an enzyme with aldosterone synthase activity.

chrome *P450* enzymes, *CYP11B1* (11β-hydroxylase), and *CYP11B2* (aldosterone synthase), determining the different catalytic activities of both enzymes (Table 7). Efficient 18-hydroxylation requires a glycine residue at position 288 and subsequent 18-oxidation requires an alanine at position 320 *(38)*.

MANAGEMENT AND TREATMENT OF ALDOSTERONE SYNTHASE DEFICIENCY

Patients with aldosterone synthase deficiency fully recover under treatment with an oral mineralocorticoid. Replacement therapy with 9α-fluorocortisol in doses of 100–250 μg/m^2/d is recommended, at least during early infancy and childhood. In addition, generous sodium supplementation may be given. Continued mineralocorticoid replacement therapy after childhood is not always necessary, as shown by the clinical observation that compensatory extraadrenal salt-conserving mechanisms mature with age.

ACKNOWLEDGMENT

The authors thank Ms. Gisela Hohmann, Susanne Olin, and Sabine Stein for expert technical assistance. This work was supported by Grant Pe 589/1-2 from the Deutsche Forschungsgemeinschaft (DFG) and by an additional grant from the Fritz-Thyssen-Stiftung.

REFERENCES

1. Quinn SL, Williams GH. Regulation of aldosterone secretion. Annu Rev Physiol 1988; 50:409–426.
2. Ogishima T, Mitani F, Ishimura Y. Isolation of aldosterone synthase cytochrome P-450 from zona glomerulosa mitochondria of rat adrenal cortex. J Biol Chem 1989; 264:10,935–10,938.
3. Yanagibashi K, Haniu M, Shively JE, Shen WH, Hall P. The synthesis of aldosterone by the adrenal cortex. Two zones (fasciculata and glomerulosa) possess one enzyme for 11β-, 18-hydroxylation, and aldehyde synthesis. J Biol Chem 1986; 261:3556–3562.
4. Miller WL. Molecular biology of steroid hormone biosynthesis. Endocr Rev 1988; 9:295–318.
5. Kawamoto T, Mitsuuchi Y, Ohnishi T, et al. Cloning and expression of a cDNA for human cytochrome P-450aldo as related to primary aldosteronism. Biochem Biophys Res Commun 1990; 173:309–316.
6. Ogishima T, Shibata H, Shimada H, et al. Aldosterone synthase cytochrome P-450 expressed in the adrenals of patients with primary aldosteronism. J Biol Chem 1991; 266:10,731–10,734.
7. Curnow KM, Tusie LM, Pascoe L, et al. The product of the CYP11B2 gene is required for aldosterone biosynthesis in the human adrenal cortex. Mol Endocrinol 1991; 5:1513–1522.
8. Kawamoto T, Mitsuuchi Y, Toda K, et al. Role of steroid 11β-hydroxylase and steroid 18-hydroxylase in the biosynthesis of glucocorticoids and mineralocorticoids in humans. Proc Natl Acad Sci USA 1992; 89:1458–1462.
9. White PC, Curnow KM, Pascoe L. Disorders of steroid 11β-hydroxylase isozymes. Endocr Rev. 1994; 15:421–438.
10. Mornet E, Dupont J, Vitek A, White PC. Characterization of two genes encoding human steroid 11β-hydroxylase (P-450 11β). J Biol Chem 1989; 264:20,961–20,967.
11. Chua SC, Szabo P, Vitek A, Grzeschnik KH, John M, White PC. Cloning of cDNA encoding steroid 11β-hydroxylase (P450c11). Proc Natl Acad USA 1987; 84:7193–7197.
12. Taymans SE, Pack S, Pak E, Torpy DJ, Zhuang Z, Stratakis CA. Human CYP11B2 (aldosterone synthase) maps to chromosome 8q24.3. J Clin Endocrinol Metab 1998; 83:1033–1035.
13. Nelson DR, Kamataki T, Waxma DJ, et al. The P450 superfamily: update on new sequences, gene mapping, accession number, early trivial names of enzyme, and nomenclature. DNA Cell Biol 1993; 12:1–55.
14. Arriza JL, Weinberger C, Cerelli G, et al. Cloning of the human mineralocorticoid receptor complementary DNA: structural and functional kinship with the glucocorticoid receptor. Science 1997; 237: 268–275.
15. Visser HKA, Cost WS. A new hereditary defect in the biosynthesis of aldosterone: urinary C21-corticosteroid pattern in three related patients with a salt-losing syndrome, suggesting an 18-oxidation defect. Acta Endocrinol Copenh 1964; 47:589–612.
16. Degenhart HJ, Frankena L, Visser HKA, Cost WS, van Seters AP. Further investigation of a new hereditary defect in the biosynthesis of aldosterone: evidence for a defect in 18-hydroxylation of corticosterone. Acta Physiol Pharmacol Neerl 1966; 4:1–2.

17. Ulick S, Gautier E, Vetter KK, Markello JR, Yaffe S, Lowe CU. An aldosterone biosynthetic defect in a salt-losing disorder. J Clin Endocrinol Metab 1964; 24:669–672.

18. Rappaport R, Dray F, Legrand JC, Royer P. Hypoaldostéronisme congénital familial par défaut de la 18-OH-déhydrogénase. Pediatr Res 1968; 2:456–463.

19. Ulick S. Diagnosis and nomenclature of the disorders of the terminal portion of the aldosterone biosynthetic pathway. J Clin Endocrinol Metab 1976; 43:92–96.

20. Ulick S. Correction of the nomenclature and mechanism of the aldosterone biosynthetic defects. J Clin Endocrinol Metab 1996; 81:1299–1300.

21. Rösler A. The natural history of salt-wasting disorders of adrenal and renal origin. J Clin Endocrinol Metab 1984; 59:689–700.

22. Peter M, Partsch CJ, Sippell WG. Multisteroid analysis in children with terminal aldosterone biosynthesis defects. J Clin Endocrinol Metab 1995; 80:1622–1627.

23. Peter M, Sippell WG. Congenital hypoaldosteronism: The Visser-Cost syndrome revisited. Pediatr Rev 1996; 39:554–560.

24. Ulick S, Wang JZ, Morton DH. The biochemical pheontypes of two inborn errors in the biosynthesis of aldosterone. J Clin Endocrinol Metab 1992; 74:1415–1420.

25. Sippell WG, Bidlingmaier F, Becker H, et al. Simultaneous radioimmunoassay of plasma aldosterone, corticosterone, 11-deoxycorticosterone, progesterone, 17-hydroxyprogesterone, 11-deoxycortisol, cortisol, and cortisone. J Steroid Biochem 1978; 9:63–67.

26. Mitsuuchi Y, Kawamoto T, Miyahara K, et al. Congenitally defective aldosterone biosynthesis in humans: Inactivation of the P-450C18 gene (CYP11B2) due to nucleotide deletion in CMO I deficient patients. Biochem Biophys Res Commun 1993; 190:864–869.

27. Geley S, Jöhrer K, Peter M, et al. Amino acid substitution R384P in aldosterone synthase causes corticosterone methyloxidase type I deficiency. J Clin Endocrinol Metab 1995; 80:424–429.

28. Nomoto S, Massa G, Mitani F, et al. CMO I deficiency caused by a point mutation in exon 8 of the human CYP11B2 gene encoding steroid 18-hydroxylase (P450$_{c18}$). Biochem Biophys Res Commun 1997; 234:382–385.

29. Peter M, Fawaz L, Drop SLS, Visser HKA, Sippell WG. Hereditary defect in biosynthesis of aldosterone: aldosterone synthase deficiency 1964–1997. J Clin Endocrinol Metab 1997; 82:3525–3528.

30. Peter M, Bünger K, Drop SLS, Sippell WG. Molecular genetic study in two patients with congenital hypoaldosteronism (types I and II) in relation to previously published hormonal studies. Eur J Endocrinol 1998; 139:96–100.

31. Portrat-Doyen S, Tourniaire J, Richard J, et al. Isolated aldosterone synthase deficiency caused by simultaneous E198D and V386A mutations in the CYP11B2 gene. J Clin Endocrinol Metab 1998; 83:4156–4161.

32. Mitsuuchi Y, Kawamoto T, Rösler A, et al. Congenitally defective aldosterone biosynthesis in humans: the involvement of point mutations of the P-450C18 gene (CYP11B2) in CMO II deficient patients. Biochem Biophys Res Commun 1992; 182:974–979.

33. Pascoe L, Curnow KM, Slutsker L, Rosler A, White PC. Mutations in the human CYP11B2 (aldosterone synthase) gene causing corticosterone methyloxidase II deficiency. Proc Natl Acad Sci USA 1992; 89:4996–5000.

34. Zhang G, Rodriguez H, Fardella CE, Harris DA, Miller WL. Mutation T318M in the CYP11B2 gene encoding P450c11AS (aldosterone synthase) causes corticosterone methyl oxidase II. Am J Hum Genet 1995; 57:1037–1043.

35. Peter M, Bünger K, Sólyom J, Sippell WG. Mutation Thr-185 Ile is associated with corticosterone methyl oxidase deficiency type II. Eur J Pediatr 1998; 157:378–381.

36. Peter M, Nikischin W, Heinz-Erian P, Fussenegger W, Kapelari K, Sippell WG. Homozygous deletion of arginine-173 in the CYP11B2 gene in a girl with congenital hypoaldosteronism (corticosterone methyl oxidase deficiency type II). Horm Res 1998; 50:222–225.

37. Fardella CE, Hum DW, Rodriguez H, et al. Gene conversion in the CYP11B2 gene encoding P450c11AS is associated with, but does not cause, the syndrome of corticosterone methyloxidase II deficiency. J Clin Endocrinol Metab 1996; 81:321–326.

38. Curnow KM, Mulatero P, Emeric-Blanchouin N, Aupetit-Faisant B, Corvol P, Pascoe L. The amino acid substitutions Ser288Gly and Val320A1a convert the cortisol producing enzyme, CYP11B1, into an aldosterone producing enzyme. Nat Struct Biol 1997; 4:32–35.

27   Mineralocorticoid Excess Syndromes

Richard D. Gordon

CONTENTS

From: *Contemporary Endocrinology: Adrenal Disorders*
Edited by: A. N. Margioris and G. P. Chrousos © Humana Press, Totowa, NJ

CONCLUSIONS
ACKNOWLEDGMENT
REFERENCES

INTRODUCTION

Mineralocorticoid excess syndromes are characterized by overactivity of amiloride-sensitive sodium channels (ASSCs) in the distal tubule and collecting duct of the kidney, and presumably in other tissues. Most of the currently recognized, and widely accepted pathophysiological sequels of that overactivity can be explained by overactivity of the renal tubular ASSCs. However, sodium pumps are ubiquitous, and important effects of intrinsically overactive ASSCs or ASSCs activated by stimulated mineralocorticoid receptors (MRs) in other tissues, such as the brain and heart, are currently under investigation *(1–4)* and likely to be identified and clarified by future studies. Activation of MRs could also lead to important effects other than stimulation of ASSCs, but this is speculative.

The clinical hallmark of the mineralocorticoid excess syndrome is hypertension aggravated by a high-salt diet and improved by strict dietary salt restriction. The biochemical hallmark is suppressed plasma–renin activity and, less commonly, hypokalemia. The most common, currently recognized cause of overactivity of the ASSC is inappropriate, relatively autonomous, overproduction of aldosterone, or "primary aldosteronism" (PAL). A very important practical, clinical discovery of recent years has been that PAL is not a rare cause of hypertension, to be suspected only when hypokalemia is present, but probably the most common specifically treatable and potentially curable cause of hypertension *(5–8)*. This has come about for several reasons. (1) Measurements of plasma aldosterone and of plasma–renin activity are now widely available, enabling their relationship to be examined in every hypertensive patient. (2) This has permitted diagnosis of primary aldosteronism in the absence of hypokalemia, indeed more common than in the presence of hypokalemia. That is, normokalemic primary aldosteronism is not rare, but common. (3) Whereas aldosterone-producing adenomas (APAs) have long been known to increase aldosterone production in response to ACTH, and in that sense not to be strictly speaking autonomous, responsiveness to angiotensin II was thought to be rare. Irony et al. *(9)* and Fontes et al. *(10)* reported only 4 of 154 and 6 of 146 patients with PAL, respectively, to have "renin-responsive" APAs. Renin-responsive adenomas were defined in terms of a 30% or greater response of aldosterone to upright posture. Aldosterone response to infused angiotensin II (AII) was not tested. However, consistent use of adrenal venous sampling (AVS, in order to identify lateralization of aldosterone production) has permitted recognition of angiotensin-responsive APAs (AII-R APA) and shown that they occur as frequently as unresponsive APAs (AII-U APA) *(7,11,12)*. This discovery has approximately doubled the number of patients with PAL who can be offered the possibility of cure by surgery.

Seventy of the 153 APAs removed in the Greenslopes Hospital Hypertension Unit between 1986, when AII-R APA was recognized *(11)* and May 1997, were AII-R based on posture testing alone, with a criterion of a 50% or greater increase in plasma aldosterone. Protocols for further investigation of patients diagnosed with PAL [for

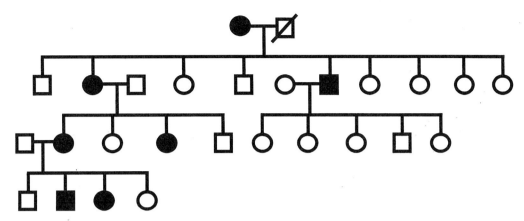

Fig. 1. A family with familial hyperaldosteronism type 11 (FH-11). Those identified as "affected" by PAL are indicated by filled symbols.

example, positive fludrocortisone suppression test (FST)] which do not include AVS in every patient will miss AII-R APAs. Many published protocols proceed to AVS only if there is no aldosterone response to posture, and CT scan does not show an apparent adenoma. Protocols that do not suggest, for patients with PAL and aldosterone unresponsive to posture, a test for glucocorticoid-suppressible hyperaldosteronism (such as a genetic test for the hybrid gene using peripheral blood DNA or a dexamethasone suppression test) will miss this specifically treatable form of PAL. The decision to screen all hypertensives for PAL using aldosterone-to-renin ratio (ARR) led to a dramatic (more than tenfold) increase in the diagnosis rate of PAL in the Hypertension Unit, Greenslopes Hospital, Brisbane, Australia *(5–7),* and more recently in the Mayo Clinic *(8).*

FAMILIAL PRIMARY ALDOSTERONISM

As PAL was becoming more frequently diagnosed in the Brisbane series, it became obvious that the apparently serendipitous discovery some years earlier of a patient with a similarly affected relative was quite significant. In this and in 21 subsequently recognized families, the glucocorticoid suppressible familial variety of hyperaldosteronism [Familial Hyperaldosteronism Type 1, (FH-I)] had been excluded *(13–15)* and by October 1999, 55 patients from 22 families with this second variety of familial hyperaldosteronism (FH-II) had been recognized in the Brisbane series of 709 patients with PAL. This variety of familial occurrence of PAL is more common than FHI, and its genetic basis is currently under investigation. Based on transmission vertically through generations, it appears to be a dominant form of inheritance in the largest family and in six others, being indeterminate so far in the other 15. Affected families include one with seven affected members in three generations, all with bilateral disease, sometimes nodular (Fig. 1). In another family, the APAs in an affected mother and daughter were biochemically different, AII-R in the mother and AII-U in the daughter. A male with bilateral adrenal hyperplasia (BAH) of giant macronodular variety had a second cousin with the diffuse variety, which showed further enlargement during 4 yr of follow-up. Their mothers, who were sisters, had each survived subarachnoid hemorrhage from bleeding berry aneurysms, another familial condition. In the family with seven affected members, mutations of the angiotensin II (ATI)-receptor gene do not explain the hyperaldosteronism *(16)*. This gene is also normal in sporadically occurring APAs *(17)*. The aldo synthase gene *(CYP11B1)* has also been closely examined and is normal in this family *(18)*. Much work remains to be done on the genetics of FH-II.

The descriptive title FH-II was chosen to distinguish this inherited variety of PAL from the apparently less-common FH-1, which was described clinically in 1966 *(19)* and elucidated genetically in 1992 *(20)*, in which the aldosterone overproduction is suppressible with dexamethasone [glucocorticoid-suppressible hyperaldosteronism (GSH); or glucocorticoid-remediable aldosteronism (GRA)] because of its dependence on ACTH. Once Lifton and coworkers *(20)* postulated and then identified a "hybrid" or "chimeric" gene, presumed to be formed during the recombination phase of meiosis caused by "crossover" of the highly homologous 11-beta hydroxylase *(CYP11β1)* and aldo synthase *(CYP11βB2)* genes, and capable of producing aldosterone *(21)*, the pathophysiology of FH-1 was largely explained, including the formation in excessive amounts of the "hybrid" steroids 18-oxo-cortisol and 18-hydroxy-cortisol *(22,23)*. These hybrid steroids are also produced in excess in the angiotensin unresponsive variety of APA *(23)*, where the tumors are composed predominantly of cells resembling *zona fasciculata (12)*. Presumably, when aldosterone is produced in cells that also have the enzymatic capacity to produce cortisol, and are responsive to ACTH and unresponsive to angiotensin II, the hybrid steroids are a byproduct.

Because, in the hybrid gene, the regulatory portion of the *CYP11β1* gene (sensitive to ACTH) is fused to the coding region of *CYP11β2* (the missing regulatory portion of which is sensitive to angiotensin II), aldosterone production is regulated by ACTH, and not by angiotensin II. According to Lifton's hypothesis, there are also two normal wild-type *CYP11β2* genes, capable of responding normally to angiotensin II, and two normal wild-type *CYP11β1* genes, capable of responding normally to ACTH. However, Stowasser and coworkers *(24)* have produced evidence that the hybrid gene continues to dominate over the wild-type aldo synthase gene (sensitive to angiotensin II) during long-term management of FH-I, at a time when angiotensin II levels are normal or raised. As well, Jamieson and coworkers *(25)* have shown that the wild-type *CYP11β1* genes do not show normal IIβ-hydroxylase activity in FH-I. Future work will clarify these points, and the original hypothesis may require some modification.

The phenotype is extremely variable in FH-I within a single pedigree *(15,26,27)*. Clinical expression varies from fatal hypertensive strokes in young males aged 20 to 40 yr to normal blood pressure, plasma potassium, aldosterone, and renin activity levels in older females. Most affected members have normal potassium levels. Litchfield et al. *(28)* postulated impaired potassium-stimulated aldosterone production as a possible contributing factor to normokalemia in FH-I. Gates et al. *(29)* have pointed out that many patients with FH-I with mild hypertension and normal biochemistry are clinically indistinguishable from essential hypertension, making a missed diagnosis of FH-I highly likely.

These discoveries of familial varieties of PAL have important implications for the understanding of hypertension in general, and particularly of its clinical diversity, its natural evolution, and the importance of other genetic factors (including gender) and environmental factors (such as dietary salt) upon the development and clinical manifestations of hypertension *(15,27)*. Whereas these two familial forms of hypertension are both examples of the "salt-sensitive variety" of hypertension, it would be a mistake to assume that they did not have relevance to the great mass of so-called essential hypertension, which is not an entity at all, but merely the large collection of patients for whom the pathophysiology has not yet been elucidated. In many of them it has never been thoroughly investigated. At the present time, it is reasonable to suggest that, apart from pheochromocytoma, renin-dependent hypertension (such as reninoma, and renal artery stenosis) and possibly coarctation of the aorta, all other forms of hypertension may be salt sensitive.

THE SYNDROME OF APPARENT MINERALOCORTICOID EXCESS (SAME, ABNORMAL CORTISOL-CORTISONE "SHUTTLE")

The understanding of the syndrome of apparent mineralocorticoid excess (SAME) as a consequence of cortisol's natural affinity for the mineralocorticoid receptor, cortisol's presence in one-thousand times the concentration of aldosterone, and deficient activity of the enzyme converting cortisol to the low-affinity cortisone, opened up a fresh avenue of enquiry into the normal and abnormal regulation of the mineralocorticoid receptor *(30–33)*. It also provided another example of a familial form of salt-sensitive hypertension, this time with a mendelian recessive form of inheritance, considerable genetic heterogeneity *(34),* and the possibility of modulation by, for example, other steroid metabolites *(35)*. It seems likely that in its various forms, this condition is not uncommon, and although usually recessive in terms of its phenotypic expression, heterozygotes may be predisposed to hypertension *(36)*.

THE SYNDROME OF PRIMARY CORTISOL RESISTANCE (SPCR)

Described by Chrousos et al. in 1982 *(37),* this condition, which can be familial, is rarely recognized even in its severe form. Less-severe forms are almost certainly more common, but usually escape diagnosis. Based on resistance at the glucocorticoid receptor (GR), the pathophysiology resembles that of the congenital adrenal hyperplasias (CAH). In CAH, the problem is impaired cortisol production because of deficiency of one or more biosynthetic enzymes, with all the sequelas of chronically elevated ACTH. Androgens and estrogens are produced in excess by the *zona reticularis* of the adrenal cortex, and 11-desoxy corticosterone (DOC) and other mineralocorticoids by the *zona fasciculata*. In SPCR, ACTH is chronically elevated, with excessive production of ACTH-dependent steroids. In this respect, with hypertension and hypokalemia developing in severe cases, SPCR is a true "mineralocorticoid excess" syndrome. As well, the very high levels of cortisol, which are characteristic of this condition, although relatively inactive at the GR, appear to be normally active at the mineralocorticoid receptor (MR), where they may exceed the capacity of the HSD enzyme to render them ineffective by conversion to cortisone. This same problem almost certainly contributes to the hypertension of Cushing's disease and all other conditions of cortisol excess, including ectopic ACTH production by neoplasms, where levels of cortisol (and DOC) are very high, and levels of renin and aldosterone secondarily suppressed by volume expansion. Studies of GRs in SPCR have demonstrated reduced numbers or reduced affinity for cortisol *(38–40)*. Whereas there appears to be a genetic basis in some patients, and the adjective "primary" is appropriate, clearly any acquired condition that reduces

GR numbers or their affinity for cortisol will result in a "secondary" form of cortisol resistance.

LIDDLE'S SYNDROME

In another experiment of nature involving genetic mutations, the intrinsic control of the ASSC can be defective, giving rise to a sodium channel behaving as though it were being stimulated by excessive mineralocorticoid. As with FH-I, a clinical syndrome described many years earlier in 1963 *(41)* and known as Liddle's Syndrome or pseudohyperaldosteronism [becaue of hypertension and hypokalemia with very low levels of renin and aldosterone in the untreated state *(42)*] was found to have a single gene pathophysiological basis in 1994 *(43,44)*. This was subsequently shown to include a number of possible genetic mutations affecting different subunits of the ASSC *(45,46)*. However, a consistent mutation within families means that families can be screened prospectively for additional affected members *(47)*. Liddle's syndrome, although not strictly caused by mineralocorticoid excess, presents with hypertension and hypokalemia and can reasonably be included in the mineralocorticoid excess syndromes. It may be more common than originally thought *(48)*. Examination of additional families with this syndrome is adding to knowledge of the regulation of the ASSC and is another example of the important interactions between clinical medicine and basic science, nowhere better seen than in the genetic syndromes. Not only does early identification of affected family members and more-enlightened patient care result, but, inevitably, surprising insights follow into the diversity of the mutational basis of a final common biochemical defect of varying severity, helping to explain biochemical and clinical diversity. For example, studying the ASSC in circulating B lymphocytes, Warnock and coworkers *(49)* can examine the characteristics of the channel in particular families, including responsiveness to amiloride and triamterene, which varies from family to family, and has implications for long-term management.

VARIED PATHOPHYSIOLOGY OF MINERALOCORTICOID-EXCESS SYNDROMES (TABLE 1)

There are thus a number of possible ways in which mineralocorticoid excess syndromes may develop (Table 1). Some of these are better understood than others, but in all cases much remains to be learned. At present, new information is flowing from the application of new techniques in molecular biology and genetics.

Hormones with high intrinsic mineralocorticoid activity such as aldosterone (most commonly) or DOC (rarely) can be produced endogenously in excess (Table 1.1). Alternatively, they or their analogs could be administered in unintentionally excessive dosage to patients without adrenal glands. Aldosterone can be overproduced in a primary or autonomous fashion, or secondary to overproduction of its principal chronic secretogog and normal regulator, renin–angiotensin, as in the rare renin-secreting tumour of the kidney (reninoma), in some cases of renal-artery stenosis and in malignant or accelerated hypertension. The syndrome of apparent mineralocorticoid excess (Table 1.2) occurs because of a genetic mutation or in response to ingestion of licorice or carbenoxolone *(31)*, which contain a substance that inhibits the enzyme converting cortisol to cortisone. Cortisol resistance at the GR exerts its effects through raised levels of cortisol affecting the MR directly and through raised levels of DOC, secondary

Table 1
Mineralocorticoid Excess Syndromes: Known and Suspected Etiologies

1. Excessive Production of Mineralocorticoid Hormones.
    (a) Aldosterone Excess
        (i) Autonomous regarding renin-angiotensin (primary)
            - abnormal regulation by ACTH in glucocorticoid-suppressible hyperaldosteronism, FH-I
            - aldosterone-producing aldrenocortical adenoma
              aldosterone-producing adrenocortical carcinoma
            - bilateral adrenocortical hyperplasia—diffuse
                                            —micronodular
                                            —macronodular
            - unilateral adrenocortical hyperplasia—diffuse
                                            —micronodular
                                            —macronodular
        (ii) In response to renin-angiotensin (secondary)
            - reninoma (primary reninism)
            - severe renal artery stenosis
            - malignant (accelerated) hypertension
    (b) II—desoxy corticosterone (DOC) excess
        (i) Autonomous (primary)
            - DOC-secreting adrenocortical adenoma
            - DOC-secreting adrenocortical carcinoma
        (ii) In response to chronically elevated ACTH (secondary)
            - 11-β hydroxylase deficiency (congenital adrenal hyperplasia-recessive inheritance)
            - 17-α hydroxylase deficiency (congenital adrenal hyperplasia-recessive inheritance)
            - Primary cortisol resistance (see also 2. below)
    (c) Cortisol-excessive levels from any source (see also 2. below)
    (d) Iatrogenic over-dosing with 9α-fluoro-hydrocortisone (florinef, fludrocortisone) or any natural or synthetic steroid with mineralocorticoid activity.
2. Loss of protection of the mineralocorticoid receptor from cortisol: deficiency of 11-β hydroxy steroid dehydrogenase (HSD) activity. The syndrome of apparent mineralocorticoid excess (SAME).
    (a) Inherited deficiency of active enzyme (autosomal recessive).
    (b) Ingested glycyrrhetinic acid (licorice or carbenoxolone) reducing the activity of the enzyme.
    (c) Cortisol excess exceeding the capacity of HSD enzyme (see also 1. above)
        Cushing's syndrome—pituitary-dependent (ACTH secreting microadenoma)
                        —pituitary-independent adrenocortical tumour or nodular hyperplasia
        Iatrogenic (steroid treatment of disease)
        Ectopic ACTH production by neoplasms
        Primary cortisol resistance
3. Genetically determined alterations in mineralocorticoid receptor structure and function.
4. Modulation of the mineralocorticoid receptor by "nonmineralocorticoid" corticosteroid metabolites or currently unidentified substances.
5. Genetic variations in the amiloride-sensitive sodium channel (ASSC) where mineralocorticoids act.
    (a) Inherited defects in negative regulatory elements (β and γ subunits)—Liddle's Syndrome (dominant inheritance).
    (b) ? Mutations in positive regulatory elements leading to increased responsiveness to standard doses of classical mineralocorticoids such as aldosterone (speculative).

to raised ACTH, also affecting the MR. There are probably other influences on the MR, some genetically determined, which await elucidation (Table 1.3). For example, at the 25th Annual International Aldosterone Conference in San Diego, CA, June 10 and 11, 1999, Geller D, Moretz M, Spitzer A, and Lifton R described a new mendelian form of human hypertension that links to the mineralocorticoid receptor gene locus on chromosome 4. Overactivity of the ASSC is inherited in an autosomal dominant fashion in Liddle's syndrome (Table 1.5).

THE SYNDROME OF HYPERTENSION AND HYPERKALEMIA WITH NORMAL GFR (SHH, PSEUDOHYPOALDOSTERONISM TYPE II, GORDON'S SYNDROME)

This is yet another currently recognized form of familial, salt-sensitive hypertension, but the genetic, and, hence, biochemical, etiology has so far eluded complete understanding. Like Liddle's syndrome, renin and aldosterone are suppressed. However, Liddle's syndrome earns its place among the mineralocorticoid excess syndromes because the ASSC, where mineralocorticoids normally exert their renal effects, is hyperactive, whereas in Gordon's syndrome, the distal nephron ASSC appears to be underactive. Possibly a problem with a sodium channel elsewhere in the nephron, it might one day qualify for inclusion in the Syndromes of Mineralocorticoid excess. For the moment, the inclusion of SHH in Table 2 does not appear justified.

Gordon's syndrome is expressed biochemically and clinically as an overactive sodium channel, but not the classic distal renal tubule sodium channel where potassium is excreted. It is a salt-sensitive, salt-overload hypertension, but there is reduced renal secretion of potassium, as if aldosterone were deficient or the distal nephron ASSC were hypofunctional. Possibly the responsible sodium channel in the kidney that causes such striking salt overload is somewhere other than in the distal nephron, where sodium is reabsorbed without chloride, and potassium excreted. Gordon and coworkers, in their investigation of the index case (50), a 10-yr-old girl presenting in Adelaide, Australia, with short stature, hypertension, and a serum potassium of 8.5 mmol/L; and subsequently in their investigation of a Brisbane, Australia family with seven affected members (51), found normal qualitative responses to blockade of endogenous aldosterone and to administration of synthetic mineralocorticoid (9α-fluro-hydrocortisone) (50,51). All features could be reversed with very strict dietary salt restriction (50–52). Clearly not explained by overactivity of the distal nephron ASSC, studies of lithium clearance suggested the possibility of a proximal tubular sodium channel overactivity, where aldosterone (suppressed by chronically low renin levels, but stimulated by hyperkalemia) does not act (53,54).

In 1997, Mansfeld et al. (55) published evidence suggesting linkage with chromosomes 17 and 1 in various families with this condition. In the well-characterized Brisbane family, linkage to C-I has been excluded, and strong linkage with the marker D17S250 on the long arm of chromosome 17 demonstrated, with all affected and no unaffected members carrying single copies of allele 8 for this microsatellite (56). This area of chromosome 17 contains an amino-acid sequence homologous with a syntenic interval on rat chromosome 10 strongly linked with hypertension (57) and linkage has recently been established between this same area and human familial essential hypertension

(58). This apparently rare form of human hypertension, which is salt-sensitive, may also be found to be genetically heterogeneous, to have a broad clinical spectrum, and to encroach on "essential hypertension."

BETTER SCREENING FOR PAL LEADING TO INCREASED INCIDENCE: THE CONCEPT OF THE ALDOSTERONE–RENIN RATIO

Conn pointed out the seminal importance of suppressed renin in the pathophysiology and diagnosis of primary aldosteronism *(59)*, and examined the interrelationship between urinary aldosterone and plasma–renin activity in this condition. However, it was only after easy access to simultaneous measurement of aldosterone and renin activity in the same plasma sample that Hiramatsu and coworkers *(60)* in 1981 demonstrated the utility and sensitivity of this interrelationship (aldosterone/plasma renin activity ratio) in screening "essential hypertensives" for PAL. They measured the ratio in 348 "unselected hypertensives," and investigated further only those with a very high ratio, using the insensitive techniques of adrenal venography and scintigraphy. They went on to remove nine APAs, an incidence of 2.6%, no doubt overlooking smaller tumors. The incidence of PAL (if bilateral hyperplasia were included) would have been at least 5%. Six of the nine patients with APA were normokalemic, and upright plasma aldosterone was within the normal range in five of the nine on at least one occasion. How can this be reconciled with hyperaldosteronism, the clinical hallmark of which hypokalemia? It can be reconciled if we think of PAL as a slowly developing condition, which ultimately produces a characteristic, florid clinical picture. However, it can be diagnosed early, to the patient's great advantage, based on consideration of the pathophysiology, and use of modern biochemical techniques. McKenna and coworkers, screening for PAL using the ratio, confirmed that a significant number of patients with PAL had normal aldosterone levels *(61)*. In the Greenslopes Hospital, Brisbane series, more than half of the 70–90 patients diagnosed per year with PAL, by screening every new hypertensive patient, were normokalemic, and more than one-third had normal aldosterone levels *(62)*. Importantly, however, aldosterone levels failed to suppress with fludrocortisone *(62)*.

An oversimplified schematic diagram (Fig. 2) can go some way to explaining the greater sensitivity of the ratio compared with either PRA or aldosterone measurements. Whereas in FH-I, the production of aldosterone is abnormally regulated and presumably inappropriately high from birth, in the common form of PAL there is probably some point later in life at which some autonomous aldosterone production begins, in one or several clones of cells within the *zona glomerulosa* or *fasciculata* of the adrenal cortex. This point is (arbitrarily) indicated in Fig. 1 by the lowermost arrow. As autonomous aldosterone production slowly increases (no attempt has been made in Fig. 1 to illustrate the probable gentle acceleration of the rate of increase), it is a long time before aldosterone leaves the broad normal range and becomes a reliable indicator of overproduction. However, the "negative-feedback" on renin secretion via sodium and volume, blood pressure, sympathetic nervous system, and atrial natriuretic peptide begins to operate gently, but immediately, and renin begins to fall, initially probably quite slowly. Renin will drop out of the normal range eventually, and certainly sooner than aldosterone will rise out of its wide normal range. However, the falling plasma–renin activity (PRA)

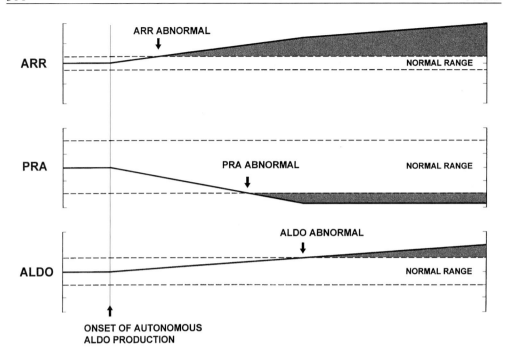

Fig. 2. Schematic diagram showing how slowly rising plasma aldosterone levels and slowly falling plasma–renin activity (PRA) levels will together cause the ratio of aldosterone-to-plasma renin activity (aldosterone-to-renin ratio, ARR) to move beyond the normal range earlier than either PRA or aldosterone do so.

level and the rising aldosterone level combine to push ARR above the normal range significantly earlier than either PRA or aldosterone themselves become recognizably abnormal.

Provided the medications that affect the ratio are either ceased or taken into account, the ARR is remarkably robust and reliable *(7,62)*. Although false-negative ratios are not uncommon, at least 90% of patients with consistently raised ratios also have abnormal FST's. Thus, false positives are rare. Other causes of salt overload such as a very high salt diet, renal impairment, nonsteroidal antiinflammatory drugs, or Gordon's syndrome can cause a falsely high ratio, because renin is suppressed, but aldosterone is suppressed less, because of continuing stimulation of aldosterone by potassium and ACTH.

Consideration of the points at which hypertension and, independently, hypokalemia might occur in Fig. 1 is difficult. Genetic and environmental factors that influence blood pressure and potassium homeostasis will be present in different combinations in different patients. The same levels of aldosterone will lead to hypokalemia in one patient but not in another, because presumably of factors such as intrinsic tubular sensitivity to aldosterone, sodium load at the distal nephron, and potassium intake. Clearly, dietary salt restriction will delay the appearance of hypertension. Levels of PRA will be less suppressed, and the raised aldosterone levels will be perfectly appropriate. Conversely, dietary salt loading will hasten the development of an abnormal ratio by suppressing renin further, and making unsuppressible aldosterone levels even less appropriate. It will accelerate the appearance of hypertension, and also of hypokalemia, by delivering more sodium to the ASSC in the distal tubule and collecting duct.

UNDERSTANDING THE EVOLUTION OF DISEASE FROM SMALL BEGINNINGS: THE CONCEPT OF "PRECLINICAL" DIAGNOSIS

The concept of preclinical diagnosis, which is illustrated by the application of the ARR to the diagnosis of PAL, applies to all forms of mineralocorticoid excess by detection of biochemical changes that can be present without symptoms or signs, and even earlier by detection of genetic abnormalities when appropriate tests are available. In the case of FH-I, the abnormal "hybrid" gene can be detected in peripheral blood DNA either by Southern blotting (20) or the faster long polymerase chain reaction (PCR) technique developed by Jonsson and coworkers (63). In the case of the SAME families, affected members can be separated from nonaffected by examination of peripheral blood DNA (33,34), but there is as yet no genetic screening test that is readily applicable to the general population of hypertensives. In FH-I, children in known families can be tested at birth using DNA from cord blood (64), and the entire population of "essential hypertensives" can theoretically be screened. A higher yield could be expected if screening was reserved for hypertensives with a strong family history of hypertension, especially if complicated by early stroke. Every patient with PAL should be screened for FHI, even if the adrenal or adrenals are abnormal on CT, because Pascoe et al. (65) reported abnormal adrenal morphology in four of seven affected members of a French family with FH-I, and adrenal nodules have been observed in some patients with FH-I in the Greenslopes Hospital, Brisbane series. Examination of the adrenal cortical tissue removed from one of the French patients with FH-I, using *in situ* hybridization, reverse transcriptase (RT)-PCR and Northern blot analysis, demonstrated expression of the hybrid gene at higher levels than $CYP11\beta1$ or $CYP11\beta2$, and in all three zones of the cortex (65).

Whereas severe hypokalemia of PAL diagnosed late can cause nocturia, muscle cramps, spontaneous tetany, or muscle weakness, which can be profound (66), the normokalemic hypertensive patient with PAL could perhaps be regarded as preclinical. The patient with PAL and mild hypertension responding to dietary salt restriction with normal blood pressure is clinically indistinguishable from other forms of hypertension.

THE CONCEPT OF APPARENTLY NONFUNCTIONING ADRENAL MASS OR MASSES

The advent of widely available, accurate ultrasonography, CT, and MRI scanning of the abdomen, often performed for abdominal pain or suspected gall bladder disease, has led to a need to formulate protocols in order to deal with unexpectedly discovered adrenal masses. Apparently clinically nonfunctioning, a proportion of these masses will be producing steroids such as aldosterone or cortisol autonomously, and suppression tests (overnight dexamethasone suppression test, IV saline load, or fludrocortisone suppression test) will be required to demonstrate this (67). Measurements of urinary noradrenaline or adrenaline are mandatory in order to exclude pheochromocytoma. Biochemical demonstration of cortical or medullary hormone production by an adrenal mass is often regarded as an indication for removal. Paradoxically, "function," in terms of capacity to concentrate an appropriate isotope (such as NP-59) on scintigraphy, is regarded by some as reassuring that cancer is unlikely, and a reason to leave the mass undisturbed.

Masses apparently nonfunctioning, even after appropriate testing, demand careful consideration in terms of immediate treatment and long-term follow-up, after discussion of all the options with the patient, and patient-guided determination of a strategy for the longer term. Because adrenal cancer carries a very bad prognosis, repeat CT scanning at intervals is important. Adrenal masses in general grow slowly. Rapid growth would make surgical removal mandatory, whereas slow growth requires a difficult and somewhat arbitrary decision on the frequency of future CT scanning and repeat biochemical testing. A decision involving a criterion of upper limit in size as an indication for removal is difficult, with no general consensus. Each patient should be regarded as a unique individual who should contribute in a major way to discussion and who will make the final decision. Because apparently nonfunctioning adrenal cancers can present as incidentalomas as small as 3.5 cm and 4.0 cm, an argument can be made for beginning to consider adrenalectomy for incidentalomas 2.5 cm or larger. A progressive increase in size is usually an indication for removal.

Quite commonly, adrenal masses are not solitary, but multiple, and may be bilateral. The concept that one or more of these masses may be functional, and one or more nonfunctional, is important, for example in the case of primary aldosteronism with one or more masses evident on CT. If the mass is solitary, there is a probability, but not a certainty, that it is an APA responsible for the PAL. Soma et al. *(68)* were among the first to report the necessity for AVS, rather than imaging, to decide appropriate treatment, and to avoid operation on "the wrong adrenal." They left the "adenoma" seen on CT behind, and removed the normal appearing adrenal, which AVS had indicated was the only source of aldosterone *(68)*. The patient was cured. The experience of the Greenslopes Hospital, Brisbane, Hypertension Unit is similar, with CT lateralization misleading on at least 12 occasions. Adrenal venous sampling is a necessary prelude to surgery.

After "exclusion" of pheochromocytoma by 24-h urinary noradrenaline and adrenaline measurement, the patient with an adrenal mass can have PAL "excluded" by demonstration that plasma–renin activity is not suppressed, and adrenal Cushing's Syndrome "excluded" by demonstration that ACTH is not suppressed, and that cortisol can be suppressed by an overnight dexamethasone suppression test with higher than normal dosage (for example, 3 mg).

THE SURGICAL TREATMENT OF MINERALOCORTICOID EXCESS

The form of mineralocorticoid excesses that is amenable to surgery (in approx one-third of cases) is PAL, provided that the diagnosis has been established by FST and the unilaterality of the disease proven by AVS, with definite aldosterone production by the side to be removed, and definite "contralateral" suppression of the other gland *(7,62,69)*. It is essential to correct for catheter placement by comparing aldosterone/cortisol ratios in presumed "adrenal venous" samples, rather than compare absolute concentrations of aldosterone *(7,62,69,70)*. It is also essential to collect a simultaneous peripheral blood or low IVC sample (below the adrenal veins) in order to compare adrenal venous with peripheral aldosterone/cortisol ratios *(7,62,69,70)*.

The difficulties of AVS include the variable anatomy (multiple veins draining each adrenal), and the radiologist's inability to know immediately whether a satisfactory adrenal venous sample has been collected. This necessitates collection of several samples on each side. The appearance on venography can be quite misleading, and attempts to obtain reliable venograms with which to judge success of sampling may produce extremely painful intraadrenal hemorrhage. Perhaps, in the future, a filter-paper or test-tube "spot" test will be devised, requiring only one drop of blood and giving an immediate answer, being sensitive only to very-high steroid concentrations. Then further, unnecessary sampling could be avoided, but further sampling undertaken if necessary.

The advent of laparoscopic abdominal surgery (applied to gall bladder and colon, for example) led to the use of laparoscopic surgery for adrenalectomy. Because of the variable anatomy, and proximity of the adrenals to major vessels, this technique should be reserved for surgeons constantly utilizing laparoscopic techniques, and who are in a position to gain significant ongoing experience with adrenalectomy. In experienced hands, it provides excellent exposure and usually takes no longer than the open technique. Unusual anatomy or significant obesity may prolong the operation *(71)* and occasionally force "conversion" to an open operation.

The question of removal of the entire adrenal vs removal of the "adenoma" is of practical importance. Because the AVS indicates only which adrenal is at fault, and cannot distinguish small-functioning adenomas (say 5 mm) from larger nonfunctioning nodules (say 10 mm), a sound policy is to remove the entire adrenal. An exception can be made in the patient with a recurrence of PAL some years after unilateral adrenalectomy for APA. If there is a nodule in the remaining adrenal on CT, and a normal-appearing separate limb, there are at least two options. One is to remove the nodule and attempt to preserve the limb, provided the blood supply can be preserved. If so, the need for replacement therapy may be avoided, but not necessarily so. There is also the small risk of yet another recurrence, requiring further surgery to effect a cure. The other option is to remove the gland entirely, making further recurrence extremely unlikely, but making replacement therapy essential.

THE CONCEPT OF HYPERPLASIA AND BENIGN AND MALIGNANT NEOPLASIA OF THE ADRENAL AS A CONTINUUM, GENETICALLY DETERMINED: ALL ADRENAL CORTICAL TISSUE IS POTENTIALLY, IF NOT ALREADY, ABNORMAL IN PRIMARY ALDOSTERONISM

Because patients with FH-II have been biochemically and clinically indistinguishable from those with apparently "sporadic" PAL, it is possible that PAL is often, if not always, genetic *(5,15,27,72)*. It is possible to define true biochemical recurrence of PAL only if the outcome of operation has been assessed within 3 mo of surgery, and a biochemical cure demonstrated *(72,73)*.

Careful long-term follow-up of patients with PAL suggests that adrenal cortical hyperplasia and adenoma causing PAL usually progress in size and function very slowly. Patients having unilateral adrenalectomy for PAL may die from other causes before sufficient time has elapsed for PAL to redevelop. However, it is reasonable to regard the entire adrenal cortex of patients with PAL with suspicion, and prudent to follow-up all patients for life, and to explain to them and to their relatives that there may be further developments. These may be (1) biochemical, without appreciable change in adrenal size; (2) morphological, with or without currently recognizable function or (fortunately rarely); (3) progression to adrenocortical cancer *(74,75),* which can be minimized by considering removal if size is increasing. Progressive slow increase in size and function of the remaining adrenal tissue after unilateral adrenalectomy or adenectomy for PAL is counterbalanced by the reduction in overall adrenal mass. After careful follow-up of 28 patients for 2 yr after unilateral adrenalectomy for PAL, the recovery from suppression of renin and of aldosterone secretion by the residual, nonautonomous tissue, occurred at variable speed *(76).* At 2 yr after operation, the mean level of aldosterone was lower, and the mean level of plasma–renin activity higher than in age and sex-matched controls *(76).* In a complementary study that included long-term follow-up, mean PRA levels were again elevated following removal of an adrenal for Conn's syndrome *(73).* The levels in patients biochemically cured by surgery were significantly higher than in those biochemically improved, in keeping with the lower-mean aldosterone levels in the cured group *(73).* In each of these studies, hypertension was either cured or significantly improved in all patients by unilateral adrenalectomy following lateralization on AVS.

Based on the published literature, the histology of adrenal tissue removed at unilateral adrenalectomy (with or without prior evidence of unilateral production of aldosterone at AVS) has been very variable. It has included an apparently solitary adenoma with hypoplastic nontumorous glomerulosa, one or more "adenomas" or "nodules" with hyperplastic nontumorous glomerulosa, and micronodular or macronodular hyperplasia. Surgical reduction of the mass of abnormal tissue, regardless of its nodularity and bilaterality, can result in a clinical and biochemical remission of PAL *(77),* which may or may not, of course, be permanent. Such a surgical approach to bilateral disease should be undertaken only after very full and frank discussion with the patient. It should take place only at the patient's request, and will at present be rarely indicated until the results of careful follow-up of such patients becomes widely known.

The natural history of hyperplasia and nodularity in other endocrine glands such as the thyroid is not dissimilar. A multinodular goiter can be composed of nodules with varying degrees of biosynthetic activity, some producing thyroxine and triiodothyronine autonomously, and slowly growing in size. If excision of only one larger nodule, or a hemithyroidectomy, is performed, the remaining tissue often gradually becomes increasingly nodular. In the case of the thyroid, however, instances of solitary "hot nodules" (analogous to APAs) are less common than in the adrenal. In the case of the parathyroid, like the adrenal, hyperfunction may be caused by a solitary adenoma, or to more than one adenoma, or to hyperplasia of one or more glands. It is not surprising that the adrenals can manifest a wide variety of morphological and functional changes involving one or both glands, and where function can be dissociated from structure, creating a wide biochemical and clinical spectrum of "disease." Ranging from minor to major, such changes are possibly common in an aging population.

PRIMARY ALDOSTERONISM AS PART OF MULTIPLE ENDOCRINE NEOPLASIA TYPE 1 (MEN 1)

There have been several reports of APA occurring in patients with MEN I *(78–80),* and at least one report of an APA demonstrating loss of heterozygosity (LOH) at the MEN I locus on C11q13 *(78).* Interestingly, that APA also demonstrated LOH at the adenomatous polyposis coli (APC) gene locus, and APC has a known association with adrenocortical cancer (81).

Whereas none of the 709 patients with PAL in the Greenslopes Hospital, Brisbane series are from families known to suffer from MEN I, a number of them have suffered from conditions that occur as part of the MEN I syndrome, as has been reported by others (82,83). Thus, 14 had primary hyperparathyroidism, 4 had pituitary adenoma (secreting ACTH in 2, growth hormone in 1, and prolactin in 1), 2 had carcinoid tumors, 12 had multinodular goiters, and 4 had lipomas.

Burgess et al. (84) reported that 12 of 33 patients from a large MEN I kindred (Tasman-1) who underwent organ imaging had adrenal lesions not associated with clinically obvious adrenal disease. However, appropriate endocrine testing was not performed in order to determine whether lesions were biochemically functional. In one patient, the adrenal lesion enlarged by 5 cm over 5.5 yr of follow-up, and three adrenocortical carcinomas had been recognized in this kindred up to 1984.

Skogseid et al. (74) reviewed the literature on adrenocortical lesions in MEN-I, which ranged from diffuse hyperplasia, through nodular hyperplasia, to carcinoma, and added 12 adrenal lesions (7 bilateral) in 33 patients with MEN I, one of which was a feminizing adrenal carcinoma developing after 4 yr of observation of bilateral hyperplasia. Because none of the five benign lesions from which DNA was obtained showed LOH at C11q13 (the carcinoma did, as well as LOH for alleles at 17p, 13p, and 11p). The authors concluded that the benign adrenal abnormalities were unrelated to the genetic lesions of MEN I. Because 58% of those with adrenal enlargement had, as well, parathyroid, pituitary, *and* endocrine pancreas involvement (compared with only 9.5% of those without adrenal enlargement), the adrenal lesions had possibly developed later than lesions in other endocrine glands. Ten of the 12 patients with adrenal enlargement had raised plasma insulin and proinsulin levels, but no hypoglycemia. The adrenal lesions were considered to be "nonfunctional on endocrine testing," which included plasma aldosterone levels in the broad normal range, but which did not include plasma–renin activity, which would have been essential in order to exclude its suppression secondary to autonomous aldosterone production. Yano and coworkers (85) also found LOH at C17q13 in adrenocortical cancers, but not in benign lesions of the adrenal.

Paired adrenal tumor and peripheral blood DNA samples from patients with PAL, using six RFLP markers straddling the MEN I locus were studied by the Greenslopes Hospital group in collaboration with Nakamura, Imai, and coworkers from the National Cancer Institute, Tokyo, Japan (86). Five of 11 informative tumors showed LOH for one or more markers. Two of these patients with APAs were from different families with FH-II. Two others had adrenocortical cancer causing PAL, and one was an apparently sporadic case of APA. This work was extended using microsatellite markers around the MEN I locus on chromosome 11q13, including PYGM, and 64 paired APA and peripheral blood DNA samples (87). Seven of 33 tumors that were informative showed LOH for one or more markers (87).

Taken together, the above findings suggest that, in at least some patients with APA, there may be loss of tumor-suppressor genes such as the gene commonly involved in the development of MEN I. The recently identified *MEN* I gene contains 10 exons and encodes a ubiquitously expressed 2.8 kb transcript (88). Further study of the predicted 610 amino acid protein product, which appears so far to be unique, should elucidate at least one mechanism for endocrine hyperplasia and neoplasia. Furthermore, structural abnormalities affecting band q13 of chromosome 11 have also been reported in some nonendocrine human tumors, such as breast and squamous-cell carcinomas *(89)*.

CONCEPT: ADRENAL HYPERPLASIA AND NEOPLASIA IS BASED ON A VARIETY OF PREDISPOSING GENETIC MUTATIONS, AND ASSOCIATED AUTONOMOUS OVERPRODUCTION OF HORMONES IS AN EPIPHENOMENON

It appears that adrenal cortical hyperplasia, which is rarely diffuse and uniform and more often associated with nodules, is common. A solitary nodule (called "adenoma" if functioning) is less common, and adrenocortical cancer (functioning or nonfunctioning) is fortunately very rare. Whether or not hormones are secreted autonomously (or semiautonomously) by this abnormal tissue is unpredictable, and may be based on the particular cell or cells of origin, monoclonality or polyclonality, and on an ability to look for and recognize the autonomous secretion.

At present, aldosterone is the hormone whose autonomous secretion is most often recognized, because of the utility and sensitivity of the aldosterone-to-renin ratio. This leads to mineralocorticoid hypertension. Cushing's syndrome leads to hypertension, an important mechanism being stimulation of mineralocorticoid receptors, and, hence, ASSCs, as aforementioned. The early recognition of pituitary-independent Cushing's syndrome of adrenal origin should also be possible because of suppressed ACTH level, and by resistance to high-dose, overnight, dexamethasone suppression testing. This requires precise measurement of cortisol in the lower range, and clear definition of normal suppression. Pituitary-independent familial Cushing's syndrome caused by primary adrenal nodular hyperplasia has been long recognizsed *(90,91)*. The nodules can be very large, producing single adrenal weights up to 100 g, as reported by Hidai et al. *(92)* and seen in one of the patients with FH-II in the Greenslopes Hospital series, who had both Cushing's syndrome and PAL *(15)*. In both patients, cortisol was hyperresponsive to ACTH, which is a well-recognized characteristic of some patients with pituitary-independent adrenal Cushing's syndrome *(90,92)*. One variety of familial Cushing's syndrome associated with pigmented nodular adrenocortical disease, and various extraadrenal manifestations, is Carney's complex or syndrome *(93,94)*. This syndrome has recently been found to be genetically heterogeneous *(95–97)*. A detailed study of the mutated gene products may provide important information on the mechanisms and consequences of unrestrained stimulation in endocrine and nonendocrine tissues.

Rarely, adrenal adenomas causing clinical PAL have also caused clinical Cushing's syndrome *(98–100)*. Double hypersecretion severe enough to be recognizable clinically appears to be rare and has been recognized in only 2 of 709 patients with PAL in the Greenslopes Hospital series. Both patients had bilateral, macronodular hyperplasia of the adrenals. However, in 17 patients with PAL, low-dose dexamethasone administered for 5 d, showed failure of cortisol to suppress in 3 patients (1 adrenal cortical cancer, 2 APA), and satisfactory suppression in the remaining 8 with APA, in 4 with BAH, and in 2 with FH-I *(101)*.

The predictable occurrence of PAL and pituitary-independent adrenal Cushing's in different members of the same family has recently been recognized in Singapore (personal communication). It is interesting to speculate: (1) why in families genetically predisposed to nodular hyperplasia of the adrenal cortex, aldosterone is secreted (FH-

II) in some and cortisol (familial Cushing's) in others; and (2) whether different, overlapping, or identical genetic mechanisms are responsible. The occurrence of adrenal tumors producing either aldosterone or cortisol in different members of the same family is suggestive of a common genetic mechanism, in at least some instances.

MINERALOCORTICOID EXCESS AND VASCULAR HYPERTROPHY AFFECTING THE HEART AND ARTERIAL SYSTEM

As noted in the Introduction, ASSCs have been demonstrated in a number of extrarenal, nonepithelial tissues, and these include vascular smooth muscle (102). This opens the exciting possibility that mineralocorticoids may have important effects on the circulatory system and blood pressure regulation that are independent of indirect, renally mediated salt and water retention. There is considerable current interest in the possibility that when hypertension is caused by aldosterone (and probably other mineralocorticoids) in excess, the degree of cardiac hypertrophy is out of proportion to the hypertension and related more directly to the level of mineralocorticoid (103). In animal models, the degree of myocardial hypertrophy and interstitial fibrosis appears to be related to mineralocorticoid levels rather than to raised blood pressure, and to be preventable by spironolactone (4). Myocardial hypertrophy and interstitial fibrosis develop and persist in the presence of mineralocorticoid excess, even when hypertension is prevented or corrected (4).

Several studies comparing patients with essential hypertension with equally hypertensive patients with PAL suggest that left ventricular hypertrophy in PAL is greater than expected for the degree of hypertension, that left ventricular end-diastolic volume is greater, and that diastolic function is poorer (104–106).

FUTURE DIRECTIONS

The glucocorticoid biosynthetic pathway is of great interest, because not only does cortisol have the capacity to simulate mineralocorticoid receptors, but a number of its precursors and their metabolites have this capacity as well. Hence, minor variations in efficiency of biosynthetic enzymes, either genetic or acquired (caused by interactions with various steroid products or other currently unknown substances), could provide slow-onset, but powerful modulation of blood pressure control. Such subtle changes are currently under investigation, for example, the conversion of 11 desoxy-cortisol to cortisol in so-called essential hypertension (107). Other subtle mineralocorticoid-related changes capable of influencing blood pressure level may include the heterozygous state of recessive disorders such as SAME (36) or of the various, currently recognizable hypertensive forms of congenital adrenal hyperplasia. It has recently been shown that the ratio of GR-alpha to GR-beta can modulate the sensitivity of mineralocorticoid tissues to aldosterone (108). A very large number of individually minor influences on the MR, and on postreceptor events, may together go a long way to defining mineralocorticoid activity, however measured, including blood pressure level. It is not surprising that the "normal range" for plasma aldosterone, still probably the major controlling mineralocorticoid agent, is so broad.

As the effects of mineralocorticoids on vascular tissues are better defined, aldosterone antagonists such as spironolactone and its derivatives, and drugs that inhibit ASSC activity such as amiloride and triamterene, may attract renewed interest in the treatment not only of hypertension, but of cardiac hypertrophy from any cause and even of cardiac failure *(109,110)*, provided that renal function is not significantly reduced.

Just as atrial and brain natriuretic peptides have done over the last decade, Leptin *(111,112)*, the newly discovered and characterized secretion of the fat organ, will attract future attention in terms of possible interactions with glucocorticoids and mineralocorticoids. It appears to interact at several levels in the hypothalamic-pituitary-adrenal axis *(113,114)*, and may impact on cardiovascular regulation by a number of mechanisms *(115,116)*.

The management of hypertension has been dramatically enhanced by the ability to diagnose primary aldosteronism in its earlier stages of development and in its milder forms. Significant further refinement is inevitable. In the same way, as genetic techniques continue to become more accessible, and careful investigation provides the necessary scientific basis, the ability to identify affected members of families with more subtle forms of SAME, Liddle's syndrome, Gordon's syndrome, or of a variety of similar pathologies yet to be defined will assume great practical importance, making possible the delay or prevention of the development of hypertension by dietary salt restriction or appropriate, specific medical therapy.

CONCLUSIONS

Knowledge of pathophysiological mechanisms (including genetic) causing altered responsiveness of the mineralocorticoid receptor continues to grow, as does knowledge of practical methods for their detection.

The syndromes of mineralocorticoid excess are excellent examples of how experiments of nature, initially described as clinical syndromes, have been defined in biochemical detail before the tools of molecular biology have demonstrated the heterogeneity of their genetic bases, and the breadth of their clinical expression. It becomes increasingly possible to say, with confidence, that many, if not most forms of hypertension are not "essential."

ACKNOWLEDGMENT

The studies performed in the Hypertension Unit, University Department of Medicine, Greenslopes Hospital, Brisbane were supported by Research Grants from the National Health and Medical Research Council of Australia, the Heart Foundation of Australia, the Australian Government Department of Veterans Affairs, and the Mayne Bequest of the University of Queensland. Sincere thanks to Bernice Opperman, who typed the manuscript.

REFERENCES

1. Krowzowski ZS, Funder JW. Mineralocorticoid receptors in rat anterior pituitary: towards redefinition of "mineralocorticoid hormone". Endocrinology 1981; 109:1221–1224.
2. Krowzowski ZS, Funder JW. Renal mineralocorticoid receptors and hippocampal corticosterone binding sites have identical intrinsic steroid specificity. Proc Natl Acad Sci USA 1983; 80:6056–6060.
3. Sasano H, Fukushima K, Sasaki I, Matsuno S, Nagura H, Krowzowski Z. Immunolocalization of mineralocorticoid receptor in human kidney, pancreas, salivary, mammary and sweat glands. Light and electron microscopy immunohistochemical studies. J Endocrinol 1992; 132:305–310.
4. Funder JW, Krowowski Z, Myles K, Sato A, Sheppard KE, Young M. Mineralocorticoid receptors, salt, and hypertension. Recent Prog Horm Res 1997; 52:247–260.

5. Gordon RD, Klemm SA, Tunny TJ, Stowasser M. Primary aldosteronism: hypertension with a genetic basis. Lancet 1992; 340:159–161.

6. Gordon RD, Klemm SA, Stowasser M, Tunny TJ, Storie WS, Rutherford JS. How common is primary aldosteronism? Is it the most frequent cause of curable hypertension? J Hypertens 1993; 11 (Suppl 5):S310–S311.

7. Gordon RD, Stowasser M, Klemm SA, Tunny TJ. Primary aldosteronism and other forms of mineralo-corticoid hypertension. In: Swales JD, ed. Textbook of Hypertension. Blackwell Scientific, Oxford, 1994, pp. 865–892.

8. Young WF. Primary aldosteronism: update on diagnosis and treatment. The Endocrinologist 1997; 7:213–221.

9. Irony I, Kater CE, Biglieri EG, Shackleton CHL. Correctible subsets of primary aldosteronism. Primary adrenal hyperplasia and renin responsive adenoma. Am J Hypertens 1990; 3:576–582.

10. Fontes RG, Kater CE, Biglieri EG, Irony I. Reassessment of the predictive value of the postural stimulation test in primary aldosteronism. Am J Hypertens 1991; 4:786–791.

11. Gordon RD, Gomez-Sanchez CE, Hamlet SM, Tunny TJ, Klemm SA. Angiotensin-responsive aldoste-rone-producing adenoma masquerades as idiopathic hyperaldosteronism (IHA: adrenal hyperplasia) or low-renin essential hypertension. J Hypertens 1987; 5 (suppl 5):S103–S106.

12. Tunny TJ, Gordon RD, Klemm SA, Cohn D. Histological and biochemical distinctiveness of atypical aldosterone-producing adenoma responsive to upright posture and angiotensin. Clin Endocrinol 1991; 34:363–369.

13. Gordon RD, Stowasser M, Tunny TJ, Klemm SA, Finn WL, Krek AL. Clinical and pathological diversity of primary aldosteronism including a new familial variety. Clin Exp Pharmacol Physiol 1991; 18:283–286.

14. Stowasser M, Gordon RD, Tunny TJ, Klemm SA, Finn WL, Krek AL. Familial Hyperaldosteronism type II: five families with a new variety of primary aldosteronism. Clin Exp Physiol Pharmacol 1992; 19:319–322.

15. Gordon RD, Stowasser M. Familial forms broaden the horizons for primary aldosteronism. Trends Endocrinol Metab 1998; 9:220–223.

16. Torpy DJ, Gordon RD, Stratakis CA. Linkage analysis of familial hyperaldosteronism type II— absence of linkage to the gene encoding the angiotensin II receptor Type I. J Clin Endocrinol Metab 1998; 83:1046.

17. Davies E, Bonnardeaux A, Plouin PF, Corvol P, Clausser E. Somatic mutations in the angiotensin II (ATI) receptor gene are not present in aldosterone-producing adenoma. J Clin Endocrinol Metab 1997; 82:611–615.

18. Torpy DJ, Gordon RD, Lin J-P, Huggard PR, Taymans SE, Stowasser M, et al. Familial hyperaldoster-one type II: exclusion of the aldosterone synthase (CYPIIB2) gene. J Clin Endocrinol Metab 1998; 83:3214–3218.

19. Sutherland DJA, Ruse JL, Laidlaw JC. Hypertension, increased aldosterone secretion and low plasma renin activity relieved by dexamethasone. Canad Med Assoc J 1996; 95:1109–1119.

20. Lifton RP, Dluhy RG, Powers M, Rich GM, Cook S, Ulick S, et al. A chimaeric 11β-hydroxylase/ aldosterone synthase gene causes glucocorticoid remediable aldosteronism and human hypertension. Nature 1992; 355:262–265.

21. Miyahara K, Kawamoto T, Mitsuuchi Y, Toda K, Imura H, Gordon RD, et al. The chimaeric gene linked to glucocorticoid-suppressible hyperaldosteronism encodes a fused P-450 protein possessing aldosterone synthase activity. Biochem Biophys Res Commun 1992; 189:885–891.

22. Ulick S, Chiu MD. Hypersecretion of a new corticosteroid, 18 hydroxy cortisol in two types of adrenocortical hypertension. Clin Exp Hypertens 1982; A4:1771–1777.

23. Ulick S, Blumenfeld JD, Atlas SA, Wang JZ, Vaughan ED. The unique steroidogenesis of the aldosteronoma in the differential diagnosis of primary aldosteronism. J Clin Endocrinol Metab 1992; 76:873–878.

24. Stowasser M, Gartside MG, Taylor WL, Tunny TJ, Gordon RD. In familial hyperaldosteronism Type I, hybrid gene-induced aldosterone production dominates that induced by wild-type genes. J Clin Endocrinol Metab 1997; 82:3670–3676.

25. Jamieson A, Ingram MC, Inglis GC, Davies E, Fraser R, Connell JMC. Altered 11β-hydroxylase activity in glucocorticoid-suppressible hyperaldosteronism. J Clin Endocrinol Metab 1996; 81:2298–2302.

26. Rich GM, Ulick S, Cook S, Wang JZ, Lifton RP, Dluhy RG. Glucocorticoid remediable aldosteronism

in a large kindred: clinical spectrum and diagnosis using a characteristic biochemical phenotype. Ann Intern Med 1992; 116:813–820.

27. Gordon RD, Klemm SA, Tunny TJ, Stowasser M, Rutherford JC. The genetics of primary aldosteronism. In: Vinson GP, Anderson DC, eds. Adrenal Glands, Vascular System and Hypertension. Journal of Endocrinology Ltd., Bristol, 1996, pp. 235–252.

28. Litchfield WR, Coolidge C, Silva P, Lifton RP, Fallo F, Williams GH, et al. Impaired potassium-stimulated aldosterone production: a possible explanation for normokalemic glucocorticoid-remediable aldosteronism. J Clin Endocrinol Metab 1997; 82:1607–1610.

29. Gates LJ, MacConnachie AA, Lifton RP, Haites NE, Benjamin N. Variation of phenotype in patients with glucocorticoid remediable Hypertension. J Med Genet 1996; 33:25–28.

30. Ulick S, Levine LS, Gunczler P, Zanconata G, Ramirez LC, Rauh W, et al. A syndrome of apparent mineralocorticoid excess associated with defects in the peripheral metabolisms of cortisol. J Clin Endocrinol Metab 1979; 49:757–764.

31. Stewart PM, Corrie JET, Shackleton CHL, Edwards CRW. Syndrome of apparent mineralocorticoid excess. A defect in the cortisol-cortisone shuttle. J Clin Invest 1988; 82:340–349.

32. Ulick S, Chan CK, Rao KD, Ledassery J, Mantero F. A new form of the syndrome of apparent mineralocorticoid excess. J Steroid Biochem 1989; 32:209–212.

33. Ferrari P, Obeyesekere VR, Li K, Wilson RC, New MI, Funder J, et al. Point mutations abolish 11β-hydroxysteroid dehydrogenase type II activity in three families with the congenital syndrome of apparent mineralocorticoid excess. Mol Cell Endocrinol 1996; 119:21–24.

34. Mune T, Rogerson FM, Nikkila H, Agarwal AK, White PC. Human hypertension caused by mutations in the kidney isoenzyme of 11 beta-hydroxysteroid dehydrogenase. Nature Genet 1995; 10:394–399.

35. Latif SA, Sheff MF, Ribeiro CE, Morris DJ. Selective inhibition of sheep kidney 11 beta-hydroxysteroid dehydrogenase isoform 2 activity by 5 alpha-reduced (but not 5 beta) derivates of adrenocorticosteroids. Steroids 1997; 62:230–237.

36. Li A, Li K, Maru S, Krozowski ZS, Batista MC, Whorwood CB, et al. Apparent mineralocorticoid excess in a Brazilian kindred: hypertension in the heterozygous state. J Hypertens 1997; 15:1397–1402.

37. Chrousos GP, Vingerhoeds A, Brandon D, Eil C, Pugeat M, De Vroede M, et al. Primary cortisol resistance. J Clin Invest 1982; 69:1261–1269.

38. Jida S, Gomi M, Moriwaki K, Yoshiharu I, Hirobe K, Matsuzaura Y, et al. Primary cortisol resistance accompanied by a reduction of glucocorticoid receptors in two members of the same family. J Clin Endocrinol Metab 1985; 60:967–971.

39. Malchoff DM, Brufsky A, Reardon G, McDermott P, Javier EC, Bergh CH, et al. A mutation of the glucocorticoid receptor in primary cortisol resistance. J Clin Invest 1993; 91:1918–1925.

40. Lamberts SW, Koper JW, Biemond P, den Holder FH, de Jong FH. Cortisol receptor resistance: the variability of its clinical presentation and response to treatment. J Clin Endocrinol Metab 1992; 74:313–321.

41. Liddle GW, Bledsoe T, Coppage WS. A familial rendal disorder simulating primary aldosteronism but with negligible aldosterone secretion. Trans Am Assoc Physic 1963; 26:199–213.

42. Gordon RD, Klemm SA, Tunny TJ. Renin in Liddle's syndrome and in the syndrome of apparent-mineralocorticoid excess. In: JIS Robertson, MG Nicholls, eds. The Renin-Angiotensin System. Gower Medical, London, UK, 1993, pp. 2:66.1–66.9.

43. Skimkets RA, Warnock DG, Bositis CM, Nelson-Williams C, Hanssons JH, Schambelan M, et al. Liddle's syndrome: heritable human hypertension caused by mutations in the β subunit of the epithelial sodium channel. Cell 1994; 79:407–414.

44. Bubien JK, Ismailov II, Berdiev BK, Cornwell T, Lifton RD, Fuller CM, et al. Liddle's disease: abnormal regulation of amiloride-sensitive Na$^+$ channels by beta-subunit mutation. Am J Physiol 1996; 270 (1 pt 1) C208–213.

45. Hansson JH, Nelson-Williams C, Suzuki H, Schild L, Shimkets R, Lu Y, et al. Hypertension caused by a truncated epithelial sodium channel gamma subunit: genetic heterogeneity of Liddle's Syndrome. Nature Genet 1995; 11:76–82.

46. Gordon RD. Heterogeneous hypertension. Nature Genet 1995; 11:6–9.

47. Findling JW, Raff H, Hansson JH, Lifton RP. Liddle's syndrome: prospective genetic screening and suppressed aldosterone secretion in an extended kindred. J Clin Endocrinol Metab 1997; 82:1071–1079.

48. Gaddalah MF, Abreo K, Work J. Liddles's syndrome, an underrecognized entity: a report of four cases, including the first report in black individuals. Am J Kidney Dis 1995; 25:829–835.

49. Bubien JK, Warnock DG. Amiloride-sensitive sodium conductance in human B lymphoid cells. Am J Physiol 1993; 265:C1175–C1183.

50. Gordon RD, Geddes RA, Pawsey CGK, O'Halloran MW. Hypertension and severe hyperkalaemia associated with suppression of renin and aldosterone and completely reversed by dietary sodium restriction. Aust Ann Med 1970; 4:287–294.

51. Gordon RD, Ravenscroft PJ, Klemm SA, Tunny TJ, Hamlet SM. A new Australian kindred with the syndrome of hypertension and hyperkalaemia has dysregulation of atrial natriuretic factor. J Hypertens 1998; 6(suppl 4):S323–S326.

52. Gordon RD. Syndrome of hypertension and hyperkalemia with normal glomerular filtration rate. Hypertension 1986; 8:93–102.

53. Klemm SA, Gordon RD, Tunny TJ, Thompson RE. The syndrome of hypertension and hyperkalemia with normal GFR (Gordon's Syndrome): is there increased proximal sodium reabsorption? Clin Invest Med 1991; 14:551–558.

54. Gordon RD, Klemm SA, Tunny TJ, Stowasser M. Gordon's syndrome: a sodium-volume-dependent form of hypertension with a genetic basis. In: Laragh JH, Brenner BM, eds. Hypertension: Pathophysioloy, Diagnosis and Management, second Ed. Raven, New York, 1995, pp. 2111–2123.

55. Mansfield TA, Simon DB, Farfel Z, Bia M, Tucci JR, Lebel M, et al. Multilocus linkage of familial hyperkalemia and hypertension, pseudohyperaldosteronism type II, to chromosomes 1q31–42 and 17p11–q21. Nature Genet 1997; 16:202–205

56. O'Shaughnessy KM, Fu B, Johnson A, Gordon RD. Linkage of Gordon's syndrome to the long arm of chromosome 17 in a region recently linked to familial essential hypertension. J Hum Hypertens 1998.

57. Hilbert P. Chromosomal mapping of two genetic loci associated with blood pressure regulation in hereditary hypertensive rats. Nature 1991; 353:521–526.

58. Julier C, Delepine M, Keavney B, Terwilliger T, Davis S, Weeks DE, et al. Genetic susceptibility to human familial essential hypertension in a region of homology with blood pressure linkage on rat chromosome 10. Hum Molec Genet 1997; 6:2077–2085.

59. Conn JW, Cohen EL, Rovner DR. Suppression of plasma renin activity in primary aldosteronism: distinguishing primary from secondary aldosteronism in hypertensive disease. J Am Med Assoc. 1964; 190:213–221.

60. Hiramatsu K, Yamada T, Yukimura Y, Komiya I, Ichikawa K, Ishihara M, et al. A screening test to identify aldosterone-producing adenoma by measuring plasma renin activity. Arch Int Med 1981; 141:1589–1593.

61. McKenna TJ, Sequira SJ, Heffernan A, Chambers J, Cunningham S. Diagnosis under random conditions of all disorders of the renin-angiotensin-aldosterone axis, including primary hyperaldosteronism. J Clin Endocrinol Metab 1991; 79:952–957.

62. Gordon RD. Primary aldosteronism. J Endocrinol Invest 1995; 18:495–511.

63. Jonsson JR, Klemm SA, Tunny TJ, Stowasser M, Gordon RD. A new genetic test for familial hyperaldosteronism type I aids in the detection of curable hypertension. Biochem Biophys Res Commun 1995; 207:565–571.

64. Stowasser M, Gartside MG, Gordon RD. A PCR-based method of screening individuals of all ages, from neonates to the elderly, for familial hyperaldosteronism type I. Aust NZ J Med 1997; 27:685–690.

65. Pascoe L, Jeunemaitre X, Lebrethon MC, Curnow KM, Gomez-Sanchez CE, Gase JM, et al. Glucocorticoid-suppressible hyperaldosteronism and adrenal tumours occurring in a single French pedigree. J Clin Invest 1995; 96:2236–2246.

66. Huang YY, Hsu BR, Tsai JS. Paralytic myopathy—a leading clinical presentation for primary aldosteronism in Taiwan. J Clin Endocrinol Metab 1996; 81:4038–4041.

67. Mantero F, Masini AM, Opocher G, Giovagnetti M, Arnaldi G. Adrenal incidentaloma: an overview of hormona data from the National Italian Study Group. Horm Res 1997; 47:284–289.

68. Soma R, Miyamori I, Nakagawa A, Matsubara T, Takasaki H, Morise T, et al. Possible association of aldosterone producing adenoma and non-functioning adrenal tumor. J Endocrinology 1989; 12:183–186.

69. Young WF, Stanson AW, Grant CS, Thompson GB, Van Heerden JA. Primary aldosteronism: adrenal venous sampling. Surgery 1996; 120:913–920.

70. Vaughan NJA, Jowett TP, Slater JOH. Wiggins RC, Lightman SL, Ma JTC, et al. The diagnosis of primary hyperaldosteronism. Lancet 1981; 1:120–125.

71. Rutherford JC, Stowasser M, Tunny TJ, Klemm SA, Gordon GD. Laparoscopic adrenalectomy. World J Surg 1966; 20:758–761.

72. Gordon RD. Primary aldosteronism: a new understanding. Clin Exp Hypertens. 1997; 19:857–870.

73. Rutherford JR, Taylor WL, Stowasser M, Gordon RD. Success of surgery in primary aldosteronism judged by residual autonomous aldosterone production. World J Surg 1998; 22:1243–1245.

74. Skogseid B, Larsson C, Lindgren P-G, Kvanta E, Rastad J, Theodorsson E, et al. Clinical and genetic features of adrenocortical lesions in multiple endocrine neoplasia type I. J Clin Endocrinol Metab 1992; 75:76–81.

75. Hamwi GJ, Serbin RA, Kruger FA. Does adrenocortical hyperplasia result in adrenocortical carcinoma? N Engl J Med 1957; 257:1153–1157.

76. Gordon RD, Hawkins PG, Hamlet S, Tunny TJ, Klemm SA, Bachmann AW. Reduced adrenal secretory mass after unilateral adrenalectomy for aldosterone-producing adenoma may explain unexpected incidence of hypotension. J Hypertens 1989; 7:S210–S211.

77. McLeod MK, Thompson NW, Gross MD, Grekin RJ. Idiopathic aldosteronism masquerading as discrete aldosterone-secreting adrenal cortical neoplasms among patients with primary aldosteronism. Surgery 1989; 106:1161–1168.

78. Beckers A, Abs R, Willems PJ, Van Der Auwera B, Kovacs K, Reznik M, et al. Aldosterone-secreting adrenal adenoma as part of multiple endocrine neoplasia type 1 (MEN I): loss of heterozygosity for polymorphic chromosome 11 deoxyribonucleic acid markers, including the MEN I locus. J Clin Endocrinol Metab 1992; 75:564–570.

79. Herd GW. A case of primary hyperparathyroidism, primary aldosteronism and Cushing's disease. Acta Endocrinol (Copenh) 1984; 107:371–374.

80. Strauch G, Vallotten MB, Touitou Y, Bricaire H. The Renin-angiotensin-aldosterone system in normotensive and hypertensive patients with acromegaly. N Engl J Med 1972; 287:795–799.

81. Seki M, Tanaka K, Kikudni-Yanoshita R, Konishi M, Fukunari H, Iwama T, et al. Loss of normal allele of the APC gene in an adrenocortical carcinoma from a patient with familial adenomatous polyposis. Human Genet 1992; 89:298–300.

82. Ballard HS, Frame B, Hartscok RJ. Familial multiple endocrine adenoma-peptic ulcer complex. Medicine 1964 43:481–516.

83. Fertig A, Webley M, Lynn JA. Primary hyperparathyroidism in a patient with Conn's syndrome. Postgrad Med J 1980; 56:45–47.

84. Burgess JR, Harle RA, Tucker P, Parameswaran V, Davies P, Greenaway TM, et al. Adrenal lesions in a large kindred with multiple endocrine neoplasia type I. Arch Surg 1996; 131:699–702.

85. Yano T, Linehan M, Anglard P, Lerman MI, Daniel LN, Stein CA, et al. Genetic changes in human adrenocortical carcinomas. J Natl Cancer Inst 1989; 81:518–523.

86. Iida A, Blake K, Tunny T, Klemm S, Stowasser M, Hayward N, et al. Allelic losses on chromosome 11q13 in aldosterone-producing adrenal tumours. Genes Chromosomes and Cancer 1995; 12:73–75.

87. Gordon R, Gartside M, Tunny T, Stowasser M. Different allelic patterns of chromosome 11q13 in paired aldosterone-producing tumours and blood DNA. Clin Exp Pharmacol Physiol 1996; 23:594–596.

88. Chandrasekharappa SC, Guru SC, Manickam P, Olufemi S-E, Collins FS, Emmert-Buck MR, et al. Positional cloning of the gene for multiple endocrine neoplasia—type 1. Science 1997; 276:404–407.

89. Lammie GA, Peters G. Chromosome 11q13 abnormalities in human cancer. Cancer Cells 1991; 3:413–420.

90. Kirschner MA, Powell RD, Lipsett MB. Cushing's syndrome: nodular cortical hyperplasia of adrenal glands with clinical and pathological features suggesting adrenocortical tumour. J Clin Endocrinol Metab 1964; 24:947–955.

91. Findlay JC, Sheeler LR, Engeland WC, Aron DC. Familial adrenocorticotropin-independent Cushing's syndrome with bilateral macronodular adrenal hyperplasia. J Clin Endocrinol Metab 1993; 76:189–191.

92. Hidai H, Fujii H, Otsuka K, Abé K, Shimazu N. Cushing's syndrome due to huge adrenocortical multinodular hyperplasia. Endocrinol J 1995; 22:555–560.

93. Carney JA, Gordon H, Carpenter PC, Shendy BV, Go VL. The complex of myxomas, spotty pigmentation, and endocrine overactivity. Medicine (Baltimore) 1985; 64:270–283.

94. Young WF, Carney JA, Musa PU, Wulffraat NM, Lens JW, Drexhage HA. Familial Cushing's syndrome due to primary pigmented adrenocortical disease. Reinvestigation 50 years later. N Engl J Med 1989; 321:1659–1664.

95. Stratakis CA, Carney JA, Lin J-P, Papanicolaou DA, Karl M, Kastner DL, et al. Carney complex,

a familial multiple neoplasia and lentigenous syndrome. Analysis of II kindreds and linkage to the short arm of chromosome 2. J Clin Invest 1996; 97:699–705.

96. Stratakis CA, Jenkins RB, Pras E, Mitsiadis CS, Raff SB, Stalboerger PG, et al. Cytogenetic and microsatellite alterations in tumors from patients with the syndrome of myxomas, spotty pigmentation, and endocrine overactivity (Carney Complex). J Clin Endocrinol Metab 1996; 81:3607–3614.

97. Basson CT, Macrae CA, Korf B, Merliss A. Genetic heterogeneity of familial atrial myxoma syndrome (Carney Complex). Am J Cardiol 1997; 79:994–995.

98. Hobma S, Hermus A, Pieters G, Smals A, Kloppenborg P. Concurrent hypercortisolism and hyperaldosteronism due to an adrenal adenoma. Klin Wschr 1990; 68:981–983.

99. Nagae A, Murakami E, Hiwada K, Kubota O, Takada Y, Ohmori T. Primary hyperaldosteronism with cortisol overproduction from bilateral multiple adrenal adenomas. Jpn J Med 1991; 30:26–31.

100. Baert D, Bobels F, Van Crombrugge P. Combined Conn's and Cushing's Syndrome: an unusual presentation of adrenal adenoma. Acta Clin Belgica 1995; 50:310–313.

101. Tunny TJ, Klemm SA, Gordon RD. Some aldosterone-producing adrenal tumours also secrete cortisol, but present clinically as primary aldosteronism. Clin Exp Pharmacol Physiol 1990; 17:167–171.

102. Van Renterghem C, Lazdunski M. A new voltage-dependent epithelial-like Na channel in vascular smooth muscle cells. Pflugers Arch 1991; 419:401–408.

103. Tanabe A, Naruse M, Naruse K, Hase M, Yoshimoto T, Tanaka M, et al. Left ventricular hypertrophy is more prominent in patients with primary aldosteronism than in patients with other types of secondary hypertension. Hypertens Res 1997; 20:85–90.

104. Rossi GP, Sacchetto A, Pavan E, Palatini P, Graniero GR, Canali C, et al. Remodelling of the left ventricle in primary aldosteronism due to Conn's adenoma. Circulation 1997; 95:1471–1478.

105. Shigematsu Y, Hamanda, Okayama H, Hara Y, Kodama K, Lohara K, et al. Left ventricular hypertigraphy precedes other target-organ damage in primary aldosteronism. Hypertension. 1997; 29:723–727.

106. Rizzoni D, Porteri E, Castellano M, Bettoni G, Muiesan ML, Muiesan P, et al. Vascular hypertrophy and remodelling in secondary hypertension. Hypertension 1996; 28:785–790.

107. Connel JM, Jamieson AJ, Davies E, Ingram M, Soro A, Fraser R. 11 beta-hydroxylase activity in glucocorticoid suppressible hyperaldosteronism: lessons for essential hypertension? Endocr Res 22:691–700.

108. Bamberger CM, Bamberger AM, Wald M, Chrousos GP, Schulte HM. Inhibition of mineralocorticoid activity by the beta-isoforms of the human glucocorticoid receptor. J Steroid Biochem Mol Biol 1997; 60:43–50.

109. Brilla CG, Schencking M, Scheer C, Rupp H. Spironolactone: renaissance of anti-aldosterone therapy in heart failure? Schweiz Rundsch Med Prax 1997; 86:566–574.

110. Pitt B, Zannad F, Remme WS, Cody R, Castaigne A, Perez A, et al. (For the Randomized Aldactone Evaluation Study investigators.) The effect of spironolactone on morbidity and mortality in patients with severe heart failure. N Engl J Med 1999; 341:708–717.

111. Zhang Y, Proenca R, Maffei M, Barone M, Leopold L, Friedman JM. Positional cloning of the mouse obese gene and its human homologue. Nature 1994; 372:425–432.

112. Caro JF, Sinha MK, Kogaczynski JW, Zhang PL, Considine RV. Leptin: the tale of an obesity gene. Diabetes 1996; 45:1455–1462.

113. Ozata M, Ozdemir IC, Licinio J. Human leptin deficiency caused by missense mutation: multiple endocrine defects, decreased sympathetic tone, and immune system dysfunction indicate new targets for leptin action, greater central than peripheral resistance to the effects of leptin, and spontaneous correction of leptin-mediated defects. J Clin Endocrinol Metab 1999; 84:3586–3695.

114. Torpy DJ, Bornstein SR, Taylor W, Tauchnitz R, Gordon RD. Leptin levels are suppressed in primary aldosteronism. Horm Metab Res, 1999; 31:533–536.

115. Shek EW, Brands MW, Hall JE. Chronic leptin infusion increases arterial pressure. Hypertension 1998; 31:409–414.

116. Suter PM, Locer R, Haler E, Vetter W. Is there a role for the ob gene product leptin in essential hypertension? Am J Hypertens 1998; 11:1305–1311.

28   Pheochromocytoma

Progress in Diagnosis, Therapy, and Genetics

*Karel Pacak, George P. Chrousos,
Christian A. Koch, Jacques W. M. Lenders,
and Graeme Eisenhofer*

Contents

INTRODUCTION

Pheochromocytomas are catecholamine-secreting tumors typically arising in about 90% of cases from adrenomedullary tissue and in about 10% of cases from extraadrenal chromaffin tissue. Those arising from extraadrenal tissue are commonly known as paragangliomas or chemodectomas, but all pheochromocytomas display similar histopathological characteristics. Paragangliomas arise mainly from chromaffin tissue adjacent to sympathetic ganglia of the neck, mediastinum, abdomen, and pelvis. Others may arise from a collection of chromaffin tissue around the origin of the inferior mesenteric artery, the organs of Zuckerkandl. Most represent sporadic tumors and only about 10% of pheochromocytomas are familial. In contrast to sporadic pheochromocytomas that are usually unicentric and unilateral, familial pheochromocytomas are often multicentric and bilateral *(1)*. Pheochromocytomas are rare endocrine tumors, which, according to different reviews and statistics account for approx 0.05% to 0.1% of patients with any degree of sustained hypertension *(2)*. However, this probably accounts for only 50% of persons harboring a pheochromocytoma, when it is considered that about half the patients with pheochromocytomas have only paroxysmal hypertension or are normotensive. Also, despite the low incidence of pheochromocytoma in patients with sustained hypertension, it must also be considered that the prevalence of sustained hypertension in the adult population of Western countries is between 15 and 20% *(3,4)*. Thus, in Western countries, the prevalence of pheochromocytoma can be estimated to

Table 1
Clinical Symptoms and Signs Characteristic for Pheochromocytoma

Symptoms	Percent	Signs	Percent
Headache	70–90	Hypertension	>98
Palpitations±tachycardia	50–70	sustained	50–60
Diaphoresis	60–70	paroxysmal	50
Anxiety	20	Orthostatic hypotension	12
Nervousness	35–40	Pallor	30–60
Chest/abdominal pain	20–50	Flushing	18
Nausea	26–43	Fever	up to 66
Fatigue	15–40	Hyperglycemia	42
Dyspnea	11–19	Vomiting	26–43
Dizziness	3–11	Convulsions	3–5
Heat intolerance	13–15		
Paresthesias/pain	up to 11		
Visual symptoms	3–21		
Constipation	10		
Diarrhea	6		

Adapted from Ram and Fierro-Carrion (3), Manger and Gifford (9), and Werbel and Ober (48).

lie between 1:6500 and 1:2500 with an annual incidence in the United States of 500 to 1600 cases per year. Despite this relatively low incidence, it must always be considered that once identified, the condition can be cured in 90% of cases, whereas left untreated, the tumor is often likely to be fatal.

CLINICAL PRESENTATION

Signs and Symptoms

The presence of pheochromocytoma is usually characterized by clinical signs and symptoms (Table 1) that result from hemodynamic and metabolic actions of circulating catecholamines, including norepinephrine, epinephrine, and dopamine. Less-frequent secretion into the blood stream of other hormones, such as gastrin, calcitonin, somatostatin, vasoactive intestinal peptide, and adrenocorticotropin may also add to clinical findings (5).

Clinical findings such as hypertension, headache, sweating, arrhythmias, and pallor are highly suggestive of pheochromocytoma. Sustained or paroxysmal hypertension is the most common clinical sign. Less than 10% of the patients typically present with persistent normal blood pressure (2,6), but this proportion can be much higher in patients who undergo periodic screening for familial pheochromocytoma (7,8). Pheochromocytoma may also present with hypotension, particularly postural hypotension or alternating episodes of high and low blood pressure (9). Thus, a careful evaluation and follow-up of the blood pressure of a patient with a pheochromocytoma before and during antihypertensive therapy should be carried out periodically.

Headache occurs in up to 90% of patients with pheochromocytoma (2,6,9,10). Headache may be mild or severe, short or long in duration, and may last for up to several days. In some patients, catecholamine-induced headache may be similar to tension headache.

Excessive generalized sweating occurs in approx 60–70% patients presenting with pheochromocytoma *(6,10)*. Other complaints are palpitations and dyspnea, weight loss despite normal appetite (caused by catecholamine-induced glycogenolysis and lipolysis), and generalized weakness *(9–12)*. Although headache, palpitations, and sweating are nonspecific symptoms, their presence in patients with hypertension should arouse immediate suspicion for a pheochromocytoma because this triad is the most frequently encountered triad of symptoms in patients with a pheochromocytoma. Some patients present with severe episodes of anxiety or panic attacks *(9)*. Palpitations, anxiety, and nervousness are more common in patients with pheochromocytomas producing epinephrine *(9)*. Less-frequent clinical manifestations include fever of unknown origin (hypermetabolic state) and constipation, secondary to catecholamine-induced decrease in intestinal motility *(6,13)*.

Clinical findings that occur in paroxysms presumably reflect episodic catecholamine hypersecretion, whereas those that are sustained may be assumed to reflect continuous excessive secretion of catecholamines.

Pheochromocytoma-induced metabolic or hemodynamic attacks may last from a few seconds to several hours, with intervals between attacks varying widely and as infrequent as once every few months. Unusual symptoms related to paroxysmal blood pressure elevation during diagnostic procedures (e.g., endoscopy, radiographical contrast agents), anesthesia, or food ingestion should promptly arouse a suspicion of pheochromocytoma.

Causes that account for episodic catecholamine secretion often remain unestablished, but in some situations may be caused by either intentional or accidental tumor manipulation. Timing of attacks may be unpredictable and attacks may also occur at rest (e.g., on awakening). Some patients may present with symptoms that occur during physical activity, trauma, or by direct tumor stimulation (pheochromocytoma of urinary bladder may cause an attack when the patient urinates). In others, symptoms occur when certain drugs are used [e.g., histamine, tyramine, guanethidine, saralasin, adrenocorticotropic hormone (ACTH), metoclopramide, methyldopa, ethanol, phenothiazine, and tricyclic antidepressants].

Estrogen and growth hormone administration have been shown to induce pheochromocytoma in experimental animals *(14,15)*. Whether these hormones contribute to the higher incidence of clinical pheochromocytoma or an increase in malignant potential is unknown.

Extraadrenal and Malignant Pheochromocytomas

Malignant pheochromocytomas account for about 10% of all adrenal pheochromocytomas *(16)*. Pheochromocytomas located in extraadrenal tissues exhibit symptoms and signs more aggressively, are more frequently malignant, are associated with a higher incidence of persistence or recurrent disease, and have a higher mortality rate than those found in the adrenal gland *(17–19)*. Pheochromocytoma in children have a lower incidence of malignancy, but tend to exhibit more aggressive development *(20)*.

Malignant tumors appear to be larger, contain more necrotic tissue, and are composed of smaller cells than benign adrenal pheochromocytoma *(2)*. However, as reviewed in detail by Clarke et al. *(21)* and Manger and Gifford *(2)*, it is impossible, to distinguish malignant from benign pheochromocytoma based on histopathological features. Capsular invasion, vascular penetration, coarse nodularity, the presence of atypical nuclei, absence of intracytoplasmic hyaline granules, and mitosis exist in both types of pheochromocytoma. Only the tumor invasion of adjacent tissues and the presence of metastatic lesions (most commonly in liver, lungs, lymphatic nodes, and bones) are consistent with the diagnosis of malignant pheochromocytoma [for review, see *(2)*]. As described by Linnoila et al. *(22)*, fewer neuropeptides are expressed in malignant than in benign pheochromocytoma cells. There are no differences in immunohistochemical expression of cathepsins, basic fibroblastic growth factor, c-*met*, and collagenase between benign and malignant pheochromocytomas *(21)*.

Analysis of telomerase activity appears to be a powerful tool for the diagnosis of malignant pheochromocytoma. Kubota et al. *(23)* recently reported on elevated levels of telomerase activity in malignant pheochromocytoma. They analyzed telomerase activity in 16 benign and 3 malignant pheochromocytomas, as well as in 16 normal adrenal medullae. No telomerase activity was detected in any of the normal adrenal medullas or the benign pheochromocytomas. All of the three malignant pheochromocytomas, however, had elevated telomerase activity. Similarly, Kinoshita et al. *(24)* examined seven pheochromocytomas for telomerase activity and found two to be telomerase-positive. None of the tumors examined were associated with metastases, but telomerase-positive tumors demonstrated reportedly clinicopathological features suggesting malignant potential.

Several studies have suggested that DNA aneuploidy or tetraploidy is associated with potential malignancy *(25,26)*. Using various antibodies, the positive reaction of monoclonal antibody MIB-1 with the nuclear protein Ki-67 that is increasingly expressed in cells through phase G1 to M, was shown to reflect proliferation in normal and tumor tissue *(21)*. Clarke et al. recently reported that MIB-1 appears to be the best indicator of metastatic pheochromocytoma's potential with a specificity of 100% and a sensitivity of 50% *(21)*.

Abundant c-*myc* gene expression in neoplasms has been often linked to poor prognosis. C-*myc* mRNA is expressed and hormonally regulated in human adrenals. Therefore, Liu et al. *(27)* investigated expression patterns of the c-*myc* gene in adrenocortical tumors and pheochromocytomas. In their study, the c-*myc* mRNA abundance in benign adrenal pheochromocytomas was similar to that in normal adrenal medulla. However, in malignant pheochromocytomas c-*myc* mRNA levels were threefold higher than in benign pheochromocytomas.

GENETICS OF PHEOCHROMOCYTOMA

In recent years, knowledge of tumor genetics has grown tremendously as a result of the advances in molecular biology. Studies of families with hereditary cancer syndromes (e.g., multiple endocrine neoplasia) have enabled linkage analyses and genomic localization of disease-associated genes. Cancer genes are classified into three functional categories: (1) unrestrained active oncogenes resulting from mutations in genes with normal cellular function (protooncogenes); (2) tumor-suppressor genes in which mutations lead to loss of function; (3) genes encoding DNA repair molecules thereby preventing replication errors within DNA. Familial cancer syndromes result from germline mutations, whereas most mutations found in sporadic tumor cells occur in somatic DNA.

Pheochromocytoma occurs in three known familial cancer syndromes: multiple endocrine neoplasia type 2 (MEN-2), von Hippel-Lindau (VHL) disease, and neurofibromatosis type 1. There are also reports of familial pheochromocytoma occurring without any established links to the above three syndromes. Genetically predisposed patients are younger at the diagnosis of pheochromocytoma and present much more frequently with bilateral or multicentric tumors than do patients with sporadic pheochromocytomas *(8)*. Extraadrenal pheochromocytoma is rarely associated with familial syndromes *(27a)*. The prevalence of malignant pheochromocytoma in familial syndromes can be as high as 20% *(27b,27c,28,28a)*.

Why is molecular genetics of pheochromocytoma important? First, further identification of mutated genes may allow clinical use of these potential diagnostic and prognostic markers in genetic, pharmacological, and other therapeutic strategies. Second, and perhaps most important for the individual patient, this knowledge helps identify a genetic predisposition to pheochromocytoma, thereby establishing an early diagnosis by regular screening and surveillance. However, because it is not yet possible to predict when and how severe a pheochromocytoma will manifest, the role of prophylactic surgery (e.g., adrenalectomy and subcapsular adrenalectomy) remains controversial.

In some patients with VHL or MEN-2, pheochromocytomas are the sole presenting tumor, justifying screening patients with pheochromocytoma for possible underlying mutations in the respective genes VHL and RET *(8,28b,29)*. Conversely, patients identified with a familial predisposition for pheochromocytoma should undergo periodic screening tests for the tumor *(8,30,31)*. Many patients with a familial predisposition for pheochromocytoma are asymptomatic when tumors are first diagnosed. In the study of Pomares et al. *(32)*, the most common clinical feature and the presenting feature in isolated pheochromocytoma was hypertension, whereas 52% of patients with MEN-2A were asymptomatic and only 35% presented with hypertension. Similar findings have been reported by others in studies that have included patients with VHL disease *(7,8)*. Thus, in patients identified with a familial predisposition for pheochromocytoma, the clinician should not rely on the presentation of the usual clinical symptoms before carrying out biochemical testing. Such testing should be carried out periodically as part of the routine screening and surveillance for the particular tumors that the patient is predisposed to. Because of the high sensitivity of the test, biochemical screening for pheochromocytoma should ideally include measurements of plasma-free metanephrines *(33)*.

Pheochromocytoma in Multiple Endocrine Neoplasia (MEN-2)

Multiple endocrine neoplasia (MEN-2) consists of three forms: (1) MEN-2A, clinically characterized by a predisposition to medullary thyroid cancer, pheochromocytoma, and parathyroid hyperplasia/adenoma; (2) MEN-2B, with an earlier onset of medullary thyroid cancer and pheochromocytoma and additional skin, mucosal, skeletal, and dysmorphic/marfanoid features; and (3) familial medullary thyroid cancer.

In MEN-2A, pheochromocytoma occurs in about 50% of patients and, on average, about 8 yr after medullary thyroid cancer with a mean age at diagnosis of 37 years *(34)*. In about 50% of affected patients, pheochromocytoma is bilateral.

MEN-2B is rarer than MEN-2A. In MEN-2B, cutaneous and mucosal neuromas and café-au-lait patches may be present requiring differentiation from neurofibromatosis type 1. Pheochromocytomas occur at an earlier age with 25% of affected patients less than 20 yr. Malignant pheochromocytoma has a low incidence in MEN-2 *(8,35)*.

Pheochromocytomas in patients with MEN-2 are characterized by a high incidence of epinephrine-producing tumors *(36–38)*. All MEN-2 patients with pheochromocytoma

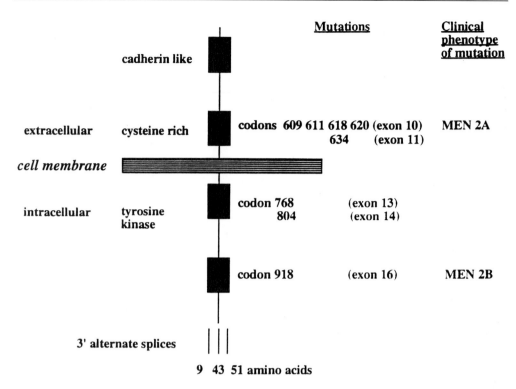

Fig. 1. The main features of the protein encoded by the *ret* protooncogene, and the sites of the mutations in the different clinical varieties of MEN-2. Constitutive activation of *ret* will ensue as a result of mutation of a cysteine in the extracellular domain (updated in ref. 34a).

that we have examined have shown elevations in plasma metanephrine (the O-methylated metabolite of epinephrine) in addition to the more common elevations in normetanephrine (the O-methylated metabolite of norepinephrine). Thus, pheochromocytomas in patients with MEN-2 exhibit a distinctly adrenergic phenotype as opposed to the more common noradrenergic phenotype in sporadic pheochromocytoma or other familial pheochromocytoma syndromes. The presence of a MEN-2 familial syndrome should, therefore, always be considered in those patients with epinephrine-producing pheochromocytomas.

Mutations in the RET/*ret* protooncogene are responsible for the dominantly inherited group of disorders in MEN-2 (Fig. 1). The name *ret* is an acronym for "rearranged during transfection." This reflects the original identification of *ret* as a chimeric oncogene formed by rearrangement during transfection assays using DNA from human lymphomas and gastric tumors. *Ret* is a cell-surface glycoprotein that is a member of the receptor tyrosine kinase family. In 1987, the gene for MEN-2 was mapped to the centromeric region of the long arm of chromosome 10 by family linkage analyses *(39)*. In 1993, Mulligan *(40)* reported on missense mutations in *ret* in unrelated kindreds with pheochromocytoma and MEN-2A. In most cases, a single highly conserved cysteine at codon 634 in the extracellular domain was mutated (Fig. 1). The restricted spectrum of these mutations is not explained by a founder effect *(41)*. The result of these missense mutations is (constitutive) *ret* dimerization at steady state, and hence activation of downstream signal transduction *(42,43)*. At least four other germline missense mutations of *ret* on chromosome 10q11.2 in MEN-2A have been identified, most of which also occurred at highly conserved cysteine residues in the extracellular domain at codons 609, 611, 618, and 620 in exons 10 and 11 *(44–47)* (Fig. 1). The risk for development of pheochromocytoma is higher in codon 634 mutations than in other exon 10 and 11 mutations *(45,48)*.

Germline *ret* mutations have also been identified in MEN-2B patients. However, more than 94% of unrelated patients have had a single methionine to threonine substitution at codon 918 in exon 16 of *ret*, the tyrosine kinase domain *(47,49–51)*. Mutations affected the tyrosine kinase catalytic site in the *intra*cellular domain of the protein *(49,50)*.

Ret's ligand is glial cell line-derived neurotrophic factor (GDNF), which was already known as a trophic factor for dopaminergic neurons. GDNF is a member of the transforming growth factor (TGF)-β family. *Ret* activation by GDNF appears to occur via a membrane-bound protein, GDNFRα, which seems to function as the ligand-binding domain of the ligand-receptor complex *(52,53)*. The second ligand for Ret is neurturin (34a). The normal function of *ret* is largely unknown. It is expressed in neural crest-derived tissue and it may play a role in kidney and gastrointestinal neuronal development. *Ret* is expressed in pheochromocytoma and in other tumors of neural crest origin, such as medullary thyroid carcinoma, and neuroblastoma. Because germline *ret* mutations may be distributed throughout the gene, some (mutations) may even inactivate *ret* *(54)*. MEN-2A and MEN-2B *ret* mutations may induce hyperplasia of the adrenal medulla chromaffin cells. However, a pheochromocytoma develops only if further mutational events, e.g., deletion of a tumor suppressor gene on the short arm of chromosome 1 (1p), occur *(39)*. To date, the so-called "second hit" is unknown, although we have unpublished laboratory data suggesting two possible mechanisms of tumor formation.

[Au:Greek alpha here, or "a"?]

Pheochromocytoma in von Hippel-Lindau (VHL) Disease

von Hippel-Lindau (VHL) disease represents another multisystem neoplastic disorder that, like MEN-2, is also inherited in an autosomal dominant fashion and also involves a predisposition to develop pheochromocytoma. On average, about 10 to 20% of patients with VHL disease develop pheochromocytoma, but this incidence varies dramatically from family to family depending on the specific mutation *(55–58)*. Despite the low incidence of VHL disease (1:36,000), the disorder is the most common cause of familial pheochromocytoma *(8)*. Because of variable expression and age and tumor-dependent penetrance, it has been proposed that all patients with familial, multiple, or early onset (<40 yr) pheochromocytoma should be examined for underlying VHL disease *(8,28,29)*. Findings that pheochromocytomas in patients with VHL disease display a distinct noradrenergic phenotype (as opposed to the adrenergic phenotype in MEN-2) provide an additional guideline for appropriate genetic testing in patients with pheochromocytoma where underlying VHL disease is suspect.

More than 150 *vhl* germline mutations have been identified and 32 of them are associated with pheochromocytoma *(27b)*. However, there are large interfamilial variations with some families having pheochromocytoma as the most-frequent complication of VHL disease *(59,60)*. The mean age at diagnosis is 28 yr, and in about 50% of cases, pheochromocytomas are bilateral *(27b)*. Most *vhl* mutations associated with pheochromocytoma also predispose to renal cell carcinoma with exception of a single ancestral mutation in southwestern Germany *(61)*.

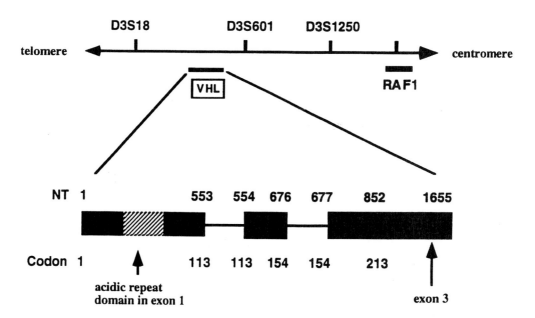

Fig. 2. Genomic organization of the *vhl* gene showing the three exons and the location of the acidic repeat domain.

The *vhl* tumor-suppressor gene is located on chromosome 3p25–26 and was isolated in 1993, five years after the initial mapping of the gene *(62)*. The cloned coding sequence is represented in three exons (Fig. 2). Pheochromocytoma is uncommon in patients with large germline mutations or deletions (nonsense mutations and frameshift insertions or deletions) because those are predicted to produce a truncated protein product. Only about 15% of patients with *vhl* associated pheochromocytoma have large germline deletions detected by Southern blot analysis. Another 2% of patients have (even) larger deletions detected by Southern pulsed field gel electrophoresis *(62–65)*. On the other hand, small intragenic mutations can be identified in about 50% of patients with *vhl* associated pheochromocytoma. These mutations are variable and include frameshift deletions and insertions, in-frame deletions, and nonsense and missense mutations. The latter account for about half of characterized intragenic mutations *(66–68)*, that is, >95% patients with *vhl* associated pheochromocytoma have missense mutations. A mutation hotspot has been described at codon 167 in exon 3 (equivalent to nt 712/713), which accounts for 9% of patients (Fig. 2) *(27b)*. The notion, according to Knudson et al. *(69)*, that a second hit is required is also suggested by the detection of chromosome 3p allele loss in pheochromocytoma from patients with codon 167 missense mutations *(70)*. There are genotype-specific *vhl* phenotypes *(27b,71)*. Pheochromocytoma-associated missense mutations may not necessarily act in a simple dominant negative manner causing a more-severe phenotype. Instead, these *vhl* mutations may have tissue-specific effects *(61)*. "Founder effects" may explain differences in regional prevalence rates, such as in the Black Forest area in southern Germany where VHL patients with the missense mutation of tyrosine to histidine at codon 98 *(Tyr98His)* have a high risk of pheochromocytoma *(8,61,72)*.

The *vhl* protein forms a stable complex with the highly conserved transcription elongation factors, elongin B, and elongin C, which regulate RNA polymerase II elongation. Formation of this heterotrimeric complex with elongin B and C appears to be the tumor-suppressor function of the *vhl* gene, because the majority of tumor-predisposing mutations of *vhl* disrupt the formation of this complex *(73–75)*. Elongin A is required to inhibit the processing of RNA polymerase II, allowing cell processing of transcription. The *vhl* gene product and elongin A compete for binding to elongin B and C via a short shared sequence motif. This sequence which is found in the third exon of *vhl* is highly mutated in VHL disease *(76)*.

Pheochromocytoma in Neurofibromatosis type 1

Neurofibromatosis type 1 is the most common familial cancer syndrome predisposing to pheochromocytoma. It affects about one in 4000 individuals. The risk of pheochromocytoma in neurofibromatosis type 1, however, is small—about 1% *(77,78)*. Neurofibromatosis type 1 is inherited as an autosomal dominant trait with variable expression. About 50% of patients have new mutations. Pheochromocytoma in patients with neurofibromatosis type 1 occur at a later age than in MEN-2 and VHL disease. The modal age at diagnosis is in the fifth decade. Onset before age 20 yr is uncommon *(78a)*. About 10% of neurofibromatosis type 1 patients with pheochromocytoma have multiple tumors.

The *nf1* gene is a large tumor-suppressor gene mapping to chromosome 17q11.2 *(79–81)*, with three genes embedded within an intron. Mutation analysis has been hindered by the large gene size (11 kb of coding sequence extending over 300 kb of genomic DNA) and number of exons so that mutations are identified in only about 15% of patients. Patients with neurofibromatosis type 1 associated pheochromocytoma show loss of the wild-type allele *(82)*. Fifty percent of mice heterozygous for one mutant *nf1* allele developed pheochromocytoma *(83)*. Neurofibromin, the *nf1* gene product, shows homology to the *ras*/GTPase-activating protein (GAP) *(84)*. P21-*ras*/GAP increases the rate of intrinsic GTP hydrolysis in the small G proteins, the *ras* genes, thereby mediating the return of the G protein switch to the "off" GDP-bound form. It can therefore control signal transduction via the *ras* pathways, thereby perhaps acting as a tumor suppressor (Fig. 3). This notion is supported by the fact that inactivating mutations in *nf1* are mainly found in the *ras*/GAP homology region. Interestingly, human somatic mutations in *nf1* have also been found in tumors generally not associated with neurofibromatosis type 1 *(85)*.

Familial Pheochromocytoma

Familial pheochromocytoma occurring without any clear link to VHL disease or MEN-2 syndromes is usually inherited as an autosomal dominant trait. However, detailed investigation may reveal subclinical evidence of VHL disease of MEN-2 *(8,86)*. *Vhl* germline mutations in the absence of other features of VHL disease have been detected by molecular genetic screening for *vhl* and *ret* mutations in some patients with familial pheochromocytoma *(74,87)*. Tissue specificity can be a feature of some *vhl* mutations as suggested by the *Tyr98His* mutation described by Brauch 1995 *(61)*. Paraganglioma, a tumor arising in extraadrenal chromaffin tissue, may be familial. However, the genetic basis of this disorder is still unknown *(88)*. Some of these tumors have been mapped/linked to chromosome 11q23 *(27a)*.

guanosine nucleotide
replacing factor

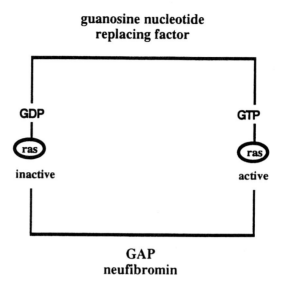

GAP
neufibromin

Fig. 3. The *p21-ras* cycle of activation and inactivation by GAP-related proteins. *p21-ras* is inactive in the GDP-bound state and is converted to an active GTP-bound state by guanosine nucleotide-replacing proteins that substitute GTP for GDP. Interaction of GAP-like proteins with *p21-ras* accelerates the conversion of *p21-ras* GTP to *p21-ras*-GDP by increasing the intrinsic GTPase activity of *p21-ras* and converting *p21-ras* to the inactive GDP-bound form. In resting cells, the majority of *p21-ras* is inactive and in the GDP-bound form (modified from ref. 88a).

Sporadic Pheochromocytoma

Somatic mutations of genes identified as causes for familial cancer syndromes have been identified in nonfamilial forms of pheochromocytoma. *Vhl* somatic mutations are uncommon in sporadic pheochromocytomas *(89,90)*. Eng et al. *(28)* detected *vhl* mutations in only 4 of 48 apparently sporadic pheochromocytomas and only one of the *vhl* mutations was confirmed as truly somatic in this study. Van der Harst et al. *(67)* recently reported on 68 patients with sporadic pheochromocytomas, 6 of which had a *vhl* germline mutation.

Analysis of *ret* mutations in sporadic pheochromocytomas has (exon 16) revealed somatic mutations in 0 to 15% of tumors *(90–94)* with the codon 918 somatic *ret* mutation (MEN-2B mutation) as the one most commonly found, in 3–10% of cases *(28,92–94)*. On the other hand, exon 10 and 11 somatic *ret* mutations (as seen in MEN-2A) only occur in <1% of tumors.

Somatic mutations/changes in *nf1* have also been described in sporadic pheochromocytomas including a finding of reduced or absent *nf1* gene expression in seven of 20 nonneurofibromatosis type 1 pheochromocytomas *(95)* suggesting that *nf1* inactivation can be involved in the pathogenesis of nonfamilial pheochromocytomas.

Allele losses at chromosome 1p, 3p, and 17p are common findings *(39,40,96–98)*. Mulligan et al. *(40)* found allele loss on chromosome 13 and 17 coincided with the location of *RB1* (retinoblastoma gene) and *p53* tumor-suppressor genes. Further delineation of allele loss and analysis of candidate genes in sporadic pheochromocytomas will not only provide an insight into the molecular pathogenesis of sporadic pheochromocytomas, but will also identify candidate susceptibility genes for familial pheochromocytoma

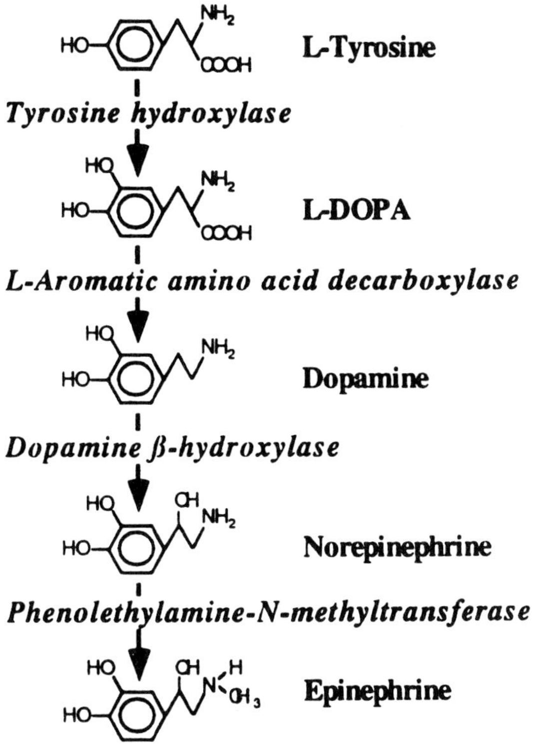

Fig. 4. Pathway of catecholamine synthesis from tyrosine to epinephrine.

kindreds in which *nf1, vh1,* or *ret* mutations are excluded. One can implicate an accumulation of mutations in several genes in both familial and sporadic pheochromocytoma. However, the specific role/function of some of these genes remains to be elucidated, i.e., details of how mutations in different biochemical pathways might interact with each other to produce tumorigenesis. Williamson et al. *(99)* found a codon 201 Gsα (protooncogene) mutation in an extraadrenal pheochromocytoma and in a primary pheochromocytoma including its metastases suggesting that Gsα may be mutated in a small proportion of pheochromocytomas in both benign and malignant phenotypes.

In summary, pheochromocytomas can arise from both germline and somatic genetic mutations. Patients identified with a germline mutations leading to a familial predisposition for pheochromocytoma require periodic screening for the tumor, regardless of appearance of signs and symptoms.

CATECHOLAMINE SYNTHESIS IN PHEOCHROMOCYTOMA

Tyrosine hydroxylase (TH) is the rate-limiting enzyme for the hydroxylation of L-tyrosine to L-dihydroxyphenylalanine and subsequent synthesis of the catecholamines, dopamine, norepinephrine, and epinephrine by the respective enzymes, aromatic amino acid decarboxylase, dopamine-β-hydroxylase, and phenolethanolamine-N-methyltransferase (PNMT) (Fig. 4). Studies at the cellular level suggest that an increase in the biosynthesis of catecholamines may follow an overexpression of the *TH* gene. Recently, Isobe et al. *(100)* demonstrated that mRNA levels for TH, aromatic L-amino acid decarboxylase, and dopamine beta-hydroxylase were much higher in tissue from pheochromocytomas than in that of normal adrenal medullas, whereas the PNMT mRNA concentration in the pheochromocytomas was lower than that in normal adrenal medullae. This difference in gene expression is likely responsible for the higher content of norepinephrine to epinephrine in tumor compared to normal adrenal tissue and predominant secretion of norepinephrine from most pheochromocytomas, and particularly extraadrenal tumors that are not close to a source of glucocorticoids. These steroids induce the activity of PNMT, the enzyme responsible for conversion of norepinephrine to epinephrine, this presumably contributing to the higher incidence of epinephrine producing adrenal than extraadrenal pheochromocytomas.

Tumer et al. *(101)* studied mRNA levels of TH, TH activity, and catecholamine content in normal human adrenals and in six sporadic pheochromocytomas, in two pheochromocytomas from patients VHL disease, in one pheochromocytoma from a patient with MEN-2B, and in one malignant extraadrenal pheochromocytoma. Similar to the study of Isobe *(100)*, there was a positive correlation between TH mRNA expression and total catecholamine content. TH mRNA was also well-correlated with TH activity. Catecholamine contents in the normal adrenal tissue were lower than in the pheochromocytomas. There were also distinctive patterns of TH mRNA expression in the different settings in which the pheochromocytomas arose; TH mRNA levels were highest in the MEN-2B pheochromocytoma and low in the VHL pheochromocytomas and in the extraadrenal malignant pheochromocytoma (compatible with a dedifferentiation of tumor tissue). This suggests that in tumor tissue small increases in TH activity result in a large increase in catecholamine levels. It also implies that tumor-specific expression of catecholamine synthesizing enzymes may provide an explanation not only of the varying clinical phenotypes, but also possibly the differentiation of pheochromocytomas into benign or malignant tumors.

In summary, synthesis of catecholamines in pheochromocytoma is dependent on the rate-limiting enzyme, tyrosine hydroxylase. Additional presence of the enzyme, phenolethanolamine-N-methyltransferase, is responsible for conversion of norepinephrine to epinephrine and adrenergic vs noradrenergic phenotypes of tumors.

BIOCHEMICAL DIAGNOSIS OF PHEOCHROMOCYTOMA

Unequivocal diagnosis of pheochromocytoma typically requires confirmation by several tests, perhaps the most important being biochemical evidence of excessive catecholamine production by the tumor. This is usually achieved from measurements of catecholamines and catecholamine metabolites in urine or plasma *(102–106)* (Table 2). However, the catecholamines, norepinephrine and epinephrine, are ubiquitously produced by the sympathoadrenalmedullary system and are not specific to pheochromocytomas. Increased levels of catecholamines and their metabolites may be produced by a variety of physiological conditions or pathological states involving sympathoadrenalmedullary activation or alterations in catecholamine disposition after their release *(107)*. Sometimes pheochromocytomas may be "silent"; that is, they may not produce catecholamines in amounts sufficient to produce a positive test result or the associated typical clinical signs and symptoms. Also, many pheochromocytomas secrete catecholamines episodically; between episodes, plasma levels, or urinary excretion of catecholamines may be normal. Thus, commonly utilized tests of plasma or urinary

Table 2
Biochemical Tests for Diagnosis of Pheochromocytoma

Biochemical Test	Assay Method	Reference Range*
1. Urine Catecholamines	HPLC	
Norepinephrine		(15–80 µg/24 h)
Epinephrine		(0–20 µg/24 h)
2. Urine Deconjugated Fractionated Metanephrines	HPLC	
Normetanephrine (sulfate conjugated plus free)		(44–540 µg/24 h)
Metanephrine (sulfate conjugated plus free)		(26–230 µg/24 h)
3. Urine Deconjugated Total Metanephrines (Sum of free plus sulfate conjugated metanephrine and normetanephrine)	Spectrofluorimetry	(0–1.2 mg/24 h)
4. Urine VMA	Spectrofluorimetry	(0–7.9 mg/24 h)
5. Plasma Catecholamines	HPLC	
Norepinephrine		(80–498 pg/mL)
Epinephrine		(4–83 pg/mL)
6. Plasma-Free Metanephrines	HPLC	
Normetanephrine (free)		(18–112 pg/mL)
Metanephrine (free)		(12–61 pg/mL)
7. Plasma Deconjugated Metanephrines	HPLC	
Normetanephrine (sulfate conjugated plus free)		(610–3170 pg/mL)
Metanephrine (sulfate conjugated plus free)		(316–1706 pg/mL)

*Reference ranges indicate lower and upper reference limits of a normal population commonly estimated from the 95% confidence intervals. Reference ranges may vary from laboratory to laboratory.

catecholamines and their urinary metabolites do not always reliably exclude or confirm the presence of a tumor (33,108–111). A more-recently developed biochemical test involving measurements of plasma-free metanephrines, the O-methylated metabolites of catecholamines, offers advantages over other tests for diagnosis of pheochromocytoma (33).

Pathways of Catecholamine Metabolism

Understanding the utility and limitations of biochemical tests for diagnosis of pheochromocytoma can benefit from an understanding of the disposition of catecholamines under normal physiological conditions, as well as in the many disease states associated with elevated catecholamines. Central to this is a basic understanding of the sites of catecholamine production and pathways of their metabolism. Norepinephrine is produced mainly in sympathetic nerves, whereas epinephrine is produced mainly within the adrenal medulla. Both catecholamines are metabolized by a multiplicity of pathways catalyzed by an array of enzymes, resulting in a considerable number of different metabolites, only some of which are routinely used for diagnosis of pheochromocytoma (Fig. 5).

Norepinephrine and epinephrine are both metabolized by monoamine oxidase to 3,4-dihydroxyphenylglycol (DHPG), the deaminated glycol metabolite (Fig. 5). Deamination to the deaminated acid metabolite, 3,4-dihydroxymandelic acid (DHMA), is not a favored pathway (112–114). DHPG is further metabolized by catechol-O-methyltransferase (COMT) to 3-methoxy-4-hydroxyphenylglycol (MHPG), a metabolite also

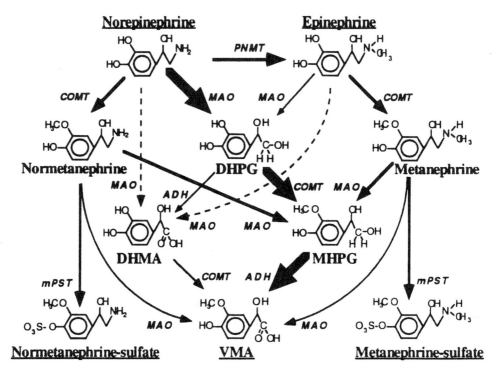

Fig. 5. Pathways of metabolism of norepinephrine (NE) and epinephrine (EPI). Enzymes responsible for each pathway are shown at the head of arrows. The solid arrows indicate more major pathways of metabolism, whereas the dotted arrows indicate pathways of negligible importance. Compounds that are routinely measured in urine or plasma for diagnosis of pheochromocytoma are underlined. Note that free normetanephrine and metanephrine are distinct metabolites from normetanephrine-sulfate and metanephrine-sulfate. The pathways of sulfate conjugation for other compounds are not shown. Abbreviations: PNMT, phenolethanolamine-N-methyltransferase; MAO, monoamine oxidase; COMT, catechol-O-methyltransferase; ADH, alcohol dehydrogenase; m-PST, monoamine preferring phenolsulfotransferase; DHPG, 3,4-dihydroxyphenylglycol; DHMA, 3,4-dihydroxymandelic acid; MHPG, 3-methoxy-4-hydroxyphenylglycol; VMA, vanillylmandelic acid.

produced to a limited extent by deamination of normetanephrine and metanephrine *(115,116)*.

In humans, 3-methoxy-4-hydroxymandelic acid—more commonly known as vanillylmandelic acid (VMA)—is the principal endproduct of norepinephrine metabolism, produced largely by oxidation of MHPG and to a lesser extent from oxidative deamination of normetanephrine and metanephrine *(117–119)* (Fig. 5). VMA is present in urine and plasma at very high concentrations (Table 3), which, like the conjugated metanephrines, makes measurement of VMA relatively simple. It is perhaps this that has made measurements of urinary VMA a time-honored, though not necessarily sensitive, biochemical test for diagnosis of pheochromocytoma.

With the exception of VMA, all the catecholamines and their metabolites are metabolized to sulfate conjugates, which represent other end products of norepinephrine metabolism typically present at higher concentrations than the free compounds (Table 3). In particular, the sulfate conjugates of the metanephrines are present in plasma and urine in concentrations more than 25-fold higher than those of the free compounds. Assays

Table 3
Concentrations of Free and Sulfate-Conjugated Norepinephrine, Epinephrine,
and Their Metabolites (mean±SEMs) in Normal Human Plasma

Compound	Free	Sulfate-Conjugated	% Free
Norepinephrine	1.38±0.08	4.88±0.43	22
Epinephrine	0.35±0.11	0.70±0.22	33
DHPG	5.53±0.20	6.09±0.33	48
Normetanephrine	0.25±0.02	9.13±0.95	3
Metanephrine	0.20±0.02	3.9±0.47	5
MHPG	14.34±0.54	25.55±2.73	26
VMA	33.65±2.33	0	100

of urine metanephrines, typically used for diagnosis of pheochromocytoma, employ a deconjugation step so that sulfate-conjugated metanephrines comprise the bulk of these measurements. Thus, these assays are largely measurements of different metabolites (i.e., sulfate conjugated derivatives) from those of the free metanephrines. The latter are present in plasma and urine at much lower and harder to detect concentrations than their sulfate-conjugated derivatives.

Differential Metabolism of Catecholamines

Although knowledge of the sources of catecholamines and the pathways of their metabolism is useful, what is perhaps more important to an understanding of the utility of catecholamines and their metabolites in the diagnosis of pheochromocytoma is an appreciation of how catecholamines are metabolized differently within neuronal and extraneuronal compartments, before and after their entry into the bloodstream and among various organs and tissues, including chromaffin cells and pheochromocytoma tumor tissue. Pheochromocytomas, like the adrenal medulla, differ from sympathetic neurons or central nervous system noradrenergic nerves in that they secrete catecholamines directly into the bloodstream. In contrast, only a small amount of the norepinephrine released from sympathetic nerves escapes neuronal and extraneuronal uptake to diffuse into the bloodstream (120–123) (Fig. 6).

Pheochromocytomas, however, differ from the adrenal medulla in that the tumors mainly secrete norepinephrine, whereas the predominant catecholamine secreted by the adrenal medulla is epinephrine. It is norepinephrine that is, therefore, more consistently elevated in patients with pheochromocytoma, although a significant, but much smaller, proportion may also show elevations in plasma or urinary epinephrine (124). Pheochromocytoma-associated elevations in only epinephrine are infrequent. Increases in epinephrine either occurring alone or in combination with norepinephrine are, however, quite common in pheochromocytomas associated with multiple endocrine neoplasia type 2 (MEN 2) (36,37). Dopamine and its metabolites are poor markers of pheochromocytoma and, although isolated cases have been described (125), pheochromocytomas that secrete only dopamine are extremely rare.

Because norepinephrine is the predominant catecholamine secreted by pheochromocytomas, an understanding of its metabolism after release and production within sympathetic nerves, as compared with after release directly into the circulation by a pheochromocytoma, is particularly important. Because monoamine oxidase is the only

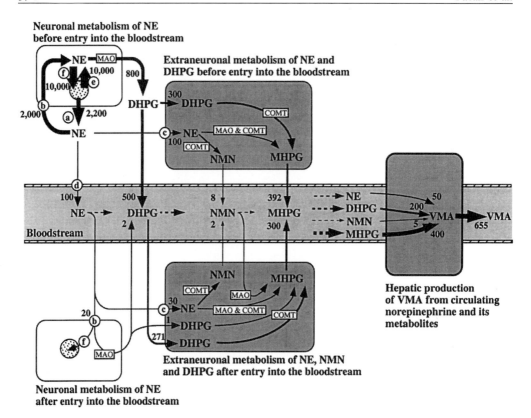

Fig. 6. Quantitative diagram showing neuronal and extraneuronal pathways of norepinephrine (NE) metabolism by monoamine oxidase (MAO) and catechol-O-methyltransferase (COMT) before and after entry of the compounds into the bloodstream and of hepatic production of vanillylmandelic acid (VMA) from circulating NE and its metabolites. Numbers at the head of arrows show relative rates of each process as derived from previously published data *(115,116,119,122,123,135)*. The diagram does not show sulfate conjugation pathways of metabolism that are particularly important for normetanephrine (NMN) and 3-methoxy-4-hydroxyphenylglycol (MHPG). The diagram also does not include the contribution of the adrenals to circulating NE (9%) and free normetanephrine (NMN) (24%). Most of the NE released by sympathetic nerves **(a)** is removed by neuronal uptake **(b)** and a much smaller amount is removed by extraneuronal uptake **(c)** so that only a small portion escapes to enter the bloodstream **(d)**. Most of the NE recaptured by sympathetic nerves is sequestered into storage vesicles by the vesicular monoamine transporter **(f)** and a smaller proportion is metabolized intraneuronally to 3,4-dihydroxyphenylglycol (DHPG). However, considerably more of the NE that is sequestered into storage vesicles or metabolized intraneuronally to DHPG is derived from transmitter leaking from storage vesicles **(e)** than from reuptake **(b)**. Very little circulating DHPG is derived from metabolism of circulating NE, whereas a significant proportion of the small amounts of circulating free NMN is formed from circulating NE. MHPG is mainly derived from O-methylation of DHPG before and after its entry into the bloodstream. VMA is mainly derived from metabolism of MHPG and DHPG in the liver.

catecholamine-metabolizing enzyme present in noradrenergic neurons, the norepinephrine metabolized within these neurons is all converted to DHPG *(126–128)* (Fig. 6). As a consequence, the DHPG appearing in plasma is almost exclusively produced in sympathetic neurons, whereas the additional presence of COMT in extraneuronal cells means that normetanephrine is exclusively a marker of extraneuronal norepinephrine metabolism *(122,127)*. Much of the DHPG formed in nerves is metabolized further to 3-methoxy-4-hydroxyphenylglcol (MHPG) by COMT in extraneuronal tissues *(115,127)*. Thus, in contrast to DHPG and normetanephrine, MHPG reflects both neuronal metabolism of norepinephrine to DHPG and extraneuronal metabolism of DHPG and normetanephrine, but is mainly derived from the DHPG produced in neurons *(115)*.

Comparison of neuronal and extraneuronal uptake has indicated that the former process is far more important than the latter for inactivation of neuronally released norepinephrine *(116,122,129)*, meaning that neuronal metabolism of recaptured norepinephrine is much more important than extraneuronal metabolism of the transmitter that escapes reuptake (Fig. 6). However, most of the norepinephrine deaminated within sympathetic nerves is not derived from recaptured transmitter, but rather from transmitter that leaks from storage vesicles into the sympathetic axoplasm *(123)*. This highly dynamic process of vesicular leakage and sequestration is the main determinant of norepinephrine metabolism and turnover, and contributes to the importance of neuronal over extraneuronal pathways for norepinephrine metabolism.

The aforementioned considerations, combined with the series nature of neuronal and extraneuronal removal mechanisms *(129)*, explain why very little of the DHPG in plasma (<1%) is derived from neuronal metabolism of circulating norepinephrine (Fig. 6). Thus, large increases in circulating norepinephrine caused by an iv infusion or release of the amine from a pheochromocytoma cause only small increases in DHPG compared with those accompanying sympathetic activation *(128,130)*. Hence, patients with pheochromocytoma and high norepinephrine levels often have normal or only slightly elevated plasma concentrations of DHPG *(103,130)*. This has led to the proposal that the relative plasma concentrations of norepinephrine to DHPG can provide additional useful information about the presence of a tumor *(130–132)*. Although there is some merit to this concept, use of the norepinephrine to DHPG ratio has not proven popular as a marker for a tumor, probably because of reports of some pheochromocytoma patients with both elevated plasma concentrations of norepinephrine and DHPG or normal norepinephrine to DHPG ratios caused by tumors that produce DHPG *(103)* or only epinephrine *(124)*. Nevertheless, findings of a high norepinephrine combined with a normal DHPG do provide supportive evidence that an increased norepinephrine is not because of sympathetic activation and might rather reflect a tumor. Whereas it cannot be ignored that both an increased norepinephrine and DHPG could reflect a tumor that produces DHPG, this pattern is more typical of a state of sympathetic activation.

In contrast to the greater importance of neuronal over extraneuronal pathways for metabolism of neuronally released norepinephrine, the reverse is the situation for metabolism of circulating norepinephrine (Fig. 6). The effects of neuronal uptake blockade with desipramine in humans indicate that only 20–30% of circulating norepinephrine is cleared by neuronal uptake, whereas for locally released norepinephrine, neuronal uptake is responsible for up to 90% and more of removal *(116,133,134)*. This, in part, reflects the series nature of neuronal and extraneuronal mechanisms operating between sites of neuronal release and the circulation, but it also influenced by organs such as the liver that play an important role in the clearance of circulating catecholamines by extraneuronal mechanisms *(119,135)*. As a result, about 20% of circulating levels of the extraneuronal metabolite, normetanephrine, are produced from circulating norepinephrine *(135,136)*, a relatively high amount compared to the less than 2% for the neuronal metabolite, DHPG. Because pheochromocytomas secrete catecholamines directly into the bloodstream, extraneuronal production of metanephrines from circulating catecholamines provides one reason why the metanephrines are better markers for a tumor than other metabolites that are largely derived from neuronal metabolism.

VMA, the major end product of norepinephrine and epinephrine metabolism, is produced almost exclusively from the hepatic extraction and metabolism of circulating catecholamines and their metabolites *(119)* (Fig. 6). This is because the enzyme responsible for formation of VMA from MHPG, alcohol dehydrogenase, is localized to the liver *(137,138)*. The substantial production of VMA from circulating DHPG and MHPG, most of which is derived from neuronal norepinephrine metabolism, explains why VMA is a relatively insensitive marker for pheochromocytoma compared with the precursor catecholamines and metanephrines *(8,139–142)*.

Production of Metanephrines within Chromaffin Tissue

At least 90% of metanephrine and up to 40% of normetanephrine are formed from epinephrine and norepinephrine within the adrenals before release of these catecholamines into the circulation *(135,136)*. This makes the adrenal medulla the single largest source of both normetanephrine and metanephrine in the body, exceeding the contribution of the liver *(135)*, which helps explain why so little of these circulating metabolites (6% for metanephrine and 20% for normetanephrine) are formed from metabolism of catecholamines after release into the circulation *(136)*. Adrenal medullary and pheochromocytoma tissue contain high quantities of the membrane-bound form of COMT *(143)*, the isoenzyme most important for O-methylation of catecholamines *(144)*. The COMT is localized within chromaffin cells so it would appear the metanephrines from these sources are derived from catecholamines leaking from storage vesicles into the chromaffin cell cytoplasm. In patients with pheochromocytoma, over 94% of the elevated plasma concentrations of metanephrines in these patients are derived from metabolism of catecholamines by the COMT within chromaffin cells and not by actions of extraadrenal COMT on catecholamines released by tumors into the circulation *(143)*. This means that production of metanephrines is an ongoing process within chromaffin cells, independent of catecholamine release, explaining why plasma metanephrines are relatively insensitive markers of sympathoadrenalmedullary activation or of a paroxysmal attack associated with large increases in catecholamine release from a pheochromocytoma *(143)*.

Sensitivity of Biochemical Tests

A problem with use of plasma or urinary catecholamines for diagnosis of pheochromocytoma is that some tumors are quiescent or encapsulated and may not secrete large amounts of catecholamines, whereas other tumors appear to secrete catecholamines episodically. Thus, plasma levels and urinary outputs of catecholamines are normal in a small, but important, proportion (5–15%) of patients with pheochromocytoma and the presence of a pheochromocytoma cannot be reliably excluded using measurements of plasma or urinary catecholamine concentrations *(8,10,33,56,108–111,145)*. In contrast, plasma-free metanephrines (either normetanephrine or metanephrine or both) are constantly produced by the actions of COMT on catecholamines leaking from storage vesicles within tumors and therefore show much more consistent increases above normal than plasma catecholamines and appear to reliably exclude the presence of all but the smallest of pheochromocytomas *(33,143)*. Where excluded, no other tests are necessary.

This means that measurements of plasma-free metanephrines avoid a missed diagnosis and minimize the need to run multiple diagnostic tests to exclude the presence of a tumor.

Because the free metanephrines are formed extraneuronally, and to a large extent within chromaffin tissues (e.g., adrenal medulla and pheochromocytoma), these metabolites are also more sensitive markers for a pheochromocytoma than the other catecholamine metabolites that are derived mainly from neuronal sources.

Urinary metanephrines are commonly measured after acid hydrolysis and thus largely represent sulfate-conjugated metanephrines. A substantial amount of the normetanephrine-sulfate is derived from sulfate conjugation of normetanephrine produced in parts of the body other than the adrenal medulla or pheochromocytoma tumor chromaffin tissue. Therefore, the sulfate-conjugated normetanephrine, as commonly measured in urine, is a less-sensitive marker of pheochromocytoma than the free normetanephrine measured in plasma. Nevertheless, fractionated measurements of urinary deconjugated normetanephrine and metanephrine (i.e., free plus sulfate conjugated metanephrines), performed by modern HPLC methods, do provide a reasonably sensitive biochemical test for diagnosis of pheochromocytoma, and these measurements may be more sensitive than measurements of catecholamines (7,111).

Specificity of Biochemical Tests

Because upper reference limits of normal of most diagnostic tests are typically established form the 95% confidence intervals of a range of values determined in a reference population, it is reasonable to expect at least a 2.5% incidence of false positives and specificity at least no greater than that set from the confidence intervals of the reference population. In practice, however, numbers of false-positive test results are often higher than would be expected from the reference population; this can be particularly problematic for the biochemical tests used to detect pheochromocytoma.

Because catecholamines and their metabolites are ubiquitously produced by the sympathoadrenalmedullary system, none of these compounds are highly specific for the presence of a pheochromocytoma. In particular, plasma and urinary catecholamines may be elevated by a variety of physiological, pharmacological, and pathological conditions (107). As yet, none of the various biochemical markers of pheochromocytoma have been shown by any rigorous study to be any more specific than the others for diagnosis of a tumor. Nevertheless, the combination of measurements of parent amines and certain metabolites can be useful in helping to distinguish elevated catecholamines caused by a tumor from elevated catecholamines secondary to sympathoadrenalmedullary activation.

Sympathoadrenalmedullary activation associated with exercise, mental stress, hypotension, hypovolemia, hypoglycemia, or certain drugs are all conditions that may elevate plasma and urinary catecholamines and cause false positive test results. During blood sampling and 24-h urine collections, these influences must be avoided. Posture is another important determinant of catecholamine release, increasing plasma norepinephrine by as much as three-fold above supine values. Therefore, collection of blood samples should be performed with the patient resting quietly supine for at least 20 min before sampling with an indwelling iv catheter previously inserted to avoid any possible acute stress associated with venepuncture.

A wide variety of pathological conditions may be associated with elevated plasma and urinary catecholamines. Congestive heart failure, renovascular hypertension, hypernoradrenergic hypertension, shock, sepsis, dumping syndrome, sleep apnea, anxiety neurosis, and panic disorder are some of the syndromes that may be associated with elevated plasma or urinary catecholamines and clinical symptoms suggestive of a pheochromocytoma.

The aforementioned physiological and pathological conditions can also lead to elevated production of metanephrines and VMA, with attendant false positives for these metabolites. However, because production of these metabolites is somewhat independent of catecholamine release from the sympathoadrenalmedullary system, their proportional increases are typically less than those in catecholamines. The metanephrines, in particular, are relatively poor markers of sympathoadrenal activation *(136,143)*. Theoretically, this should make the metanephrines less prone to false-positive results in physiological and pathological states associated with sympathoadrenalmedullary activation. However, there are other factors to consider that may additionally contribute to false-positive test results for these tests. Deficiencies or pharmacological inhibition of MAO increases both urinary deconjugated and plasma-free metanephrines caused by impaired breakdown of the metabolite by MAO and increased shunting of metabolism through O-methylation pathways *(146,147)*. Severe renal failure can be particularly problematic in patients with pheochromocytoma, making urine test results unreliable or urine collection impossible *(148)*. In these patients, biochemical diagnosis typically requires assays of plasma catecholamines and metanephrines. However, the sympathetic nervous system can be activated in these patients resulting in elevated norepinephrine levels. Also, end products of catecholamine metabolism, that depend on elimination by the kidneys—such as the sulfate conjugated metanephrines—tend to build up in plasma to very high levels *(149)*. Reduced renal perfusion in states such as congestive heart failure and hypertension with impaired renal function can also reduce the circulatory clearance of metabolic end products leading to increased plasma concentrations independent of any effect of sympathetic activation.

The clinician should be sensitive to the fact that biochemical test results present a range of values and should not be simply considered as either negative (within the normal range) or positive (above the normal range). Rather, the magnitude of an increase above the upper reference limits should also be considered when specificity is an issue. For example, a patient presenting with suggestive symptoms and a plasma norepinephrine concentration of over 2500 pg/mL (14.8 pmol/mL), approx five times above the upper reference limit of normal, is far more likely to have a pheochromocytoma than a patient with the same symptoms and a plasma norepinephrine concentration just above the upper reference limits. The few conditions where plasma norepinephrine can reach such high levels (e.g., hypernoradrenergic hypertension, end stage congestive heart failure, circulatory shock) are easily excluded. In patients with pheochromocytoma, plasma concentrations of free metanephrines typically show much higher relative increases above the upper reference limits than observed for tests of catecholamines, urinary metanephrines and VMA. This indicates that at the higher limits more specific for a tumor, measurements of plasma-free metanephrines provide better proof of a pheochromocytoma than other available tests.

Glucagon-Stimulation and Clonidine-Suppression Tests

Glucagon-stimulation and clonidine-suppression tests, used appropriately in the right situation, are additional interventional test procedures that can help improve the accuracy of plasma levels of catecholamines in the diagnosis of pheochromocytoma. Glucagon stimulation is perhaps the most specific provocative test for diagnosis of pheochromocytoma. The glucagon is given in the dose of 1.0 mg intravenously. The catecholamine response to glucagon is very fast so that timing of blood collection is crucial. A threefold increase in plasma norepinephrine levels 2 min after glucagon administration indicates a pheochromocytoma with a high degree of specificity (150). The sensitivity of the test in patients with pheochromocytoma who have normal plasma norepinephrine levels is only 62%, but increases to 81% if carried out in patients with elevated baseline levels of plasma norepinephrine. The value of the test, therefore, resides in its specificity rather than its sensitivity. Also, in patients with adrenal incidentalomas, the glucagon-stimulation test has been reported not to offer any additional advantage in diagnosis of pheochromocytoma over standard biochemical tests of catecholamines (151).

Clonidine, as a centrally acting alpha$_2$ adrenoceptor agonist, inhibits release of norepinephrine from sympathetic nerves, but not from pheochromocytomas. Thus, the clonidine suppression test is particularly useful in patients with increased plasma norepinephrine, in whom it is unclear whether the increase is caused by sympathetic activation or catecholamine release from a tumor (152). Clonidine is administered in a dose of 0.3 mg/70 kg orally and complete lack of a decrease in norepinephrine (below 500 pg/mL) 3 h after the drug is highly suggestive of a pheochromocytoma, whereas a substantial decrease in plasma norepinephrine indicates a source of the amine from sympathetic nerves (150,153). Perhaps a problem with the test is that there are no clear-cut guidelines for the degree of decrease or the level of plasma norepinephrine reached that constitutes a positive or negative test result.

As reported by Grossman et al. (150), the glucagon test has 100% specificity with 81% sensitivity and the clonidine test a 67% specificity and 97% sensitivity. Grossman and colleagues concluded that if both tests are used, a conclusive result can be obtained in about 80% of the patients. However, it should also be considered that it is not always appropriate to carry out both tests in the same patient. A clonidine-suppression test carried out in a patient with a normal plasma norepinephrine is likely to be of little value (154), whereas the glucagon-stimulation test carried out in the same patient may evoke catecholamine release in an otherwise silent tumor. Using the aforementioned pharmacological tests, the clinician should also be aware of the possibility of glucagon-induced rapid and marked increase in blood pressure and clonidine-induced hypotension and bradycardia, especially when a patient is taking beta adrenoceptor blockers. The risk of a hypertensive crisis can be reduced by administering either a dihydropyridine (e.g., 10 mg nifedipine orally) 30 min before glucagon administration or a α-adrenergic blockading agent, such as phenoxybenzamine (155).

Possible interference from medications must also be considered. Tricyclic antidepressants may be particularly problematic. These drugs not only inhibit norepinephrine reuptake, and thus increase the norepinephrine to DHPG ratio (this can be suggestive of a pheochromocytoma), but they also substantially reduce sympathetic outflow through actions within the brain (134,156). Elevated plasma norepinephrine in this situation is thus maintained not by increased sympathetic outflow, but by blockade of norepinephrine removal at neuroeffector sites. Suppression of sympathetic activity with clonidine is no longer possible and a false-positive test is imminent.

In summary, biochemical testing is particularly important for the initial workup of a patient suspected of harboring a pheochromocytoma. Choice of appropriate biochemical testing procedures, their sequence of use and the interpretation of test results can benefit considerably from an understanding of the disposition and metabolism of catecholamines among different cellular compartments and in various clinical conditions where differential diagnosis may be important.

PHEOCHROMOCYTOMA IMAGING

Computed Tomography and Magnetic Resonance Imaging

A variety of imaging techniques are available for localization of a pheochromocytoma. In most institutions, computed tomography (CT) of the abdomen, either with or without contrast, provides the initial method of localizing pheochromocytoma. CT can be used to localize adrenal tumors 0.5–1.0 cm or larger and extraadrenal tumors 2 cm or larger *(157,158)*. Although 90% of pheochromocytomas are located in the adrenals, a CT scan of the entire abdomen is preferable so that in patients with normal adrenals, localization of an extraadrenal tumor is possible without additional delay. Administration of iv contrast media for CT scanning is preferred, but these agents have been suggested to evoke norepinephrine release from tumors. A study in which the nonionic contrast medium iohexol was used did not, however, find any support for this notion *(159)*. Nevertheless, administration of phenoxybenzamine and atenolol before administration of contrast agents remains customary and provides a precautionary measure against hypertensive paroxysms and annlythmias.

Although CT may localize about 95% of pheochromocytomas, magnetic resonance imaging (MRI) with or without gadolinium enhancement is the most reliable method and may identify more than 95% of tumors and is superior to CT in detecting extraadrenal tumors (almost 100% sensitivity) and familial adrenal pheochromocytoma *(157,158,160)*. MRI may also be used as the initial imaging procedure when there is pregnancy or allergy to the contrast materials used for CT scans.

Because of widespread use of CT in diagnostic medicine, it is important to distinguish between functionally and nonfunctionally incidentally discovered adrenal or extraadrenal masses. If there are no clinical signs or symptoms and biochemical tests are negative, a high suspicion exists that an incidentally discovered mass is nonfunctional *(161)*. Regular follow-up is necessary for masses less than 3 cm in size, surgery should be considered for larger ones.

Metaiodobenzylguanidine (MIBG) Imaging

In rare cases, pheochromocytoma cannot be localized by CT or MRI studies. This may be because of very small tumor size or unusual locations of a tumor such as in the heart or neck. In such cases, whole-body scanning using metaiodobenzylguanidine (MIBG) labeled with radioiodine (^{123}I or ^{131}I) should be considered.

After iv injection, MIBG is concentrated in peripheral sympathetic neurons, the adrenal medulla, and tumors by neuronal uptake, a high energy, temperature, and sodium-dependent mechanism [for review, see *(13)*]. MIBG specifically concentrates in catecholamine storage vesicles and enables whole-body screening. MIBG enables an excellent visualization of body areas with excess catecholamine concentrations, yielding nearly 100% specificity *(162–164)*. Nevertheless, occasional reports of false-positive tests with MIBG *(165)* illustrate the need to support a positive MIBG imaging result with other evidence of a pheochromocytoma. Also, as reviewed by Manger and

Gifford, MIBG can be accumulated in other tumors such as carcinoid, medullary thyroid carcinoma, and small-cell lung carcinoma (157).

MIBG labeled with ^{131}I provides negative results in up to 15% of patients with proven pheochromocytomas (166). Much better sensitivity is, however, available with MIBG labeled with [123]I (167,168). Another advantage of ^{123}I-labeled MIBG over ^{131}I-labeled MIBG is its additional utility for imaging by single-photon emission computed tomography (SPECT). The accumulation of MIBG can be decreased by a number of classes of drugs: (1) agents that cause depletion of storage vesicle contents, such as sympathomimetics, reserpine, and labetolol; (2) agents that inhibit neuronal uptake, including cocaine, tricyclic antidepressant, and tranquilizers; and (3) other drugs such as calcium channel blockers and α- and β-adrenergic receptor blockers [for review, see (169)]. The frequently used α-adrenergic receptor blocking agent, phenoxybenzamine, probably interferes with MIBG uptake only at high doses (169).

In patients with MEN-2A, who present with clear clinical suspicion of having a pheochromocytoma, CT of the adrenals is the first choice to localize a pheochromocytoma. However, if bilateral adrenal involvement is not revealed, MIBG should be performed (32,170). At present, arteriography is no longer indicated.

Positron Emission Tomographic Imaging

A new promising method, positron emission tomography (PET), has the ability to detect pathologic tissue based on physiologic and biochemical processes within the abnormal tissue (171). Recently, [^{18}F]-fluorodeoxyglucose has been used as a marker of tumor activity, based on its increased uptake caused by the higher rate of glycolysis in tumor tissue as compared with most normal tissues (172,173). [^{18}F]-fluorodeoxyglucose or [^{11}C]-hydroxyephedrine localize well in pheochromocytoma, but their use at this stage is experimental and directed toward situations where other more readily available imaging studies fail to reveal the source of excessive catecholamine production (174).

In summary, imaging studies are particularly useful in locating a pheochromocytoma once its presence has been established by clinical screening and biochemical testing. CT and MRI are highly sensitive as first-choice imaging procedures for localizing a tumor, whereas MIBG offers higher specificity.

DIAGNOSTIC PROCEDURAL RECOMMENDATIONS

Initial Biochemical Testing

With issues of sensitivity and specificity in mind, as well as consideration of the potential dangers of a pheochromocytoma and the rarity of the tumor, the most important consideration in choice of initial biochemical test is the reliability of the test for exclusion of pheochromocytoma. In pheochromocytoma, a missed diagnosis because of a false-negative test result can have catastrophic consequences for the patient. In contrast, a single false-positive test result can be refuted by further tests. Therefore, a suitably sensitive biochemical test remains the first choice in the initial workup of the patient suspected to be harboring a pheochromocytoma. With most available biochemical tests, however, confirming the absence of a tumor can be more problematic than confirming the presence of a tumor.

Because of the high sensitivity of the test, our recommendation is to use HPLC measurements of plasma-free normetanephrine and metanephrine. This test should preferably be combined with HPLC measurements of plasma catecholamines collected under appropriately controlled circumstances for further interpretation of any elevations in plasma-free metanephrines. To circumvent false-positive test results, appropriate consideration should always be given to interference with assay results by any drugs that the patient may be receiving. In centers where measurements of plasma-free metanephrines are not available, we recommend that initial biochemical tests for exclusion of a pheochromocytoma should include either HPLC measurements of plasma or 24-h urine deconjugated (free + sulfate conjugated) normetanephrine and metanephrine combined with measurements of plasma or urinary catecholamines. Because of a lower sensitivity, a finding of a normal 24-h urinary output of VMA is of little practical use in initial exclusion of a pheochromocytoma. Although, some have proposed the use of spot urine metanephrine tests, with values corrected for creatinine *(106)*, these additional creatinine measurements introduce another potential confounding variable into the equation. Measurements in urine should always be performed on carefully collected 24-h specimens.

If plasma-free metanephrines have been run, and they are well within the normal range, then it is highly unlikely that the patient has anything but a very small tumor (<2 cm) and there should be little need to run further tests. On the other hand, normal results for each of the other biochemical tests, even when performed in combination, are still possible in a small percentage of patients with a pheochromocytoma. Thus, if plasma-free metanephrines have not been run, but the other above test results are all normal, then although unlikely it is still possible that the patient has a pheochromocytoma. If suggestive signs or symptoms persist, repeat biochemical testing may be appropriate.

Secondary Diagnostic Tests

If tests of plasma-free metanephrines or any of the above combination of test results are positive, then the clinician must consider further tests to exclude or prove the existence of a pheochromocytoma. At this stage, it is again important to consider any potential associated clinical conditions or influences of medications that may cause a false-positive test result (see previous section on SPECIFICITY). Additional considerations include the magnitude of increase above normal of biochemical test results along with the pattern of alterations in biochemical parameters that may be used together to make some kind of qualitative assessment of the likelihood that the patient has a tumor. From this, a strategy for further testing can be developed, including imaging studies to localize the tumor, provocation tests, and further biochemical tests. Ultimately, it is a combination of biochemical and radiological tests combined with clinical assessment of symptoms, signs, and associated conditions that provides the clinician with sufficient evidence to establish or refute the diagnosis.

Ruling out Sympathoadenalmedullary Activation

Use of the clonidine-suppression test is particularly useful when there is suspicion that elevated plasma levels of norepinephrine are secondary to sympathetic activation rather than a pheochromocytoma. In situations such as this, it might be more practical to carry out a clonidine-suppression test before imaging studies. Patterns of biochemical test results that are more suggestive of sympathoadrenalmedullary activation than a tumor (such as occurs in hypernoradrenergic hypertension, renovascular hypertension, congestive heart failure, panic disorder, dumping syndrome, and other conditions), include proportionally larger elevations above the upper reference limits of normal of plasma norepinephrine or epinephrine than of plasma normetanephrine or metanephrine. In sympathetic activation, increases in plasma DHPG parallel the increases in norepinephrine typically reflect increased neuronal uptake of norepinephrine, indicative of a sympathoneuronal source of the elevated norepinephrine. This pattern of biochemical test results combined with a negative clonidine suppression test result (i.e., a substantial decrease in plasma norepinephrine after clonidine) is highly suggestive of sympathetic activation rather than a tumor, and, unless imaging studies suggest otherwise, a pheochromocytoma can be excluded and no further tests should be necessary.

Localizing the Tumor

If plasma or urine levels of catecholamines and metanephrines are extremely high or suppression tests and/or stimulation tests are positive (i.e., plasma norepinephrine does not decrease after clonidine, plasma norepinephrine shows a substantial increase after glucagon), and if the biochemical pattern of test results are indicative of a tumor rather than sympathetic activation, then it is important to localize the tumor for subsequent surgical removal.

In most cases of positive initial biochemical test results, where clinical suspicion of a pheochromocytoma remains reasonable, a CT or MRI scan of the entire abdomen may be immediately appropriate. A finding of an adrenal or abdominal mass, together with typical clinical signs and symptoms and highly elevated catecholamines and their metabolites and an appropriate pattern of changes in metabolites and catecholamine precursors (i.e., larger relative increases in plasma-free metanephrines than catecholamines and/or normal plasma DHPG levels), is not sufficient to justify surgery since metastic disease must be ruled out. Therefore, MIBG scintigraphy, preferably using the ^{123}I-labeled compound is important next step in diagnostic work, up before surgical removal of the tumor.

In rare cases, where imaging studies are all negative, but where suspicion of a pheochromocytoma remains high, it may be appropriate to consider a vena caval sampling procedure to establish the source of the high circulating levels of catecholamines or metanephrines.

Identifying the "Silent" Pheochromocytoma

In occasional cases of sporadic pheochromocytoma and in some incidentalomas, but quite frequently during routine screening of VHL and MEN-2 patients, a small adrenal mass may be present without any of the symptoms and signs associated with a pheochromocytoma (8,56,145). In these patients, the pheochromocytoma is "silent" and may not produce catecholamines in amounts sufficient to cause typical symptoms or a positive test result for plasma or urinary catecholamines, urinary VMA, or urinary total metanephrines. These patients, however, typically show some elevation of either plasma-free normetanephrine (VHL patients) or both plasma-free normetanephrine and metanephrine or only metanephrine (MEN-2 patients). Should this not be sufficient reason to operate, then it is important to follow these patients carefully over time, because as the tumor(s) enlarge, the plasma-free metanephrines increase providing stronger reason to operate. Use of glucagon-stimulation tests and other imaging techniques with higher specificity than CT, such as MIBG scintigraphy, may also be useful to identify a silent pheochromocytoma. However, the likelihood of false-negative results for the glucagon-stimulation test and MIBG scanning, particularly in cases of small tumors, point to the need for careful follow-up studies in patients suspected of harboring a silent pheochromocytoma.

In summary, the combination of clinical screening, biochemical testing, and imaging studies, when used appropriately, provide a useful and reliable approach to establishing the absence or presence of a pheochromocytoma. Avoidance of false-negative results is critical to the initial workup of a patient suspected of harboring a pheochromocytoma. Initial findings of a positive biochemical test can be confirmed or refuted by further biochemical and imaging studies.

MANAGEMENT OF PHEOCHROMOCYTOMA

Preoperative Management of Pheochromocytoma

To minimize operative and postoperative complications, appropriate medical treatment is an important part of the management of pheochromocytoma. The preoperative medical treatment is directed at controling hypertension, including hypertensive crisis during the removal of pheochromocytoma, to maintain stable blood pressure during surgery, and to minimize adverse effects during anesthesia and other clinical signs and symptoms caused by high plasma catecholamine levels.

Maintenance of adequate blood pressure control for 2 wk before the operation is an important aspect of management once a tumor is diagnosed. At first, treatment should be initiated with the noncompetitive α-adrenoceptor blocker phenoxybenzamine (Dibenzyline). The initial dose of long-acting phenoxybenzamine is usually 10 mg twice a day and is increased until the clinical manifestations are controlled or side effects appear. Mostly, a total daily dose of 1 mg/kg is sufficient. Other antihypertensive agents, such as the α-adrenergic receptor blockers, prazosin or doxazosine, have not been established to be sufficiently safe. Available evidence continues to support the use of phenoxybenzamine as the drug of choice (175).

Hypertensive crises that can manifest as severe headache, visual disturbances, acute myocardial infarction, congestive heart failure, or cerebrovascular accident are appropriately treated with an iv bolus of 5 mg phentolamine (Regitine). Phentolamine has a very short half-time, therefore, if necessary, the same dose can be repeated every 2 min until hypertension is adequately controlled or phentolamine is given as a continuous infusion (100 mg of phentolamine in 500 mL of 5% dextrose in water). A continuous iv infusion of sodium nitroprusside (preparation similar to phentolamine) or in some cases nifedipine (10 mg orally or sublingually) can also be used to control hypertension. Sufficient attention should also be given to the possibility that some drugs, such as tricyclic antidepressants, metoclopramide, and naloxone, can cause hypertensive crisis in patients with pheochromocytoma (9).

In patients with clinical manifestations caused by β-adrenoceptor stimulation (e.g., tachycardia or arrhythmias, angina, nervousness, and so on) β-adrenergic receptor blockers such as propranolol, atenolol, or metoprolol are indicated. β-adrenoceptor blockers, however, should never be employed before α-adrenoceptor blockers are administered because unopposed stimulation of α-adrenoceptors and loss of β-adrenoceptor-mediated vasodilatation may cause a serious and life-threatening elevation of blood pressure. Labetelol, a combined α- and β-adrenoceptor blocker, is not preferred because in some patients it may cause hypertension perhaps by its greater effect on beta than α-adrenoceptors (176).

α-methyl-para-tyrosine (metyrosine) inhibits the synthesis of catecholamines by blocking tyrosine hydroxylase. In some clinical centers, this drug is used in those patients who have persistent catecholamine-induced clinical manifestations including hypertension despite treatment with α and β adrenergic drugs. The initial dose is 250 mg every 6 h, up to a total dose of 2–4 g daily [for review, see (177,178)].

As reviewed in detail by Bravo and Gifford (9), to ensure adequate preoperative preparation, several criteria should be fulfilled: (1) blood pressure not greater than 160/90 mm Hg; (2) orthostatic hypotension not exceeding 80/45 mm Hg; and (3) no more than one ventricular extrasystole every 5 min and EKG without nonspecific ST segment elevations or depression and T-wave inversions. If necessary, hypovolemia may be corrected by iv infusion of appropriate fluids perioperatively to avoid hypotension. Pressor agents are not usually effective in the presence of severe and persistent hypovolemia. Because of excessive insulin release, previously inhibited by high-circulating catecholamines, postoperative hypoglycemia may occur and can be successfully treated with 5% dextrose. Despite successful surgery, 25% of patients remain hypertensive (157).

Surgical removal of intraadrenal pheochromocytomas may be successfully carried out by laparoscopy, a procedure that minimizes catecholamine-induced hemodynamic changes during operation, postoperative morbidity, hospital stay, and expense compared to conventional transabdominal adrenalectomy (179,180). Because of the high incidence of bilateral adrenal disease in familial pheochromocytoma, partial adrenalectomies have been advocated in these patients in order to preserve adrenal function and avoid the morbidity associated with medical adrenal replacement (181).

In patients with familial or metastatic pheochromocytoma, it is important to know whether the tumor involves one or both adrenal glands or metastases are present. In cases of unilateral or bilateral localization, the pheochromocytomas are removed first and treatment of other conditions that coexist with familial pheochromocytoma (e.g., medullary thyroid cancer, hyperparathyroidism) follows. When metastatic disease is found, medical therapy is the initial treatment of choice.

Malignant Pheochromocytoma

Malignant pheochromocytoma requires more aggressive treatment than that used for metastic pheochromocytoma. Except for traditional antihypertensive therapy, there are few studies describing the role of cytotoxic therapy in treatment of malignant pheochromocytoma [for review, see (182)]. However, such treatment should be initiated only in patients in whom the quality of life is affected or metastatic lesions are aggressive and affect local surrounding tissue. As described by Averbach et al., combination chemotherapy with cyclophosphamide, vincristine, and dacarbazine produces a complete or partial response rate of clinical and radiologic signs in 57% of patients and biochemical response based on 24-h urinary measurement of catecholamines, metanephrines, and VMA in 79% of patients (182). Painful skeletal metastatic lesions are treated with external radiation.

Pheochromocytoma in Pregnancy

Pheochromocytoma in pregnancy is a rare, but one of the most serious, conditions with a high maternal mortality if unrecognized before delivery. Maternal mortality amounts to nearly 50%, but an early diagnosis and treatment decrease mortality to nearly 10% *(183–185)*. A special difficulty in recognizing a pheochromocytoma during pregnancy is the potential confusion of signs attributable to preeclampsia. The biochemical diagnosis is similar as in nonpregnant patients because the "normal" values of catecholamines and its metabolites are similar in pregnancy. An MRI, rather than CT, is the first choice for localizing the tumor in pregnancy. In the first half of pregnancy, the tumor should be removed after the usual preparation of the mother with phenoxybenzamine. After 24 wk, the patient should be treated medically and surgery should be postponed until fetal maturity has been reached, at which stage a cesarean section is called for. Removal of the pheochromocytoma should be carried out at the time of cesarean section.

In summary, if diagnosis of pheochromocytoma is made correctly and early (the tumor is frequently under detected) and no metastatic disease is present, the condition is usually curable by tumor resection. The 5-yr survival of patients operated for benign pheochromocytoma is 95%, whereas that for malignant pheochromocytoma is 36–50% *(157)*. However, left untreated, pheochromocytomas have a high probability of eventually proving fatal.

REFERENCES

1. Webb TA, Sheps SG, Carney JA. Differences between sporadic pheochromocytoma and pheochromocytoma in multiple endocrine neoplasia, type 2. Am J Surg Pathol 1980; 4:121–126.
2. Manger WM, Gifford RW. Clinical and Experimental Pheochromocytoma. Blackwell Science, Cambridge, MA, 1996.
3. Epstein FH, Eckhoff RD. The epidemiology of high blood pressure—geographic distributions and etiologic factors. In: Stamler J, Stamler R, Pullman TN eds. The epidemiology of hypertension. Grune and Stratton, New York, 1967, pp. 155–166.
4. Page LB. Epidemiologic evidence on the etiology of human hypertension and its possible prevention. Am Heart J 1976; 91:527–534.
5. Goldfien A. Basic Endocrinology. Appleton and Lange, Norwalk, CT, 1998, pp. 370.
6. Ram CV, Fierro-Carrion GA. Pheochromocytoma. Semin Nephrol 1995; 15:126–137.
7. Casanova S, Rosenberg-Bourgin M, Farkas D, et al. Pheochromocytoma in multiple endocrine neoplasia type 2 A: survey of 100 cases. Clin Endocrinol 1993; 38:531–537.
8. Neumann HP, Berger DP, Sigmund G, et al. Pheochromocytomas, multiple endocrine neoplasia type 2, and von Hippel-Lindau disease. N Engl J Med 1993; 329:1531–1538.
9. Bravo EL, Gifford RW. Pheochromocytoma. Endocrinol Metab North Am 1993; 22:329–341.
10. Stein PP, Black HR. A simplified diagnostic approach to pheochromocytoma. A review of the literature and report of one institution's experience. Medicine 1991; 70:46–66.
11. Gifford RW, Kvale WF, Maher FT, Roth GM, Priestley JT. Clinical features, diagnosis, and treatment of pheochromocytoma. A review of 76 cases. Mayo Clin Proc 1964; 39:281–302.
12. Kvale WF, Roth GM, Manger WM, Priestley JT. Pheochromocytoma. Circulation 1956; 14:622–630.
13. Bouloux PG, Fakeeh M. Investigation of pheochromocytoma. Clin Endocrinol (Oxf) 1995; 43:657–664.
14. Moon HD, Koneff AA, Li CC, Simpson ME. Pheochromocytomas of adrenals in male rats chronically injected with pituitary growth hormone. Proc Soc Exp Biol Med 1956; 93:74–77.
15. Lupulescou A. Less pheochromocytomes experimentaux. Ann Endocrinol 1961; 22:459–468.
16. Scott HW Jr, Oates JA, Nies AS, Burko H, Page DL, Rhamy RK. Pheochromocytoma: present diagnosis and management. Ann Surg 1976; 183:587–593.
17. Goldfarb DA, Novick AC, Bravo EL, Straffon RA, Montie JE, Kay R. Experience with extra-adrenal pheochromocytoma. J Urol 1989; 142:931–936.
18. van Heerden JA, Roland CF, Carney JA, Sheps SG, Grant CS. Long-term evaluation following resection of apparently benign pheochromocytoma(s)/paraganglioma(s). World J Surg 1990; 14:325–329.

19. O'Riordain DS, Young WF Jr, Grant CS, Carney JA, van Heerden JA. Clinical spectrum and outcome of functional extraadrenal paraganglioma. World J Surg 1996; 20:916–21; discussion.

20. Daneman A. Adrenal neoplasms in children. Semin Roentgenol 1988; 23:205–215.

21. Clarke MR, Weyant RJ, Watson CG, Carty SE. Prognostic markers in pheochromocytoma. Hum Pathol 1998; 29:522–526.

22. Linnoila RI, Lack EE, Steinberg SM, Keiser HR. Decreased expression of neuropeptides in malignant pheochromocytomas: an immunohistochemical study. Hum Pathol 1988; 19:41–50.

23. Kubota Y, Nakada T, Sasagawa I, Yanai H, Itoh K. Elevated levels of telomerase activity in malignant pheochromocytoma. Cancer 1998; 82:176–179.

24. Kinoshita H, Ogawa O, Mishina M, et al. Telomerase activity in adrenal cortical tumors and pheochromocytomas with reference to clinicopathologic features. Urol Res 1998; 26:29–32.

25. Lewis PD. A cytophotometric study of benign and malignant pheochromocytomas. Virchows Arch B Cell Pathol 1971; 9:371–376.

26. Hosaka Y, Rainwater LM, Grant CS, Farrow GM, van Heerden JA, Lieber MM. Pheochromocytoma: nuclear deoxyribonucleic acid patterns studied by flow cytometry. Surgery 1986; 100:1003–1010.

27. Liu J, Voutilainen R, Kahri AI, Heikkila P. Expression patterns of the c-myc gene in adrenocortical tumors and pheochromocytomas. J Endocrinol 1997; 152:175–181.

27a. Milunsky J, DeStefano AL, Huang XL, Baldwin CT, Michels VV, Jako G, Milunsky A. Familial paragangliomas: linkage to chromosome 11q23 and clinical implications. Am J Med Genet 1997; 72:66–72.

27b. Walther MM, Reiter R, Keiser HR, et al. Clinical and genetic characterization of pheochromocytoma in von Hippel-Lindau families: comparison with sporadic pheochromocytoma gives insight into natural history of pheochromocytoma. J Urol 1999; 162:659–664.

27c. Tisherman SE, Tisherman BG, Tisherman SA, Dunmore S, Levey GS, Mulvihill JJ. Three-decade investigation of familial pheochromocytoma. An allele of von Hippel-Lindau disease? Arch Intern Med 1993; 153:2250–2556.

28. Carney JA, Sizemore GW, Sheps SG. Adrenal medullary disease in multiple endocrine neoplasia type 2: pheochromocytoma and its precursors. Am J Clin Pathol 1976; 66:279–290.

28a. Wilson RA, Ibanez ML. A comparative study of 14 cases of familial and nonfamilial pheochromocytomas. Hum Pathol 1978; 9:181–188.

28b. Eng C, Crossey PA, Mulligan LM, et al. Mutations in the RET protooncogene and the von Hippel-Lindau disease tumour suppressor gene in sporadic and syndromic pheochromocytomas. J Med Genet 1995; 32:934–937.

29. Richard S, Beigelman C, Duclos JM, et al. Pheochromocytoma as the first manifestation of von Hippel-Lindau disease. Surgery 1994; 116:1076–1981.

30. Gagel RF, Tashjian AH Jr, Cummings T, et al. The clinical outcome of prospective screening for multiple endocrine neoplasia type 2a. An 18-year experience. N Engl J Med 1988; 318:478–484.

31. Calmettes C, Ponder BA, Fischer JA, Raue F. Early diagnosis of the multiple endocrine neoplasia type 2 syndrome: consensus statement. European Community Concerted Action: Medullary Thyroid Carcinoma. Eur J Clin Invest 1992; 22:755–760.

32. Pomares FJ, Canas R, Rodriguez JM, Hernandez AM, Parrilla P, Tebar FJ. Differences between sporadic and multiple endocrine neoplasia type 2A pheochromocytoma. Clin Endocrinol 1998; 48:195–200.

33. Lenders JW, Keiser HR, Goldstein DS, et al. Plasma metanephrines in the diagnosis of pheochromocytoma. Ann Intern Med 1995; 123:101–109.

34. Howe JR, Norton JA, Wells SA. Prevalence of pheochromocytoma and hyperparathyroidism in multiple endocrine neoplasia type 2A: results of long-term follow-up. Surgery 1993; 114:1070–1077.

34a. Eng C. RET proto-oncogene in the development of human cancer. J Clin Oncol 1999; 17:380–393.

35. Wilson RA, Ibanez ML. A comparative study of 14 cases of familial and nonfamilial pheochromocytomas. Hum Pathol 1978; 9:181–188.

36. Vistelle R, Grulet H, Gibold C, et al. High permanent plasma adrenaline levels: a marker of adrenal medullary disease in medullary thyroid carcinoma. Clin Endocrinol 1991; 34:133–138.

37. Hamilton BP, Landsberg L, Levine RJ. Measurement of urinary epinephrine in screening for pheochromocytoma in multiple endocrine neoplasia type II. Am J Med 1978; 65:1027–1032.

38. Sato T, Kobayashi K, Miura Y, Sakuma H, Yoshinaga K. High epinephrine content in the adrenal tumors from Sipple's syndrome. Tohoku J Exp Med 1975; 115:15–19.

39. Mathew CG, Chin KS, Easton DF, et al. A linked genetic marker for multiple endocrine neoplasia type 2A on chromosome 10. Nature 1987; 328:527–528.

40. Mulligan LM, Kwok JB, Healey CS, et al. Germ-line mutations of the RET protooncogene in multiple endocrine neoplasia type 2A. Nature 1993; 363:458–460.

41. Gardner E, Mulligan LM, Eng C. Haplotype analysis of MEN2 mutations. Hum Mol Genet 1994; 3:1771–1774.

42. Santoro M, Carlomagno F, Romano A, et al. Activation of RET as a dominant transforming gene by germline mutations of MEN 2 and MEN 2B. Science 1995; 267:381–383.

43. Asai N, Iwashita T, Matsuyama M, Takahashi M. Mechanism of activation of the ret proto-oncogene by multiple endocrine neoplasia 2A mutations. Mol Cell Biol 1995; 15:1613–1619.

44. Donis-Keller H, Dou S, Chi D. Mutations in the RET proto-oncogene are associated with MEN 2A and FMTC. Hum Mol Genet 1993; 2:851–856.

45. Mulligan LM, Eng C, Healey CS. Specific mutations of the RET proto-oncogene are related to disease phenotype in MEN 2A and FMTC. Nat Genet 1994; 6:70–74.

46. Eng C, Clayton D, Schuffenecker I, et al. The relationship between specific RET proto-oncogene mutations and disease phenotype in multiple endocrine neoplasia type 2. International RET mutation consortium analysis. JAMA 1996; 276:1575–1579.

47. Mulligan LM, Marsh DJ, Robinson BG, et al. Genotype-phenotype correlation in multiple endocrine neoplasia type 2: report of the International RET Mutation Consortium. J Intern Med 1995; 238:343–346.

48. Schuffenecker I, Billaud M, Calendar A. RET proto-oncogene mutations in French MEN 2A and FMTC families. Hum Mol Genet 1994; 3:1939–1943.

49. Eng C, Smith DP, Mulligan LM. Point mutation within the tyrosine kinase domain of the RET proto-oncogene in multiple endocrine neoplasia type 2B and related sporadic tumors. Hum Mol Genet 1994; 3:237–241.

50. Carlson KM, Dou S, Chi D. Single missense mutation in the tyrosine kinase catalytic domain of the RET proto-oncogene is associated with multiple endocrine neoplasia type 2B. Proc Natl Acad Sci 1994; 91:1579–1583.

51. Gordon Cm, Majzoub JA, Marsh DJ, et al. Four cases of mucosal neuroma syndrome: multiple endocrine neoplasm 2B or not 2B? J Clin Endocrinol Metab 1998; 83:17–20.

52. Jing S, Wen D, Yu Y, et al. GDNF-induced activation of the ret protein tyrosine kinase is mediated by GDNFR-alpha, a novel receptor for GDNF. Cell 1996; 85:1113–1124.

53. Trupp M, Arenas E, Fainzilber M, et al. Functional receptor for GDNF encoded by the c-ret protooncogene. Nature 1996; 381:785–788.

54. Romeo G, Ronchetto P, Luo Y. Point mutations affecting the tyrosine kinase domain of the ret proto-oncogene in Hirschsprung's disease. Nature 1994; 367:377–378.

55. Lamiell JM, Salazar FG, Hsia YE. von Hippel-Lindau disease affecting 43 members of a single kindred. Medicine 1989; 68:1–29.

56. Karsdorp N, Elderson A, Wittebol-Post D, et al. Von Hippel-Lindau disease: new strategies in early detection and treatment. Am J Med 1994; 97:158–168.

57. Choyke PL, Glenn GM, Walther MM, Patronas NJ, Linehan WM, Zbar B. von Hippel-Lindau disease: genetic, clinical, and imaging features. Radiology 1995; 194:629–642.

58. Linehan WM, Lerman MI, Zbar B. Identification of the von Hippel-Lindau (VHL) gene. Its role in renal cancer. JAMA 1995; 273:564–570.

59. Maher ER, Yates JR, Harries R, et al. Clinical features and natural history of von Hippel-Lindau disease. Q J Med 1990; 77:1151–1163.

60. Richard S, Chaveau D, Chretien Y. Renal lesions and pheochromocytoma in von Hippel-Lindau disease. Adv Nephrol 1994; 23:1–27.

61. Brauch H, Kishida T, Glavac D, et al. Von Hippel-Lindau (VHL) disease with pheochromocytoma in the Black Forest region of Germany: evidence for a founder effect. Hum Genet 1995; 95:551–556.

62. Latif F, Tory K, Gnarra J. Identification of the von Hippel-Lindau disease tumor suppressor gene. Science 1993; 260:1317–1320.

63. Richards FM, Phipps ME, Latif F. Mapping the von Hippel-Lindau disease tumor suppressor gene: identification of germline deletions by pulsed field gel electrophoresis. Hum Mol Genet 1993; 2:879–882.

64. Yao M, Latif F, Orcutt ML. Von Hippel-Lindau disease: identification of deletion mutations by pulsed field gel electrophoresis. Hum Genet 1993; 92:605–614.

65. Richards FM, Crossey PA, Phipps ME. Detailed mapping of germline deletions of the von Hippel-Lindau disease tumor suppressor gene. Hum Mol Genet 1994; 3:595–598.

66. Crossey PA, Richards FM, Foster K. Identification of intragenic mutations in the von Hippel-Lindau disease tumor suppressor gene and correlation with disease phenotype. Hum Mol Genet 1994; 3:1303–1308.

67. van der Harst E, de Krijger RR, Dinjens WN, et al. Germline mutations in the vhl gene in patients presenting with pheochromocytomas. Int J Cancer 1998; 77:337–340.

68. Ritter MM, Frilling A, Crossey PA, et al. Isolated familial pheochromocytoma as a variant of von Hippel-Lindau disease. J Clin Endocrinol Metab 1996; 81:1035–1037.

69. Knudson AG Jr, Strong LC. Mutation and cancer: neuroblastoma and pheochromocytoma. Am J Hum Genet 1972; 24:514–532.

70. Whaley JM, Naglich J, Gelbert L. Germline mutations in the von Hippel-Lindau tumor suppressor gene are similar to somatic von Hippel-Lindau aberrations in sporadic renal cell carcinoma. Am J Hum Genet 1994; 55:1092–1102.

71. Atuk NO, Stolle C, Owen JA, Carpenter JT, Vance ML. Pheochromocytoma in von Hippel-Lindau disease: clinical presentation and mutation analysis in a large, multigenerational kindred. J Clin Endocrinol Metab 1998; 83:117–120.

72. Gross DJ, Avishai N, Meiner V, Filon D, Zbar B, Abeliovich D. Familial pheochromocytoma associated with a novel mutation in the von Hippel-Lindau gene. J Clin Endocrinol Metab 1996; 81:147–149.

73. Duan DR, Pause A, Burgess WH, et al. Inhibition of transcription elongation by the VHL tumor suppressor protein. Science 1995; 269:1402–1406.

74. Neumann HP, Eng C, Mulligan LM, et al. Consequences of direct genetic testing for germline mutations in the clinical management of families with multiple endocrine neoplasia, type II. JAMA 1995; 274:1149–1151.

75. Aso T, Lane WS, Conaway JW, Conaway RC. Elongin (SIII): a multisubunit regulator of elongation by RNA polymerase II. Science 1995; 269:1439–1443.

76. Maher ER, Kaelin WG. von Hippel-Lindau disease. Medicine 1997; 76:381–391.

77. Riccardi VM. Neurofibromatosis: past, present, and future. N Engl J Med 1991; 324:1283–1285.

78. Huson SM, Compston DA, Harper PS. A genetic study of von Recklinghausen neurofibromatosis in south east Wales. II. Guidelines for genetic counselling. J Med Genet 1989; 26:712–721.

78a. Walther MM, Herring J, Enquist E, Keiser HR, Linehan WM. Von Recklinghausen's disease and pheochromocytomas. J Urol 1999; 162:1582–1586.

79. Viskochil D, Buchberg AM, Xu G, et al. Deletions and a translocation interrupt a cloned gene at the neurofibromatosis type 1 locus. Cell 1990; 62:187–192.

80. Wallace MR, Marchuk DA, Andersen LB, et al. Type 1 neurofibromatosis gene: identification of a large transcript disrupted in three NF1 patients. Science 1990; 249:181–186.

81. Cawthon RM, Weiss R, Xu GF, et al. A major segment of the neurofibromatosis type 1 gene: cDNA sequence, genomic structure, and point mutations. Cell 1990; 62:193–201.

82. Xu W, Mulligan LM, Ponder MA, et al. Loss of NF1 alleles in pheochromocytomas from patients with type I neurofibromatosis. Genes Chromo Cancer 1992; 4:337–342.

83. Jacks T, Shih TS, Schmitt EM. Tumor predisposition in mice heterozygous for a targeted mutation in nf1. Nat Genet 1994; 7:353–361.

84. Ballester R, Marchuk D, Boguski M, et al. The NF1 locus encodes a protein functionally related to mammalian GAP and yeast IRA proteins. Cell 1990; 63:851–859.

85. Li Y, Bollag G, Clark R, et al. Somatic mutations in the neurofibromatosis 1 gene in human tumors. Cell 1992; 69:275–281.

86. Mulvihill JJ, Ferrell RE, Carty SE, Tisherman SE, Zbar B. Familial pheochromocytoma due to mutant von Hippel-Lindau disease gene. Arch Intern Med 1997; 157:1390–1391.

87. Crossey PA, Eng C, Ginalska-Malinowska M, et al. Molecular genetic diagnosis of von Hippel-Lindau disease in familial pheochromocytoma. J Med Genet 1995; 32:885–886.

88. Vargas MP, Zhuang Z, Wang C, Vortmeyer A, Linehan WM, Merino MJ. Loss of heterozygosity on the short arm of chromosomes 1 and 3 in sporadic pheochromocytoma and extra-adrenal paraganglioma. Hum Pathol 1997; 28:411–415.

88a. Vogelstein B, Kinzler KW (eds.). The genetic basis of human cancer. McGraw-Hill, New York, 1998.

89. Bar M, Friedman E, Jakobovitz O, et al. Sporadic pheochromocytomas are rarely associated with germline mutations in the von Hippel-Lindau and RET genes. Clin Endocrinol 1997; 47:707–712.

90. Hofstra RM, Stelwagen T, Stulp RP, et al. Extensive mutation scanning of RET in sporadic medullary thyroid carcinoma and of RET and VHL in sporadic pheochromocytoma reveals involvement of these genes in only a minority of cases. J Clin Endocrinol Metab 1996; 81:2881–2884.

91. Komminoth P, Roth J, Muletta-Feurer S, Saremaslani P, Seelentag WK, Heitz PU. RET proto-oncogene point mutations in sporadic neuroendocrine tumors. J Clin Endocrinol Metab 1996; 81:2041–2046.

92. Chew SL, Lavender P, Jain A, et al. Absence of mutations in the MEN2A region of the ret proto-oncogene in non-MEN 2A pheochromocytomas. Clin Endocrinol 1995; 42:17–21.

93. Lindor NM, Honchel R, Khosla S, Thibodeau SN. Mutations in the RET protooncogene in sporadic pheochromocytomas. J Clin Endocrinol Metab 1995; 80:627–629.

94. Beldjord C, Desclaux-Arramond F, Raffin-Sanson M, et al. The RET protooncogene in sporadic pheochromocytomas: frequent MEN 2-like mutations and new molecular defects. J Clin Endocrinol Metab 1995; 80:2063–2068.

95. Gutmann DH, Geist RT, Rose K, Wallin G, Moley JF. Loss of neurofibromatosis type I (NF1) gene expression in pheochromocytomas from patients without NF1. Genes Chromo Cancer 1995; 13:104–109.

96. Khosla S, Patel VM, Hay ID, et al. Loss of heterozygosity suggests multiple genetic alterations in pheochromocytomas and medullary thyroid carcinomas. J Clin Invest 1991; 87:1691–1699.

97. Tsutsumi M, Yokota J, Kakizoe T, Koiso K, Sugimura T, Terada M. Loss of heterozygosity on chromosomes 1p and 11p in sporadic pheochromocytoma. J Natl Cancer Inst 1989; 81:367–370.

98. Moley JF, Brother MB, Fong CT, et al. Consistent association of 1p loss of heterozygosity with pheochromocytomas from patients with multiple endocrine neoplasia type 2 syndromes. Cancer Res 1992; 52:770–774.

99. Williamson EA, Johnson SJ, Foster S, Kendall-Taylor P, Harris PE. G protein gene mutations in patients with multiple endocrinopathies. J Clin Endocrinol Metab 1995; 80:1702–1705.

100. Isobe K, Nakai T, Yukimasa N, Nanmoku T, Takekoshi K, Nomura F. Expression of mRNA coding for four catecholamine-synthesizing enzymes in human adrenal pheochromocytomas. Eur J Endocrinol 1998; 138:383–387.

101. Tumer N, Brown JW, Carballeira A, Fishman LM. Tyrosine hydroxylase gene expression in varying forms of human pheochromocytoma. Life Sci 1996; 59:1659–1665.

102. Bravo EL, Tarazi RC, Gifford RW, Stewart BH. Circulating and urinary catecholamines in pheochromocytoma. Diagnostic and pathophysiologic implications. N Engl J Med 1979; 301:682–686.

103. Duncan MW, Compton P, Lazarus L, Smythe GA. Measurement of norepinephrine and 3,4-dihydroxyphenylglycol in urine and plasma for the diagnosis of pheochromocytoma. N Engl J Med 1988; 319:136–142.

104. Chen F, Slife L, Kishida T, Mulvihill J, Tisherman SE, Zbar B. Genotype-phenotype correlation in von Hippel-Lindau disease: identification of a mutation associated with VHL type 2A. J Med Genet 1996; 33:716–717.

105. Manu P, Runge LA. Biochemical screening for pheochromocytoma. Superiority of urinary metanephrines measurements. Am J Epidemiol 1984; 120:788–790.

106. Heron E, Chatellier G, Billaud E, Foos E, Plouin PF. The urinary metanephrine-to-creatinine ratio for the diagnosis of pheochromocytoma. Ann Intern Med 1996; 125:300–303.

107. Goldstein DS. Stress, Catecholamines, and Cardiovascular Disease. Oxford University Press, New York, 1995.

108. Sinclair D, Shenkin A, Lorimer AR. Normal catecholamine production in a patient with a paroxysmally secreting pheochromocytoma. Ann Clin Biochem 1991; 28:417–419.

109. Stewart MF, Reed P, Weinkove C, Moriarty KJ, Ralston AJ. Biochemical diagnosis of pheochromocytoma: two instructive case reports. J Clin Pathol 1993; 46:280–282.

110. Bravo EL. Evolving concepts in the pathophysiology, diagnosis, and treatment of pheochromocytoma. Endocr Rev 1994; 15:356–368.

111. Shawar L, Svec F. Pheochromocytoma with elevated metanephrines as the only biochemical finding. J La State Med Soc 1996; 148:535–538.

112. Eisenhofer G, Goldstein DS, Stull R, Ropchak TG, Keiser HR, Kopin IJ. Dihydroxyphenylglycol and dihydroxymandelic acid during intravenous infusions of noradrenaline. Clin Sci 1987; 73:123–125.

113. Eriksson BM, Persson BA. Liquid chromatographic method for the determination of 3,4-dihydroxyphenylethylene glycol and 3,4-dihydroxymandelic acid in plasma. J Chromatogr 1987; 386:1–9.

114. Kawamura M, Kopin IJ, Kador PF, Sato S, Tjurmina O, Eisenhofer G. Effects of aldehyde/aldose reductase inhibition on neuronal metabolism of norepinephrine. J Auron Nerv Syst 1997; 66:145–148.

115. Eisenhofer G, Pecorella W, Pacak K, Hooper D, Kopin IJ, Goldstein DS. The neuronal and extraneuronal origins of plasma 3-methoxy-4-hydroxyphenylglycol in rats. J Auton Nerv Syst 1994; 50:93–107.

116. Eisenhofer G, Friberg P, Rundqvist B, et al. Cardiac sympathetic nerve function in congestive heart failure. Circulation 1996; 93:1667–1676.

117. Blombery PA, Kopin IJ, Gordon EK, Markey SP, Ebert MH. Conversion of MHPG to vanillylmandelic acid. Implications for the importance of urinary MHPG. Arch Gen Psychiatry 1980; 37:1095–1098.

118. Märdh G, Änggard E. Norepinephrine metabolism in man using deuterium labelling: origin of 4-hydroxy-3-methoxymandelic acid. J Neurochem 1984; 42:43–46.

119. Eisenhofer G, Aneman A, Hooper D, Rundqvist B, Friberg P. Mesenteric organ production, hepatic metabolism, and renal elimination of norepinephrine and its metabolites in humans. J Neurochem 1996; 66:1565–1573.

120. Eisenhofer G, Goldstein DS, Kopin IJ. Plasma dihydroxyphenylglycol for estimation of noradrenaline neuronal reuptake in the sympathetic nervous system in vivo. Clin Sci 1989; 76:171–182.

121. Eisenhofer G, Esler MD, Meredith IT, et al. Sympathetic nervous function in human heart as assessed by cardiac spillovers of dihydroxyphenylglycol and norepinephrine. Circulation 1992; 85:1775–1785.

122. Eisenhofer G. Plasma normetanephrine for examination of extraneuronal uptake and metabolism of noradrenaline in rats. Naunyn Schmiedebergs Arch Pharmacol 1994; 349:259–269.

123. Eisenhofer G, Rundqvist B, Friberg P. Determinants of cardiac tyrosine hydroxylase activity during exercise-induced sympathetic activation in humans. Am J Physiol 1998; 43:R626–R634.

124. Lenders JWM, Willemsen JJ, Beissel T, Kloppenborg PWC, Thien T, Benrad TJ. Value of the plasma norepinephrine/3,4-dihydroxyphenylglycol ratio for the diagnosis of pheochromocytoma. Am J Med 1992; 92:147–152.

125. Ferrante A, Bellantone R, Barbarino A, et al. Paroxystic hypertension in a long-term hemodialyzed patient. Successful adrenalectomy for a dopamine-producing pheochromocytoma. J Endocrinol Invest 1995; 18:656–662.

126. Graefe KH, Henseling M. Neuronal and extraneuronal uptake and metabolism of catecholamines. Gen Pharmacol 1983; 14:27–33.

127. Eisenhofer G, Goldstein DS, Ropchak TG, Nguyen HQ, Keiser HR, Kopin IJ. Source and physiological significance of plasma 3,4-dihydroxyphenylglycol and 3-methoxy-4-hydroxyphenylglycol. J Auton Nerv Syst 1988; 24:1–14.

128. Goldstein DS, Eisenhofer G, Stull R, Folio CJ, Keiser HR, Kopin IJ. Plasma dihydroxyphenylglycol and the intraneuronal disposition of norepinephrine in humans. J Clin Invest 1988; 81:213–220.

129. Eisenhofer G, Smolich JJ, Esler MD. Disposition of endogenous adrenaline compared to noradrenaline released by cardiac sympathetic nerves in the anaesthetized dog. Naunyn Schmiedebergs Arch Pharmacol 1992; 345:160–171.

130. Brown M. Simultaneous assay of noradrenaline and its deaminated metabolite, dihydroxyphenylglycol, in plasma: a simplified approach to the exclusion of pheochromocytoma in patients with borderline elevation of plasma noradrenaline concentration. Eur J Clin Invest 1984; 14:67–72.

131. Atuk NO, Hanks JB, Weltman J, Bogdonoff DL, Boyd DG, Vance ML. Circulating dihydroxyphenylglycol and norepinephrine concentrations during sympathetic nervous system activation in patients with pheochromocytoma. J Clin Endocrinol Metab 1994; 79:1609–1614.

132. Nakada T, Sasagawa I, Kubota Y, Suzuki H, Ishigooka M, Watanabe M. Dihydroxyphenylglycol in pheochromocytoma: its diagnostic use for norepinephrine dominant tumor. J Urol 1996; 155:14–18.

133. Eisenhofer G, Esler MD, Meredith IT, Ferrier C, Lambert G, Jennings G. Neuronal re-uptake of noradrenaline by sympathetic nerves in humans. Clin Sci 1991; 80:257–263.

134. Esler MD, Wallin G, Dorward PK, et al. Effects of desipramine on sympathetic nerve firing and norepinephrine spillover to plasma in humans. Am J Physiol 1991; 260:R817–R823.

135. Eisenhofer G, Rundqvist B, Aneman A, et al. Regional release and removal of catecholamines and extraneuronal metabolism to metanephrines. J Clin Endocrinol Metab 1995; 80:3009–3017.

136. Eisenhofer G, Friberg P, Pacak K, et al. Plasma metadrenalines: do they provide useful information about sympatho-adrenal function and catecholamine metabolism? Clin Sci 1995; 88:533–542.

137. Märdh G, Luehr CA, Vallee BL. Human class I alcohol dehydrogenases catalyze the oxidation of glycols in the metabolism of norepinephrine. Proc Natl Acad Sci USA 1985; 82:4979–4982.

138. Märdh G, Dingley AL, Auld DS, Vallee BL. Human class II (pi) alcohol dehydrogenase has a redox-specific function in norepinephrine metabolism. Proc Natl Acad Sci USA 1986; 83:8908–8912.

139. Peaston RT, Lai LC. Biochemical detection of pheochromocytoma: Should we still be measuring urinary HMMA? J Clin Pathol 1993; 46:734–737.

140. Tormey WP, FitzGerald RJ. Pheochromocytoma: a laboratory experience. Ir J Med Sci 1995; 164:142–145.

141. Mornex R, Peyrin L. The biological diagnosis of pheochromocytoma. Bull Mem Acad R Med Belg 1996; 151:269–277.

142. Peaston RT, Lennard TW, Lai LC. Overnight excretion of urinary catecholamines and metabolites in the detection of pheochromocytoma. J Clin Endocrinol Metab 1996; 81:1378–1384.

143. Eisenhofer G, Keiser H, Friberg P, et al. Plasma metanephrines are markers of pheochromocytoma produced by catechol-O-methyltransferase within tumors. J Clin Endocrinol Metab 1998; 83:2175–2185.

144. Roth JA. Membrane-bound catechol-O-methyltransferase: a reevaluation of its role in the O-methylation of the catecholamine neurotransmitters. Rev Physiol Biochem Pharmacol 1992; 120:1–29.

145. Aprill BS, Drake AJ, Lasseter DH, Shakir KM. Silent adrenal nodules in von Hippel-Lindau disease suggest pheochromocytoma. Ann Intern Med 1994; 120:485–487.

146. Eisenhofer G, Finberg JP. Different metabolism of norepinephrine and epinephrine by catechol-O-methyltransferase and monoamine oxidase in rats. J Pharmacol Exp Ther 1994; 268:1242–1251.

147. Lenders JWM, Eisenhofer G, Abeling NGGM, et al. Specific genetic deficiencies of the A and B isozymes of monoamine oxidase are characterized by distinct neurochemical and clinical phenotypes. J Clin Invest 1996; 97:1010–1019.

148. Box JC, Braithwaite MD, Duncan T, Lucas G. Pheochromocytoma, chronic renal insufficiency, and hemodialysis: a combination leading to a diagnostic and therapeutic dilemma. Am Surg 1997; 63:314–316.

149. Peyrin L, Cottet-Emard JM, Pagliari R, Cottet-Emard RM, Badet C, Mornex R. Plasma methoxyamines assay: a practical advance for the diagnosis of pheochromocytoma. Pathol Biol 1994; 42:847–854.

150. Grossman E, Goldstein DS, Hoffman A, Keiser HR. Glucagon and clonidine testing in the diagnosis of pheochromocytoma. Hypertension 1991; 17:733–741.

151. Bernini GP, Vivaldi MS, Argenio GF, Moretti A, Sgro M, Salvetti A. Frequency of pheochromocytoma in adrenal incidentalomas and utility of the glucagon test for the diagnosis. J Endocrinol Invest 1997; 20:65–71.

152. Bradley T, Gewertz BL, Scott WJ, Goldberg LI. Dopamine receptor blockade does not affect the natriuresis accompanying sodium chloride infusion in dogs. J Lab Clin Med 1986; 107:525–528.

153. Bravo EL, Gifford RW Jr. Current concepts. Pheochromocytoma: diagnosis, localization and management. N Engl J Med 1984; 311:1298–1303.

154. Elliott WJ, Murphy MB. Reduced specificity of the clonidine suppression test in patients with normal plasma catecholamine levels. Am J Med 1988; 84:419–424.

155. Elliott WJ, Murphy MB, Straus FH, Jarabak J. Improved safety of glucagon testing for pheochromocytoma by prior alpha-receptor blockade. A controlled trial in a patient with a mixed ganglioneuroma/pheochromocytoma. Arch Intern Med 1989; 149:214–216.

156. Eisenhofer G, Saigusa T, Esler MD, Cox HS, Angus JA, Dorward PK. Central sympathoinhibition and peripheral neuronal uptake blockade after desipramine in rabbits. Am J Physiol 1991; 260:R824–R832.

157. Manger WM, Gifford RW Jr. Pheochromocytoma: current diagnosis and management. Clev Clin J Med 1993; 60:365–378.

158. Fink IJ, Reinig JW, Dwyer AJ, Doppman JL, Linehan WM, Keiser HR. MR imaging of pheochromocytomas. J Comput Assist Tomogr 1985; 9:454–458.

159. Mukherjee JJ, Peppercorn PD, Reznek RH, et al. Pheochromocytoma: effect of nonionic contrast medium in CT on circulating catecholamine levels. Radiology 1997; 202:227–231.

160. Schmedtje JF Jr, Sax S, Pool JL, Goldfarb RA, Nelson EB. Localization of ectopic pheochromocytomas by magnetic resonance imaging. Am J Med 1987; 83:770–772.

161. Kloos RT, Gross MD, Francis IR, Korobkin M, Shapiro B. Incidentally discovered adrenal masses. Endocr Rev 1995; 16:460–484.

162. Sisson JC, Frager MS, Valk TW, et al. Scintigraphic localization of pheochromocytoma. N Engl J Med 1981; 305:12–17.

163. Saad MF, Frazier OH, Hickey RC, Samaan NA. Intrapericardial pheochromocytoma. Am J Med 1983; 75:371–376.

164. Shulkin BL, Shapiro B. Current concepts on the diagnostic use of MIBG in children. J Nucl Med 1998; 39:679–688.

165. Letizia C, De Toma G, Massa R, et al. False-positive diagnosis of adrenal pheochromocytoma on iodine-123-MIBG scan. J Endocrinol Invest 1998; 21:779–783.

166. Shapiro B, Copp JE, Sisson JC, Eyre PL, Wallis J, Beierwaltes WH. Iodine-131 metaiodobenzylgua-nidine for the locating of suspected pheochromocytoma: experience in 400 cases. J Nucl Med 1985; 26:576–585.

167. Lynn MD, Shapiro B, Sisson JC, et al. Pheochromocytoma and the normal adrenal medulla: improved visualization with I-123 MIBG scintigraphy. Radiology 1985; 155:789–792.

168. Tsuchimochi S, Nakajo M, Nakabeppu Y, Tani A. Metastatic pulmonary pheochromocytomas: positive I-123 MIBG SPECT with negative I-131 MIBG and equivocal I-123 MIBG planar imaging. Clin Nucl Med 1997; 22:687–690.

169. Solanki KK, Bomanji J, Moyes J, Mather SJ, Trainer PJ, Britton KE. A pharmacological guide to medicines which interfere with the biodistribution of radiolabeled meta-iodobenzylguanidine (MIBG). Nucl Med Commun 1992; 13:513–521.

170. Clesham CJ, Kennedy A, Lavender JP, Dollery CT, Wilkins MR. Meta-iodobenzylguanidine (MIBG) scanning in the diagnosis of pheochromocytoma. J Hum Hypertens 1993; 7:353–356.

171. Niederhuber JE. Future of positron-emission tomography in oncology. Ann Surg 1998; 227:324–325.

172. Adams S, Baum R, Rink T, Schumm-Drager PM, Usadel KH, Hor G. Limited value of fluorine-18 fluorodeoxyglucose positron emission tomography for the imaging of neuroendocrine tumours. Eur J Nucl Med 1998; 25:79–83.

173. Trauss LG, Conti PS. The applications of PET in clinical oncology. J Nucl Med 1991; 32:623–48.

174. Arnold DR, Villemagne VL, Civelek AC, Dannals RF, Wagner HN Jr, Udelsman R. FDG-PET: A sensitive tool for the localization of MIBG-negative pelvic pheochromocytoma. Endocrinologist 1998; 8:295–298.

175. Russell WJ, Metcalfe IR, Tonkin AL, Frewin DB. The preoperative management of pheochromocy-toma. Anaesth Intensive Care 1998; 26:196–200.

176. Briggs RS, Birtwell AJ, Pohl JE. Hypertensive response to labetalol in phaeochromocytoma. Lancet 1978; 1:1045–1046.

177. Brogden RN, Heel RC, Speight TM, Avery GS. alpha-Methyl-p-tyrosine: a review of its pharmacol-ogy and clinical use. Drugs 1981; 21:81–89.

178. Werbel SS, Ober KP. Pheochromocytoma. Update on diagnosis, localization, and management. Med Clin North Am 1995; 79:131–153.

179. Fernandez-Cruz L, Taura P, Saenz A, Benarroch G, Sabater L. Laparoscopic approach to pheochro-mocytoma: hemodynamic changes and catecholamine secretion. World J Surg 1996; 20:762–768.

180. Vargas HI, Kavoussi LR, Bartlett DL, et al. Laparoscopic adrenalectomy: a new standard of care. Urology 1997; 49:673–678.

181. Walther MM, Keiser HR, Choyke PL, Rayford W, Lyne JC, Linehan WM. Management of hereditary pheochromocytoma in von Hippel-Lindau kindreds with partial adrenalectomy. J Urol 1999; 161:395–398.

182. Averbuch SD, Steakley CS, Young RC, et al. Malignant pheochromocytoma: effective treatment with a combination of cyclophosphamide, vincristine, and dacarbazine. Ann Intern Med 1988; 109:267–273.

183. Schenker JG, Granat M. Pheochromocytoma and pregnancy: an updated appraisal. Aust N Z J Obstet Gynaecol 1982; 22:1–10.

184. Antonelli NM, Dotters DJ, Katz VL, Kuller JA. Cancer in pregnancy: a review of the literature. Part I. Obstet Gynecol Surv 1996; 51:125–134.

185. Oishi S, Sato T. Pheochromocytoma in pregnancy: a review of the Japanese literature. Endocr J 1994; 41:219–225.

Index